D1496481

Infection Management for Geriatrics in Long-Term Care Facilities

INFECTIOUS DISEASE AND THERAPY

Series Editor

Burke A. Cunha

Winthrop-University Hospital
Mineola, and
State University of New York School of Medicine
Stony Brook, New York

1. Parasitic Infections in the Compromised Host,
   edited by Peter D. Walzer and Robert M. Genta
2. Nucleic Acid and Monoclonal Antibody Probes:
   Applications in Diagnostic Methodology, *edited by*
   Bala Swaminathan and Gyan Prakash
3. Opportunistic Infections in Patients with the Acquired
   Immunodeficiency Syndrome, *edited by*
   Gifford Leoung and John Mills
4. Acyclovir Therapy for Herpesvirus Infections, *edited by*
   David A. Baker
5. The New Generation of Quinolones, *edited by*
   Clifford Siporin, Carl L. Heifetz, and John M. Domagala
6. Methicillin-Resistant *Staphylococcus aureus*: Clinical
   Management and Laboratory Aspects, *edited by*
   Mary T. Cafferkey
7. Hepatitis B Vaccines in Clinical Practice, *edited by*
   Ronald W. Ellis
8. The New Macrolides, Azalides, and Streptogramins:
   Pharmacology and Clinical Applications, *edited by*
   Harold C. Neu, Lowell S. Young, and Stephen H. Zinner
9. Antimicrobial Therapy in the Elderly Patient, *edited by*
   Thomas T. Yoshikawa and Dean C. Norman
10. Viral Infections of the Gastrointestinal Tract:
    Second Edition, Revised and Expanded, *edited by*
    Albert Z. Kapikian
11. Development and Clinical Uses of *Haemophilus b*
    Conjugate Vaccines, *edited by Ronald W. Ellis*
    and Dan M. Granoff
12. *Pseudomonas aeruginosa* Infections and Treatment,
    edited by Aldona L. Baltch and Raymond P. Smith

13. Herpesvirus Infections, *edited by Ronald Glaser and James F. Jones*
14. Chronic Fatigue Syndrome, *edited by Stephen E. Straus*
15. Immunotherapy of Infections, *edited by K. Noel Masihi*
16. Diagnosis and Management of Bone Infections, *edited by Luis E. Jauregui*
17. Drug Transport in Antimicrobial and Anticancer Chemotherapy, *edited by Nafsika H. Georgopapadakou*
18. New Macrolides, Azalides, and Streptogramins in Clinical Practice, *edited by Harold C. Neu, Lowell S. Young, Stephen H. Zinner, and Jacques F. Acar*
19. Novel Therapeutic Strategies in the Treatment of Sepsis, *edited by David C. Morrison and John L. Ryan*
20. Catheter-Related Infections, *edited by Harald Seifert, Bernd Jansen, and Barry M. Farr*
21. Expanding Indications for the New Macrolides, Azalides, and Streptogramins, *edited by Stephen H. Zinner, Lowell S. Young, Jacques F. Acar, and Harold C. Neu*
22. Infectious Diseases in Critical Care Medicine, *edited by Burke A. Cunha*
23. New Considerations for Macrolides, Azalides, Streptogramins, and Ketolides, *edited by Stephen H. Zinner, Lowell S. Young, Jacques F. Acar, and Carmen Ortiz-Neu*
24. Tickborne Infectious Diseases: Diagnosis and Management, *edited by Burke A. Cunha*
25. Protease Inhibitors in AIDS Therapy, *edited by Richard C. Ogden and Charles W. Flexner*
26. Laboratory Diagnosis of Bacterial Infections, *edited by Nevio Cimolai*
27. Chemokine Receptors and AIDS, *edited by Thomas R. O'Brien*
28. Antimicrobial Pharmacodynamics in Theory and Clinical Practice, *edited by Charles H. Nightingale, Takeo Murakawa, and Paul G. Ambrose*
29. Pediatric Anaerobic Infections: Diagnosis and Management, Third Edition, Revised and Expanded, *Itzhak Brook*

30. Viral Infections and Treatment, *edited by Helga Ruebsamen-Waigmann, Karl Deres, Guy Hewlett, and Reinhold Welker*

31. Community-Aquired Respiratory Infections, *edited by Charles H. Nightingale, Paul G. Ambrose, and Thomas M. File*

32. Catheter-Related Infections: Second Edition, *Harald Seifert, Bernd Jansen and Barry Farr*

33. Antibiotic Optimization: Concepts and Strategies in Clinical Practice (PBK), *edited by Robert C. Owens, Jr., Charles H. Nightingale and Paul G. Ambrose*

34. Fungal Infections in the Immunocompromised Patient, *edited by John R. Wingard and Elias J. Anaissie*

35. Sinusitis: From Microbiology To Management, *edited by Itzhak Brook*

36. Herpes Simplex Viruses, *edited by Marie Studahl, Paola Cinque and Tomas Bergström*

37. Antiviral Agents, Vaccines, and Immunotherapies, *Stephen K. Tyring*

38. Epstein-Barr Virus, *Alex Tselis and Hal B. Jenson*

39. Infection Management for Geriatrics in Long-Term Care Facilities, Second Edition, *edited by Thomas T. Yoshikawa and Joseph G. Ouslander*

Infection Management for Geriatrics in Long-Term Care Facilities

Second Edition

edited by

Thomas T. Yoshikawa

Charles R. Drew University of Medicine and Science
Los Angeles, California, U.S.A.

Joseph G. Ouslander

Emory University School of Medicine
The Birmingham/Atlanta VA Geriatric Research,
Education, and Clinical Center
Atlanta, Georgia, U.S.A.

informa

healthcare

New York London

Infection management for
geriatrics in long-term
c2007.

2009 07 31

Informa Healthcare USA, Inc.
270 Madison Avenue
New York, NY 10016

International Standard Book Number-10: 0-8493-9893-2 (Hardcover)
International Standard Book Number-13: 978-0-8493-9893-3 (Hardcover)

Visit the Informa Web site at
www.informa.com

and the Informa Healthcare Web site at
www.informahealthcare.com

To our wives, Catherine Yoshikawa and Lynn Ouslander,
for their love and support.

Preface to the Second Edition

The second edition of *Infection Management for Geriatrics in Long-Term Care Facilities* continues with the tradition of the first edition in providing a book with quick and easy access to key information on the diagnosis, treatment, control, and prevention of infections and infectious diseases—issues in the long-term care setting. All chapters have been carefully reviewed, and new or updated information has been inserted as appropriate by our team of internationally and nationally recognized authors.

The chapters are consistent in their format so that the reader can anticipate and easily find the desired information. We have also added a new feature to this edition by beginning each chapter with a section of "Key Points," which consists of a summation of the important information or issues described in that particular chapter.

In contrast to the first edition, which had three major sections, the editors have reorganized the second edition into four major sections: Principles of Aging, Long-Term Care, and Infection; Principles of Managing Infections in Long-Term Care Facilities; Common Infections in Long-Term Care Facilities; and Emerging and Drug-Resistant Pathogens. In addition, we have added new chapters including "Role of Functional Assessment in Evaluating and Managing Infections in Long-Term Care"; "Conjunctivitis, Otitis, and Sinusitis"; "Human Immunodeficiency Virus Infection in the Nursing Home"; and "Severe Acute Respiratory Syndrome". The emergence of newer pathogens, especially in frail older persons; the evolving field of geriatric assessment; and the changing dynamics, expectations, policies, and role(s) of long-term care facilities required that the editors add these new topics. Finally, we added a new appendix (Appendix C), which summarizes the minimum criteria for initiating antibiotics in residents of long-term care facilities.

We have maintained the emphasis on inserting tables and figures to allow the reader to quickly grasp data, information, or concepts. The references have been updated where indicated, and the editors have reduced the number of references in each chapter compared with the first edition in order to focus on the most important literature on the topic. Moreover, we have added another feature, "Suggested Reading," which lists two or three of the key references that the reader can review to gain greater details about the subject matter.

The second edition of *Infection Management for Geriatrics in Long-Term Care Facilities* is a valuable and clinically useful reference for health-care providers, pharmacists, epidemiologists, infection control professionals, and administrators who interact and care for elderly residents in long-term care facilities, as well as infectious disease specialists, general internists, family physicians, and geriatric fellows who will have many occasions to visit, consult, and administer to these persons.

Thomas T. Yoshikawa
Joseph G. Ouslander

Preface to the First Edition

With the increasing growth of the aging population—especially those aged 85 years and older—over the next 40 years, there will be a parallel demand for long-term care. Such a demand is inevitable, given the changes, diseases, disabilities, and socioeconomic factors associated with growing old. When such age-related factors in an older person create a need for care, services, and support that cannot be met by family and other caregivers, the need arises for long-term care outside the home environment. Although there are different types of and venues for long-term care, nursing homes (nursing facilities) remain the dominant sites for providing care for chronically and functionally disabled and cognitively impaired older persons. Thus, the nursing homes serves as the prototype long-term care facility that manages chronically disabled elderly.

As more and more care is provided in long-term care facilities, inherent risks and problems arise when the population is very old, frail, and disabled. The population at risk resides in a closed institutional setting; the ratio of health-care staff to residents may be suboptimal, and quick and easy access to diagnostic, therapeutic, and preventive interventions is limited. One of the most common risks (and complications) of long-term care is infection. Infection (or presence of a fever) is often the reason a long-term care facility resident is sent to an emergency department or transferred to an acute care facility. However, the clinical diagnosis of an infection in a frail, elderly long-term care facility resident may be quite difficult, given the atypical clinical manifestations of infection in the very old, limited availability of a clinician on site in the long-term care facility to examine the resident, and lack of quick access to diagnostic laboratory and radiological tests. Moreover, once a presumptive diagnosis of infection is made, the decision for an appropriate therapeutic approach may be complex. Issues of advanced directives and/or desires of the resident/family regarding the extent of diagnostic and therapeutic interventions must be considered. Can the resident be treated in the long-term care facility or is transfer to an acute care facility more appropriate? Does the long-term care facility have the resources and appropriately trained personnel to treat the resident within the long-term care facility? If treatment is initiated in the long-term care facility, what antibiotics and dosages should be used? In addition, other clinical infectious disease issues to be considered when caring for residents in a long-term care facility include the following: What are the most common infections in this setting? What is the role of a long-term care facility nurse in managing infections? What ethical factors need to be considered? What should be done when an outbreak of an infection occurs? Are there drug-resistant pathogens in this setting, and how should these be managed?

Infection Management for Geriatrics in Long-Term Care Facilities addresses these and many other important questions and issues related to the diagnosis, treatment, prevention, and control of infections in elderly residents of long-term care facilities. The book was written by internationally and nationally recognized experts in the area of infections, geriatrics, and long-term care. The editors are clinicians who have a long record of patient care, education and training, and research in the fields of geriatrics, gerontology, and long-term care. They are editor-in-chief and deputy editor, respectively, of the *Journal of the American Geriatrics Society*—the leading journal in the field of aging.

The book is divided into three major sections. The first is devoted to the principles of aging, long-term care, and infection, with chapters discussing the demographics of long-term care; the differences between acute care and long-term care; epidemiology and special aspects of infections in long-term care; host resistance changes with aging; the interrelationship between aging, nutrition, and immunity; altered clinical manifestations of infections with aging; ethical considerations in managing infections in this setting; the role of nursing in managing infections in a long-term care facility; principles of infection control in a long-term care facility; identification and management of outbreaks in a long-term care facility; and rational approach to using antibiotics in residents of a long-term care facility. The second section focuses on the most common and important infectious disease problems encountered in a long-term care facility. These include urinary tract infection; influenza and other respiratory viruses; pneumonia and bronchitis; tuberculosis; infected pressure ulcers; selected skin infections, i.e., herpes zoster, cellulitis, and scabies; infectious diarrhea; viral hepatitis; and vaccination. The third and final section addresses the problem of emerging drug-resistant pathogens in long-term care facilities, with detailed information on pathogenetic and molecular mechanisms for antibiotic resistance; methicillin-resistant *Staphylococcus aureus*; glycopeptide (primarily vancomycin)-resistant enterococci; gram-negative bacteria; and selected fungi (e.g., *Candida*). An appendix is included, with definitions of common infections in a long-term care setting and guidelines for the evaluation of fever and infections in long-term care facilities.

The book is formatted for easy and quick access to key information; there are numerous figures and tables that summarize important data and the most relevant and up-to-date references are provided. Clinicians will find this book informative, easy to read, and helpful in managing their long-term care facility residents who have fever and infection. *Infection Management for Geriatrics in Long-Term Care Facilities* is an essential resource for all health-care providers and administrators involved with the care of elderly residents in long-term care facilities.

Thomas T. Yoshikawa
Joseph G. Ouslander

Acknowledgment

We are grateful to Ms. Patricia Thompson for her assistance in the typing and retyping of the manuscripts.

Contents

Preface to the Second Edition . . . . *v*
Preface to the First Edition . . . . *vii*
Acknowledgment . . . . *xi*
Contributors . . . . *xxv*

PART I: PRINCIPLES OF AGING, LONG-TERM CARE, AND INFECTION

1. **Demographics and Economics of Long-Term Care** *1*
   A. Jefferson Lesesne and Joseph G. Ouslander
   Key Points 1
   Introduction 2
   Demand for Nursing Facility Care 2
   Economics of LTC 8
   Evolving Changes in LTC 11
   References 12

2. **Epidemiology and Special Aspects of Infectious Diseases in Aging** *15*
   Thomas T. Yoshikawa
   Key Points 15
   Conceptual Basis for Importance of
     Infection and Aging 15
   Special Aspects of Infections in the Elderly 17

Suggested Reading 19
References 19

3. **Evaluation of Infections in Long-Term Care
   Facilities Versus Acute Care Hospitals** *21*
   Arnel M. Joaquin
   Key Points 21
   Introduction 21
   When to Transfer Long-Term Care Facilities Residents
      to an Acute Care Setting 25
   Summary 27
   Suggested Reading 27
   References 28

4. **Role of Functional Assessment in Evaluating and
   Managing Infections in Long-Term Care** *31*
   Barbara J. Messinger-Rapport and Robert M. Palmer
   Key Points 31
   Introduction 32
   Importance of Functional Assessment During
      Transitions of Care 37
   Functional Assessment in LTC 42
   Process of Functional Assessment 43
   Infection Control and Function 46
   Summary 46
   Suggested Reading 47
   References 47

5. **Impaired Immunity and Increased Risk of Infections in
   Older Adults: Impact of Chronic Disease
   on Immunosenescence** *49*
   Steven C. Castle, Koichi Uyemura, and Takashi Makinodan
   Key Points 49
   Introduction 50
   Immunosenescence 50
   Impaired Immunity Due to the Impact of Chronic
      Illness on an Aging Immune System
      (Immunosenescence) 57
   Inflammatory Mediators and Immunity 59
   Impact of Age and Chronic Illness–Related
      Impaired Immunity on Infections 62

Concluding Remarks 66
Suggested Reading 67
References 68

6. **Nutrition and Infection** *71*
   Kevin P. High
   Key Points 71
   Introduction 72
   Prevalence and Causes of Malnutrition
      in Older Residents of LTCFs 72
   Assessment of Nutritional Status and Consequences of
      Malnutrition in Long-Term Care Residents 75
   Nutritional Interventions to Reduce Infection
      and Improve Outcomes in LTCF Residents 77
   Specific Syndromes Where Nutritional Supplementation
      May Be of Benefit 79
   Drug–Nutrient Interactions 82
   Conclusions 82
   Suggested Reading 84
   References 84

7. **Ethical Issues of Infectious**
   Disease Interventions *87*
   Elizabeth L. Cobbs
   Key Points 87
   Introduction 87
   Elements of Ethics 88
   Everyday Ethics 90
   The Doctor–Patient Relationship 91
   Goals of Care and Advance Care Plans 91
   Interventions: Burdens and Benefits 92
   Quality of Life 93
   Health Promotion 94
   Health-Care Decision Making 94
   Role of the Interdisciplinary Team 97
   Role of the Medical Director 98
   Advanced Dementia 98
   Human Immunodeficiency Virus/Acquired
      Immunodeficiency Syndrome 99
   End-of-Life Care 99
   Infection Control Practices 100

Cost Concerns 100
Research Issues 101
The Future 101
Suggested Reading 102
References 102

**PART II: PRINCIPLES OF MANAGING INFECTIONS IN
LONG-TERM CARE FACILITIES**

8. Clinical Manifestations of Infections *105*
Dean C. Norman and Megan Bernadette Wong
Key Points 105
Introduction 106
Atypical Presentations of Infection 107
Fever 108
Conclusion 111
Suggested Reading 111
References 111

**9. Establishing an Infection
Control Program** *115*
Lona Mody
Key Points 115
Background 116
Unique Challenges to Infection Control 116
Regulatory Aspects of Infection Control 118
Components of Infection Control 119
Infection Control Practitioner 127
Review Committee 127
Resources for Infection Control Practitioners
and Suggested Reading 128
References 128

**10. Epidemiologic Investigation of Infectious Disease Outbreaks
in Long-Term Care Facilities** *131*
Chesley L. Richards, Jr. and William R. Jarvis
Key Points 131
Introduction 132
Characteristics of Long-Term Care Facilities 132
Risk Factors for Outbreaks in LTCFs 133

Key Aspects of Infectious Disease Outbreak
  Investigation 134
Selected Infectious Disease Outbreaks 141
Conclusions 145
Suggested Reading 146
References 146

11. **An Approach to Antimicrobial Therapy** *149*
  Jay P. Rho
  Key Points 149
  General Issues of Antimicrobial Therapy 149
  Optimizing the Use of Antimicrobial Agents in the
    LTCF 151
  Drug Factors to Consider in Prescribing Antimicrobial
    Therapy 155
  Potentially Useful and Safe Antimicrobial Agents for
    LTCF Residents 159
  Suggested Reading 164
  References 164

**PART III: COMMON INFECTIONS IN LONG-TERM
CARE FACILITIES**

12. **Urinary Tract Infection** *169*
  Lindsay E. Nicolle
  Key Points 169
  Introduction 170
  Epidemiology and Clinical Relevance 170
  Clinical Manifestations 175
  Diagnostic Approach 177
  Therapeutic Interventions 180
  Infection Control Measures 184
  Prevention 185
  Suggested Reading 187
  References 187

13. **Influenza and Other Respiratory Viruses** *191*
  Ghinwa Dumyati
  Key Points 191
  Introduction 192
  Influenza 192
  Respiratory Syncytial Virus 201

Parainfluenza 204
Coronavirus 206
Rhinovirus 208
Human Metapneumovirus 209
Suggested Reading 210
References 210

14. **Pneumonia and Bronchitis** *215*
Joseph M. Mylotte
Key Points 215
Nursing Home–Associated Pneumonia 215
Bronchitis 228
Suggested Reading 229
References 229

15. **Tuberculosis** *233*
Shobita Rajagopalan
Key Points 233
Introduction 233
Epidemiology and Clinical Significance 234
Pathogenesis 235
Clinical Manifestations 236
Diagnosis 236
Treatment 237
Prevention 244
Infection Control 244
Suggested Reading 247
References 247

16. **Infected Pressure Ulcers** *251*
Steven C. Reynolds and Anthony W. Chow
Key Points 251
Epidemiology and Clinical Relevance 252
Pathogenesis of Infected Pressure Ulcers 257
Clinical Manifestations 258
Diagnostic Approach 259
Therapeutic Interventions 264
Infection Control Measures 270
Prevention 272
Suggested Reading 274
References 274

17. **Herpes Zoster, Cellulitis, and Scabies** *277*
    Kenneth E. Schmader and Jack Twersky
    Key Points 277
    Herpes Zoster 278
    Cellulitis 284
    Scabies 290
    Suggested Reading 295
    References 295

18. **Infectious Diarrhea** *297*
    Abbasi J. Akhtar and Made Sutjita
    Key Points 297
    Epidemiology and Clinical Relevance 298
    Clinical Manifestations 300
    Diagnostic Approach 301
    Therapeutic Intervention 305
    Infection Control Measures 307
    Prevention 308
    Suggested Reading 308
    References 308

19. **Hepatitis in Long-Term Care Facilities** *311*
    Darrell W. Harrington and Peter V. Barrett
    Key Points 311
    Introduction 311
    Epidemiology and Clinical Relevance 312
    Clinical Manifestations and Complications
       of Viral Hepatitis 320
    Therapeutic Interventions 323
    Infection Control and Prevention 326
    Conclusion 331
    Suggested Reading 332
    References 332

20. **Conjunctivitis, Otitis, and Sinusitis** *335*
    Deborah Moran, Made Sutjita, and Kathleen Daretany
    Key Points 335
    Conjunctivitis 336
    Otitis Media 338
    Otitis Externa 340

Sinusitis 342
Suggested Reading 345
References 345

21. **Human Immunodeficiency Virus Infection
    in the Nursing Home** *349*
    Allen S. Funnyé
    Key Points 349
    Introduction 349
    General Epidemiology 350
    Epidemiology in Older Adults 352
    Long-Term Care Facilities 356
    Pathogenesis of HIV in the Elderly 358
    Clinical Issues in Nursing Home
       AIDS Residents 359
    Treatment of HIV Infection in the Nursing Home 361
    Psychosocial Concerns and Prevention 366
    Suggested Reading 367
    References 367

22. **Vaccinations** *369*
    *Rex Biedenbender, Stefan Gravenstein, and
    Arvydas Ambrozaitis*
    Key Points 369
    Infection, Aging, and Immune Response 370
    Vaccine Utilization in Long-Term Care Facilities 370
    Efforts to Increase Vaccine Utilization 371
    Influenza 371
    Pneumococcal Disease 376
    Varicella Vaccine 386
    Vaccination of Health-Care Workers in LTCFs 387
    Summary 387
    Suggested Reading 388
    References 388

PART IV: EMERGING AND DRUG-RESISTANT PATHOGENS

23. **Methicillin-Resistant *Staphylococcus aureus*** *391*
    Thomas T. Yoshikawa and Larry J. Strausbaugh
    Key Points 391
    Introduction 392

Epidemiology and Clinical Relevance 392
Clinical Manifestation 396
Diagnostic Approach 398
Therapeutic Interventions 399
Infection Control Measures 400
Prevention 406
Suggested Reading 406
References 407

24. **Vancomycin (Glycopeptide)-Resistant Enterococci in the**
   Long-Term Care Setting *411*
   Suzanne F. Bradley
   Key Points 411
   Epidemiology and Clinical Relevance 411
   Clinical Manifestations 415
   Diagnostic Approach 416
   Therapeutic Interventions 418
   Infection Control Measures 419
   Prevention 423
   Suggested Reading 424
   References 424

25. **Gram-Negative Bacteria** *427*
   Vinod K. Dhawan
   Key Points 427
   Epidemiology and Clinical Relevance 428
   Clinical Syndromes 434
   Diagnostic Approach 434
   Therapeutic Interventions 435
   Prevention 439
   Suggested Reading 440
   References 440

26. **Fungal Infections** *445*
   Carol A. Kauffman and Sara A. Hedderwick
   Key Points 445
   Introduction 445
   Epidemiology and Clinical Relevance 446
   Clinical Manifestations 448
   Diagnostic Approach 452

Therapeutic Interventions 455
Infection Control Measures 460
Prevention 461
Suggested Reading 462
References 462

27. **Severe Acute Respiratory Syndrome** *465*
Mark B. Loeb
Key Points 465
Introduction 465
SARS: Epidemiology and Clinical Relevance 466
Microbiology 467
Clinical Disease 468
Diagnosis 469
Treatment 470
Prevention 471
Suggested Reading 471
References 471

PART V: IMPORTANT SOURCE REFERENCES

**Appendix A: Definitions of Common Infections
in Long-Term Care Facilities** *473*
Conditions Applicable to Definitions 473
Respiratory Tract Infection 473
Urinary Tract Infection 474
Skin Infections 475
Gastrointestinal Tract Infection 475
Comments 476

**Appendix B: Guide to Evaluating Fever and Infection
in Long-Term Care Facilities** *477*
Clinical Evaluation 477
Laboratory Tests 478
Indications for Transfer to an Acute Care
Facility 480

**Appendix C: Minimum Criteria for the Initiation of
Antibiotics in Residents of Long-Term Care
Facilities: Results of a Consensus Conference** *481*
Skin and Soft Tissue Infections 481

Respiratory Infections 481
Urinary Tract Infection 482
Fever in Which the Focus of Infection is
    Unknown 483

Index *485*
About the Editors *501*

Contributors

Abbasi J. Akhtar Divisions of Gastroenterology and Infectious Disease, Department of Internal Medicine, Charles R. Drew University of Medicine and Science, and Martin Luther King, Jr.–Charles R. Drew Medical Center, Los Angeles, California, U.S.A.

Arvydas Ambrozaitis Clinic of Infectious Diseases and Microbiology, Vilnius University, Vilnius, Lithuania

Peter V. Barrett Department of Medicine, Harbor-UCLA Medical Center, Torrance, California, U.S.A.

Rex Biedenbender Division of Geriatrics, The Glennan Center for Geriatrics and Gerontology, Department of Medicine, Eastern Virginia Medical School, Norfolk, Virginia, U.S.A.

Suzanne F. Bradley Divisions of Infectious Diseases and Geriatric Medicine, Veterans Affairs Ann Arbor Healthcare System, The University of Michigan Medical School, Ann Arbor, Michigan, U.S.A.

Steven C. Castle Department of Veterans Affairs, Geriatric Research Education and Clinical Center, Veterans Affairs Greater Los Angeles Healthcare System, UCLA School of Medicine, Los Angeles, California, U.S.A.

Anthony W. Chow Division of Infectious Diseases, Department of Medicine, University of British Columbia, and Vancouver Hospital Health Sciences Center, Vancouver, British Columbia, Canada

Elizabeth L. Cobbs   Departments of Medicine and Health Care Sciences, George Washington University, Veterans Affairs Medical Center, Washington, D.C., U.S.A.

Kathleen Daretany   Center for Psycho-Oncology Research, Dartmouth-Hitchcock Medical Center, Dartmouth College, Lebanon, New Hampshire, U.S.A.

Vinod K. Dhawan   Division of Infectious Diseases, Department of Internal Medicine, Charles R. Drew University of Medicine and Science, Martin Luther King, Jr.–Charles R. Drew Medical Center, and UCLA School of Medicine, Los Angeles, California, U.S.A.

Ghinwa Dumyati   Department of Infectious Diseases, University of Rochester School of Medicine and Dentistry, Rochester, New York, U.S.A.

Allen S. Funnyé   Department of Internal Medicine, Charles R. Drew University of Medicine and Science, and Martin Luther King, Jr.–Charles R. Drew Medical Center, Los Angeles, California, U.S.A.

Stefan Gravenstein   Division of Geriatrics, The Glennan Center for Geriatrics and Gerontology, Department of Medicine, Eastern Virginia Medical School, Norfolk, Virginia, U.S.A.

Darrell W. Harrington   Department of Medicine, Harbor-UCLA Medical Center, Torrance, California, U.S.A.

Sara A. Hedderwick   Department of Infectious Diseases, Royal Victoria Hospital, Belfast, Northern Ireland, U.K.

Kevin P. High   Sections of Infectious Diseases and Hematology/Oncology, Department of Medicine, Wake Forest University School of Medicine, Winston Salem, North Carolina, U.S.A.

William R. Jarvis   Division of Pediatric Infectious Diseases, Emory University School of Medicine, Atlanta, Georgia, U.S.A.

Arnel M. Joaquin   Division of Geriatrics, Department of Internal Medicine, Charles R. Drew University of Medicine and Science, and Martin Luther King, Jr.–Charles R. Drew Medical Center, Los Angeles, California, U.S.A.

Carol A. Kauffman   Division of Infectious Diseases, Department
of Internal Medicine, Veterans Affairs Ann Arbor Healthcare
System, University of Michigan Medical School, Ann Arbor,
Michigan, U.S.A.

A. Jefferson Lesesne   Division of Geriatric Medicine and Gerontology,
Department of Medicine, Wesley Woods Center of Emory University,
Atlanta, Georgia, U.S.A.

Mark B. Loeb   Departments of Pathology and Molecular Medicine, and
Clinical Epidemiology and Biostatistics, McMaster University,
Hamilton, Ontario, Canada

Takashi Makinodan   Department of Veterans Affairs, Geriatric
Research Education and Clinical Center, Veterans Affairs Greater
Los Angeles Healthcare System, UCLA School of Medicine,
Los Angeles, California, U.S.A.

Barbara J. Messinger-Rapport   Section of Geriatric Medicine,
Department of General Internal Medicine, Cleveland Clinic Foundation,
Cleveland, Ohio, U.S.A.

Lona Mody   Division of Geriatric Medicine, University of
Michigan Medical School, Geriatrics Research, Education, and
Clinical Center, Veterans Affairs Ann Arbor Healthcare System,
Ann Arbor, Michigan, U.S.A.

Deborah Moran   Department of Internal Medicine, Charles R. Drew
University of Medicine and Science, and Martin Luther King, Jr.–Charles
R. Drew Medical Center, Los Angeles, California, U.S.A.

Joseph M. Mylotte   Department of Medicine, School of
Medicine and Biomedical Sciences, State University of New York,
Buffalo, New York, U.S.A.

Lindsay E. Nicolle   Departments of Internal Medicine and Medical
Microbiology, University of Manitoba, Winnipeg, Manitoba, Canada

Dean C. Norman   Department of Medicine, David Geffen School of
Medicine at UCLA, and Veterans Affairs Greater Los Angeles Healthcare
System, Los Angeles, California, U.S.A.

Joseph G. Ouslander   Division of Geriatric Medicine and Gerontology, Department of Medicine, Wesley Woods Center of Emory University, Emory University School of Medicine, Birmingham/Atlanta Veterans Affairs Geriatric Research, Education, and Clinical Center, Atlanta, Georgia, U.S.A.

Robert M. Palmer   Section of Geriatric Medicine, Department of General Internal Medicine, Cleveland Clinic Foundation, Cleveland, Ohio, U.S.A.

Shobita Rajagopalan   Division of Infectious Disease, Department of Internal Medicine, Charles R. Drew University of Medicine and Science, and Martin Luther King, Jr.–Charles R. Drew Medical Center, Los Angeles, California, U.S.A.

Steven C. Reynolds   Division of Infectious Diseases, Department of Medicine, University of British Columbia, and Vancouver Hospital Health Sciences Center, Vancouver, British Columbia, Canada

Jay P. Rho   Inpatient Pharmacy, Kaiser Foundation Hospital Los Angeles, and School of Pharmacy, University of Southern California, Los Angeles, California, U.S.A.

Chesley L. Richards, Jr.   Geriatric Research, Education, and Clinical Center (GRECC), Atlanta Veterans Affairs Medical Center, and Emory University School of Medicine, Atlanta, Georgia, U.S.A.

Kenneth E. Schmader   Center for the Study of Aging and Human Development and Division of Geriatrics, Department of Medicine, Duke University Medical Center, and Geriatric Research, Education, and Clinical Center, Durham Veterans Affairs Medical Center, Durham, North Carolina, U.S.A.

Larry J. Strausbaugh   Portland Veterans Affairs Medical Center and Oregon Health Sciences University School of Medicine, Portland, Oregon, U.S.A.

Made Sutjita   Division of Infectious Disease, Department of Internal Medicine, Charles R. Drew University of Medicine and Science, and Martin Luther King, Jr.–Charles R. Drew Medical Center, Los Angeles, California, U.S.A.

Jack Twersky   Center for the Study of Aging and Human Development and Division of Geriatrics, Department of Medicine, Duke University Medical Center, and Geriatric Research, Education, and Clinical Center, Durham Veterans Affairs Medical Center, Durham, North Carolina, U.S.A.

Koichi Uyemura   Department of Veterans Affairs, Geriatric Research Education and Clinical Center, Veterans Affairs Greater Los Angeles Healthcare System, UCLA School of Medicine, Los Angeles, California, U.S.A.

Megan Bernadette Wong   University of California–Los Angeles, Los Angeles, California, U.S.A.

Thomas T. Yoshikawa   Office of Research, Charles R. Drew University of Medicine and Science, Los Angeles, California, U.S.A.

1

Demographics and Economics of Long-Term Care

A. Jefferson Lesesne

Division of Geriatric Medicine and Gerontology, Department of Medicine, Wesley Woods Center of Emory University, Atlanta, Georgia, U.S.A.

Joseph G. Ouslander

Division of Geriatric Medicine and Gerontology, Department of Medicine, Wesley Woods Center of Emory University, Emory University School of Medicine, Birmingham/Atlanta Veterans Affairs Geriatric Research, Education, and Clinical Center, Atlanta, Georgia, U.S.A.

KEY POINTS

1. Disability, chronic diseases, dementia with behavioral symptoms and associated conditions such as incontinence, and lack of family and social support are predictors of need for LTC.
2. Medicare and Medicaid expenditures for LTC services continue to increase with the aging of the population.
3. Post-acute care in skilled nursing facilities is growing, and as a result there is an increased risk of infections and resistant organisms in this setting.
4. Changes in Medicare payment for post-acute care have changed the relationship of facilities to primary care providers, because the cost of medications, therapies, and diagnostic tests are bundled into a payment to the facility.
5. Assisted living facilities are growing as a niche in the LTC market often reducing the need for traditional nursing home beds but

providing care for frail elderly in a setting with minimal medical and nursing supervision.

6. Medicare Part D will have major implications on the nature of drug prescribing for the LTC population.

INTRODUCTION

Long-term care (LTC), as defined by Kane and Kane (1) is "a set of health, personal care, and social services delivered over a sustained period of time to persons who have lost or never acquired some degree of functional capacity." LTC includes a broad range of services for chronically disabled individuals over an extended period of time. Venues for care are predominantly nursing homes, assisted living facilities, senior housing, and personal dwellings. Coordination of care among these sites remains a challenge. The nursing facility remains the predominant institutional setting for LTC. In 2002, there were approximately 15,000 certified facilities with 1.8 million beds (2). This is nearly three times the number of acute care hospitals and twice the number of hospital beds. An aging society will place ever-increasing demands for services and costs associated with LTC. This chapter will review the relevant demographic and economic factors affecting primarily nursing facilities with a brief discussion of the growth of post-acute and assisted-living facility care.

DEMAND FOR NURSING FACILITY CARE

There are three main factors contributing to the demand for nursing home care: (1) the number of frail older adults with physical functional disabilities and/or mental health problems that preclude independent living or community-based care; (2) the available social support system; and (3) available, accessible, and affordable community-based LTC resources (Table 1). Of people reporting LTC needs as measured by requiring assistance with activities of daily living, 57% are aged 65 and older. The National Health Interview Survey in 2003 revealed that those aged 85 and older were more than six times likely to need help with personal care needs as those aged 65 to 74 (Fig. 1). Among those 85 and above, 21% resided in nursing facilities in 1995. In 1996, The Agency for Health-Care Policy and Research (now the Agency for Healthcare Research and Quality) concluded in a consensus panel that moderate to severe dementia was present in the population: 2% age 65 to 69, 4% age 70 to 74, 8% age 75 to 79, and 16% age 85 and over (3). Another study concluded that 47% of persons aged 85 had some degree of dementia (6). Figure 2 depicts the projected rise in those with dementia over the next 50 years. The older, more cognitively impaired individual is more likely to need assistance with activities of daily living and therefore need some form of LTC.

However, predicting the need for LTC is problematic when there is uncertainty about the future of certain diseases. For example, the cost of

Table 1   Factors Affecting the Need for Nursing Home Admission

Characteristics of the individual
  Age, sex, race
  Marital status
  Living arrangements
  Degree of mobility
  Ability to perform basic and instrumental activities of daily living
  Urinary incontinence
  Memory impairment
  Mood disturbance
Behavioral symptoms associated with dementia
  Tendency for falls
  Clinical prognosis
  Income
  Payment eligibility
  Need for special services
Characteristics of the support system
  Family capability
    Health and function of spouse (if married)
    Availability of responsible relative (usually adult child)
    Family structure of responsible relative
    Employment status of responsible relative
  Physician and other health-care provider availability
  Amount of care received from family and others
Community resources
  Formal community resources (Table 2)
  Informal support systems
  Presence of LTC institutions
  Characteristics of LTC institutions

Source: From Ref. 4.

care for Alzheimer's disease is estimated to be about $100 billion per year. The Alzheimer's Association estimates that approximately 14 million people will suffer with this condition by the middle of the 21st century. If a cure is developed or treatment is greatly improved, this alone could dramatically alter the predictions about who will need LTC (8).

Much of LTC in the United States is carried out by family and friends, especially wives and daughters. About half of Medicare beneficiaries live with their spouse, 16% live with their children, and 29% live alone (9). A survey of informal caregivers indicated that nearly 75% are women, while 40% are spouses, and 35% are adult children (10). Among informal caregivers, 12% are aged 65 and older, and 15% report physical or mental health concerns due to caregiving (11). The average age of the informal caregiver is 60, with 50% employed full time. Two-thirds of those who work outside the home reported conflicts with work and caregiving. Of older adults

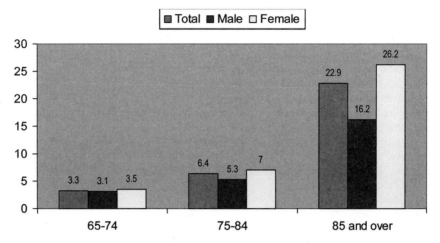

Figure 1 Percent of adults aged 65 and over who require help with personal care needs, January–September 2003. *Source*: From Ref. 5.

aged 75 and above, approximately 20% of men and 50% of women live alone. About one-third of those who live alone has no children. The older population now tends to have fewer children and is more geographically disbursed than previous generations (12). The significance of informal caregiving is evident by the fact that 50% of older adults with LTC needs and no family support reside in nursing facilities, compared with 7% of those with family caregivers (13).

The geriatric population will see unprecedented growth with the aging of the baby boomer generation, and this growth will greatly increase the

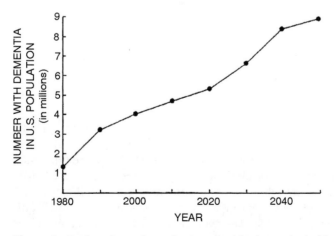

Figure 2 Projected number of persons with dementia in the U.S. population. *Source*: From Ref. 7.

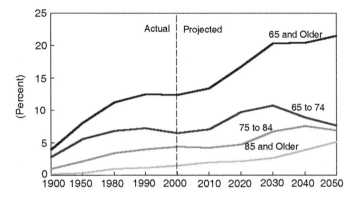

Figure 3 People aged 65 and older as a share of the U.S. population, selected years, 1900–2050. *Source*: From Ref. 14.

likelihood of needing LTC. In 2002, there were 33.6 million (12%) Americans aged 65 and older, and this is expected to increase to 18% by 2025. By the year 2050, 20% of the U.S. population will be 65 and older, and the 85-and-older population, those most likely to need LTC, will represent 5% of the U.S. population (Fig. 3). A portion of the increase is due to increased life expectancy. Males aged 65 could expect to live 15 years in 1995 and they can expect to live 18 years by 2030 (Fig. 4). Some estimates project the number of people aged 65 and older with functional limitations

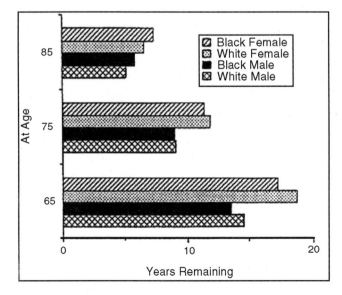

Figure 4 Life expectancy in the geriatric population. *Source*: From Ref. 15.

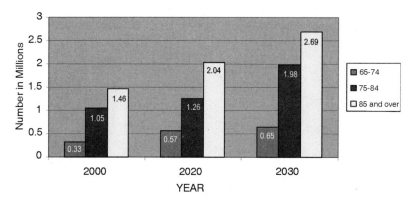

Figure 5 Nursing home population by age. *Source*: From Ref. 16.

to be approximately 20 million to 30 million by 2040. These demographic shifts will substantially increase the need for nursing home care. Figure 5 shows the projected growth of the nursing home population by age.

There are many community services available to frail older adults, which have been demonstrated to delay or prevent nursing facility admission for some people (Table 2). These services tend to be fragmented and in many cases not reimbursable by most insurance or governmental funding sources. Additionally, there is poor integration of care in the acute and long-term settings. The primary funding sources of Medicare and Medicaid have differing eligibility requirements and coverage rules that prevent integration. There is also fear of financial loss on the part of commercial carriers because of inadequate risk adjustment for chronically ill or disabled people. Social health maintenance organizations attempt to add community services and short-term nursing home care to a traditional health maintenance organizations health plan. The Program for All-inclusive Care for the Elderly (PACE) is designed for frail older adults, who are eligible for Medicaid and nursing home certifiable. The PACE program attempts to help frail older adults remain in the community (17). Many states are also developing their own initiatives to provide better community care and delay nursing home admission. Although the number of such programs is increasing, many frail older adults will reach a point where institutional care is the most appropriate alternative.

The growth in the number of assisted-living facilities has had a substantial impact on LTC over the last several years. Although there is no clear definition of what constitutes an assisted-living facility, these venues provide some level of LTC for their residents. The Center for Medicare and Medicaid Services data indicate that the number of Medicare beneficiaries residing in nursing facilities has declined while the number residing in assisted-living facilities has increased (Fig. 6). A national study of assisted-living

Table 2 Examples of Formal Community Services Available
Outside of Nursing Homes

Housing
  Senior apartments
  Residential care facilities
  Assisted living
  Foster care
  Life care or CCRC
Health promotion activities
  Wellness programs
  Exercise classes
  Family and patient education
  Nutrition consultation
  Meal programs
  Volunteer programs
Outreach
  Screening clinics
  Mobile vans
  Discharge planning
  Case management
  Information and referral
  Meals on wheels
  Transportation
  Emergency response system
  Respite care
Outpatient centers
  Geriatric clinics
  Psychosocial counseling
  Rehabilitation
  Adult day care
Home health
  Home health agencies
    Medicare-certified
    Private
    Visiting nurse associations
  Hospice
  Homemaker and chore
  Home infusion therapies
  Durable medical equipment
Acute inpatient units
  Geriatric
  Rehabilitation
  Psychiatric
  Alcohol/substance abuse

Abbreviation: CCRC, continuing care retirement community.

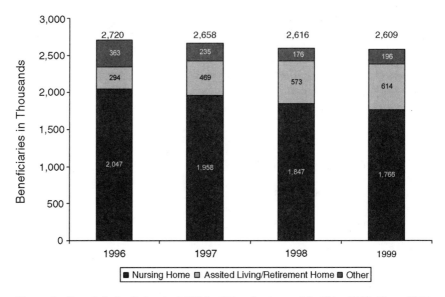

Figure 6 Beneficiaries living in LTC facilities, by type of facility, 1999. Since 1996, the number of beneficiaries living in traditional nursing homes and other facilities has declined, while use of other types of assisted living arrangements has increased.

facilities estimated that there were approximately 11,500 facilities with 650,000 beds providing services to 560,000 residents (18). This survey included facilities with at least 11 beds, providing 24-hour oversight, and serving at least two meals per day. The major difference in this industry is that it tends to be comprised more of real-estate developers and hotel managers than health-care providers. This management culture may have important implications for how infection control and other health-care issues are addressed and managed.

The rates of nursing home usage vary with age and race. There are a greater number of whites than blacks, and more women than men, in nursing facilities. Nearly 25% of white women reside in a nursing home by age 85. The number of those aged 65 and over, who stay overnight in a nursing home, fell by 8% from 1985 to 1995 (19). This decline may have resulted from a decline in disability rates of the elderly, increased usage of home health services, and the growth in assisted living facilities. One study based on national LTC surveys indicated that disability rates for those aged 65 and older decreased by 1.3% per year from 1982 to 1994 (20). All of these tend to delay or prevent placement in a nursing home.

ECONOMICS OF LTC

Financing for LTC in the United States is primarily provided through private funding and governmental assistance programs, including Medicare and

Table 3 Long-Term Care Expenditures for the Elderly, by Source of Payment, 2004 (in Billions of Dollars)

Payment source	Institutional care		Home care		Total	
	$	%	$	%	$	%
Medicaid	36.5	39.5	10.8	25.4	47.3	35.0
Medicare	15.9	17.2	17.7	41.6	33.6	24.9
Private insurance	2.4	2.5	3.3	7.7	5.6	4.2
Out of pocket	35.7	38.6	8.3	19.5	44.0	32.6
Other	2.0	2.2	2.5	5.8	4.4	3.3
Total	92.4	100	42.5	100	134.9	100

Source: From Ref. 21.

Medicaid. Private funding can include personal resources and may include a component of LTC insurance. There are also "Medigap" insurance policies to cover the copayment required by Medicare. LTC costs as a percentage of personal health-care expenditures have increased from 4% in 1960 to 10% in 2002. Approximately $135 billion was spent on LTC, including home care, in 2004. Medicare accounted for nearly 25% and Medicaid 35% (Table 3). States are the major financiers of LTC for older adults, whereas the federal government finances most acute care. Many Americans are unprepared for LTC expenditures because they believe it is a Medicare benefit.

Medicare

Medicare is a governmental insurance program that covers the cost of acute hospitalization for those aged 65 and older. In addition, Medicare covers outpatient services (Part B) as well as post-acute hospital care for up to 100 days, following a 3-day hospitalization, based on medical complexity (Table 4) and/or progress in rehabilitation (Part A, linked to the acute hospital stay). Currently, there are approximately 40.5 million Medicare beneficiaries, and in 2002 the annual budget was $252 billion. Forty-seven percent of Medicare expenditures go to hospitals, with another 20% covering physician services and 6% going to nursing home care (2).

Medicare expenditures for home health increased nearly 10-fold from 1987 to 1995 (22). In response, Congress enacted the 1997 Balanced Budget Act, which greatly reduced these payments and initiated a significant effort to reduce fraud and abuse. Many states have developed strategies to help their Medicaid recipients maximize their Medicare home health benefits in an effort to conserve state Medicaid dollars. Medicare also limits its funding for LTC by only covering postacute or "subacute" skilled care. Medicare provides postacute skilled care for 100 days following an acute hospitalization of three or more days. To qualify the patient requires daily skilled

Table 4 Examples of Admission Criteria to Subacute (Medicare Skilled) Units

Intravenous antibiotics
Physical therapy 6–7 times/week
Occupational therapy 5 times/week
Weaning oxygen therapy for respiratory conditions
Tracheal suctioning at least 2 times/shift
Respiratory therapy treatment 3 times/day or more frequently
Capillary blood glucose monitoring 2 times/day with insulin coverage
Injectable medications every 8 hr or 2 times/day
Wound care daily
Enteral tube feeding
Laboratory test monitoring every 2–3 days
Renal dialysis with monitoring
Bladder training
Pain management (parenteral)
Skilled nursing observation of congestive heart, liver, or renal failure

nursing care or rehabilitation services for the condition that was treated in the hospital (Table 4).

Funding for postacute care from Medicare has transitioned to a prospective payment system (PPS) based on resident problems identified in the Minimum Data Set. Under the PPS model, a capitated reimbursement is made to the nursing home for care of particular care needs following an acute hospitalization. The reimbursement is calculated based on the Minimum Data Set and then translated into resource utilization groups (RUGs) similar to the DRG (diagnostic related group) payment system for acute hospitals. An important component is that all ancillary services (rehabilitation therapy, laboratory services, medications, etc.) are now bundled into the payment. This has profound implications for the relationship between nursing homes and physicians, because under PPS the nursing home bears the cost of physician-ordered laboratory tests, medications, and therapies.

Medicaid

Medicaid is a federally sponsored, state-administered program to provide health insurance for the indigent. It covers both acute hospital care and outpatient services for those who qualify based on means testing. There is an LTC component that covers nursing home care on a means-tested basis. This program insures 41 million people (11% elderly) at an annual cost of $246 billion. Forty-three percent of expenditures go to nursing homes (2). Each state administers the program differently, so there is a great amount of variability in terms of benefits covered.

The vast majority of nursing home care is paid for out of pocket or by Medicaid, which has led to a phenomenon known as "spend down."

Individuals and families will deplete a person's assets until they can pass the means test for Medicaid funding for LTC. Given the fact that nursing home care can cost as much as $40,000 to $60,000 per year, it does not take older adults very long to qualify for Medicaid. As a result, Medicaid has become in effect the payer of last resort for institutional LTC. This has inspired many state Medicaid agencies to develop and work with programs that prevent or delay the need for institutional care.

Private Funding

Private LTC insurance only covered 6% of nursing home and home care costs in 1995 (12). The number of policies sold has recently seen a dramatic increase from 300,000 in 1988 to nearly 700,000 in 2001 (23). There is a wide range of coverage available through these policies; however, most provide some type of home care component to avoid or delay nursing home coverage. Several states have promoted the purchase of LTC insurance by providing a mechanism to protect assets from Medicaid eligibility requirements equal to the amount of LTC coverage.

EVOLVING CHANGES IN LTC

The LTC industry has seen substantial growth of postacute care in the United States over the last decade. As the population ages and hospital lengths of stay are shortened, more medically complex patients with greater nursing home care needs are being discharged from hospitals to nursing facilities. Often they are not functionally able or medically stable enough to return home. Subacute units in nursing facilities have become a place where these residents can convalesce prior to their ultimate discharge. For these units to succeed there need to be adequate reimbursement, availability of skilled nurses, and quality medical care, as well as adequate ancillary services. Management of infectious diseases for which treatment was initiated in an acute hospital, as well as new nosocomial infections that occur in postacute patients, is a major challenge in the nursing home setting.

Regulations that set standards for staffing ratios will help improve care quality in nursing homes (24). Nursing homes will also benefit from a survey process that provides education and is outcomes based rather than a punitive process to identify misconduct. Additionally, unfunded government mandates are difficult to implement and drain resources. Improved reimbursement will help insure adequate staffing of nurses and therapists as well as improve the availability of ancillary services. Improving nursing education and professional opportunities will also help to attract and retain quality staff. This is also true for physicians, nurse practitioners, and physician assistants. Nurse practitioners and physician assistants can be instrumental in managing infections in the nursing home, thereby reducing the need for acute hospitalizations. Innovative programs are essential to improve the job and quality of care provided by nurse's aides. These staff members provide more than 90% of hands-on care in nursing homes and must be involved in the early identification of infectious illness as well as other acute conditions.

Reimbursements that are adjusted for risk and complexity will help provide quality care in the most appropriate setting. The RUGs system is a step in this direction. Medicare Part D will improve the coverage of the costs of many medications for a substantial number of long-stay nursing home residents but will change the nature of prescribing for this population. Outcome monitoring based on quality indicators will continue to evolve and will provide incentives for improving quality care in the nursing home (25). Center for Medicare and Medicaid Services, through its quality improvement organizations based in each state, is making intensive efforts to impact several of these quality indicators in order to improve the overall quality of nursing home care. Finally, the growth of integrated care systems made up of hospitals, primary care providers, LTC facilities, and community-based partners will also improve the quality of care transitions and have financial implications. These systems must have shared visions, goals, and financial incentives to providing good care. They also implement care standards as well as develop information systems that can improve the critical transition of elderly patients and their medical information across care settings. All of these features will reduce practice variability and medical errors, and improve the quality of LTC in the future.

REFERENCES

1. Kane RA, Kane RL. Long Term Care: Principles, Programs, and Policies. New York: Springer, 1987.
2. U.S. Department of Health and Human Services, Centers for Medicare and Medicaid Services, Office of Research, Development, and Information, October 2004. (CMS publication no. 03455.).
3. Stone RI. LTC for the elderly with disabilities: current policy, emerging trends, and implications for the twenty-first century. Milbank Memorial Fund, 2000.
4. Kane RL, Ouslander JG, Abrass IB. Essentials of clinical geriatrics. 3rd ed. New York: McGraw-Hill, 1994.
5. National Health Interview Survey, January–September, 2003.
6. Costa PT, Williams TF, Albert MS. Recognition and initial assessment of Alzheimer's disease and related dementias. Clinical practice guideline No. 19. Washington, D.C.: Agency for Health Care Policy and Research, 1996. (AHCPR publication no. 97–0702.).
7. National Institute on Aging and U.S. Bureau of census. Prevalence Estimates and Projections.
8. Demography is not destiny. Natl Acad Aging Soc. Washington, D.C., 1999;51.
9. CMS, Office of Research, Development, and Information. Data from the Medicare Current Beneficiary Survey (MCBO), 2000.

10. Administration on Aging. Informal Caregiving: Compassion in Action. Washington, D.C., 1998.
11. National Alliance for Caregiving and the American Association of Retired Persons. Family caregiving in the U.S., 1997; 8:41.
12. Kane RL, Ouslander JG, Abrass IB. Essentials of clinical geriatrics. 2nd ed. New York: McGraco-Hill, 2004:25.
13. National Academy on Aging. Facts on LTC. Washington, D.C., 1997. (Available at http://geron.org/NAA/ltc.html).
14. U.S. interim projections by age, sex, race, and Hispanic origin. "Projected Population of the United States, by Age and Sex: 2000 to 2050," March 2004. Congressional Budget Office, Bureau of the Census. (Available at WWW. census. gov/ipc/WWW/usinterimproj/natprojtab02a.pdf).
15. Havlik RJ, Suzman R. Health status—Mortality. In: Havlik RJ, Liu MG, Kovar MG, et al, eds.: Health Statistics on Older Persons, United States, 1986. Viral and Health Statistics, Series 3, No. 25. DHHS Publ. No (PHS)87-1409. Public Health Service, U.S. Government Printing Office, 1987.
16. Who will pay for the baby boomers' long-term care needs? Expanding the role of private LTC insurance, American Council on Life Insurance, 1998.
17. Pacala J, Kane R, Atherly A, Smith M. Using structured implicit review to assess quality of care in the Program of All-inclusive Care for the Elderly (PACE). J Am Geriatr Soc 2000; 48:903–910.
18. Hawes C, Rose M, Phillips CD, Iannacchione V. A National Study of Assisted Living for the Frail Elderly: Results of a National Telephone Survey of Facilities. Beachwood, OH: Menorah Park Center for the Aging, 1999.
19. Bishop CE. Where are the missing elders? The decline in nursing home use 1985 and 1995. Health Aff 1999; 18:146–155.
20. Manton K, Corder L, Stallard E. Chronic disability trends in the elderly in the United States. Natl Acad Sci USA 1997; 94:2593–2598.
21. Congressional Budget Office Testimony. The Cost and Financing of Long-Term Care Services. The Congress of the United States, 2005.
22. Kenney G, Rajan S, Soscia S. State spending for Medicare and Medicaid home care programs. Health Aff 1998; 17:201–212.
23. Congressional Budget Office based on data from the America's Health Insurance Plans. Financing Long-Term Care for the Elderly. CBO, The Congress of the United States, 2004.
24. Wunderlich GS, Kohler PO, eds. Improving the Quality of LTC: A Report of the Institute of Medicine. Washington, D.C.: National Academy Press, National Academy of Sciences, 2001.
25. Zimmerman DR, Karon SL, Arling G. Developments and testing of nursing home quality indicators. Health Care Financ Rev 1995; 16:107–127.

2

Epidemiology and Special Aspects of Infectious Diseases in Aging

Thomas T. Yoshikawa

*Office of Research, Charles R. Drew University of Medicine and Science,
Los Angeles, California, U.S.A.*

KEY POINTS

1. Aging is associated with increased risk for infectious diseases and their complications.
2. Age-related functional disabilities increase the susceptibility to infections, and, conversely, infectious diseases will lead to significant functional incapacities in older adults.
3. Clinical manifestations of infections in the frail elderly nursing home resident may be atypical or absent.
4. Fever may be absent, normal, or subnormal in elderly nursing home residents with serious infections.
5. Age-related changes in pharmacokinetics and pharmacodynamics should be carefully considered whenever antibiotics (or any drug) are prescribed in older patients or nursing home residents.

CONCEPTUAL BASIS FOR IMPORTANCE OF INFECTION AND AGING

Modern infectious diseases evolved once the germ theory of medicine was established (1). The impact of the germ theory was enormous and led to the development and implementation of antisepsis, antimicrobial therapy,

vaccination, sanitation, and public health measures. For industrialized
nations such as the United States, these practices and processes reduced
mortality in the latter half of the 20th century—primarily in children—
which was predominantly due to infections. This resulted in the increase
in life expectancy that has occurred during the last 50 years (see Chapter 1), as
well as a change in the major causes of death in developed countries.
Whereas infectious diseases were the leading causes of death up to the early
part of the 20th century in the United States, heart disease, cancer, and
stroke now head the list of top causes of death. However, in less developed
countries throughout the world, infections still remain the primary cause of
mortality, accounting for one-third of all deaths worldwide (1).

As life expectancy increases, there is concomitant growth in the number
of aging adults, including those requiring long-term care (see Chapter 1).
With aging comes physiological changes that include alterations in the host
immune system and acquisition of diseases, disabilities, and functional
limitations—all of which place the frail elderly person at significant risk
for infectious diseases and their complications (see Chapter 5). Moreover,
these and other factors contribute substantially to the increased morbidity
and mortality associated with infections in elderly persons (Table 1) (2).
The infections that are especially relevant because of higher incidence, prevalence, morbidity, and mortality with aging are listed in Table 2 (3). Many
of these infections are very important in the long-term care facility (LTCF)
setting. More recently, it has become apparent that infectious diseases—like
many other age-related disorders—have a dual relationship with the functional capacity and abilities of older adults (4). Age-related functional
disabilities increase the susceptibility to infections, and, conversely, infectious diseases will lead to significant functional incapacities in aging adults.
Such an association becomes even more apparent in the very old and very
frail person residing in an LTCF. Thus, residents in LTCFs, such as a
nursing home, who are generally already functionally disabled, experience
the greatest susceptibility to infectious diseases as well as the highest risk

Table 1 Factors Contributing to Increased Morbidity and Mortality
of Infections in Elderly Persons

Age-related decrease in physiological reserve capacity
Chronic comorbidities/diseases
Diminished host immune response
Delayed or inadequate response to antimicrobial therapy
Delays in diagnosis and treatment
Greater risk and incidence of health-care facility–associated infections
Higher rates of adverse drug reactions
Poor tolerance to invasive diagnostic and therapeutic interventions

Source: From Ref. 2.

Table 2 Important Infectious Diseases in the Geriatric Population

Urinary tract infection
Respiratory tract infection (pneumonia and bronchitis)
Tuberculosis
Skin and soft tissue infections (e.g., infected pressure ulcer, cellulitis,
    and herpes zoster)
Intra-abdominal infections (cholecystitis, diverticulitis, appendicitis,
    and infectious diarrhea)
Bacterial meningitis
Infective endocarditis

Source: From Ref. 3.

for death and further disability and functional incapacity following an infection. Only through research, which is then translated to bedside care, will we be able to address this conundrum if we are to improve the health, quality of life, and quality of care in the population at highest risk for adverse and poor outcomes.

SPECIAL ASPECTS OF INFECTIONS IN THE ELDERLY

Clinical Manifestations

Infection is now well known to be an important cause of morbidity and mortality in elderly persons. However, the clinical diagnosis of infectious disease in older patients is often difficult and overlooked. The clinical manifestations of infections in the frail and elderly LTCF resident may be atypical or absent (see Chapter 8). Fever may not be detectable in older persons with serious infections (5). In frail LTCF residents, studies have shown that baseline body temperatures may be subnormal, and febrile responses to an infection may occur but go unrecognized because the "fever" fails to reach a predetermined criterion [e.g., 101°F (38°C)]. In such cases, a change in body temperature of at least 2°F from baseline should be interpreted as a possible "febrile" response (6). It has also been proposed that the absolute criterion for fever should be lowered in frail elderly persons, that is, 99°F (37.2°C) for oral temperature and 99.5°F (37.5°F) for rectal temperature (7).

Increased Susceptibility to Infections

The increased susceptibility of older people to select infections may be a multifactorial process. A "normal" process of aging is the phenomenon of immune dysregulation or dysfunction (see Chapter 5). It is most likely the interrelationships between age-related immune dysregulation and age-associated chronic diseases that affect immune processes place the older, frail LTCF resident at high risk for infectious diseases (8). In addition, other factors, such as nutrition (see Chapter 6), and chronic use of antibiotics (see Chapter 11), have an impact on the risk, severity, and types of infections found in the geriatric population. The risk or severity of an infection can be simply illustrated in an equation that includes innate microbial factors (virulence), quantity of exposure to microorganisms, and host resistance:

$$\text{Infection (risk/severity)} \approx \frac{\text{virulence} \times \text{inoculum size}}{\text{host resistance}}$$

This relationship states that infection risk or severity is directly proportional to the virulence of the pathogen and quantity of organisms and inversely proportional to the integrity of host resistance (9).

Certainly, frail LTCF residents are being exposed more to highly virulent organisms by virtue of several pathogens having resistance to multiple antibiotics [e.g., methicillin-resistant *Staphylococcus aureus* (Chapter 23), vancomycin-resistant enterococci (Chapter 24). The quantity of microorganisms to which these residents are exposed can be enormous, especially when they experience aspiration pneumonia, intra-abdominal infections, and infected skin/soft tissues (e.g., pressure ulcers). In addition, the age-related changes in immune function and the immune dysregulation associated with underlying chronic diseases reduce the elderly LTCF residents' resistance to infection.

Antimicrobial Therapy

Chapter 11 provides an in-depth discussion of the principles and approach to prescribing antibiotics for elderly patients with suspected or confirmed infections. Nevertheless, it is important to consider the age-related changes in pharmacokinetics and pharmacodynamics whenever any drug is prescribed to an elderly patient. Dose adjustments and the pharmacological properties of a drug must be carefully determined because of the age-associated alterations in volume of distribution, reductions in renal function, and potential sensitivity of select organs to certain drugs. Moreover, because the vast majority of older patients are taking some type of prescribed or over-the-counter medication, potential drug interactions as well as adverse side effects must be carefully evaluated before and during administration of an antibiotic (e.g., divalent ion-containing antacids, such as calcium carbonate, may affect the absorption of many quinolones). Adverse drug events occur more often in the elderly and increase with the number of drugs prescribed (10). It is imperative, therefore, that careful monitoring for adverse events in elderly patients or residents be performed regularly during administration of antibiotics or any other drugs. Because elderly persons may not exhibit typical manifestations of drug side effects as described by the drug information packet, it is important to be aware that unexplained changes in cognitive function, behavior, or physical capacity may be attributable to medications, However, close monitoring is especially difficult in LTCFs because of the high level of disability and inability to communicate in many of the residents in these institutions, the limited number of visits made by physicians and other health providers, and lack of immediate availability of laboratory tests in such facilities. Given these limitations, prescribing antibiotics to LTCF residents will require careful thought, appropriate indications, and judicious selection (see Appendix C).

SUGGESTED READING

High KP, Bradley S, Loeb M, Palmer R, Quagliarello V, Yoshikawa T. A new paradigm for clinical investigation of infectious syndromes in older adults: assessment of functional status as a risk factor and outcome measure. Clin Infect Dis 2005; 40:114–122.

Yoshikawa TT. Epidemiology and unique aspects of aging and infectious diseases. Clin Infect Dis 2000; 30:931–933.

REFERENCES

1. Kuppersmith D. Three Centuries for Infectious Disease. In: An Illustrated History of Research and Treatment. Greenwich, CT: Greenwich Press, 1998.
2. Yoshikawa TT. Epidemiology and unique aspects of aging and infectious diseases. Clin Infect Dis 2000; 30:931–933.
3. Yoshikawa TT. Important infections in elderly persons. West J Med 1981; 135: 441–445.
4. High KP, Bradley S, Loeb M, Palmer R, Quagliarello V, Yoshikawa T. A new paradigm for clinical investigation of infectious syndromes in older adults: assessment of functional status as a risk factor and outcome measure. Clin Infect Dis 2005; 40:114–122.
5. Norman DC. Fever in the elderly. Clin Infect Dis 2000; 31:148–151.
6. Castle SC, Yeh M, Toledo S, Norman DC. Lowering the temperature criterion improves detection of infections in nursing home residents. Aging Immunol Infect Dis 1993; 4:67–76.
7. Norman DC, Yoshikawa TT. Fever in the elderly. Infect Dis Clin North Am 1996; 10:93–99.
8. Castle SC. Clinical relevance of age-related immune dysfunction. Clin Infect Dis 2000; 31:578–585.
9. Yoshikawa TT, Norman DC. Aging and Clinical Practice: Infectious Diseases. Diagnosis and Treatment. New York: Igaku-Shoin, 1987.
10. Wong FS, Rho JP. Drug dosing and life-threatening drug reactions in the critically ill patient. In: Yoshikawa TT, Norman DC, eds. Acute Emergencies and Critical Care of the Geriatric Patient. New York: Marcel Dekker, Inc., 2000:31–47.

3

Evaluation of Infections in Long-Term Care Facilities Versus Acute Care Hospitals

Arnel M. Joaquin

Division of Geriatrics, Department of Internal Medicine, Charles R. Drew University of Medicine and Science, and Martin Luther King, Jr.–Charles R. Drew Medical Center, Los Angeles, California, U.S.A.

KEY POINTS

1. The primary care professional (PCP) should recognize that medical decisions in long-term care facilities might be made with limited information and resources.
2. Change in functional status and behavior may be the only sign that infection is present in a resident.
3. Use of routine protocols for resident assessment and communication of information between nursing staff and PCP is essential.
4. The PCP should be aware of the existence of advance directives that the resident has executed, as this will often determine the course of action one will take.
5. Transfers to the emergency room should be done judiciously, as it is not always associated with better outcome.

INTRODUCTION

Long-term care facilities (LTCFs) include nursing homes (NH), assisted-living facilities, and other facilities where chronic care is provided to residents. This chapter will mainly focus on NH when referring to LTCF. NH are typically staffed with skilled health professionals that include nursing, physical and occupational therapists, respiratory therapists, dieticians, physicians, nurse practitioners, and physician assistants, among others. The physician and often the nurse practitioner or physician assistant are the PCP responsible for making medical decisions in their setting. Infection, particularly urinary tract infections, pneumonia, and skin and soft tissue infections, in the LTCF is a common problem (1–3).

Residents of a nursing home are typically the frail elderly who are immunocompromised. Nursing home infections also behave like hospital infections in most respects, and this is addressed in other parts of this chapter. There are variations in capability, but infections in the LTCF can be treated in-house, and more unstable patients are transferred out to the acute hospital setting. Registered nurse (RN) turnover, corporate structure of the NH, and other social and environmental factors may affect the decisions whether to treat a patient in the NH or in an acute hospital setting (4). A PCP needs to recognize the difference between an acute care setting and an NH where there are certain limitations to resources, as indicated in Table 1. As often happens, a physician may not be present at the time of symptom presentation and would have a need to make judgments based on verbal reports, as well as limited information on the chart, to determine the appropriate action. It is not always appropriate for the physician to instruct a nurse to transfer a resident to the emergency room for evaluation, and residents and family members may express dissatisfaction when residents are transferred in and out of the nursing facility. A multidisciplinary approach in the LTCF setting will help guide the appropriate course of action.

Acute Care vs. Long-Term Care Facilities

Staffing and Resources

NH have licensed and unlicensed nursing staffs that provide the majority of care. Staffing varies from one LTCF to another, determined partly by type

Table 1 Differences Between Acute Care Facility and Long-Term Care Facility

Parameter	Acute care facility	Long-term care facility
Patient population	Young and old	Predominantly old
Setting	High technology	Home-like
Goals	Acute disease treatment	Comfort, support
Length of stay	Days, weeks	Months, years
Physician role	Primary	Secondary, limited
Infection definition	Clinical + tests	Clinical + limited tests
Resources for infection control	Broad	Variable and often limited
Isolation capability	Broad	Limited to none

Source: From Ref. 5.

of organization and case mix. There are guidelines in LTCF regarding appropriate nursing staff, and it is generally accepted that the higher the ratio of nurse aids and licensed nurse to residents, the better the outcome. In a study done by the Centers for Medicare and Medicaid Services, as required by Omnibus Budget Reconciliation Act of 1990, on the appropriateness of establishing minimum staffing ratios in NH, threshold levels of nursing ratio were established, which correlated with better outcome (6). Certified nursing assistants (CNAs) provide the majority of hands-on care, including grooming, washing, ambulation, feeding, dressing, and overall supervision of residents. An optimal ratio based on the above study would be no greater than 1:12. Optimal licensed nursing (RN + licensed practical nurse) ratio would be approximately 1:30 with registered nursing ratio of not more than 1:120.

PCP typically visit their patients on a monthly basis and more often as medically necessary. To facilitate the visit, input of information from the different disciplines is typically necessary to obtain a complete assessment of the resident. A PCP should always communicate with a CNA or an RN to discuss behavior, medical symptoms and signs, functional status, and other issues.

Many skilled nursing facilities have the capability to perform stat laboratory procedures as well as portable X-rays for infection evaluation, especially of the most common infections in the NH. The PCP needs to recognize the limitations of ordering these tests in the NH. Some technicians are not available on weekends and holidays, or results may take longer than in the acute hospital setting. Clinical judgment as to the appropriate course of action to take is essential to avoid an adverse outcome. Empirical treatment may be justified in a stable patient prior to arrival of laboratory and X-ray results. Consultants are very rarely available, and complicated infectious disease cases may need to be transferred to the acute facility to be seen by an infectious disease consultant.

Intravenous (IV) fluids, antibiotics (both IV and oral), and nebulizers are usually available in most NHs, and many urinary tract infections and pneumonias may be treated successfully without the need for an acute hospital transfer (7).

Recognition of Infection

Nursing home residents are all under the supervision of licensed nursing staff, but monitoring of individual residents is variable depending on their functional status and medical comorbidities. Some residents get vital signs monitored frequently, and others may have them performed monthly or at longer intervals. Subtle temperature changes, behavioral changes, and overt symptoms may go unnoticed until the infection is more manifest. Presence of infection may present with typical manifestations, with the presence of high fever, chills, cough, and pulmonary congestion. However, infections may also present with symptoms and signs that are considered atypical, such as a fall, behavioral change, lethargy, and loss of appetite (see also Chapter 8). CNAs are the first providers to have the opportunity to identify infection, as they interact closely with the residents and ordinarily should be able to identify small changes in mental status or functional decline that could signal an underlying infection. The CNAs should report these observations to the licensed nurse on duty. The nurse is then expected to obtain vital signs and perform a nursing assessment so that this information, along with any recent pertinent history, can be given to the PCP when one is contacted.

The residents' family members are also good sources of information for the health-care professionals. Family members may elicit specific verbal complaints from the resident, or they may also notice some subtle change in their relative. Physical therapists, occupational therapists, and other skilled professionals in contact with the resident may report changes to the nursing staff for appropriate attention. On occasion, they may even call the PCP directly.

The Initial Evaluation of Suspected Infection

The PCP is not required to be in the nursing home on a daily basis. Thus, quite often the PCP is notified of changes in the residents' condition by phone. The nurse on duty usually completes the initial assessment in the facility after being notified of a change in status by a CNA, a family member, or a member of the multidisciplinary team. The nurse reports the findings to the PCP. Depending on the clinical stability of the resident, the PCP may give orders for stat laboratory and X-rays to be done, if available at the facility. The licensed nurse often can make a determination whether a call to the paramedics (911) is warranted, which may be done without prior authorization from the physician. However, a nonemergency transfer to the emergency room or urgent care needs authorization from a physician for the transportation to be covered by the residents' health insurance.

If a patient is judged to be clinically stable by both the licensed nurse and PCP, initial management may be done while waiting for laboratory and X-ray results. Initiation of IV or oral antibiotics may be done if clinically warranted, prior to the above results. Negative laboratory and X-ray results would prompt further investigation.

Complete blood counts are most helpful when abnormal. Values of total white blood cell (WBC) count equal to or above 15,000 cells/mm^3, or a left shift even with normal WBC count is higly associated with bacterial infection (8). Abnormal WBC, while suggestive of infection, does not necessarily mean that the resident needs to be transferred to an acute care facility. It is useful in following the resident's response to antibiotics.

Urinalysis and urine culture are also frequently ordered and treated if associated with symptoms, such as low-grade fever, confusion, functional decline, and incontinence. However, limited studies suggest that they are not always associated with urinary tract infection (9). Bacteriuria, on the other hand, is present in up to 50% of non-catheterized female resident of LTCFs and may be observed and not treated with antibiotics (10).

Blood cultures, sputum cultures, skin, and soft tissue cultures may be necessary to guide the treatment of the LTCF resident. Hospital and nursing home pathogens are similar and these cultures are more useful in instances when polymicrobial infections are present. Stool cultures are helpful in cases of diarrhea to rule out bacterial gastroenteritis. Some pathogens that may be isolated include *C. dificile*, *C. perfringens*, *S. aureus*, *Salmonella*, *Shigella*, *C. jejuni*, and *E. coli* (11).

Use of pulse oximetry is acceptable provided that the HCP are fully aware of its limitations on assessing ventilatory failure. A normal pulse oximetry is difficult to interpet in LTCF residents with baseline functional and mental deficits. However, a saturation of less than 90% with a respiratory rate of >25 is suggestive of impending respiratory failure (12). The HCP may still attempt some urgent interventions, such as a aggressive suctioning, chest physical therapy, bronchodilators to improve the residents condition. Success of these measures is dependent on several factors. Nursing staff in a LTCF would need to determine their own comfort level based on their knowledge of the resident's medical problems, and their own staffing level.

If residents are treated in the nursing home, the physician can instruct the nurse to monitor patients more frequently, with provision for less frequent monitoring as patients' condition improves (see also Chapter 14).

Infection Control

Infection in the nursing home is a significant problem. Outbreaks frequently occur, and the rates of infection are high. Current infection control strategies in the acute care setting may not be appropriate or practical for most LTCFs. Despite extensive regulations that include requirement for infection control, LTCFs do not provide enough resources and personnel for this activity. Unfortunately, there are not enough data on the cost effectiveness of infection control intervention in LTCFs (2). Much of infection control activities focus on data gathering and not on intervention. It is said that "interventional epidemiology" may be the next phase of development of the field of infection control. This would shift emphasis from data collection to data-driven intervention in LTCFs (see also Chapter 9) (13).

WHEN TO TRANSFER LONG-TERM CARE FACILITIES RESIDENTS TO AN ACUTE CARE SETTING

Except for 911 calls or paramedic transfers to the emergency rooms, physicians' decisions to transfer a patient to an acute facility for evaluation may depend not only on the clinical information available but also on other factors as well. Reports in the literature suggest that there are considerable variations in community practice. The rate of hospitalization for pneumonia in LTCFs is 9% to 51% (14). Factors include the clinical skill of the RN giving the report, the physicians' availability to visit the nursing home, the length of time the resident has seen the physician as the resident's primary care, etc. Residents may also have advanced directives that preclude them from being transferred to an acute facility. For-profit facilities and chain-affiliated facilities have a two to three times higher number of hospitalizations for infections than nonprofit and nonchain affiliated facilities (15).

The expense and inconvenience to the resident may be considerable when transfers are not properly used. The reasons for and frequency of transfers of LTCF residents to the emergency department for evaluation vary considerably by practice and location (Table 2) (16,17). The ability to evaluate, monitor, and safely treat an NH resident is often a key question confronting the practitioner. As a matter of policy, most NH address the issue of advanced directives, including a residents' preference for level of care in case of an acute problem. Physicians should review these issues from time to time with residents and their families, as they may change depending on several variables.

Communication between nursing home and physicians may be facilitated by using protocols that would enable the nursing staff to organize and collect their information prior to calling the physicians. It is appropriate for the licensed nurse to call the physician in order to have an efficient communication. Published protocols are available (17,19).

There is evidence that the advantage of an acute hospital transfer (closer patient monitoring, access to diagnostic resources, more treatment

Table 2 Reasons to Transfer a Long-Term Care Facilities Resident to an Emergency Department for Suspected Infection in the Absence of Advanced Directives

---

Abrupt change in vital signs or mental status associated with suspected infection

---

Inability to maintain adequate hydration and nutrition

In nurse's judgment, the resident is not stable and practitioner not able to make onsite evaluation

Infections that are not responding to initiated treatment

Need for intravenous antibiotic or other necessary treatment that cannot be administered at the facility

Inability to obtain critical laboratory or radiological studies in the LTCF setting in a timely manner

Required infection control measures cannot be adequately implemented in the facility

Family concerns that adequate care is not being provided in the facility and requests transfer for more aggressive intervention

---

Abbreviation: LTCF, long-term care facility.
Source: From Ref. 18.

options) may be negated by such factors as development of pressure ulcers, adverse events from drugs, and complications from procedures (20).

Even though distinction is made between an acute care facility and a nursing home in the early part of this chapter, nursing homes require the physician or the physician's designee to be available 24 hours a day for routine and emergency orders. Proper endorsement of residents' problems to covering physicians is important to avoid confusion and unwanted or unnecessary intervention. Facilities should develop continuous quality improvement projects to review the entire evaluation and transfer process of residents to monitor the efficacy of current policies and procedures. Information of transfers and hospital admissions should be collected to assess whether there are procedures that can be implemented or current policies modified to improve the efficiency of the system in use. The facility medical director should be involved in the development, implementation, and review of all protocols to assure efficiency of assessments and information control procedures in collaboration with the infection control nurse and director of nursing. Data should also be collected on antibiotic resistance patterns, if possible.

SUMMARY

Evaluation and treatment of infection in the nursing home is a challenging endeavor and should be done with the help of the interdisciplinary team. Availability of resources, including laboratory tests, radiologic procedures, specialty consultants, and nursing staff, are often limited and vary from nursing home to nursing home. Common infections, such as urinary tract infection and pneumonia, may be treated effectively in the nursing home. The decision to transfer to an acute care facility is affected by several factors and is made easier by establishing advanced directives upon admission to the nursing home, if possible. Nursing home administration should be involved in the development, review, and implementation of all infection control and treatment protocols.

SUGGESTED READING

American Medical Directors Association (AMDA). Common Infections in the Long-Term Care Setting. Columbia (MD): American Medical Directors Association (AMDA); 2004; 34 [21 References].

Besdine RW, Rubenstein LZ, Snyder L. Medical Care of the Nursing Home Resident: What Physicians Need to Know. Philadelphia: American College of Physicians, 1996.

Ouslander JG, Morley J, Osterweil D. Medical Care in the Nursing Home. 2nd ed. New York: McGraw-Hill, 1997.

REFERENCES

1. Mylotte JM, Goodnaugh S, Naughton BJ. Pneumonia versus aspiration pneumonitis in nursing home residents: diagnosis and management. J Am Geriatr Soc 2003; 51:17–23.
2. Richards C. Infections in residents of long-term care facilities: an agenda for research. Report of an expert panel. J Am Geriatr Soc 2002; 50:570–576.
3. Capitano B, Leshem OA, Nightingale CH, Nicolau DP. Cost effect of managing methicillin-resistant *Staphylococcus aureus* in a long-term care facility. J Am Geriatr Soc 2003; 51:10–16.
4. Zimmerman S, Gruber-Baldini AL, Hebel JR, Sloane PD, Magaziner J. Nursing home facility risk factors for infection and hospitalization: importance of registered nurse turnover, administration, and social factors. J Am Geriatr Soc 2002; 50:1987–1995.
5. Yoshikawa TT, Norman DC. Infection control in long term care. Clin Geriatr Med 1995; 11:467–480.
6. http://www.cms.hhs.gov/medicaid/reports/rp1201home.asp (accessed August 2005).
7. Naughton BJ, Mylotte J, Ramadan F, Karuza J, Priore RL. Antibiotic use, hospital admissions, and mortality before and after implementing guidelines for nursing home-acquired pneumonia. J Am Geriatr Soc 2001; 49:1020–1024.
8. Bentley D, Bradley S, High K, Schoenbaum S, Taler G, Yoshikawa T. Practice Guideline for Evaluation of Fever and Infection in Long-Term Care Facilities. J Am Geriatr Soc 2001; 49:210–222.
9. Berman P, Hogan DB, Fox RA. The Atypical Presentation of Infection in Old Age. Age Ageing 1987; 16:201–207.
10. Nicolle LE. Urinary tract infections in long-term care facilities. Infect Control Hosp Epidemiol 1993; 4:220–225.
11. Bennet RG. Diarrhea among residents of long-term care facilities. Infect Control Hosp Epidemiol 1993; 14:397–404.
12. Mylotte JM, Naughton B, Saludades C, Maszarovics Z. Validation and application of the pneumonia prognosis index to nursing home residents with pneumonia. J Am Geriatr Soc 1998; 46:1538–1544.
13. Garcia R, Barnard B, Kennedy V. The fifth evolutionary era in infection control: interventional epidemiology. Am J Infect Control 2000; 28:30–43.
14. Muder RR. Management of nursing home-acquired pneumonia: unresolved issues and priorities for future investigation. J Am Geriatr Soc 2000; 48:95–96.
15. Jones JS, Dwyer PR, White LJ, Firman R. Patient transfer from nursing home to emergency department. Outcomes and policy implications. Acad Emerg Med 1997; 4:908–915.
16. Hutt E, Ecord M, Eilertsen TB, Frederickson E, Kramer AM. Precipitants of emergency room visits and acute hospitalization in short-stay Medicare nursing home residents. J Am Geriatr Soc 2001; 50:223–229.
17. Ouslander JG, Osterweil D, Morley J. Medical Care in the Nursing Home. 2nd ed. New York: McGraw-Hill, 1997.
18. Yoshikawa TT, Ouslander JG. Infection Management for Geriatrics in Long Term Care Facilities. New York: Marcel Dekker, Inc., 2002.

19. AMDA. Protocols for Physician Notification: Assessing Patients and Collecting Data on Nursing F patients: A Guide for Nurses on Effective Communication with Physicians. Columbia, MD: American Medical Directors Association, 2000:1–33.
20. Boockvar KS, Gruber-Baldini AL, Burton L, Zimmerman S, May C, Magaziner J. Outcomes of infection in nursing home patients with and without early hospital transfer. J Am Geriatr Soc 2005; 53:590–596.

4

Role of Functional Assessment in Evaluating and Managing Infections in Long-Term Care

Barbara J. Messinger-Rapport and Robert M. Palmer
Section of Geriatric Medicine, Department of General Internal Medicine,
Cleveland Clinic Foundation, Cleveland, Ohio, U.S.A.

KEY POINTS

1. Infection can initiate a vicious cycle, where the nursing home resident declines in cognition, nutritional status, mobility, conditioning, and self-care ability during an infection, predisposing the resident to further infection and functional decline.
2. Clinical tools to measure function exist in the long-term care setting. Some functions are assessed by physicians, but functional assessment data collected by staff for regulatory requirements are useful clinically as well. Functional assessment information is used to trigger resident assessment protocols that address functional decline.
3. Existing risk assessment tools for falls, pressure ulcers, malnutrition, and other events in the nursing home may also be helpful in developing care plans to improve function.
4. Polypharmacy may lead to inadequate treatment of infection, functional decline, adverse reactions, and antimicrobial resistance.
5. Infection control measures need to take into account resident cognitive and physical function as well as the clinical and psychosocial effects of isolation measures.

INTRODUCTION

Infections are common in long-term care (LTC) and impact the resident's functional status, risk of mortality, and quality of life. Mortality risks of infections, particularly with respiratory and urinary tract infections, have been studied both in the nursing home and upon admission to the hospital in older adults. Functional status before and after infection has been studied less extensively but may be as important to the older and frail resident (1). Impaired baseline functional status increases susceptibility to infection. Susceptibility, as shown in Figure 1, includes intrinsic factors social factors, and treatment factors. Susceptibility incorporates functional status indirectly in terms of mobility, nutritional status, cognition, and frailty (Table 1). Impaired functional status is often seen with aging-related changes in immunity, increasing numbers of comorbid conditions, greater impairment in mobility and nutrition, frequent exposure to ill individuals (both staff and residents), and exposure to multiple antibiotics and instrumentation. A vicious cycle occurs of impaired functional status predisposing to infections and infections worsening functional status. This cascade of functional decline has important health-care implications, as impaired functional status lowers quality of life and increases costs of health care, the probability of recurrent infection, and the risk of mortality. Periodic assessment of the resident's

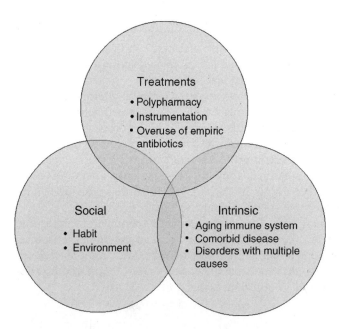

Figure 1   Paradigm for susceptibility to infectious disease in long-term care.

Table 1 Factors Increasing Susceptibility for Infection in Long-Term Care

Factor	Description	Examples
Intrinsic	Aging immune system	Decreased T-cell function
	Comorbid diseases	Diabetes mellitus
		Congestive heart failure
		Chronic pulmonary disease
		Inflammatory bowel disease
		Chronic kidney disease
		Cancers
	Disorders with multiple causes	Impaired mobility
		Malnutrition
		Dysphagia
		Dementia
		Frailty (sarcopenia)
Social	Habit	Alcohol
		Tobacco
	Environment	Cohabitation
		Exposure to ill staff, visitors
		Travel
		Pet therapy
		Ventilation system defects
		Kitchen practices
Treatment	Polypharmacy	Concomitant use of polyvalent cation drugs (iron, calcium, magnesium, aluminum supplements) or sucralfate with fluoroquinolones may impair antibiotic efficacy. The outcome includes a partially treated infection, more drug resistance, and need for further antibiotic treatment
	Overuse of empirical antibiotics	Broad-spectrum antibiotics for urinary infections prior to culture results
	Instrumentation	Indwelling bladder catheters

function in the nursing home offers an opportunity to interrupt this cascade of decline through interventions to improve quality of life, reduce the risk of future infections, and identify the goals of care with the patient and family.

This chapter summarizes the process of functional assessment in LTC. The interplay between function and infection is illustrated in a clinical example of an elderly couple residing in a nursing home. The example underscores the subtleties of the presentation of infection in elderly residents and highlights the spectrum of clinical assessment tools, the role of polypharmacy, the interventions for improving functional status, and the relevant regulatory and administrative considerations in the LTC setting.

Impact of Function on Prognosis, Therapy, and Quality of Life: Case Studies in LTC

The on-call physician received a report about a 96-year-old blind, deaf, diabetic gentleman with a moist cough for one day and a temperature of 98.8°F. Pulse was 84 per minute, blood pressure was 130/80 mmHg, and respiratory rate was 16 per minute. There was no edema, and pulse oximetry recorded 95% on room air. The physician opted for symptomatic treatment with an expectorant, believing that the resident's symptoms were of short duration and that the resident was otherwise clinically stable. However, the resident had fallen the day before. The "falls protocol" of vital signs, cognitive performance, and mobility monitoring had been initiated by nursing for the next three days and the requisite review by the falls team occurred. Vital signs two days after the fall (one day following the onset of the cough) revealed a temperature of 100.3°F, with normal pulse, blood pressure, and respirations. The interdisciplinary "falls team" also uncovered changes in behavior and function. Prior to the fall, the resident was confined to a chair but could ambulate a few steps with one-person assistance; the resident was oriented to person and surroundings and was continent of urine about half the time. The gentleman's mobility was generally limited by severe arthritis and profound visual deficit. The incremental attention the gentleman received from the team after the fall revealed important changes in the functional status: the resident was a little more irritable and restless, had a stronger odor in urine, finished about 50% of meals, and was less conversant. The team brought these changes to the attention of the resident's LTC physician. The medical evaluation included a chest X-ray that demonstrated a left lower lobe infiltrate and a normal white blood count. Antibiotic therapy was given and oral fluids were encouraged for several consecutive nursing shifts. By day 3 of antibiotic therapy, the resident was afebrile, calm, more consistently continent, and more participatory in activities. A brief course of physical therapy restored the resident's ability to assist the nursing aids in his own care and to maneuver in the room. The gentleman regained baseline level of functioning and remained stable over the next three months.

This gentleman roomed with his 92-year-old wife, who had hypertension and coronary heart disease. At baseline the wife was able to dress herself and the husband with assistance, to assist the husband with meals, to wander independently without a gait-assist device, and to push the husband's wheelchair throughout the facility. The woman was usually continent. Like the husband, the wife had an acute change in behavior one day, specifically wandering less throughout the facility and interacting less with the staff and the husband. By the third day, the woman appeared to be very uncomfortable when prompted to walk, when the woman's right hip was flexed, and when the right lower quadrant was palpated. The woman's temperature was 100.3°F, blood pressure was 160/90 mmHg, heart rate was 104 per minute, and respiratory rate was 22 per minute. Emergent evaluation by abdominal computed tomography scan confirmed a diagnosis of acute diverticulitis, and intravenous fluids and antibiotic therapy were initiated in the hospital. Subsequently, the woman developed symptoms of heart failure and a diagnosis of an acute myocardial infarction. Angioplasty and stent placement were technically successful and postinfarct ejection fraction was normal. However, the patient was very "confused" and agitated in the hospital, resulting in the use of physical and chemical restraints, and ate poorly. The patient returned to the LTC setting, comfortable and afebrile but no longer responsive to the husband's attentions and unable to perform daily activities. The woman did not get out of bed unless transferred by two individuals and ate minimally even when hand-fed. Cardiac and gastrointestinal evaluations were unremarkable. A functional and medical reassessment was performed by the health-care team. Physical and occupational therapy were unsuccessful in improving the patient's mobility. Newly prescribed sedating medications were discontinued, as they had contributed to a hypoactive delirium. Psychiatric services assessed the patient for possible depression, but a trial of an antidepressant did not improve the woman's apathy, anorexia, or immobility. The woman continued to lose weight and stay in bed. After discussion with the team about the patient's poor prognosis, the patient and family requested hospice for the wife as well as counseling services for the husband. The patient expired three months after hospitalization.

Both cases highlight many of the physical and cognitive changes that occur during infection, as well as the complex presentation and consequences of infection in elders. A depiction of the symptoms of infection and the cascading loss of function is shown in Figure 2. In both cases, symptoms and signs of infection were blunted. The older gentleman with pneumonia did not have a high fever, tachycardia, tachypnea, or leukocytosis. Instead, the gentleman had malaise, irritability, urinary incontinence, and anorexia. These symptoms were recognized as a nonspecific prodrome and delirium only after evidence for an infection appeared.

Pneumonia and urinary tract infections commonly present with delirium, although delirium can also mask other processes, such as a myocardial infarction, and coexist with any infectious, metabolic, or inflammatory process, particularly in an elder with sensory deprivation, poor intake, and cognitive impairment. Poor intake and insensible fluid losses due to fever can cause hypotension, reduce brain perfusion, worsen delirium if present, and precipitate renal insufficiency and coronary ischemia. Anorexia before and during an infection can lead to diminished nutritional status, reduction in muscle mass, and subsequent impairment in immune function. Aspiration is more likely with delirium, as is urinary incontinence. Urinary incontinence may result from delirium by compromising the ability to

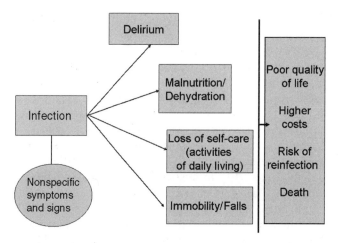

Figure 2 Impact of infections on patient care outcomes.

communicate toileting needs or through deconditioning that limits ability to ambulate and toilet. Irritated, damp skin and prolonged immobility may result in pressure ulcers, translating into increased metabolic needs and higher risk for infection. The difficulty of early diagnosis and the rapid cascade of functional decline before, during, and after infection compromises the ability of an elder to survive an infection and to return to baseline functioning.

With the elderly gentleman, a "sentinel fall" preceded the diagnosis of an infection. In this case there were no injuries, but he was certainly at risk for such complications as head injury and hip fracture. A fall exemplifies the nonspecific presentation of illness arising in elderly residents and signals the need for a careful assessment of its causes and consequences. LTC facilities employ an assessment protocol following a resident's fall. In one clinical trial, a resident assessment within seven days following a fall did not reduce the risk of future falls but did reduce the risk of subsequent hospitalization and the number of hospital days (2).

Comorbid illnesses may contribute to functional decline in elderly residents and certainly altered the outcome for the elderly woman described above. The wife's cardiac event depleted the woman's homeostatic reserves, further compromising the ability to recover from the diverticulitis. Perhaps the heart failure resulted from intravenous fluid hydration in the setting of diastolic dysfunction and evolving coronary ischemia, or the coronary event preceded the infection but was unrecognized because of nonspecific symptoms. Comorbid diseases (for example, diabetes mellitus) can both be exacerbated by infections and worsen functional outcomes. Diabetic control typically worsens during an infection. Resulting hyperglycemia increases the risk of intravascular depletion, urinary incontinence, and impaired immunity. Urinary retention due to neuropathy is more likely during an infection when associated with immobility (exacerbated by chemical or physical restraints), anticholinergic medications, constipation, or narcotic use. Other comorbid illnesses, such as cancer, mood disorders, and chronic infections, also adversely affect immune function.

Polypharmacy increases the risk of functional decline by causing adverse drug effects and interactions. Common adverse effects to specific agents include sedation, confusion, dry mouth, and anorexia, which in turn can lead to cognitive impairment, undernutrition, immobility and deconditioning, and falls. Even medications that are given for appropriate indications (e.g., diverticulitis; myocardial infarction) can be problematic in elderly residents: angiotensin-converting enzyme inhibitors, beta-blockers, high-dose statins, platelet inhibitors, and some antibiotics used for treating diverticulitis increase the potential of adverse interactions with other medications. Table 2 lists medications, and suggested alternatives, that have potentially important adverse effects in older adults during an infection. Additionally, chronic medications need to be reassessed during antibiotic therapy. For example, quinolones are often prescribed in the LTC setting, and their absorption is significantly impaired if polyvalent cations, such as sucralfate, or iron, calcium, magnesium, or aluminum supplements, are coadministered. Blood levels of digitalis may increase when broad-spectrum antibiotics reduce the gut flora and permit increased intestinal absorption of digoxin.

IMPORTANCE OF FUNCTIONAL ASSESSMENT DURING TRANSITIONS OF CARE

Residents of long-term care facilities are in fact heterogeneous in function. They may be cognitively impaired but physically robust, cognitively intact but physically impaired, or both physically and cognitively impaired. Transitions in care settings are common as residents often transfer from a long-term stay to the hospital during an acute illness, from the hospital back to a long-term care bed, from a skilled stay in a nursing facility to the community, or from the community to the nursing facility either for temporary respite or permanent residence. Functional assessment of these elderly residents before and after transitions in care setting is important to identify residents who are vulnerable to functional decline during an infection, to evaluate the effect of the infection upon function, and to monitor impact of interventions to restore function following an infection.

Many tools or scales are available for use in the functional assessment of elderly patients as they proceed through the transitions of care. The Katz index of the basic activities of daily living (BADL) is a tool used in all settings—the community, the nursing facility, and the acute care hospital—to describe

(*Text continues on page 41.*)

Table 2 Examples of Potential Adverse Effects of Pharmaceuticals on Function and Geriatric Syndromes

Domain	Drug	Indication	ADE	Additional ADE	Alternative
Cognition	Quinolones	Antibiotic, typically for respiratory and urinary infections	Delirium, hallucinations, paranoia	Increased risk hypoglycemia, inhibit metabolism at CYP 1A, lower seizure threshold, prolong QT interval on EKG	Lower dose; consider second-generation cepaphalosporin or macrolide, if appropriate
	Amantadine	Influenza therapy	Delirium	Falls	Oseltamivir (preferred), rimantadine
	Antihistamines (diphenhydramine, hydroxyzine)	Sinus congestion or allergy	Delirium, sedation	Constipation, urinary retention	Consider nonsedating antihistamines (loratadine or fexofenadine). Consider nasal corticosteroid, antihistamine eye drop, skin moisturizer, and fewer immersion baths (to reduce pruritis from dry skin)
Nutrition	Macrolides	Antibiotic, typically for respiratory infections	Anorexia, nausea, vomiting (typically with erythromycin)	Prolonged QT interval on EKG. Increased digoxin serum levels and inhibition of drugs	Avoid concurrent use with Quinolones, antipsychotics, or tricyclic

		metabolized at the CYP 3A complex (not azithromycin). Hearing loss (erythromycin ≥ 4 g/day)	antidepressants, or Class 1A or III antiarrhythmics. Lower dose of antibiotic. Hold statins (except pravastatin or fluvastatin), lower doses of CCBs
Warfarin	Anticoagulation to prevent thrombo-embolic events	Erratic intake may lead to either ineffectiveness or increased risk of bleeding	Increased risk of thromboembolic event if excessive dietary vitamin K; increased bleeding with insufficient vitamin K or with certain medications; major substrate of 2C8/9 and a moderate inhibitor of 2C8/9	Reassess need for warfarin in debilitated patient with poor or erratic intake. Monitor PT/INR closely if adding medications which inhibit or induce warfarin metabolism
Metronidazole	*Clostridium difficile* and other anaerobic infections	Anorexia, nausea, vomiting, metallic taste. Also glossitis, stomatitis, or vaginitis with candidiasis	Neuropathy with prolonged usage. Treat for candidal overgrowth	Lowest dose for shortest duration

(Continued)

Table 2 Examples of Potential Adverse Effects of Pharmaceuticals on Function and Geriatric Syndromes (*Continued*)

Domain	Drug	Indication	ADE	Additional ADE	Alternative
Mobility	Benzodiazepines	Antianxiety	Increased fall risk	Delirium, sedation	Identify cause. Reduce polypharmacy, modify environment. Behavioral therapy and/or short course of low-dose antipsychotic if delirium present
Polyphar-macy	Quinolones and polyvalent cation drugs[a]	Inadequate absorption	See cognition and quinolones		Hold polyvalent cation drugs during antibiotic therapy

[a]Polyvalent cation drugs: calcium, magnesium, aluminum, and iron supplements, plus sucralfate.

Abbreviations: ADE, adverse drug event; CCB, calcium channel blocker; EKG, electrocardiogram; PT, prothrombin time; INR, international normalized ratio.

such simple personal activities as eating, dressing, bathing, transferring, toileting and continence, and eating (3). Among adults aged 65 years and over in the community, approximately 13% are impaired in at least one or more BADL (4). In the nursing home, three-quarters of residents are dependent in three or more BADL (5).

More complex personal activities are captured by the Lawton and Brody scale of instrumental activities of daily living (IADL) (Table 3). Scoring systems were developed for these scales for use in research, and they can be adapted to clinical use as needed. For example, each activity can be described as independent (zero point) or not independent (one point). Alternatively, each activity can be independent (zero point), assisted (one point), or dependent (two points).

Although the usual IADLs are less relevant to most long-term nursing home residents, they are important for service planning for those treated for an infection in the hospital and those rehabilitating in the nursing facility. For example, a return to independent living at home is likely after short-term rehabilitation in a skilled nursing facility, when the patient is able to take medications, prepare foods, and perform household chores without personal assistance. However, approximately 17% of older adults decline in functional ability between admission and discharge from a medical hospitalization, not including the 18% who declined shortly prior to admission and did not recover function (6). A community-dwelling elder who declines during a hospitalization for infection in multiple activities of daily living

Table 3 Basic and Instrumental Activities of Daily Living

BADL
    Bathing
    Dressing
    Transferring
    Toileting
    Continence
    Eating
IADL
    Transportation
    Shopping
    Cooking
    Using the telephone
    Managing money
    Taking medications
    Cleaning
    Laundry

Abbreviations: BADL, basic activities of daily living; IADL, instrumental activities of daily living.

and IADL often requires nursing facility rehabilitation. Once in the nursing facility, appropriate assessment and intervention can help them recover function, particularly in the BADL, and return to the community with plans to assist them in their performance of IADL, such as homemaker and personal aide services, until recovery is completed.

FUNCTIONAL ASSESSMENT IN LTC

Although the BADL and IADL are an integral part of resident assessment, much more functional assessment is clinically necessary and is mandated by state and federal regulation. Regulatory requirements require assessment of cognitive and physical functioning upon admission to the facility and at prescribed periods, usually every three months, during the LTC stay. A significant change in function, as in the example above, triggers a reassessment in order to develop a new plan of care. The assessment includes several domains of functioning and health, such as BADL, mood and behavior; clinical events, such as falls and fracture; interval infections, such as pneumonia, urinary tract, *Clostridium difficile* diarrhea, and antibiotic-resistant infections; comorbidities, such as heart failure; cognitive skills; and advance directives. The functional portion of the regulatory assessment described above and synopsized in Table 4 is encompassed within the Minimum Data Set (MDS) now in version 2.0, with version 3.0 in development. Functional assessment tools are listed in Table 5 and described below. Ongoing functional assessment, when coupled with redesign of a care plan, provides an opportunity to intervene with functional decline and thus improve or at least maintain function. Additionally, with interdisciplinary input, ongoing functional assessment helps clinicians and families establish goals of care and choose modalities of treatment aligned with these goals.

Table 4 Functional Assessment in the Minimum Data Set 2.0

Section	Aspect of function	Examples
B	Cognitive patterns	Memory, cognitive skills for daily decision making
C	Communication	Hearing ability, modes of expression, speech clarity
D	Vision	Limitations in function due to vision
E	Mood and behavior	Verbal and behavioral expressions of distress
F	Psychosocial	Relationships
G	Physical functioning	Activities of daily living
H	Continence	Bowel, bladder
I	Nutritional status	Weight change

Table 5 Examples of Commonly Used Assessment Tools in Long-Term Care

Function	Measurement tool
Physical	Activities of daily living—monitored by nurses and nurses aides
	Abnormal involuntary movement scale—monitored by nurses or clinicians
	Functional independence measurement—monitored by therapist
	Berg balance—monitored by therapist
	MDS 2.0—section G
Cognitive	Orientation to self, date, and place: assessed daily by CNA, nurses, therapists
	Mini–Mental State Examination, Short Portable Mental Status Questionnaire; Geriatric Depression Scale (short form); Cornell Depression Scale. These are commonly used tests that may be performed by nurse, physician, psychologist, social worker
	MDS 2.0—mood, cognitive skills for daily living, communication ability, individual behavior symptoms, social skills
Quality of life	Resident and family council meetings
	Symptom-specific scales (e.g., faces pain scale)
	MDS 3.0 when available
Fall risk (7)	History of previous fall
	Morse fall scale
	Timed up and go
Early malnutrition (8)	Mini–nutritional assessment
Pressure ulcer risk (9)	Braden scale
	Norton scale

Abbreviations: MDS, Minimum Data Set; CNA, certified nursing assistants.

PROCESS OF FUNCTIONAL ASSESSMENT

The initial history for each nursing home resident typically includes a description of level of function prior to admission, including the BADL and IADL as described by the resident and/or family. The physical examination on admission documents functional status. Functional ability might include mobility (as tested by a get-up-and-go maneuver), hearing (by a whisper test), visual acuity (with a Snellen card), visual fields (by confrontation), and cognition (using tests listed in Table 5 and described below), in addition to standard physical examination aspects, such as strength and joint range of motion. Physicians may request further evaluation by speech, physical, and occupational therapists, and therapy may be initiated immediately to try to reverse a decline in function.

Ongoing monitoring of physical function is often performed by the certified nursing assistants (CNAs). These individuals perform the hands-on care and have the responsibility to report changes to the charge nurse. The CNA is able to report changes in strength, joint mobility, skin condition, and BADL. They are instructed to permit and encourage the resident's independence, even if the task takes more time if done by the resident than if done by the CNA. Walking to meals, or even just leaving the wheelchair outside the dining room, may help maintain conditioning and function.

The responsibility for assessing the degree of change, and the implications of change, falls upon the nursing staff. Some deficits may be more difficult to discern; for instance, visual and hearing deficits often evolve slowly and staffs accommodate to the disabilities without being conscious of a true change. Some functional deficits, when identified early, are amenable to intervention. If there is a decline in function, the patient may be referred for therapy. Therapists assess and monitor physical functioning with the BADL, but also with such scales as the Berg balance scale and the functional independence measure (10). Opportunities to improve function after assessment include training in adaptive equipment to become independent in dressing and feeding, training with a gait-assist device, and balance training to reduce the incidence of falls. Therapies must be indicated by a physician as "medically necessary." Therapy for an LTC resident not receiving Medicare Part A skilled services is usually covered by Medicare Part B.

Residents who are at risk of losing BADL by virtue of a decline in strength or range of motion but have not actually declined in function are considered to be in a vulnerable transition. These residents are candidates for a restorative program (11). Restorative care services are nursing interventions that assist or promote independent function but are not implemented by a licensed therapist. A nurse can design a program involving dressing, toileting, range of motion, ambulation, or dietary plans in order to reconstitute the threatened skill. Interventions can also address cognitive skills for daily living, behavior modification, recreation and spiritual needs. A restorative program typically provides restorative care or activities for 15 minutes or more per day and continues as long as the resident is making progress towards attaining specific goals. The facility covers the cost of the restorative program as part of its mission in caring for the elder. Medicaid and Medicare-certified facilities may capture costs related to these services by using resource utilization groups. Outcomes must be documented in the MDS or, if too small to be captured by the MDS, by appropriate measurements used both to identify the initial deficit and to measure the outcome following intervention.

Cognition is monitored in general terms by the CNAs and nurses who provide direct care to the resident. Orientation deficits are usually identified by nursing home personnel. Diurnal fluctuation, such as becoming agitated at night, can be missed if communication between shifts is poor. The social worker, advanced practice nurse, psychologist, or physician can perform more quantitative measures of cognition, such as the Mini–Mental Status Examination, which is scored from 0 to 30 and includes memory, attention, calculation, orientation, language, executive function, and visuospatial function. The Short Portable Mental Status Questionnaire has only 10 questions but is more limited in scope (10). Evaluation for delirium using the Confusion Assessment Method could be performed (12). The plan for treating a cognitive disorder is multifactorial, involving some or all of the following: pharmaceutical consultation to reduce polypharmacy, physician or consultant prescription of a cognition-enhancing medication, speech therapy to offer geriatric cognitive therapy if the deficits are mild, social and recreational services to identify activities that are cognitively stimulating.

Depressive or anxious symptoms are often identified and documented by the nursing staff. A mood disorder can be diagnosed by the physician or a clinical consultant. Scales, such as the short-form Geriatric Depression Scale, have predictive validity for identifying older patients at risk for functional decline. For residents with more than mild dementia, the Geriatric Depression Scale has less sensitivity and specificity. The Cornell scale, which incorporates patient and caregiver information, can be used by the psychologist or social worker to identify and monitor depression in a cognitively impaired individual (10). The plan for treating a mood disorder is also multifactorial, involving some or all of the following: therapy services to improve mobility, activities director to increase socialization, counseling, removal of medications that may adversely alter mood, and pharmaceutical antidepressive therapy.

Behavior monitoring, as well as monitoring of potentially adverse reactions to antipsychotic medications (movement disorder, etc.), is performed by nursing personnel and is documented. Regulations may affect monitoring patterns. For instance, federal regulations require review of adverse effects of antipsychotics every six months. Scales can be used (for example, the Abnormal Involuntary Movement scale) to monitor potential adverse drug effects. Findings are typically recorded in the Medication Administration Record. Nonpharmaceutical means of treating agitated behavior, such as decreasing stimuli, providing a reassuring routine, offering favorite foods, and nonpharmaceutical therapies such as pet, music, aroma, or touch, among others are encouraged.

Functional assessment in LTC also includes measuring risks for sentinel events, such as falls, pressure ulcers, and weight loss or malnutrition. Examples of risk measurements are included in Table 5. The choice of measurement may be that of the individual facility or mandated by a multi-facility corporation. Sentinel events often signal a medical problem and an associated or impending loss of function. Certain sentinel events are included among the quality indicators reviewed by the state and federal government. Identification of a high-risk individual by means of either a sentinel event or a high-risk score on a risk measure can lead to new care plans and multidisciplinary interventions and can potentially avert a loss of function. For example, a person identified as a high fall risk may receive increased attention to potentially sedating medications or a trial of physical and occupational therapy. Any subsequent fall would trigger a multidisciplinary review and lead to further interventions for the resident and possibly for the facility.

INFECTION CONTROL AND FUNCTION

The interplay between resident function and infection control is complex but not well reported. An example is mobility. Good mobility reduces the risk of atelectasis and deconditioning and decreases the risk of respiratory infections and sarcopenia. However, after acquiring an infection, a physically robust but cognitively impaired person may be less likely to follow hygienic practices and more likely to spread the infection to other residents and staff. A resident with adenoviral eye infection, for instance, is less likely to cooperate with hand washing and eye rubbing, resulting in an epidemic in the facility. Extra attention from the staff is often required in order to keep a cognitively impaired but mobile resident in the staff's room during an infection. Moving the resident to a special isolation room during the course of an infection could make the resident more confused leading to further disruptive behavior.

Residents with limited mobility and infectious conditions requiring isolation, such as methicillin-resistant *Staphylococcus aureus* respiratory infection or *C. difficile* diarrhea, may be easier to manage than more mobile residents. However, they may receive less clinical monitoring by nursing staff and diminished psychosocial support from family because of the greater restrictions on personal contacts. Such problems as pressure ulcers and depression may worsen in isolation in cognitively impaired individuals because symptoms are less likely to be detected. Interventions to improve mobility, such as physical or occupational therapy, might be less aggressive and less effective when limited in a resident's room rather than in the therapy department.

SUMMARY

The interplay between infection and functional status in LTC is complex. Risks such as exposure to ill residents and staff, receipt of empirical antibiotics and instrumentation (for example, urinary bladder catheterization), poor mobility, and other medical conditions intersect to increase the risk of infection (Fig. 1). The cascade of infection, beginning with the often subtle presentation and alteration in function (Fig. 2), may rapidly proceed to impaired cognition, malnutrition, immobility, falls, and loss of self-care ability. Without recognition of change and prompt intervention, function may not be restored, raising the risk of a lower quality of life, higher health-care costs, recurrent infection, and death.

Clinical tools to measure function exist in the LTC setting, many of which are collected by staff to complete the MDS. Use of these tools triggers resident assessment protocols that can address functional decline. Risk assessments of falls, pressure ulcers, malnutrition, and other events may also be helpful in developing care plans to improve function. Transfers of care may be optimized when careful functional assessment is performed to ensure that appropriate services are provided by the receiving facility, whether the hospital, nursing facility, or home in the community. Periodic review of medications used in LTC, particularly when initiating antibiotics or in the setting of a sentinel event, such as a fall, is important. Antibiotics may not be effective in the setting of certain medications (e.g., quinolones with polyvalent cations) or may make levels of certain medications toxic (Table 2). Minimization of empiric antibiotics and instrumentation may reduce antibiotic-resistant infections. Infection control measures need to take into account resident cognitive and physical function as well as the clinical and psychosocial effects of isolation measures. Importantly, organized geriatric interventions in a variety of settings—home, hospital, office, and long-term care institution—have demonstrated improved functional status of older patients, suggesting that at least some disability is preventable.

SUGGESTED READING

High K, Bradley S, Loeb M, et al. A new paradigm for clinical investigation of infectious syndromes in older adults: assessing functional status as a risk factor and outcome measure. J Am Geriatr Soc 2005; 53(3):528–535.

REFERENCES

1. High K, Bradley S, Loeb M, Palmer R, Quagliarello V, Yoshikawa T. A new paradigm for clinical investigation of infectious syndromes in older adults: assessing functional status as a risk factor and outcome measure. J Am Geriatr Soc 2005; 53:528–535.
2. Rubenstein LZ, Robbins AS, Josephson KR, Schulman BL, Osterweil D. The value of assessing falls in an elderly population. A randomized clinical trial. Ann Intern Med 1990; 113:308–316.
3. Katz S. Assessing self-maintenance: activities of daily living, mobility, and instrumental activities of daily living. J Am Geriatr Soc 1983; 31:721–727.
4. Older Americans 2004: Key Indicators of Well-Being. Washington, D.C.: U.S. Government Printing Office; November 2004.
5. Jones A. The national nursing home survey: 1999 summary. National Center for Health Statistics. Vital Health Stat 2002;13(152). www.cdc.gov/nchs/data/series/sr_13/sr13_152.pdf.

6. Covinsky KE, Palmer RM, Fortinsky RH, et al. Loss of independence in activities of daily living in older adults hospitalized with medical illnesses: increased vulnerability with age. J Am Geriatr Soc 2003; 51:451–458.
7. Perell KL, Nelson A, Goldman RL, Luther SL, Prieto-Lewis N, Rubensein LZ. Fall risk assessment measures: an analytic review. J Gerontol A Biol Sci Med Sci 2001; 56(A):M761–M766.
8. Lauque S, Arnaud-Battandier F, Mansourian R, et al. Protein-energy oral supplementation in malnourished nursing-home residents. A controlled trial. Age Ageing 2000; 29:51–56.
9. Wipke-Tevis DD, Williams DA, Rantz MJ, et al. Nursing home quality and pressure ulcer prevention and management practices. J Am Geriatr Soc 2004; 52:583–588.
10. Teresi JA, Lawton MP, Holmes DH, Ory M, eds. Measurement in Elderly Chronic Care Populations. New York: Springer Pub. Co., 1997.
11. Resnick B, Fleishell A. Developing a restorative care program. Am J Nurs 2002; 102:91–95.
12. Inouye SK, van Dyck CH, Alessi CA, Balkin S, Segal AP, Horwitz RI. Clarifying confusion: the confusion assessment method. A new method for detection of delirium. Ann Intern Med 1990; 113:941–948.

5

Impaired Immunity and Increased Risk of Infections in Older Adults: Impact of Chronic Disease on Immunosenescence

Steven C. Castle, Koichi Uyemura, and Takashi Makinodan
Department of Veterans Affairs, Geriatric Research Education and Clinical Center, Veterans Affairs Greater Los Angeles Healthcare System, UCLA School of Medicine, Los Angeles, California, U.S.A.

KEY POINTS

1. Immunosenescence, due to normal aging process, affects primarily T-cell function with accumulation of memory cells in the immune tissues (frequently CD8+CD28−) that do not proliferate well, and tend to produce more type 2 (IL-10) and less type 1 cytokines (IL-2, IFN-γ).

2. The majority of studies on immune function in older adults have been done in very healthy older adults, or inbred laboratory mice, and the changes described may not have a direct relevance on the marked increase in all types of infections found in older adults.

3. Changes in immune function due to interaction of chronic illness and changes of immunosenescence due to normal aging likely result in a shift to impaired immunity that involves other cell types, including APCs, natural killer cells, and neutrophils.

4. Impaired immunity, sometimes described as immune risk phenotype, has been shown to correlate better with disease burden than chronologic age.

5. Much attention has been given to inflammatory mediators and increased mortality in older adults, primarily due to cardiovascular death, but little is known how inflammatory mediators contribute to the development of impaired immunity and the associated severe infections and poor response to vaccination that could be reversed.

INTRODUCTION

Immunosenescence, the state of dysregulated immune function associated with aging, has been extensively studied in very healthy older adults and inbred mice raised in pathogen-free environments. Clearly identified changes associated with the aging process have been demonstrated, but the changes themselves alone are not likely responsible for the significant increased risk and severity of infections in the older adult population. This is underscored by the variable and high risk of nosocomial infections in older adults residing in long-term care facilities (LTCFs). Of note, in 1999, surveillance of LTCF-acquired infections by the National Nosocomial Infections Surveillance system reported a high incidence of infections of 3.82 infections per 1000 resident-days of care, but with significant variability (1). Data vary widely depending on the type of facility, nature of the residents, definitions used for infections, and type of data analysis. The prevalence of infection rates ranged from 1.6% to 32.7%, and overall incidence rates ranged from 1.8 to 13.5 infections per 1000 resident-days of care, with equal variability for specific infections, such as urinary tract or pneumonia. Questions raised from these reports are as follows: (i) what patient or facility factors contribute to this wide variability of incidence of infections? (ii) can anything be done to reduce the risk of infection by preventive treatment of patients? and (iii) what impact could changes in infection control policy have on infection rate for a given facility?

If the goal is to prevent serious infections in older adults, the field of geriatric immunology/infectious disease is faced with a tremendous challenge of studying a very diverse population of chronically ill older adults, in addition to the study of very healthy older adults. Grouping individuals by disease severity or by level of impairment of specific components of immunity may assist in advancing our ability to improve host defense in an at-risk population (2).

IMMUNOSENESCENCE

Studies of Aging Exclude the Impact of Disease

Immunosenescence is defined as the state of dysregulated, reduced immune function that is associated with functional, structural, and metabolic changes primarily in the T-cells, and it contributes to the increased susceptibility of older adults to infection and possibly to autoimmune disease and cancer (3). This chapter will focus on the relevance that age-related immune dysregulation has toward susceptibility to infectious disease, though there is growing awareness of how chronic age-related illness and the state of "inflammaging" associated with chronic inflammatory disease likely interact to create an impaired immune state that contributes to the significant shift in infections to older adults (2,4). This review will not address the role that dysregulated immunity plays in common age-related illness themselves, including atherosclerosis, Alzheimer's dementia, diabetes mellitus, and osteoporosis.

The immune system can be divided into innate and acquired components (Fig. 1), and recent advances in the field have focused attention on the interaction between these two components. Extensive studies in very healthy older adults have identified modest age-related decline in immunity, and, furthermore, these studies have been essentially limited to phenotypic and functional changes in T-cells of the acquired immune component (5).

In an attempt to standardize laboratory methods and isolate age-related changes from external changes of disease and medications, studies over the past 15 years have included only the very healthy older adults. This has been accomplished by the exclusion of subjects with evidence of disease or use of medications, by applying rigorous criteria as defined by the SENIEUR protocol (6). This concept of distinguishing nature (genetic)

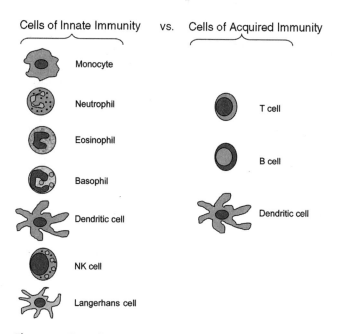

Cells of Innate Immunity   vs.   Cells of Acquired Immunity

Monocyte

Neutrophil

Eosinophil

Basophil

Dendritic cell

NK cell

Langerhans cell

T cell

B cell

Dendritic cell

Figure 1   Key effector cells of the innate versus acquired immune response. Note that dendritic cells play pivotal roles in both innate and acquired immunity.

versus nurture (environment) has long been debated and tends to distinguish the subtle differences in the fields of gerontology (the study of aging) and geriatrics (the care of the aged). The SENIEUR protocol criteria exclude subjects with unhealthy lifestyle choices; the presence of infection, inflammation, malignancy, or other immune disorders; and abnormal organ function, as well as anyone on medications for treatment of a defined disease (7). These stringent criteria exclude 90% of subjects aged 65 or older, 25% of younger subjects, and virtually 100% of the population residing in LTCF (5). Although it would appear that the original intent of the SENIEUR protocol was to develop a reference population, it has been applied to exclude subjects with almost any external/environmental exposure, which limits our understanding of mechanisms of vulnerability to infections in the at-risk population with underlying chronic diseases. Yet, despite extensive studies on possible mechanisms for age-related changes in T-cell phenotype and function in a very healthy population, no compelling scientific evidence has shown that these changes have direct relevance to the common infections seen in the aged population (3,5,6).

Overview of Components of Immune Response

Immune response consists of two interactive components: an innate and an acquired response. Innate immunity provides a first line of defense against many common microorganisms. It has a cellular component, made up of neutrophils, macrophages, epithelial cells, eosinophils, basophils, natural killer cells, and dendritic cells (DCs). These immune cells detect the presence of foreign protein by several receptors that bind to molecules secreted by or carried on the surface of the pathogen. DCs are the predominant antigen-presenting cells (APCs) involved in the initial innate inflammatory response. In response to the pathogen, DCs produce bursts of inflammatory proteins that not only kill the pathogen but also produce other proteins called cytokines that recruit and promote the further differentiation of other DCs. However, when the innate immune system cannot recognize and/or eliminate an infectious organism, the acquired immune system provides a resourceful second line of defense.

Acquired immunity utilizes lymphocytes (T and B cells) with specific cell-surface receptors generated by random recombination of gene segments. These recombinations and pairings of different variable chains produce a wide repertoire of lymphocytes with specific unique receptors that can recognize virtually any infectious organism or pathogen. Therefore, the acquired immune system has the unique characteristic of specificity of response to a given antigen. Furthermore, another unique feature of acquired immunity is establishment of memory cells, which enables a rapid response upon subsequent rechallenge with the same antigen. The distinctive cells of innate and acquired immunity are shown in Figure 1. Because it is necessary to clonally expand antigen-specific lymphocytes to a novel pathogen, acquired immunity requires four to seven days to generate appropriate number of cells to counter the infection as shown in Figure 2. Yet, cells of the innate immune system interact to play a pivotal role in the initiation and subsequent direction of acquired immune responses.

To initiate an acquired immune response, T cells must be activated by APCs. The degree or quality of interaction of lymphocytes and APC can influence the type and magnitude of immune response. If a foreign or infectious organism is encountered by APCs and presented to a particular T cell bearing the appropriate receptor, the T cells undergo clonal expansion and differentiate into effector cells that can eliminate the infectious organism. However, when APCs present self-antigens to lymphocytes bearing receptors that recognize such self-antigens, these lymphocytes are eliminated through a process called apoptosis (programmed cell death). Hence, it is at this key interface between innate and acquired immunity that regulation of turning on or off of an immune response occurs (3,5,8,9).

Cytokines have been classified as pro- or anti-inflammatory cytokines, depending on their effects on immune function, but the distinction depends on the setting (3,8,9). Furthermore, these cytokines often act in networks or

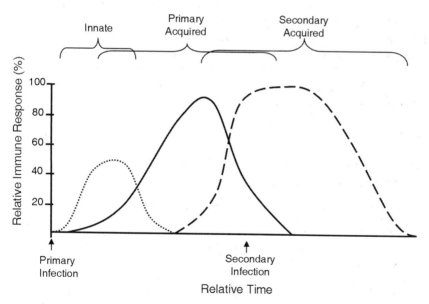

Figure 2 Kinetics of immune response: innate versus acquired immunity. Innate immune responses occur immediately after initial encounter with a pathogen. A more vigorous primary acquired immune response follows the innate response. Memory cells, generated by the primary acquired immune response, respond quickly and decisively following a second infection by the same pathogen.

cascades to regulate their complex biological activities. Interaction between the different immune constituent cell types of host defense is carried out by the strength and balance of cytokine signals. The ability of effector cells to differentiate or respond to specific signals is likely affected by aging and chronic illness. In general, activation of acquired immunity that involves cell-mediated immune response, which is protective against most infectious agents, is described as a T-helper 1 (Th1 or Type 1) response and is associated with production of high levels of the cytokines interleukin-2 (IL-2) and interferon-gamma (IFN-γ). In contrast, a T-helper 2 (Th2 or Type 2) response, which is associated with allergic or parasitic infections but not associated with clearance of most bacterial or viral infections, is associated with production of high levels of IL-10, IL-4, and IL-5. The relative concentrations of proinflammatory cytokines, defined as those that upregulate a Th1 response, or anti-inflammatory cytokines that are important in turning off a Th1 response are influenced by gene activation of effector immune cells and allow further specificity of the eventual outcome of an inflammatory response. Note that these distinctions of pro- and anti-inflammatory are from immunologists' perspective and often are confused with the discussion of inflammatory mediators that increase with aging and age-related diseases. This will be discussed later.

Mature DCs are required for efficient activation of influenza-specific cytotoxic T cells (10). Consequently, the differentiation of regulatory APC at the site of inflammation is important in determining the quality of the subsequent immune response that takes place in regional lymph nodes and likely are impacted by changes in the microenvironment caused by both aging and chronic disease-associated changes in circulating inflammatory mediators (11). Circulating inflammatory mediators could be a more likely cause for impaired vaccine response in older adults with significant disease burden.

Summary of Changes in Acquired Immunity from Aging (Immunosenescence)

Changes in T-Cell Function in Healthy Older Adults

The overall impact of age on host immunity is thought to occur primarily along two mechanisms. The first is replicative senescence that may limit T-cell clonal expansion (Hayflick phenomenon or loss of telomerase activity/telomere length, and may be related more to repeated exposure to antigen than age). The second is developmental changes associated with involution of the thymus that precedes dysfunction of the T-cell component of adaptive immunity. Studies have shown a decrease in telomere length with age in T and B cells; however, it was demonstrated that there is no significant change in telomerase activity (11). Although this study may not have included individuals with repeated exposure to antigen (characteristic of chronic illness), it suggests that age-specific changes are more due to developmental changes in T cells. Several recent reviews have summarized extensive studies on changes in T cell function with aging (3,11). The age-related decline in T cell function is preceded by involution of the thymus gland, with dramatic decline in thymic hormone levels. In addition, changes in bone marrow stem cells have also been described, which are distinct from thymic changes. These changes are thought to result in a shift in the phenotype of circulating T cells, with a decrease in the number of naïve T cells and a relative accumulation of memory T cells. The memory cells that persist include T cells, primarily CD8+, with impaired proliferative and effector capacity, that may also be as a result of repeated viral (primarily) exposure, known as chronic antigenic stress (4). Hence, due to thymic involution, repeated antigenic exposure, and alteration in susceptibility to apoptosis (increased for CD4+, decreased for CD8+), thymic and lymphoid tissues become populated by anergic memory CD8+CD28−T-cells. These anergic T cells contribute to the impaired immune response to infections and increased propensity for autoimmune disorders and are associated with a shift in cytokine propensity toward a Th2 anti-inflammatory response, as evidenced by an increase in IL-10 production (3,4,8,12,13). One study on 153 residents of an assisted living facility in Rochester, Minnesota, demonstrated that nearly half of the residents failed to generate an antibody response to any of the trivalent components of an influenza vaccine, and this correlated with both the age and the expansion of CD8+CD28− T cells (14). This combination of increase in CD8+ but decrease in CD4+T-cells, with impaired proliferative response, has been called the immune risk phenotype. Immune risk phenotype was found to be associated with increased IL-6, and, together with the presence of cognitive impairment, predicted 58% of deaths in adults over the age of 85 in a four-year longitudinal study in Sweden (15).

Significant age-related alteration is more often identified if the immune assay system requires cell-to-cell interaction. For instance, little age difference is found when T cells are stimulated by fixed anti-CD3 antibody, instead of systems that require T cell stimulation by APC, and this may be related to membrane changes in T cells discussed below (3,4). Age-related changes in T cell cytokines, other than IL-2 and IL-10, have demonstrated a much more varied response, especially cytokines IFN-γ and IL-4, which may relate to species differences between human and mouse studies and the type of stimulation (4,5,16). The relative anergic state of T cells from aged individuals is likely a result of altered postreceptor signal transduction, including calcium metabolism, phosphorylation of tyrosine kinases, and protein kinase C translocation to the nucleus (likely a key factor involved in the shift toward a Th2 response) that may be due to changes in membrane composition. Surface receptors appear to be organized in structures called lipid rafts, and alteration in cholesterol and sphingolipid composition found with aging may be associated with impaired polarization of lipid rafts on the

T-cell surface, resulting in an impaired ability to interact with APC, with impairment being more pronounced on CD4+ T cells (4). These membrane changes could be a result of changes in the microenviroment, including the hormonal milieu and exposure to free radicals, as well as other inflammatory mediators (discussed later). Finally, despite the rather universal changes in T cell response with age, the relevance is unclear. Although in vitro support of antibody response by T cells has been shown to be impaired with age, impaired proliferative response to specific antigen or a mitogen, even after adjusting for relative sensitivity to mitogen, failed to correlate with impaired antibody response to influenza immunization (16).

Changes in B Cells in Healthy Older Adults

Age-related changes in B cells are much less clear, but appear to have similarities to T cell changes. B cells from older individuals show impaired activation and proliferation that could also be related to changes in costimulatory molecule expression (8). Both primary and secondary antibody responses to vaccination have been found to be impaired. The specificity and efficacy of antibodies produced in older adults is lower than in younger populations (8,11). In one longitudinal study of young and older adults demonstrated that the proliferative responses to influenza antigen upon yearly immunization were lower in older adults, as was the percentage of older adults with protective antibody titers (16).

Changes in Innate Immunity

Studies to date have shown that (i) age-related changes in immunity have been largely limited to the T cells of acquired immunity, with intact APC function in healthy older adults and (ii) infection rates are increased in chronically ill older adults. It is surmised that chronic illness can impair both innate and acquired immunity. Innate immunity is critical to both the number of immunocompetent units and the magnitude of the immunological burst upon activation. These changes, induced by chronic illness, could be the key mechanism involved in the onset of impaired immune competence beyond normal age-related changes (2). Otherwise, with healthy aging, evidence has suggested that innate immunity remains intact or is upregulated in very healthy aging. The frequently reported nonspecific increase of proinflammatory substances produced by the innate immune system and downregulation of acquired immunity may reflect a compensatory event by either component, but their causality is unclear (2,8,17).

Changes in Neutrophils with Aging

For many years, there have not been significant findings on age-associated decline in neutrophil function, but this may have much to do with the challenge of studying neutrophil functions. Studies have been focused on possible alterations in their ability to seek out and migrate toward pathogens, phagocytize, and kill the invading organisms in older adults. Cytoskeletal and membrane changes impact on key neutrophil functions, including adherence and membrane fluidity, and are vulnerable to changes in the microenvironment that occur with aging and especially in age-related diseases (18). Phagocytic ability of neutrophils has been reported to be significantly lower in older adults (19). Other studies have reported that tumor necrosis factor (TNF)-α in particular causes a higher suppression of CD18-mediated, fibronectin-primed superoxide release in neutrophils from older adults. In addition, neutrophils from healthy older adults are more susceptible to oxidative stress and apoptosis (18). In looking for a central theme for these age-related changes in neutrophils, impaired signaling elicited by various membrane receptors as well as changes in lipid rafts has been found in healthy older adults. This has resulted in the alteration of second messenger pathways (p42/p44 MAPK), which will be discussed in the section on T cells (18).

Changes in Dendritic Cells with Aging

Increased number of DCs generated in vitro from circulating monocytes of very healthy older adults in comparison with younger adults has been reported. Similarly, the DCs generated in vitro from healthy older adults were effective in restoring the proliferative capacity of T cells from older adults and in preventing the development of apoptosis in T cells grown to senescence (no longer able to proliferate) in culture (13,16). Likewise, the antigen-presenting capacity of circulating APC (including DC) is actually greater in APC from healthy older adults, in comparison with younger adult controls, and is associated with increased production of IL-12 and IL-10 (12).

IMPAIRED IMMUNITY DUE TO THE IMPACT OF CHRONIC ILLNESS ON AN AGING IMMUNE SYSTEM (IMMUNOSENESCENCE)

Despite nearly 90% involution of the T-cell generating thymus by age 40, true opportunistic infections are not seen among older adult patients, even those with significant chronic disease. This suggests that there is likely compensation for lost immunological tissue of the thymus gland. However, bacterial infections (i.e., pneumonia, urinary tract, and skin and soft tissue infections) are a common problem in older adults. Other infections include viral infections (i.e., reactivation of herpes zoster and significantly increased morbidity and mortality associated with influenza virus) and infections that are related to microbial colonization with *Clostridium difficile*, and methicillin-resistant *Staphylococcus aureus* in severely ill individuals treated with antibiotics (11). In addition, changes in immunity create difficulty in detecting both active (primary and reactivation) and inactive tuberculosis.

Response to vaccination, which requires intact cell-mediated immunity to drive the humoral response, is clearly diminished in many different older adult populations, as well as in aged laboratory animals. An example of how chronic illness further impairs immunity is that both aging and impaired renal function reduce the response to hepatitis B vaccine in renal failure patients. Findings showed that 86% of patients with serum creatinine at or below 4 mg/dL had a protective antibody titer following hepatitis B immunization, in comparison with only 37% of individuals with a serum creatinine above 4 mg/dL. Likewise, age independently was inversely associated with antibody response. Hence, immunization of patients with chronic renal insufficiency before serum creatinine exceeds 4 mg/dL is essential (20).

It is known that T-cell–dependent immune response declines gradually with age. A review of more than 200 scientific articles that evaluated healthy older adults, who were selected by the SENIEUR protocol (7), showed that the magnitude of decline in T-cell–dependent immune response with age is modest, i.e., approximately 25% in healthy older adults (12), relative to that of the aging mouse model (3,4). In contrast, the T-cell–dependent immune response of frail older adults is impaired by two to three times compared to healthy older adults, of ages comparable to those of frail older adults (12). Moreover, the greater impairment in immunity in vulnerable older adults is associated with a decline in induction of proinflammatory IL-12 response and increased anti-inflammatory IL-10 (2,12). These results suggest that changes in the immune tissue microenvironment may play an important role in age-related decline in T-cell–dependent immune response in humans. This is not unexpected, for the aging mouse model had shown previously that the age-related decline in T-cell–dependent immune response is caused by changes occurring in both the immune cells (intrinsic changes) and the immune tissue microenvironment (extrinsic changes) (21).

One study (22) analyzed changes in various physiologic functions with age from 469 studies involving more than 54,000 older adults. The comprehensive review included 43 immunologic studies of 372 individuals. The study found that the mean annual rate of decline with age in immune functions was greater than the average rate of decline of all other physiologic functions that were assessed. The study concluded that the deterioration in immune function in older adults was due not only to biologic aging but also to the presence of chronic disease. This review underscores the need to evaluate frail older adults, in addition to healthy older adults.

Recently, the influence of chronic disease burden on T-cell immunity has been investigated (2), using the cumulative illness rating scale (CIRS). CIRS is an instrument that measures disease burden in individuals with various chronic diseases but with no evidence of acute deterioration or infection. T-cell immunity was based on phytohemagglutinin-induced proliferation and production of immunoinhibitory IL-10 and immunoenhancing IL-12. The study showed that decrease in T-cell proliferation, increase in production of

IL-10, and decrease in production of IL-12 are linearly correlated with increase in chronic disease burden (i.e., increased CIRS score), but not with increase in chronologic age, between 51 and 95 years.

Preliminary studies in a nursing home population with chronic illness suggest a potential mechanism and target of immune enhancement strategies. These findings showed elevated APC functional capacity of healthy older adults. In contrast, APCs from vulnerable older adults possess impaired antigen presenting capacity, impaired DC differentiation, and reduced production of proinflammatory cytokine IL-12 (2,12). Hence, DCs could reflect a physiologic vulnerability of the immune microenvironment as a result of underlying chronic inflammatory diseases and perhaps the increase in inflammatory mediators discussed below. This could hasten the rate of immunosenscence to below a threshold level, thereby impairing immunity. This is particularly an attractive hypothesis, because the differentiation of DCs has been identified as a key variable in the stimulation of effector T-cell function. DCs are thus an important target for immunotherapeutic adjuvants to improve antigen delivery and to boost immunity. Therefore, a greater focus should be placed on the role of DC as targets for improved vaccine response of older adults in the highest risk vaccine categories. A model of how aging and chronic illness impact specific components of innate and acquired immunity and ultimately the response to infectious exposure is summarized in Figure 3.

INFLAMMATORY MEDIATORS AND IMMUNITY

The finding that impaired immunity is correlated more with comorbidity than age in older adults suggests that changes in the composition of inflammatory mediators that occur in the immune tissue microenvironment of older adults could play an important role in accelerating the gradual age-related decline in Type 1 immune response caused by changes in T cells. The regulation and interaction of cytokines produced by cells of innate immunity are very complex. The relative timing and quantities of the cytokines of innate immunity are crucial to the priming of the acquired immune response. Studies suggest that there is a nonspecific increase in production of proinflammatory proteins in the aged population, which is associated with increased mortality (17,23). Low-level, nonspecific autoimmunity throughout different tissues, as well as an impaired immune responsiveness to infectious pathogens, is common in older adults with significant chronic illness. Studies on age-related changes in proinflammatory cytokines have had varied findings, most likely related to the complex nature of cytokine networks. However, most studies have shown an increase in plasma or serum levels of IL-6, IL-8, IL-10, and TNF-α and a decrease in IL-1 (3,8). A recent review describes 14 studies that report increases in IL-6 with aging. IL-6 itself has been shown to be inhibitory to mycobacteriostatic activities in

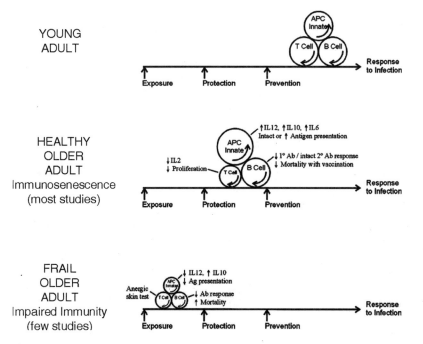

Figure 3 Diagram of response to infection as affected by aging and chronic disease. This model shows the response to infection as the distance driven by the immune "car" with the vigor of the three main immune components represented by size, with the response of younger adults as the standard. In healthy older adults, the immune response drives far enough to provide protection but may not provide prevention of infection, due to a decline in T-cell function (accumulation of memory T cells in place of more plastic naïve T cells, with a decline in IL-2 and impaired proliferative response to stimulation). B-cell function is altered but remains effective with impaired primary antibody response but an intact secondary antibody, with a decline in mortality with vaccination. This maintenance of immune competence may be due to enhanced antigen presenting cell function (increased IL-12 and IL-6 despite increased anti-inflammatory IL-10, with enhanced antigen presentation). In frail older adults, the immune "car" does not even provide protection from infection, as there is a decline in both innate (increased IL-10, decreased IL-12, and antigen presentation) and acquired immunity (T-cell and skin test anergy, impaired antibody response), resulting in loss of immune competence (increase risk and severity of infection, loss of protection from immunization). *Abbreviations*: APC, antigen presenting cell; Ab, antibody; Ag, antigen.

macrophages (24). Chronic illness likely contributes to further dysregulation of immune response. A study comparing IL-2 and IL-6 levels in young adults, healthy older adults, and "almost-healthy" older adults (individuals who did not meet the SENIEUR protocol because of no history of regular exercise or the use of medications for conditions, such as hypertension or osteoarthritis) reported lower levels of IL-2 and higher levels of IL-6 in the "almost-healthy" older adult population (6). Hence, although most articles measuring plasma or serum levels classify IL-6 as proinflammatory, immunologically it has anti-inflammatory properties and clearly is distinct from TNF-α and IL-1 (24).

Longitudinal studies suggest that higher circulating levels of IL-6 and other inflammatory mediators are associated with and are predictive of functional disability and increased mortality in older adults who had no functional impairment at entry into these longitudinal studies (23). An association also exists between physical activity and lower levels of serum IL-6. Moreover, higher serum IL-6 levels have been reported in many chronic diseases, with slight (27% to 72% increase in relative risk) but significant increase in coronary heart disease, stroke, and congestive heart failure in subjects 70 to 79 years of age without evidence of cardiovascular disease at baseline. Of note, these inflammatory markers, IL-6, TNF-α, C-reactive protein (CRP), especially serum IL-6, possess a relative risk equal to or higher than traditional risk factors as predictors of cardiovascular disease. Given these strong epidemiologic findings, IL-6 appears to be associated with many chronic diseases, including Alzheimer's disease and emphysema. However, it remains unclear what increased serum IL-6 levels represent. High plasma levels of TNF-α and IL-6 in healthy older adults and in patients with Type 2 diabetes mellitus are associated with increased truncal fat mass, and that of the TNF-α, in particular, could contribute to sarcopenia or the loss of muscle mass with age. However, the association with disease is more likely from a hormonal effect of IL-6, mediated by catabolic changes in somatic muscle, rather than on immunological causes. Very few studies have been done comparing how circulating levels of IL-6 or other markers of inflammation correlate with traditional measures of cell-mediated immunity. In one study, only 1 out of 32 Alzheimer's disease patients demonstrated a decline in production of IL-6 and TNF-α associated with severe dementia, in comparison with IL-6 and TNF-α levels among mild to moderately demented patients (24).

Preliminary reports suggest that increases in inflammatory mediators, especially increases in IL-6 and IL-10, are associated with poor outcome in some infections, including severe community-acquired pneumonia and Q fever (25,26). In addition, association of IL-10 polymorphism has been shown with severity of illness in community-acquired pneumonia (27), and persistent increased levels of IL-10 and soluble TNFR-I one week after development of pneumococcal pneumonia correlated with older age (24). Clearance of inflammatory mediators in the sputum (IFN-γ, TNF-α, IL-6, IL-8) has been reported to be early markers of clearance of pulmonary tuberculosis (28). Finally, there is evidence that proinflammatory cytokines can be modulated with medication, as IL-6 levels were attenuated in severe pneumonia requiring mechanical ventilation by the addition of glucocorticoids, and IL-6 and CRP were reduced by the addition of aspirin in subjects with chronic stable angina.

The relationship between aging, inflammatory mediators, response to infection, and the progression of chronic inflammatory diseases is important but very complicated. There is likely a final common pathway interaction of these factors that impact on the microenvironment of an acute response to infection, and the characteristic of this final common pathway response could have an impact on the ability to control infection and the progression of underlying chronic disease and wasting.

Other confounding medical conditions that may alter immunity include stress and depression (29) and such primary diseases as heart failure, kidney disease, or liver disease. These conditions make it difficult to identify causation of impaired host defense. Research involving chronically ill individuals is extremely challenging due to the large variability and potential confounding variables that cannot be easily analyzed. Regardless, the ability to detect a patient who has crossed or is below a certain threshold of impaired immunity would enable the clinical geriatrician to boost specific components of the immune response to vaccination or to prevent recurrence of an infection. Therefore, a recommended strategy for further investigation would be targeted interventions of immunity, disease severity, development of sarcopenia, impaired mobility, and malnutrition (Fig. 4)—all of which could contribute to adverse health outcomes and further decline in immunity and progression of chronic illness.

IMPACT OF AGE AND CHRONIC ILLNESS–RELATED IMPAIRED IMMUNITY ON INFECTIONS

Impact of Age and Chronic Illness on Influenza

Age-related changes in immunity likely have the most clinical relevance toward an impaired response to influenza infection and/or immunization to influenza. An estimated 90% of the 10,000 to 40,000 deaths attributed to influenza infections annually in the United States occur in persons 65 years of age or older. The national health objective for the year 2000 was to achieve a >90% coverage rate for influenza vaccination of noninstitutionalized elders, and the 2000 Advisory Committee on Immunization Practices have broadened the recommendation for vaccination to adults 50 to 64 years of age. In 2002, via a random-digit telephone survey, 36.4% of respondents aged 50 to 64 years and 66.4% of respondents ≥65 years reported having received the influenza vaccine in the prior 12 months (30). The Centers for Disease Control and Prevention states that when the antigenic match between vaccine and circulating virus is close, infection is prevented in 70% to 90% of subjects less than 65 years of age, compared with only 30% to 40% in those 65 years of age or older (31). A past review of studies on antibody response to influenza found that 10 (33%) studies identified a decline in antibody response in an aged population, 16 (53%) studies

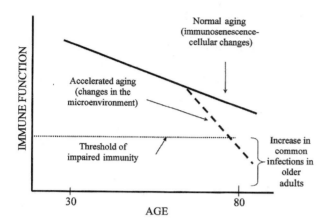

Figure 4 Model of age-associated gradual decline in immune function and the accelerated decline in immune function resulting in impaired immunity and increased risk of common infections. This model shows the decline in immune function as a gradual linear decline due to intrinsic cellular changes called immunosenescence. Some individuals will experience an accelerated decline due to the extrinsic effect on immune cells as a consequence of chronic diseases. This results in crossing a threshold of "impaired immunity" that is distinct and more directly responsible for the increase in common infections of older adults, in comparison with the effect of immunosenescence only. Detection of the inflection point would be a key clinical tool.

reported no change, and 4 (13%) showed an increased response. This variability is related to both differences between populations and differences in defining a protective antibody response. As stated previously, one study of 153 residents in assisted living facilities in Rochester, Minnesota, demonstrated that nearly half failed to generate an antibody response to any of the trivalent components and that this correlated with both the age and the expansion of CD8+CD28− T cells (14). For instance, a general medicine outpatient population (mean age 80 years) that (i) did not have any history of major medical illness, (ii) did not take immunosuppressive medications, (iii) did not smoke or report abuse of alcohol, and (iv) reported no hospitalizations or any episode of pneumonia in the past year was found to have comparable immune cell subsets, response to vaccines (i.e., tetanus, diphtheria, and pneumococcal), and proliferative response to a wide range of mitogenic stimulation, in comparison with a young adult population (31a). Another attempt at identifying changes in vaccine response used stimulation of whole blood cultures preinfluenza and two days postinfluenza vaccination in SENIEUR protocol older adults. This study suggests a slight low-grade inflammation with impaired upregulation of inflammation following vaccination with a decline in stimulated IL-6 and IL-10 (32). The use of whole blood cultures is one way of identifying changes in the microenvironment but is limited by variability in cell numbers. Interpreting the significance of these immune studies in relation to influenza infection is complicated, given the low attack rate and challenge in confirming actual influenza infection. This is also the case in assessing antibody response, because older individuals often have higher prevaccination antibody levels, in comparison with younger individuals who have had less exposure to infection and prior vaccination. Even if antibody response was intact, it may not provide the same level of protection as in younger individuals. Thus, for example, in a study reported on 72 vaccinated older adults, who later were confirmed to have influenza infection, 60% had antibody titers greater than or equal to 1:40, and 31% had titers greater than or equal to 1:640, four weeks postvaccination (33). The vaccine response is low in this population, even when vaccine response appears adequate, but protection from infection is still lower than in younger adults. This is likely related to the quality of the antibody produced in neutralizing viral pathogenesis by older adults. Nevertheless, despite the low efficacy in prevention of infections, it needs to be emphasized that vaccination in people 65 years of age and older has been effective in reducing adverse events. In this older population, vaccination reduced the incidence of hospitalization due to pneumonia by 50% to 60%, and mortality was reduced by 80%. In a three-year study of more than 75,000 community-dwelling older adults, there was a 46% (range of 39–54%) reduction in all-cause mortality associated with individuals who received influenza vaccination. Although antibody response to vaccination (both magnitude and duration) is impaired in persons 65 years of age and older, protective benefit to host defense could occur because cytolytic T-lymphocyte killing efficiency against virally infected cells and the duration of activity were reported to be intact in older subjects (16,31).

Underlying chronic illness could dramatically increase the risk of influenza infection and impair the response to vaccination. The presence of one or two chronic illnesses (such as emphysema, diabetes mellitus, or chronic renal insufficiency) is associated with a 40- to 150-fold increase in the incidence rate for influenza pneumonia (8). Whether chronic illness medication or other related external conditions further compromise immune competence has not been elucidated. One study on vaccine response in nursing home residents demonstrated that only 50% of residents had an adequate response (i.e., a four-fold increase in antibody titers). Furthermore, the response to vaccination did not correlate with nutritional status or dehydroepiandosterone levels (3). Another study in a nursing home setting reported that only 36% of 137 vaccinated residents demonstrated a rise in antibody titer, and there was no correlation with age, body mass index, or functional status, as measured by the Barthel index (34). One study of 154 individuals found that nonresponders to influenza vaccine were characterized by higher levels of anti-cytomegalovirus IgG and higher percentage of CD57+CD28− T cells (exposure to cytomegalo virus) and increased serum levels of TFN-α and IL-6 (35). Intervention studies have suggested a boost in vaccine response with supplementation of dehydroepiandrosterone-sulfate at 50 mg/day for four consecutive days before immunization versus placebo (36). One study failed to show an improved vaccine response to influenza vaccine with a nutrient supplement four months before and after vaccination in 119 nursing and residential home residents who completed the study. The supplement included vitamins A, C, D3, E, folate, and selenium (37). Another large study in Great Britain of more than 24,000 patients, aged over 75 years, suggested robust protection from respiratory and cardiovascular deaths in vaccinated patients when influenza was circulating in the community (38).

Conversely, exercise and psychosocial factors have been shown to modulate immune response to influenza vaccine. There was a graded boost in immune response of peripheral blood mononuclear cells that correlated to level of exercise. Another small study reported greater mean fold increases in trivalent antibody response [A/New Caldeonia/20/99 (H1N1) and A/Pananma/2007/99 (H3N2) and a greater Granzyme B activity to A/Pananma/2007/99] with an exercise routine at 65% to 75% heart rate reserve sustained for 25 to 30 minutes, three times per month for 10 months (39). These data suggest that regular and vigorous exercise can improve immune response to influenza vaccine. Finally, a Chilean study of 60 healthy community-dwelling older adults did show increased natural killer cell activity, less decline in stimulated IL-2 production by peripheral blood mononuclear cells, and a significant reduction in infections after four months (13% vs. 22%, $P = 0.02$) when given a dietary supplement of 31 g of protein, 120 IU of vitamin E, 3.8 µg of B12, 400 µg of folate, 10^9 colony-forming units of *Lactobacillus paracasei*, and 6 g of fructo-oligosaccharides (40).

Impact of Age and Chronic Illness on Pneumonia

The risk and severity of pneumococcal pneumonia and tuberculosis increase with age. The incidence of pneumococcal infection is high in the first two years of life, then declines through adulthood, and finally increases dramatically in people over 75 years of age. Rates of bacteremia and meningitis from the pneumococcal infection are higher in older adults, and mortality rises with advanced age, approaching 80% in those over 85 years of age. In fact, unlike all other age groups, mortality from pneumococcal pneumonia has actually increased in those over 75 years of age since the antibiotic era (1950 vs. 1985). Clearly, disease burden plays a crucial role in risk and severity of infection. A four-year study demonstrated that in adults 65 years or older, death due to pneumonia, influenza, and chronic lung disease was particularly high in nursing home residents (52.1 per 1000), and higher among senior housing residents (4.2 per 1000) than community residents (2.6 per 1000) (41).

Efficacy of the pneumococcal vaccine in preventing infection has been difficult to demonstrate in randomized control trials but has been reported to be 50% to 80% effective in case series studies. Five years after vaccination, the efficacy remains about 70% for those under 75 years of age, but 53% in subjects 75 to 85 years of age, and only 22% effective in those over 85 years of age (42). Of note, one study found that antibody response to pneumococcal vaccination in preventing pneumonia recurrences, following hospitalization for community-acquired pneumonia in nonimmunocompromised adults (50–85 years of age), correlated inversely with the risk of recurrent pneumonia 32 months after vaccination. A lower risk was seen with a four fold rise in antibody titers post vaccination (42). An outbreak of multidrug-resistant *Streptococcus pneumoniae* (serotype 23F) occurred in a nursing home in rural Oklahoma in 1996. Risk of infection was associated with recent use of antibiotics (relative risk, 3.6; 95% CI, 1.2–10.8), and only 4% of residents had received pneumococcal vaccine (43).

The overall case rate for tuberculosis declined 26% in the United States between 1992 and 1997, with the highest number of cases reported in the 25- to 44-year-old age group, which could reflect human immunodeficiency virus (HIV) epidemic. Prior to this epidemic, tuberculosis case rates had an upward inflection point at 75 years of age, due to both reactivation and primary cases of residents in institutional settings, whereas community cases may go undetected (8). The disease in older adults remains largely distinct from tuberculosis associated with HIV infection, and the majority of cases remain isoniazide sensitive. Differences in presentation include more subtle presentation (less pronounced cough, night sweats, or X-ray findings), and skin testing is difficult to interpret due to a waning of delayed hypersensitivity (i.e., false negative for inactive and active disease) but a more pronounced booster effect (i.e., false positive for conversion).

Mouse studies on tuberculosis show an age-related increase in susceptibility, with minor shifts in the immune response. Briefly, it appears that in older animals there is a delayed recruitment of CD4+ T cells, with less IFN-γ production. Hence, the infection tends to disseminate more and eventual containment is reduced. Adoptive transfer studies show that transfer of young T cells into old animals could reverse much of these changes (17).

CONCLUDING REMARKS

Reduced immune system performance contributes to increased risk of infections in older adults. Recent findings show that reduced immune functions in older adults caused by changes intrinsic to immune cells (i.e., immunosenescence from primarily genetic changes) is nominal, compared with changes extrinsic to immune cells (i.e., impaired immunity from chronic illness and environmental changes). Hence, immunosenescene predisposes to impaired immunity from progressive disease but is clearly distinct from immunosuppression, as is seen in HIV, cancer, and immunosuppressive medications. The significance of these findings is that successful intervention is more likely with environmental than genetic changes. This is supported by the relative ease in enhancing immune response of older adults through nutritional intervention, in contrast to intervention with stem cells.

The challenge we now are faced with is threefold: (i) to identify simple clinical predictors of impaired immunity associated with chronic age-related diseases; (ii) to identify immune cell(s) that are most vulnerable to microenvironmental changes, perhaps as a result of increase inflammatory mediators; and (iii) to develop intervention models with high specificity in dealing with older adults with significant comorbidities. As to identifying a clinical predictor of impaired immunity, IL-6 and/or IL-10 are likely candidates based on recent epidemiological and experimental studies. As to identifying immune cells that are highly sensitive to changes in the environment, DCs, which play a pivotal role in both innate and adaptive immune responses, are likely candidates. As to developing intervention models with high specificity, much work will be needed, for there has been no systematic study on immunologic consequence of modulating individual comorbidity. It would appear, therefore, that future studies on the impact of age and chronic illness-related impaired immunity on risk of infections will require, unlike past studies, a team approach involving geriatricians/gerontologists, immunologists, infectious disease specialists, and epidemiologists.

ACKNOWLEDGMENTS

The U.S. Department of Veterans Affairs, through the Geriatric Research Education and Clinical Center program, provides ongoing research support as well. Sources of financial support: U.S. Department of Veterans Affairs, Geriatric Research Education and Clinical Center (GRECC) and Research Service, and National Institute of Aging (RO3AG18497).

SUGGESTED READING

Bruunsgaard H, Pedersen BK. Age-related inflammatory cytokines and disease. Immunol Allergy Clin North Am 2003; 23:5–39.

Fulop T, Larbi A, Wikby A, Mocchegiani E, Hirokawa K, Pawlec G. Dysregulation of T cell function in the elderly: scientific basis and clinical implications. Drugs Aging 2005; 22:589–603.

Murasko DM, Bernstein ED, Gardner EM, et al. Role of humoral and cell-mediated immunity in protection from influenza disease after immunization of healthy elderly. Exp Gerontol 2002; 37:427–439.

Wikby A, Ferguson F, Forsey R, et al. An immune risk phenotype, cognitive impairment, and survival in very late life: impact of allostatic load in Swedish octogenarian and nonagenerian humans. J Gerontol A Biol Sci Med Sci 2005; 60A:556–565.

REFERENCES

1. Stevenson KB. Regional data set of infection rates for long-term care facilities: description of a valuable benchmarking tool. Am J Infect Control 1999; 27:20–26.
2. Castle S, Uemura K, Rafi A, Akande O, Makinodan T. Reduced immunity of elders with chronic illness correlates with cumulative illness rating scale, but not age. J Am Geriatr Soc 2005; 53:1565–1569.
3. Pawelec G. Immunosenescence: impact in the young as well as the old? Mech Ageing Dev 1999; 108:1–7.
4. Fulop T, Larbi A, Wikby A, Mocchegiani E, Hirokawa K, Pawlee G. Dysregulation of T cell function in the elderly: scientific basis and clinical implications. Drugs Aging 2005; 22:589–603.
5. Wick G, Grubeck-Loebenstein B. The aging immune system: primary and secondary alterations of immune reactivity in the elderly. Exp Gerontol 1997; 32:401–413.
6. Mysliwska J, Bryl E, Foerster J, Mysliwski A. The upregulation of TNFa production is not a generalised phenomenon in the elderly between their sixth and seventh decades of life. Mech Ageing Dev 1999; 107:1–14.
7. Ligthart GJ, Corberand JX, Fournier C, Galanaud P, Hijmans W, Kennes B. Admission criteria for immunogerontological studies in man: the SENIEUR protocol. Mech Ageing Dev 1984; 28:47–55.
8. Burns EA, Goodwin JS. Immunodeficiency of aging. Drugs Aging 1997; 11: 374–397.
9. Banchereau J, Steinman RM. Dendritic cells and the control of immunity. Nature 1998; 392:245–252.
10. Kaufman CA, Hedderwick SA, Bradley SF. Antibiotic resistance: issues in long-term care. Infect Med 1999; 16:122–128.
11. Hodes RJ, Fauci AS, eds. Report of Task Force on Immunology and Aging. National Institutes of Aging and Allergy and Infectious Disease: U.S. Department of Health and Human Services, March 1996.
12. Castle S, Uyemura K, Crawford W, Wong W, Klaustermeyer WB, Makinodan T. Age-related impaired proliferation of peripheral blood mononuclear cells is associated with an increase in both IL-10 and IL-12. Exp Gerontol 1999; 34:243–252.
13. Steger MM, Maczek C, Grubeck-Loebenstein B. Peripheral blood dendritic cells reinduce proliferation in in vitro aged T cell populations. Mech Ageing Dev 1997; 93:125–130.
14. Goronzy JJ, Fulbright JW, Crowson CS, Poland GA, O'Fallon WM, Weyand CM. Value of immunological markers in predicting responsiveness to influenza vaccination in elderly individuals. J Virol 2001; 75:12,182–12,187.
15. Wikby A, Ferguson F, Forsey R, et al. An immune risk phenotype, cognitive impairment, and survival in very late life: impact of allostatic load in Swedish octogenarian and nonagenerian humans. J Gerontol A Biol Sci Med Sci 2005; 60A:556–565.
16. Murasko DM, Bernstein ED, Gardner EM, et al. Role of humoral and cell-mediated immunity in protection from influenza disease after immunization of healthy elderly. Exp Gerontol 2002; 37:427–439.
17. Orme I. Mechanisms underlying the increased susceptibility of aged mice to tuberculosis. Nutr Rev 1995; 53(S4):S35–S40.

18. Larbi A, Douziech N, Fortin C, Linteau A, Dupuis G, Fulop T Jr. The role of MAPK pathway alterations in GM-CSF-modulated human neutrophil apoptosis with aging. Immun Aging 2005; 2(1):6.
19. Lord JM, Butcher S, Killampali V, Lascelles D, Salmon M. Neutrophil ageing and immunosenescence. Mech Ageing Dev 2001; 122:1521–1535.
20. Fraser GM, Ochana N, Fenyves D, et al. Increasing serum creatinine and age reduce the response to hepatitis B vaccine in renal failure patients. J Hepatol 1994; 21:450–454.
21. Price GB, Makinodan T. Immunologic deficiencies in senescence II. Characterization of extrinsic deficiencies. J Immunol 1972; 108:413–417.
22. Sehl ME, Yates FE. Kinetics of human aging: I. Rates of senescence between ages 30 and 70 years in healthy people. J Gerontol A Biol Sci Med Sci 2001; 56:A198–A208.
23. Elousa R, Bartali B, Ordovas JM, Corsi AM, Laurentani F, Ferrucci L. InCHIANTI Investigators. Association between physical activity, physical performance and inflammatory biomarkers in an elderly population. J Gerontol A Biol Sci Med Sci 2005; 60A:760–767.
24. Bruunsgaard H, Pedersen BK. Age-related inflammatory cytokines and disease. Immunol Allergy Clin North Am 2003; 23:15–39.
25. Fernandez-Serrano S, Dorca J, Coromines M, Carratala J, Guidol F, Manresa F. Molecular inflammatory responses measured in blood of patients with severe community-acquired pneumonia. Clin Diagn Lab Immunol 2003; 10:813–820.
26. Glynn P, Coakley R, Kilgallen I, Murphy N, O'Neill S. Circulating interleukin 6 and interleukin 10 in community acquired pneumonia. Thorax 1999; 54:51–55.
27. Gallagher PM, Lowe G, Fitzgerald T, et al. Association of IL-10 polymorphism with severity of illness in community acquired pneumonia. Thorax 2003; 58:154–156.
28. Ribeiro-Rodrigues R, Resende Co T, Johnson JL, et al. Sputum cytokine levels in patients with pulmonary tuberculosis as early markers of mycobacterial clearance. Clin Diagn Lab Immunol 2002; 9:818–823.
29. Trzonkowski P, Mysliwska J, Godlewska B, et al. Immune consequences of the spontaneous pro-inflammatory status in depressed elderly patients. Brain Behav Immun 2004; 18:135–148.
30. Centers for Disease Control and Prevention. Public health and aging: influenza vaccination coverage among adults aged = or >50 years and pneumococcal vaccination coverage among adults aged = or >65 United States, 2002. MMWR Morb Mortal Wkly Rep 2003; 52(41):987–992.
31. Fukuda F, Bridges CB, Brammer TL, Izurieta HS, Cox NJ. Prevention and control of influenza: recommendations of the Advisory Committee on Immunization Practices (ACIP). MMWR 1999; 48:1–23.
31a. Carson PJ, Nichol KL, O'Brien J, Hilo P, Janoff EN. Immune function and vaccine responses in healthy advanced elderly patients. Archives of Internal Medicine 2000; 160(13):2017–2024.
32. El Yousfi M, Mercier S, Breuille D. The inflammatory response to vaccination is altered in the elderly. Mech Ageing Dev 2005; 126:874–881.
33. Gravenstein S, Drinka PJ, Duthie EH, et al. Efficacy of an influenza hemagglutinin–diphtheria toxoid conjugate vaccine in elderly nursing home subjects during an influenza outbreak. J Am Geriatr Soc 1994; 42:245–251.

34. Potter JM, O'Donnel B, Carman WF, Roberts MA, Scott DJ. Serological response to influenza vaccination and nutritional and functional status of patients in geriatric medical long term care. Age Ageing 1999; 28:141–145.
35. Trzonkowski P, Mysliwska J, Szmit E, et al. Association between cytomegalovirus infection, enhanced proinflammatory response and low level of anti-hemagglutinins during the anti-influenza vaccination: an impact of immunosenescence. Vaccine 2003; 21:3826–3836.
36. Danenberg HD, Ben-Yehuda A, Zakay-Rones Z, Gross DJ, Friedman G. Dehydroepiandrosterone treatment is not beneficial to the immune response to influenza in elderly subjects. J Clin Endocrinol Metab 1997; 82:2911–2914.
37. Allsup SJ, Shenkin A, Gosney MA, et al. Can a short period of micronutrient supplementation in older institutionalized people improve response to influenza vaccine? A randomized, controlled trial. J Am Geriatr Soc 2004; 52:20–24.
38. Armstrong BG, Mangtani P, Fletcher A, et al. Effect of influenza vaccination on excess deaths occurring during periods of high circulation of influenza: cohort study in elderly people. BMJ 2004; 329:660–664.
39. Kohut ML, Cooper MM, Nickolaus MS, Russell DR, Cunnick JE. Exercise and psychosocial factors modulate immunity to influenza vaccine in elderly individuals. J Gerontol A Biol Sci Med Sci 2002; 57A:M557–M562.
40. Bunout D, Barrera G, Hirsch S, et al. Effects of a nutritional supplement on the immune response and cytokine production in free-living Chilean elderly. J Parenter Ent Nutr 2004; 28:348–354.
41. Menec V, MacWilliam L, Aoki FY. Hospitalizations and deaths due to respiratory illnesses during influenza seasons: a comparison of community residents, senior housing residents, and nursing home residents. J Gerontol A Biol Sci Med Sci 2002; 57A:M629–M635.
42. Hedlund J, Ortqvist A, Kndradsen HB, Kalin M. Recurrence of pneumonia in relation to antibody response after pneumococcal vaccination in middle-aged and elderly adults. Scand J Infect Dis 2000; 32:281–286.
43. Nuorti JP, Butler JC, Crutcher JM, et al. An outbreak of multidrug-resistant pneumococcal pneumonia and bacteremia among unvaccinated nursing home residents. N Engl J Med 1998; 338:1861–1868.

6

Nutrition and Infection

Kevin P. High

*Sections of Infectious Diseases and Hematology/Oncology,
Department of Medicine, Wake Forest University School of Medicine,
Winston Salem, North Carolina, U.S.A.*

KEY POINTS

1. Malnutrition is prevalent in residents of LTCFs because of disability, medications, poor dentition/swallowing, system barriers (such as inadequate staffing) and prevalent comorbidities (such as diabetes mellitus, cancer, and depression).
2. Simple assessments of nutritional status (e.g., body mass index $<24\,\text{kg}/\text{m}^2$, weight loss $>5\%$ in three months, weight $<90\%$ of ideal body weight) are available and should trigger more thorough nutritional evaluations.
3. *Prevention*: although high-quality data are often lacking, there is some evidence to support the use of commercial protein/calorie supplements, multivitamins, vitamin E not to exceed a dose of $200\,\text{mg}/\text{day}$, zinc $15\,\text{mg}/\text{day}$, and selenium $100\,\mu\text{g}/\text{day}$ to reduce the risk of infection in LTCF residents. Megadose therapy for any micronutrient should be avoided; there are data that toxic outcomes can result form oversupplementation of vitamins A, D, and E.
4. *Treatment*: there are few data suggesting benefit for any specific nutritional intervention once infection has occurred in an LTCF resident.
5. Drug–nutrient interactions are common, particularly with antibiotics.

INTRODUCTION

Aging is associated with a decline in immune competence (see Chapter 5) and an increased risk of infection (1). Nutritional factors have been shown to play a significant role in age-associated immune dysfunction (2), and the prevalence of malnutrition among older adults is greatest in residents of long-term care facilities (LTCFs) (3). Although reversal of underlying nutritional deficits is an attractive and inexpensive option for reducing morbidity and mortality in elderly residents in long-term care, there are few randomized, controlled trials of sufficient power with clearly defined clinical endpoints to allow firm recommendations. Most studies utilize surrogate markers of nutrition or immune function (i.e., reversal of previously documented vitamin deficiency, increases in serum albumin, or vaccine responses). With this limitation clearly stated at the outset, this chapter will review the prevalence, causes, methods of detection, and clinical relevance of malnutrition in residents of LTCFs and provide evidence-based suggestions to boost immune response and reduce the risk of infection in this at-risk population.

PREVALENCE AND CAUSES OF MALNUTRITION IN OLDER RESIDENTS OF LTCFs

Global malnutrition, i.e., deficiency of protein and calories, is the most common form of malnutrition in older adults, but prevalence estimates depend upon the variable used to define malnutrition. If one considers reduced daily intake to reflect malnutrition, the proportion of elderly adults who are malnourished ranges from 2% to 33% in both healthy, free-living elderly adults and residents of LTCFs. However, using nutritional parameters, such as anthropometric measures or laboratory determinations (i.e., serum albumin, total lymphocyte count), the estimated incidence of global malnutrition in healthy older adults is 3% versus 15% to 66% in institutionalized populations (4).

Residents of LTCFs are at greater risk for global malnutrition for two basic reasons: reduced nutritional intake and increased metabolic demands. LTCF regulations require that meals meet specific nutritional standards, but serving the meal does not guarantee that it will be consumed (Table 1). Most LTCF residents have significant disabilities that reduce their ability to feed themselves or properly chew and swallow. Many residents may be depressed or have anorexia secondary to comorbid conditions or drugs. Further, the environment of LTCFs may not be conducive to caloric intake for residents used to "grazing," i.e., eating small amounts throughout the day, to maintain caloric intake. Scheduled times for meals, a short duration of time to complete the meal, and reduced preferences for "institutional" ways of preparing food, all contribute to reduced caloric intake in residents

Table 1 Barriers to Voluntary Nutrient Consumption in Older Residents of Long-Term Care Facilities

Physical conditions
    Disability (inability to feed oneself)
    Medications (see Table 6)
    Poor dentition/swallowing
    Gastrointestinal disorders (e.g., peptic ulcer disease, gastroesophageal reflux, constipation)
    Restrictive diets

    Cachexia/anorexia of underlying disease (e.g., cancer, infection)
    Increased metabolic demands (e.g., wound healing, renal disease)
    Metabolic disorders (poorly controlled diabetes mellitus, thyroid disease)

Cultural/psychosocial
    Food preferences (based on religious or cultural norms)
    Social isolation

    Bereavement
    Depression

System barriers
    Inadequate staffing
    Lack of food between meals (inability of elderly to "graze")

    Restrictive meal times

of LTCFs. A major factor predisposing LTCF residents to malnutrition is a lack of adequate staffing to feed all residents at mealtime. A recent study of nearly 2000 subjects demonstrated that inability to feed oneself and low staff levels increased the risk of malnutrition in LTCF residents (5). Finally, cognitively impaired patients may not perceive hunger and thirst in the same way, thus further limiting their consumption of protein and calories.

For many of the same reasons, specific nutritional deficiencies are also more common in residents of LTCFs (Table 2). Vitamins A, B_6, B_{12}, D, and E and the trace elements zinc and selenium are most often found to be deficient in residents of LTCFs with prevalence estimates of 40% to 50% for some micronutrients. Specific risk factors for micronutrient deficiencies in elderly LTCF residents include reduced oral intake (vitamins A, B_6, D, E, and zinc), increased metabolic requirements (e.g., zinc for wound healing), decreased exposure to sunlight (vitamin D), and a high prevalence of atrophic gastritis (vitamin B_{12}). Like protein/calorie malnutrition, the prevalence of micronutrient deficiencies varies with the technique used to measure the nutrient. For example, vitamin A, a fat-soluble vitamin that is stored in the liver, is essential for proper immune function and the integrity of skin and mucous membranes. A French study (6) showed that the prevalence of vitamin A deficiency in LTCF residents was 2%, 6%, 21%, or 55% depending on whether serum levels, corneal cytology, urinary excretion after a given oral load of vitamin A, or evaluation of oral intake, respectively, was used as the determinate of "deficiency." Furthermore, there is significant debate as to what the "recommended" daily amount of vitamins or minerals should be in older adults (7). Recommendations have

Table 2 Common Nutritional Deficiencies in Older Residents of Long-Term Care
Facilities

Nutrient	Prevalence	Comment
Protein/calories	17–65%	Manifested by wasting, low BMI, low serum albumin, lymphopenia
Vitamin A	2–20%	Deficiency more common if measured by dietary intake or corneal cytology than by serum levels
Vitamin B_6 (pyridoxine)	28–49%	Particularly important when LTCF residents placed on isoniazid for tuberculosis prophylaxis/therapy
Vitamin B_{12}	0–20%	Atrophic gastritis is common in elderly
Vitamin D	20–48%	Decreased sunlight exposure and dairy product intake
Vitamin E	5–40%	Supplementation documented to improve some vaccine responses in older adults
Zinc	0–21%	Zinc supplementation to speed wound healing probably only helpful in residents who are zinc deficient.

Abbreviations: BMI, body mass index; LTCF, long-term care facility.
Source: Refs. 1, 6.

previously focused on "average" intake in large population studies rather
than the optimal level for subjects in a given setting. Obviously, these
recommendations are usually handicapped by a lack of data as to what is
"optimal." Finally, recent data suggest that energy requirements predicted
by frequently cited methods (such as the Harris–Benedict equation) do
not accurately reflect the metabolic needs of elderly subjects, by overestimat-
ing metabolic needs in 20% and underestimating metabolic needs in 35%
of LTCF residents (8). The accuracy of the Harris–Benedict equation predicting metabolic need is not improved by adding a commonly employed
"stress factor." Thus, estimating metabolic or specific micronutrient needs
in LTCF residents is difficult based on current techniques.

Anorexia in older adults is a complex state, and malnutrition is not
due merely to poor provision of nutrients (9). Undernutrition is often a
consequence of physiology or choice, rendering interventions less likely to
succeed. Specific examples include incurable cancer, a competent patient's
refusal to eat or take supplements and end-stage diseases, such as severe
congestive heart failure or chronic obstructive pulmonary disease. One
important cause of malnutrition in older LTCF residents that deserves special focus is psychiatric disorders, particularly depression, which accounts
for 22% to 32% of cases of significant weight loss in older LTCF residents.

Table 3 Mnemonic for Identifying Causes of Weight Loss in Older Residents of Long-Term Care Facilities

---

Medications
Emotional problems (depression)
Anorexia tardive (nervosa); alcoholism
Late-life paranoia
Swallowing disorders
Oral factors
No money (insufficient funds in medical facilities for palatable, individualized diets and consultant dietitian)
Wandering and other dementia-related behavior
Hyperthyroidism, hyperparathyroidism, hypoadrenalism
Enteric problems (malabsorption)
Eating problems (inability to feed oneself)
Low-salt, low-cholesterol diets
Social problems (ethnic food preferences, isolation, "disgusting" food habits of other residents)

Source: Ref. 12.

Recognition of depression and other reversible causes or undernutrition is critical (Table 3). One study specifically addressed this problem in LTCFs (3) by identifying 15 modifiable causes for undernutrition in LTCF residents (Table 4). Most of the suggested remedies could be accomplished with minimal or no additional cost; others, such as increasing or retraining staff, require significant resources. However, as outlined in the following sections, there is potential for significantly better outcomes for LTCF residents if malnutrition is recognized and addressed.

ASSESSMENT OF NUTRITIONAL STATUS AND CONSEQUENCES OF MALNUTRITION IN LONG-TERM CARE RESIDENTS

Although it might seem easy, identifying at-risk or malnourished LTCF residents can take considerable effort. Many identification methods are too complex to be readily applied in most LTCFs. However, a review of the relevant literature suggests that there are a number of readily available indicators that correlate with more sophisticated measures of nutritional status, and may help identify those at risk. Recently, one study (10) confirmed that the weight and body mass index (BMI; weight for height in kg/m^2) measures available in the Minimum Data Set closely correlate with more sophisticated measures and bioelectrical impedance analysis. Several studies have documented that a recent loss of >5% of body weight, a weight <90% ideal body weight for age/gender, and complaints of anorexia correlate with malnutrition (3,4,11). Another simple measure recently established to predict mortality in

Table 4 Reversible Causes of Malnutrition and Suggested Remedies

Cause	Method of identification	Corrective action
Staff unawareness	Lack of documentation in chart by MD, RN, or RD	Staff education
Inappropriate use of restricted diets	Patient receiving a restricted diet no longer indicated	Replace by ad lib diet
Use of drugs that impair desire or ability to eat	Review of medications	Discontinue or replace offending drug
Unmet need for eating assistance or self-help eating devices	Observation and caloric count	Provide assistance or devices
Suboptimal technique of eating assistance	Observation	Retrain the nursing aide
Suboptimal dining environment	Observation	Improve the environment
Prescription of maintenance instead of repletion dietary intakes (oral or enteral)	$<1.5 \times$ RDA of calories and protein prescribed	Increase prescription to $1.5 \times$ RDA calories and protein
Inadequate nutritional support during intercurrent illness	Weight and/or albumin decline during illness; inadequate nutrition support	Evaluation of intercurrent illness
Unrecognized febrile illness	Daily temperatures reveals elevations	Identify and treat infections
Unmet need for modified diet	Clinical review	Prescribed indicated modified diet
Inadequate management of tube-feeding complications	Prescribed tube-feeding volume not being administered or absorbed	Correct management of complication
Poor dental care	Oral examination	Prompt dental care
Unmet need for dysphagia evaluation	Clinical signs suggest dysphagia; evaluation not requested	Consult speech pathology for swallowing evaluation
Suboptimal treatment of dysphagia	Recommendations of speech pathology not being followed	Staff education

Abbreviations: MD, Medical doctor; RN, Registered nurse; RD, Registered dietitian; RDA, Recommended daily allowance.
Source: Ref. 7.

LTCF residents is mid-arm circumference (MAC) (12). A MAC of < 26 cm is associated with a fourfold increase in mortality risk, and a MAC of 26–29 cm with a threefold risk when compared with those with a MAC ≥29 cm.

There is a strong correlation between physical impairment and risk for malnutrition; elderly subjects (from the community or nursing home) who at the time of hospitalization have prevalent malnutrition are much more likely to be dependent in at least one the following activities of daily living: bathing, dressing, transfer, toileting, or eating (13). Interestingly, of the comorbid conditions examined—congestive heart failure, dementia, chronic obstructive pulmonary disease, cancer, and diabetes mellitus—only diabetes mellitus was related to nutritional status and was negatively associated with malnourishment (13). Several laboratory parameters also indicate a likelihood for malnutrition; serum albumin (<4.0 g/dL), total cholesterol (<160 mg/dL), total lymphocyte count (<1500/mm^3), and hemoglobin (<13 g/dL) all should raise the possibility of malnutrition in an LTCF resident.

Nutritional factors are strongly predictive of subsequent hospitalization, disability, and mortality. One recent study specifically focusing on LTCF residents evaluated 350 randomly selected patients and determined the value of 96 medical, functional, socioeconomic, and nutritional variables for predicting severe (life-threatening) complications. Only 5 of the 96 variables were predictive, of which 3 were nutritional (serum albumin, BMI, and amount of weight loss in the prior year) with the other 2 being renal function and functional status (activities of daily living). In a subsequent cohort of 110 residents, the authors found that these five variables could predict life-threatening events with a sensitivity of 88% and a specificity of 65% (14).

Importantly, even well-nourished elderly residents of LTCFs are likely to become malnourished during an acute hospitalization and are more likely to become so than older adults who live in the community (15). If they do become malnourished during an acute hospital stay, those elderly are more likely to require discharge to a nursing or rehabilitation facility [relative risk (RR) 2.3; 95% confidence interval (1.1–4.6)], experience in-hospital death [RR 8.0 (2.8–22.6)], and death outside the hospital within 90 days [RR 2.9 (1.4–6.1)]. Important and at times unavoidable interventions, such as "NPO" (nothing per oral) orders without adequate replacement nutrition, contribute to this outcome, but care to avoid unnecessarily long durations of NPO orders should be taken.

NUTRITIONAL INTERVENTIONS TO REDUCE INFECTION AND IMPROVE OUTCOMES IN LTCF RESIDENTS

Although elderly LTCF residents are frequently malnourished and poor nutritional status is associated with an increased risk of adverse outcomes, there are relatively few supplementation trials specifically addressing LTCF residents. Most trials that have been published suffer from a lack of clinical endpoints (i.e., incident disease) and have been underpowered to detect such benefits. Most studies use surrogate marker endpoints, such as increased caloric intake, increased weight, improved nutritional assessment scores, or serum levels of micronutrients. A few demonstrate trends toward reduced infection or improved vaccine responses, but, frequently, other small studies are contradictory. No single clinical trial of a nutritional intervention has ever shown improved survival in elderly LTCF residents.

Commercial Formulas/Protein-Energy Supplements

Early data (reviewed in Ref. 3) suggested that commercially available nutritional supplements enhance caloric intake and increase serum albumin and transferrin, but the effect on physical function or infection risk was not assessed. There is a "common sense" notion that nutritional supplements should benefit malnourished older residents of LTCFs, but clear benefit has been difficult to demonstrate. However, two recent studies have suggested that this is the case. The first, a meta-analysis of 31 randomized controlled trials of protein/energy supplements given to hospitalized or community-dwelling seniors, showed a mortality of just less than 10% in the supplemented group, and nearly 14% in the control groups (an absolute RR reduction of 33% with a number needed to treat of only 25 to save one life) (16). Infectious morbidity and mortality were not specifically analyzed in that study. Though the focus of the meta-analysis was not specifically LTCF residents, the findings may apply, but that is not guaranteed. Many "common sense" interventions are not successful in LTCF residents—a good example of this is the inability of feeding tubes and enteral nutrition to improve outcomes in dementia patients.

One recent study did specifically target nursing home residents and infection as an outcome. Upper respiratory tract infection (URI) and influenza vaccine responses were the a priori outcomes of a trial in assisted- and independent-living residents (17) in a unique trial in which both the control and intervention groups received protein/calorie supplementation, and the intervention group also received an experimental formula of vitamins/ zinc/selenium/specific carbohydrates/lipid components of long- and medium-chain fatty acids. There was no clear benefit for immunization responses, but URI symptoms were reduced in the experimental group over a six-month follow-up. There were a large number of dropouts in that study, many due to weight gain or gastrointestinal complaints, and the utility of that specific or any commercial formula to conclusively reduce infection remains uncertain.

Vitamin and/or Mineral Supplements

There have been many studies of micronutrient supplementation in elderly subjects; most of these have been performed in free-living elderly rather than residents of LTCFs. When studies have focused on LTCF resident, they are often underpowered and frequently show contradictory results. However, some unifying principles can be gleaned from review of the interventions reported to date. Clearly, micronutrient supplements can enhance vitamin and mineral intake in LTCF residents, and increase serum levels of many micronutrients. Furthermore, compliance with such supplementation is excellent and inexpensive. Trace minerals, primarily zinc and selenium, have shown the most consistent positive effects, increasing postvaccine antibody titers, raising CD4 cell numbers and reducing the risk of respiratory infection in some studies, whereas vitamin supplementation with vitamins A or C, or β-carotene, has little or no effect (Table 5). Vitamin E has shown variable effects, but, overall, supplementation up to 200 IU/day is probably safe and may be effective for reducing common colds and other mild upper respiratory tract infections. High doses of vitamin A, β-carotene, and vitamin E should be avoided due to recent data suggesting harm (22,23).

One large, well-designed study of vitamin/mineral supplementation highlights the potential benefits and limitations of current data. A total of 725 LTCF residents in 25 facilities were randomized in a factorial design to receive trace elements (zinc 20 mg + selenium 100 mg), three vitamins [C 120 mg, E 15 mg, and β-carotene 6 mg (=1000 retinol equivalents)], both or neither for two years (19). Mortality was high in all four groups (~30%) and not different between groups, but this reduced the number of subjects with complete follow-up. There was no effect on delayed-type hypersensitivity responses, but a greater proportion of subjects in the trace element groups (vitamins + trace elements or trace elements alone) had protective antibody titers after influenza vaccination ($P < 0.05$). Surprisingly, vitamins alone appeared to have had a negative effect on antibody titers ($P < 0.05$). There was no effect on urogential tract infections, but a trend toward reduced incidence of respiratory tract infections ($P = 0.06$), again in both trace element groups, but not in those receiving vitamins alone. These data confirm the findings of a smaller, prior study by the same investigators (19), but in the earlier study, the reduction in respiratory infections in the zinc + selenium groups reached statistical significance. The dose of vitamin E in the multivitamin supplement used in both studies (18,19) was quite modest, 15 mg/day. A randomized trial of vitamin E supplementation at a dose of 200 mg/day in LTCF residents showed a significant benefit by reducing URI, particularly common colds, but no benefit with regard to influenza vaccine response (20). Similarly, disappointing results were reported from a trial in LTCF residents using a brief (eight weeks) multivitamin supplement in an effort to increase influenza vaccine responses (21).

SPECIFIC SYNDROMES WHERE NUTRITIONAL SUPPLEMENTATION MAY BE OF BENEFIT

Although there are few prevention studies reported in LTCF residents with overall infection as an outcome variable, there are even fewer studies

Table 5 Selected Recent Micronutrient Supplementation Trials in Older Residents of Long-Term Care Facilities

Author(s)/ reference	Total no./ (no. on suppl)	Time/trial type	Nutrient(s)	Comment
Girodon et al. (18)	81 (61)	2 yr/R, P, F	Zn^{2+} + selenium or vitamins A, C, E or both	$\Uparrow$ Serum selenium levels in Zn^{2+} + selenium group and both groups; $\Downarrow$ infectious episodes in the groups receiving Zn^{++} + selenium, but not vitamins alone
Girodon et al. (19)	725 (543)	2 yr/R, P, F	Zn^{2+} + selenium or vitamins A, C, E or both	$\Uparrow$ Serum micronutrient levels, but no effect on DTH responses; improved responses to influenza vaccine in Zn^{++} + selenium groups, borderline reduction in respiratory infection in Zn^{++} + selenium groups ($P = 0.06$), no effect of vitamins alone
Meydani et al. (20)	671 (311)	1 yr/R, P	MVI or MVI + 200 IU/day vitamin E	451 completed the study; no change in the number of days with infection, but fewer colds (RR 0.80) and overall URIs (RR 0.88) in vitamin E recipients; almost 50% of enrollees were zinc deficient and remained so throughout the study
Allsup et al. (21)	118 (61)	8 wk/R, P	MVI/M or placebo	Primary outcome was influenza vaccine response; no difference between groups in this trial of brief supplementation

Abbreviations: R, randomized; P, placebo-controlled; F, factorial; DTH, delayed-type hypersensitivity; MVI, multivitamin; MVI/M, multivitamin/mineral; RR, relative risk; URIs, upper respiratory tract infection; $\Uparrow$, increased; $\Downarrow$, decreased.

outlining the effect of nutritional supplementation to treat or prevent specific infections. These few studies are highlighted in this section.

Influenza and Respiratory Syncytial Virus

Prevention of URI and promotion of influenza vaccine responses are common outcomes reported in the vitamin and mineral supplement studies highlighted earlier and in Table 5, but the incidence of serious respiratory clinical illness due to pneumonia, influenza, or respiratory syncytial virus (RSV) is rarely reported. One recent study did examine a nutritional intervention and specifically measured influenza and RSV as an outcome (24). During two different influenza seasons (2000 and 2001), nursing home patients were enrolled in the randomized study comparing ginseng extract (CVT-E002) to placebo. Placebo recipients had a higher risk of confirmed influenza (odds ratio 7.73, $P = 0.033$), and the combined endpoint of confirmed influenza or RSV (odds ratio 10.5, $P = 0.009$). The CVT-E002 was administered as a 200 mg dose twice daily for 12 weeks during the influenza season. This remains the only report of ginseng extract's effect on influenza or RSV in LTCF residents, but if confirmed, this intervention has the potential to markedly impact health in this population.

Pressure Ulcers

There is considerable debate over whether nutritional supplementation can prevent or speed the healing of pressure ulcers, but at the present time data do not allow a specific recommendation other than to provide adequate calories (30–35 kcal/kg) and protein (1–1.25 gm/kg) to avoid negative nitrogen balance (25). Zinc at a dose of 220 mg/day is widely used with poor supporting data, but may be effective if patients are zinc deficient at baseline.

Urinary Tract Infections

One nutritional intervention has been reasonably well studied for the prevention of urinary tract infection (UTI) in elderly subjects, cranberry juice consumption (reviewed in Ref. 26) (see also Chapter 12). Although there has been only one study in LTCF residents, there has been one reasonably sized, randomized trial in community elderly and another small crossover study that demonstrated benefit in the elderly. There are also a variety of studies in younger patients. However, there are valid criticisms against all these studies. The endpoint in many of these trials was bacteriuria, not urinary tract infection. Because asymptomatic bacteriuria in the elderly is common and does not require therapy, the clinical relevance of these studies is unclear in LTCF residents. The only LTCF study was reported only in abstract form and had several major flaws; both cranberry juice (220 mL/day) and capsules of cranberry juice extract were used, and the control group was historical.

There may be other benefits of cranberry juice (26). One possible cause for reducing UTIs with cranberry juice could be a reduction in malodorous urine, a common trigger for urinalysis and urine culture for institutionalized elderly. In addition, a small study of patients with urostomies who consumed 160 to 330 mL/day of cranberry juice experienced improvement in the skin surrounding the stoma. This could be of benefit in LTCF residents with incontinence and immobility who are at risk for skin breakdown, but no substantive trial testing this hypothesis has been performed.

DRUG–NUTRIENT INTERACTIONS

The elderly LTCF resident is likely to be receiving multiple prescription drugs, and nutrient–drug interactions can cause serious adverse effects. In a recent study of residents in three LTCFs in New York (27), residents consumed approximately five drugs per patient and, on average, were at risk for 1.4 to 2.7 drug–nutrient interactions per month. With specific regard to infection, nutrient–drug interactions are most likely with antibiotic administration. Tetracyclines and fluoroquinolones may be poorly absorbed when antacids, divalent cations (e.g., calcium), or tube feedings are provided. Certain antifungal compounds, particularly itraconazole, may be poorly absorbed with concomitant administration of antacids or histamine-type II (H_2) antagonists/proton pump inhibitors.

More likely than nutrients altering drug metabolism, drugs are likely to alter nutrient intake (Table 6). The most commonly prescribed drugs that frequently cause anorexia and decreased nutrient intake are antibiotics, antidepressants and other psychiatric drugs, digoxin, and anti-inflammatory agents. A critical part of nutritional care for elderly LTCF residents is frequent, thorough review of all medications with discontinuation of non-essential therapies.

CONCLUSIONS

Residents of LTCFs are often at risk of malnutrition and reversible causes of malnutrition are common. Most at-risk residents can be initially identified by information readily available (weight and BMI), which should trigger more extensive evaluation. Once identified, data support correction of underlying medical causes, particularly depression, and the use of nutritional supplements to increase calorie and protein intake in LTCF residents to reverse weight loss. However, the role of such supplements for preventing infection is less well defined by currently available data. Current data support the use of trace mineral supplements (up to

Table 6 Drugs that Cause Anorexia in Older Adults

Anorectic agents
  Cardiovascular drugs
    Digoxin
    Amiodarone
    Procainamide
    Quinidine
    Spironolactone
  Gastrointestinal drugs
    Cimetidine
    Interferon
  Psychiatric drugs
    Phenothiazines
    Butyrphenones
    Lithium
    Amitriptyline
    Impramine
    Fluoxetine and other selective serotonin-reuptake inhibitors
  Anti-infective drugs
    Most antibiotics
    Metronidazole
    Griseofulvin
  Nutrient supplements
    Iron sulfate
    Potassium salts
    Vitamin D (in excess)
  Antineoplastics
    Cyclophosphamide and most others
  Antirheumatic drugs
    Nonsteroidal anti-inflammatory agents
    Colchicine
    Penicillamine
  Pulmonary drugs
    Theophylline
  Malabsorptive agents
    Laxatives
    Cholestyramine
    Methotrexate
    Colchicine
    Neomycin
    Ganglionic blockers
  Agents that increase metabolism
    Theophylline
    L-Thyroxine (in excess)
    Thyroid extract
    Tri-iodotyrosine (in excess)
    D-Pseudoephedrine

20 mg/day Zn^{2+}-sulfate and 100 μg/day selenium sulfide) in most LTCF elderly because the expense and risk of adverse effects is small, and there appears to be a reduced risk of respiratory infection. Vitamin supplements have variable effects. Vitamin E at 200 mg/day may be of value in LTCF residents, but higher doses of vitamin E and vitamin A/β-carotene supplementation should be avoided due to adverse effects. Specific nutritional supplementation may be of value in certain infectious diseases, such as ginseng extract for influenza and RSV or cranberry juice for UTIs, but these data must be viewed as preliminary. Finally, physicians should be aware of the potential for antibiotic–nutrient interactions and the effect of medications on anorexia and nutrient intake.

SUGGESTED READING

Girodon F, Galan P, Monget AL, et al. Impact of trace elements and vitamin supplementation on immunity and infections in institutionalized elderly patients: a randomized controlled trial. MIN. VIT. AOX. Geriatric network. Arch Intern Med 1999; 159:748–754.

Mitchell BL, Ulrich CM, McTiernan. Supplementation with vitamins or minerals and immune function: can the elderly benefit? Nutr Res 2003; 23:1117–1139.

REFERENCES

1. High KP. Infection as a cause of age-related morbidity and mortality. Ageing Res Rev 2004; 3:1–14.
2. Wick G, Grubeck-Loebenstein B. Primary and secondary alterations of immune reactivity in the elderly: impact of dietary factors and disease. Immunol Rev 1997; 160:171–184.
3. Abbasi AA, Rudman D. Undernutrition in the nursing home: prevalence, consequences, causes and prevention. Nutr Rev 1994; 52:113–122.
4. Sullivan DH. Undernutrition in older adults. Ann Long-Term Care 2000; 8:41–46.
5. Woo J, Chi I, Hui E, Chan F, Sham A. Low staffing level is associated with malnutrition in long-term residential care homes. Eur J Clin Nutr 2005; 59: 474–479.
6. Azais-Braesco V, Moriniere C, Guesne B, et al. Vitamin A status in the institutionalized elderly. Critical analysis of four evaluation criteria: dietary vitamin A intake, serum retinol, relative dose-response test (RDR) and impression cytology with transfer (ICT). Int J Vitam Nutr Res 1995; 65:151–161.
7. Bendich A. Criteria for determining recommended dietary allowances for health older adults. Nutr Rev 1995; 53:S105–S110.
8. Roubenoff R, Giacoppe J, Richardson S, Hoffman PJ. Nutrition assessment in LTCFs. Nutr Rev 1996; 54:S40–S42.
9. Morley JE. Anorexia and weight loss in older persons. J Gerontol A Biol Sci Med Sci 2003; 58A:131–137.

10. Blaum CS, O'Neill EF, Clements KM, Fries BE, Fiatarone MA. Validity of the Minimum Data Set for assessing nutritional status in nursing home residents. Am J Clin Nutr 1997; 66:787–794.

11. Sullivan DH, Johnson LE, Bopp MM, Roberson PK. Prognostic significance of monthly weight fluctuations among older nursing home residents. J Gerontol A Biol Sci Med Sci 2004; 59A:633–639.

12. Allard JP, Ashdassi E, McArthur M, et al. Nutrition risk factors for survival in the elderly living in Canadian LTCFs. J Am Geriatr Soc 2004; 2:59–65.

13. Covinsky KE, Martin GE, Beyth RJ, Justice AC, Sehgal AR, Landefeld CS. The relationship between clinical assessments of nutritional status and adverse outcomes in older hospitalized medical patients. J Am Geriatr Soc 1999; 47: 532–538.

14. Sullivan DH, Walls RC. The risk of life-threatening complications in a select population of geriatric patients: the impact of nutritional status. J Am Coll Nutr 1995; 14:29–36.

15. Sullivan DH, Sun S, Walls RC. Protein-energy undernutrition among elderly hospitalized patients. A prospective study. JAMA 1999; 281:2013–2019.

16. Milne AC, Potter J, Avenell A. Protein and energy supplementation in elderly people at risk from malnutrition. Cochrane Database Syst Rev 2002(3): CD003288.

17. Langkamp-Henken B, Bender BS, Gardner EM, et al. Nutritional formula enhanced immune function and reduced days of symptoms of upper respiratory tract infection in seniors. J Am Geriatr Soc 2004; 52:3–12.

18. Girodon F, Lombard M, Galan P, et al. Effect of micronutrient supplementation on infection in institutionalized elderly subjects: a controlled trial. Ann Nutr Metab 1997; 41:98–107.

19. Girodon F, Galan P, Monget AL, et al. Impact of trace elements and vitamin supplementation on immunity and infections in institutionalized elderly patients: a randomized controlled trial. MIN. VIT. AOX. Geriatric network. Arch Intern Med 1999; 159:748–754.

20. Meydani SN, Leka LS, Fine BC, et al. Vitamin E and respiratory tract infections in elderly nursing home residents: a randomized controlled trial. JAMA 2004; 292:828–836. (Erratum in: JAMA 2004; 292:1305.).

21. Allsup SJ, Shenkin A, Gosney MA, et al. Can a short period of micronutrient supplementation in older institutionalized people improve response to influenza vaccine? A randomized, controlled trial. J Am Geriatr Soc 2004, 52:20–24.

22. Miller ER, Pastor-Barriuso R, Dalal D, Riemersma RA, Appel LJ, Guallar E. Meta-analysis: high-dosage vitamin E supplementation may increase all-cause mortality. Ann Intern Med 2005; 142:37–46.

23. Melhus H, Michaelsson K, Kindmark A, et al. Excessive dietary intake of vitamin A is associated with reduced bone mineral density and increased risk for hip fracture. Ann Intern Med 1998; 129:770–778.

24. McElhaney JE, Gravenstain S, Cole SK, et al. A placebo-controlled trial of a proprietary extract of North American ginseng (CVT-E002) to prevent acute respiratory illness in institutionalized older adults. J Am Geriatr Soc 2004; 52:13–19.

25. Chernoff R. Policy: nutrition standards for treatment of pressure ulcers. Nutr Rev 1996; 54:S43–S44.
26. Raz R, Chazan B, Dan M. Cranberry juice and urinary tract infection. Clin Infect Dis 2004; 38:1413–1419.
27. Lewis CW, Frongillo EA Jr, Roe DA. Drug–nutrient interactions in three long-term-care facilities. J Am Diet Assoc 1995; 95:309–315.

7

Ethical Issues of Infectious Disease Interventions

Elizabeth L. Cobbs

*Departments of Medicine and Health Care Sciences,
George Washington University, Veterans Affairs Medical Center,
Washington, D.C., U.S.A.*

KEY POINTS

1. Ethical issues occur everyday in LTCFs.
2. Physicians play an important role in supporting LTCF resident autonomy.
3. Advance care planning and advance directives serve to articulate the goals of care.
4. LTCF residents who are decisionally incapable should have a health-care proxy to speak on their behalf.
5. Systemic practices that deal with ethical dimensions in LTCFs help physicians do the "right thing."

INTRODUCTION

Long-term care facilities (LTCFs) provide care to dependent persons with a variety of needs and expectations, and, in a shifting medical marketplace, ethical issues are part of the daily routine. LTCFs continue to play an important role in posthospital care where short-term-stay residents may receive rehabilitation services or continuing treatment for medical illnesses, such as osteomyelitis. Improvement in function and health is the usual goal, and discharge to the community is often expected. The other larger group of residents living in LTCFs is composed of frailer individuals who are likely to require nursing home care for the rest of their lives. The nursing home is their home. Their expectations for medical care vary, as do their abilities to make decisions and express treatment preferences. A subset of those LTCF residents is near the end of life and desire primarily palliative care.

In addition to their medical heterogeneity, LTCF residents are at increased risk for infectious diseases because of physiological changes associated with aging, the impact of chronic conditions, and the effects of institutional living. Infection is a frequent cause of transfer to the hospital, and hospital transfer is a frequent response to the medically ill resident in the LTCF, although practice varies.

To serve this diverse group of residents, the LTCF is expected to provide timely and appropriate medical care, while at the same time soffering a comfortable, personalized residence. The dual task of meeting the medical needs of a diverse group of residents and providing a homelike environment that delivers a pleasing quality of life for dependent frail persons creates the setting for a number of ethical dilemmas faced by LTCF practitioners.

ELEMENTS OF ETHICS

Knowledge of medical ethics helps physicians and other practitioners to do the right thing in the long-term care environment, where competition between medical and humanistic agendas is typical. In addition to understanding the ethical principles at play, physicians must have effective communication skills in order to resolve these competing demands (1). Several ethical elements are common in LTCFs.

Autonomy

Autonomy refers to self-determination without overbearing external influence, a prized attribute in American society. Autonomy is a ubiquitous ethical concern in the LTCF, because all those who live in this setting do so, as their ability to function independently has been compromised. Promotion of autonomy while striving to meet the needs of dependent LTCF residents within a medical model requires a reworking of the definition of autonomy. Perception and experience of autonomy are influenced by many factors, including culture. The Milwaukee Hmong community, for example, perceives dementia not as a chronic disease that robs a person of autonomy but as a natural part of the life cycle. Individuals suffering from dementia are cared for in their sons' homes and rarely display such difficult behaviors as combativeness and wandering (2). Interestingly, resident autonomy in

LTCFs is often expressed through a pattern of living rather than through discrete decisions.

Beneficence and Nonmaleficence

Beneficence refers to doing good, and in the practice of medicine this translates to doing the right thing for the patient. Defining the "right thing" for residents living with chronic functional impairments has undergone a shift, with increased focus on the resident's right to self-determination and articulation of goals of care. The process of weighing the burdens and benefits of possible medical interventions as perceived by the resident has become standard practice in medical decision-making with LTCF residents.

Closely related to beneficence is the admonition to do no harm, known as nonmaleficence. Nonmaleficence has taken on greater importance as the burdens of common treatment options, such as hospitalization, are recognized, and options for prompt and effective out-of-hospital treatments increase. Adverse events as a result of health-care interventions are increasingly being studied. Adverse drug events, for example, occur frequently and are often preventable (3). Even infection control measures, such as patient isolation to prevent nosocomial transmission of infectious disease, has been shown in hospitals to be associated with an increase in adverse events (4). A number of approaches have been tried to reduce error and harm in LTCF residents. Federal regulation has aimed to promote nonmaleficence as in the 1987 passage of the Omnibus Reconciliation Act, which resulted in a decrease in the use of physical and chemical restraints in the care of LTCF residents. Quality improvement is a technique that aims to reduce errors in the systems of care and is widely used in LTCFs.

Fidelity

Fidelity embraces trust and confidentiality and is a foundation for the doctor–patient relationship. The doctor–patient relationship remains fundamental to the care of residents in LTCFs; however, some compromises to this relationship are inevitable because many LTCF residents have significant cognitive impairment. In addition, issues of trust pertain to relationships with other members of the interdisciplinary team (IDT) and impact on the resident's sense of autonomy.

Justice

Justice refers to the equitable distribution of resources and treatments and is especially relevant when the interests of residents, staff, institutions, and families conflict with each other. Competing demands for staff attention and resources create the need for individuals and systems to negotiate settlements to conflicts so that the needs of residents and others in the LTCF community are most equitably served.

EVERYDAY ETHICS

The need for everyday ethical principles to guide LTCF practice is derived from the complexity of the organizations, their objectives, and the many participants in processes of LTCF life. The LTCF environment aims to blend two very different cultures: the autonomous, individually controlled home and the heavily regulated, physician-directed medical facility. The use of physician orders to direct basic elements of resident life, such as diet, activity level, or permission to self-medicate, puts forth an overarching framework of medical paternalism. Affirmation of self occurs with expressions of autonomy as in residents' activities that express personal values and preferences.

At times, the mission of the LTCF and the interests of the residents conflict. The residents are the customers of the facility, yet LTCFs have been criticized for a lack of attention to the values and preferences of the individual resident. With limited staffing, residents may compete with each other for staff time and attention. An acutely ill resident may require extra care and attention from the staff, at times creating a shortage of staff to attend to the needs of other residents. Decisions about whether to hospitalize a resident are influenced by these competing interests, as well as by institutional financial incentives. Conflicts may also occur between the needs and preferences of the staff and residents as in the urging of reluctant staff members to accept the flu vaccine in order to protect the residents.

Conflict can also be found between staff and facility, and the facility and outside organizations. Families and significant others are important members of the LTCF community and contribute to the caregiving process. Families, however, may add to the conflict of competing interests. LTCFs benefit from a system of regular conflict resolution that effectively and consistently resolves conflicts between competing interests and values.

The LTCF resident faces many obstacles to maintaining a self that is capable of autonomous action. Providing opportunities for choice and exertion of control over the environment and participation in the decision-making process have been shown to positively influence resident life. Effective communication and negotiation are means to achieve the best possible outcomes for the resident as well as the staff and the institution. The LTCF must create systems that encourage consistent decisions by residents to maximize autonomy, despite resident disability and the context of the medical model.

Many common infection control decisions have ethical dimensions that require choices between competing concerns or values. Common issues include whether to isolate residents colonized with resistant organisms, whether an ill health-care worker should be allowed to work, and whether to investigate clusters of infections. Additional issues have to do with when to treat, what to treat, whether to hospitalize, how to communicate with residents and families, what to do when treatment attempts become burdensome and residents refuse, how to improve staff behaviors that protect resident safety and health, and when not to treat.

THE DOCTOR–PATIENT RELATIONSHIP

Over the last several decades, the paternalistic model of medical care in the United States has given way to an increased emphasis on patient autonomy. The typical LTCF resident has a chronic illness conferring significant cognitive impairment and/or physical frailty that will endure through the rest of the resident's life. LTCF residents are likely to benefit from the "enhanced autonomy" model, in which an active exchange of ideas and negotiation takes place with the goal of achieving the best possible decision for the resident (5). In many cases, goals of care will be discussed with health-care proxies speaking on behalf of residents to make known their preferences for health-care interventions.

The unequal balance of power in the doctor–patient relationship is exaggerated in the LTCF. Typically, the doctor has an advantage in the balance of power by having knowledge of medicine and of the patient, whereas the patient often has little knowledge of either the doctor or medicine. In the LTCF, the balance of power tips even further toward the physician. Physician orders in the medical chart determine many elements of residents' lives. Choice of physicians may be limited to a few staff doctors or others who are willing to be credentialed and to practice within the LTCF. Access to the doctor is often determined primarily by institutional routine, where the nurses serve as gatekeepers of physician access.

On this uneven "playing field," physicians must find ways to build trust with their patients so that difficult decisions can be made that afford the greatest possible autonomy and beneficence. Resident rights, such as the right to be given information about proposed or potential treatments and alternatives and the right to refuse treatment, serve as safeguards to counterbalance this enhanced physician power. Conflict between patient (or proxy) and doctor over treatment choices may occur when they disagree about values and when trust is lacking. Cultural factors may play a role. Agreement over the desirability of treatments depends on the ability of the physician and patient to reach a shared understanding of the patient's values and goals for care in the context of the medical treatment options.

GOALS OF CARE AND ADVANCE CARE PLANS

The development of individualized goals of care for each resident is a process that creates the best mechanism to maximize autonomy, quality of life, and desirable medical outcomes (6). In the process of developing goals of care, a comprehensive biopsychosocial assessment is performed. This assessment provides a framework for the integration of disease factors with psychosocial factors and other resident characteristics. This assessment yields measures of resident functional capacity and points out where interventions to improve function and enhance independence might be placed.

The values' history, including information about the resident's preferences, hopes, fears, basis for meaning, spirituality, and personal goals, is integrated with the biopsychosocial assessment. The physician and resident (or health-care proxy) aim to reach a shared understanding of the resident's health status, care needs, preferences, options for future treatment interventions, and likely outcomes. From this assessment, an advance care plan or a blueprint of goals and plans for care can be developed. In this way, LTCF residents of widely differing decisional capacity, health status, and personal preferences have deliberately articulated, personally generated (to the extent possible) advance care plans for care to guide treatment decisions.

The health values of the seriously ill vary considerably from person to person, and they cannot be easily predicted from the person's current state of health. There is no substitute for involving the resident (or health-care proxy in the event of resident decisional incapacity) in developing goals for care. Physicians who fail to develop advance care plans with their LTCF residents are in danger of making serious treatment decision errors (7). Practitioners can expect considerable variation in preferences for care based on a variety of factors, including ethnicity (8).

An example of an infectious disease where goals of care and advance care plans have played an important role is the treatment of pneumonia in frail LTCF residents. In some cultures, health-care proxies and physicians often decide to forego antibiotic treatment for LTCF residents with severe dementia, frailty, and dehydration who contract pneumonia (9). Regional and international variation exists in practices around developing goals of care and medical decision-making for seriously ill, frail LTCF residents. Many institutions have developed structured approaches to advance care planning, including prioritization of goals of care. One scheme is shown in Table 1 (10).

INTERVENTIONS: BURDENS AND BENEFITS

Diagnostic and treatment interventions may confer both benefits and burdens on the LTCF resident. Resident (or health-care proxy) decisions to accept or decline treatment may in part be determined by the perceived burdens of treatment interventions. Less burdensome options may sometimes exist. Intravenous antibiotic therapy for a resident with dementia who pulls out the intravenous line on a daily basis brings the burden of repeated needlesticks and perhaps physical restraints. For an extremely debilitated resident, even transportation for a diagnostic test may be exceedingly

Table 1 An Example of a Scheme to Prioritize Goals of Care

Priority level	Intensive care	Comprehensive care	Basic care	Palliative care	Comfort care only
First priority	Prolong life	Maintain physical and cognitive function	Maintain physical and cognitive function	Maximize comfort	Maximize comfort
Second priority	Maintain physical and cognitive function	Prolong life	Maximize comfort	Maintain physical and cognitive function	
Third priority	Maximize comfort	Maximize comfort	Prolong life	Prolong life	

Source: From Ref. 10.

burdensome because of discomfort from prolonged waiting and a bumpy ride in a wheelchair van or fear of uncertainty while in a strange environment. Practitioners often can devise alternative plans that minimize treatment burdens, sometimes with help from the IDT and outside consultants to maximize resident comfort, control, and dignity. Informed consent should be sought from the resident (or health-care proxy) before embarking on a burdensome course of diagnostic testing or treatment intervention.

Trials of treatment interventions may be helpful when the resident (or health-care proxy) is ambivalent about whether to decline or accept an intervention. A time-limited trial (e.g., of tube feeding or hemodialysis) with the opportunity to reassess at a planned interval might be offered. After assessing the benefits and burdens, a decision may be made to continue or discontinue treatment.

QUALITY OF LIFE

Quality measures in LTCFs span several domains, including quality of life, quality of care, and residents' rights. Quality of life is an important goal of care in the nursing home. Some evidence shows that overall quality of life has improved for men and women older than 85 living in LTCFs (11). Nursing home leaders and patient care advocates report the three most important components of quality of life items to be dignity, self-determination and participation, and accommodation of resident needs. Achievement of these is found in the daily fabric of nursing home life, especially in the choice and control that residents have over routine activities of daily living. Residents attach great importance to choice and control over such matters as bedtime, rising time, food, roommates, care routines, use of money, use of the telephone, trips out of the nursing home, and initiating contact with the physician.

Measurement of quality of life of cognitively impaired residents may be difficult; however, even persons with significant cognitive impairment can often answer questions about their quality of life (12). Health-care proxies may know little about a resident's satisfaction with care. Physicians and nurses appear to have limited insight into the health-related quality of life of nursing home residents and probably should not be used as proxies when resident-based assessments can be obtained. Physicians may be able to affect perceived quality of life by making themselves more accessible to residents for questions and by negotiating and communicating directly with residents about proposed interventions that require trips out of the nursing home (e.g., consultation, diagnostic studies).

HEALTH PROMOTION

Health promotion remains an important dimension of health care in LTCFs. Immunizations are a particular focus of effective health promotion and are safe for even frail residents. Influenza is an important cause of epidemic and endemic respiratory illness in LTCFs and results in considerable morbidity and mortality. The annual vaccination of residents and staff is the most effective way to prevent influenza and its complications.

Although vaccination rates continue to fall short of public health targets, resident and staff vaccination programs (such as standing orders) can improve the rate of vaccination. Pneumococcal vaccine and annual tuberculin skin testing are also recommended. Ethical challenges occur when vaccine shortages precipitate reexamination of allocation practices and the use of such alternative vaccinations as the intranasal live, attenuated influenza vaccine within health-care institutions (13). Other health promotion activities, such as regular activities to maintain the highest level of mobility and function possible, are important in preventing deep venous thromboses, pressure ulcers, and other conditions associated with immobility.

HEALTH-CARE DECISION MAKING

Efforts to enhance autonomous decision-making have received considerable attention in recent years, particularly since the Patient Self Determination Acts became effective in 1991. The Patient Self Determination Acts is a federal statute that requires patients be informed of their right to participate in medical decision-making and to write advance directives.

Decisional Capacity

Assessment of decisional capacity may be complex. Decisional capacity is decision specific and may vary over time. The resident with decisional capacity must demonstrate the ability to choose among various therapeutic goals, understand and communicate relevant information, and reasonably apply that information to decision-making in keeping with those goals. Substantial numbers of residents of LTCFs may have been excluded from participating in discussions about care preferences because of an inability to determine decisional capacity (14). Guidelines for determining decisional capacity have been developed (15). It is rare that a resident lacks all ability to participate in health-care decision-making. When a resident is judged to lack decision-making capacity around a certain issue, the health-care proxy should be consulted to speak on behalf of the resident.

Advance Directives

Advance directives are designed to preserve resident autonomy through future states of decisional incapacity. Advance directives are written documents that reflect residents' preferences for health-care proxies and care, as articulated through developing goals of care and advance care plans. All residents (or their health-care proxies) should be offered the opportunity to execute advance directives. Most LTCFs offer printed educational materials and processes for recording advance directives.

LTCF residents should be encouraged to identify a health-care proxy to speak on their behalf in the event of decisional incapacity. A durable power of attorney is one mechanism for the LTCF resident to identify a health-care proxy in the event of resident decisional incapacity. Forms for completing durable power of attorney designation are easily obtained and do not require notary or attorney participation for completion.

Often the next of kin will serve as health-care proxy in event of resident decisional incapacity. The physician should be aware of the legal standing of the health-care proxy, to be sure that the authority to speak on behalf of the resident is indeed delegated to the person acting in that capacity. Differences in health-care proxy completion rates across different ethnic groups appear to be related to reversible barriers, such as lack of knowledge and the perceived irrelevance of advance directives. Other kinds of health-care proxies include court-appointed guardians or conservators.

In the event the LTCF resident lacks decisional capacity, the physician should communicate with the health-care proxy when medical decisions need to be made. Should the decisional incapacity resolve and the resident regain decisional capacity, as in the case of a resolving delirium, the health-care proxy would step back and the LTCF resident resume primary health-care decision-making. In this way, the autonomy of the resident is best preserved, despite the occurrence of cognitive or functional deficits that render decisional-incapacitation, either temporarily or permanently.

Advance directives may also contain language about preferences and goals for care and advance care plans. These preferences may evolve over time if the medical condition or functional capacity of the resident worsens. Nondepressed, nondemented residents of LTCFs generally exhibit stable preferences for treatment when asked about cardiopulmonary resuscitation, intravenous antibiotics, mechanical ventilation, and artificial nutrition. They distinguish clearly between time-limited trials and indefinite treatment plans. They generally favor receiving intravenous antibiotics and limited mechanical ventilation (16). In advanced chronic illness when death is expected, advance care plans are likely to articulate primary goals of care centered on achieving comfort and dignity, in recognition that curative and disease-modifying treatment options are no longer available or where the burdens of attempting such treatment are judged to outweigh the potential benefits to the resident. Under such circumstances, residents (or their health-care proxies) may direct health-care professionals to implement treatment interventions to relieve symptoms (e.g., pain, dyspnea) but not to attempt to reverse medical problems or prolong life. In such cases, advance directives might direct care that forgoes hospitalization (unless uncomfortable symptoms cannot be controlled in the nursing home), intravenous fluids, antibiotic treatment, and laboratory studies in favor of remaining in the LTCF and receiving treatments aimed at the relief of suffering.

Decision to Hospitalize

Decisions about whether to hospitalize residents with infectious problems arise frequently in LTCFs. There is a wide variation in transfer rates among different LTCFs related to patient mix, clinical care resources, and advance care plans (17). Pneumonia is the leading cause of hospitalization among nursing home residents, with a mortality in some studies of 40% to 50%. In the past, acute care facilities and LTCFs offered distinctly different types of health services. Currently, treatment capabilities overlap. Differences between acute and long-term care settings may include numbers and types of practitioners, sources of financial reimbursement, and philosophy of approach to the management of chronic diseases.

The desirability and appropriateness of transfers of LTCF residents to hospitals provoke debate because of concern about cost, and also because of adverse effects of hospitalization. Physically frail LTCF residents are the most likely to be hospitalized, but they may also be the least likely to benefit from hospitalization (18). Iatrogenic complications and emotional trauma for residents and families have been cited as adverse effects of hospitalization. Advancing age, lower admission mini–mental state examination scores, and lower preadmission instrumental activities of daily living functional characteristics are independent risk factors for functional decline during hospitalization of older persons. Treatment of pneumonia in the LTCF may produce better outcomes for some patients than if they were hospitalized (19). Many patient, institutional, and physician factors affect this decision. Goals of care and the institution's capacity to provide appropriate diagnostic and treatment interventions in a timely fashion are of particular importance. The physician's obligation is to determine the course that best serves the needs and goals of each resident.

Right to Refuse Care

Residents who have the capacity to make decisions about health-care matters have the right to refuse care. A major reason LTCF residents refuse a recommended care intervention is that they misconstrue or misunderstand the recommendation. Because much communication in LTCFs is accomplished through the IDT, the physician's response to a resident refusing care ought to include a personal visit under comfortable, private, unhurried circumstances to discuss the proposed treatment with the resident (or health-care proxy). If outright disagreement between decisionally capable resident and physician continues, this is likely because of a difference in values. The refusal of amputation of a gangrenous extremity is sometimes encountered in LTCFs. Some regard the prospect of amputation as a fate worse than death (20). It is often helpful to involve other members of the IDT to better understand the reasons for the refusal and to try to create alternative plans for care that would be acceptable to the resident and also yield the best available outcomes from the physician's perspective.

ROLE OF THE INTERDISCIPLINARY TEAM

Effective IDTs are essential to the provision of high-quality care in LTCFs and can alleviate many of the ethical dilemmas that occur on a daily basis. The most prevalent providers in LTCFs are nursing aides, and they render the majority of the direct care to residents. The ability of the nursing aide to recognize a change in the resident's status and bring it to the attention of the medical practitioner permits the earliest possible identification of an infectious problem. This system of surveillance compensates for the atypical presentation that commonly characterizes illnesses of the frail LTCF resident. Nurses view advocacy as a responsibility of their practice, where advocacy is rooted in the concept of individual rights. Social workers also practice an advocacy role, supporting three elements of autonomy: free action (supporting residents' choices), decision-making (helping residents deliberate effectively), and continuity (maintaining a sense of self). Geriatric nurse practitioners help to achieve optimal coordination of care and reduce emergency department and acute care utilization costs as well as overall costs for some managed care programs for LTCF residents. The key to effective IDT functioning is good communication that facilitates the flow of information to the team member who is best able to recognize its significance and respond appropriately.

ROLE OF THE MEDICAL DIRECTOR

The medical director bears responsibility for the overall quality of care provided in the LTCF. Along with the director of nursing and the facility administrator, the medical director should develop a basic ethics policy framework. Effective implementation of ethics policies requires a shared vision by the leadership, adequate support for the process, and explicit guidelines for the staff and practitioners, residents and families. A mechanism to resolve disputes should be developed. Ethics committees have fulfilled this role in some facilities.

Measuring outcomes that reflect quality of care in LTCFs is an important dimension of quality management for which the medical director has oversight. The Minimum Data Set has provided some quality indicators for LTCFs (such as pressure ulcers, use of psychotropic medications, falls), but other measures need to be developed. Needs for pain relief and spiritual support are not routinely addressed by the Minimum Data Set and resident assessment protocol triggers.

Indicators are likely to vary for different subsets of LTCF residents. Key indicators for the care of terminally ill residents include communication of advance directives, attention to pain management, and relief of dyspnea. For residents who desire antibiotic treatment for infectious diseases, early empirical antibiotic therapy has an important impact on the outcomes of pneumonia; thus, the percent of residents who received antibiotics within four hours of diagnosis of infection might be a worthwhile quality indicator.

ADVANCED DEMENTIA

Dementia is an important condition affecting more than half the residents of LTCFs. Although residents with dementia may live many years, the disease is not curable, is inexorably progressive, and eventually ends in death. Decisions about treatment in advanced dementia are best implemented through development of the goals of care, as described above. Health-care proxies often adjust the goals of care as the disease and the resident's level of disability progress. When the burdens of treatment loom larger than the benefits to the resident, health-care proxies often choose to shift the emphasis of care to proactive interventions designed to enhance pleasure and quality of life, as in freedom from restraints.

Guidelines to support decision-making about whether to treat or not treat pneumonia in demented psychogeriatric nursing home patients have proved useful in some settings (21). When the goals of care are totally focused on achieving comfort and death is expected, as in a patient with very advanced dementia, it is not uncommon for families and surrogates to forego treating with antibiotics.

HUMAN IMMUNODEFICIENCY VIRUS/ACQUIRED IMMUNODEFICIENCY SYNDROME

Since the treatment advances of the mid 1990s, the outlook for those living with human immunodeficiency virus/acquired immunodeficiency syndrome (HIV/AIDS) has brightened considerably. Long-term care options may be needed for patients who fail antiretroviral therapy or who have significant neuropsychiatric disease. The HIV/AIDS residents have a variety of reasons for needing long-term care, including the need for 24-hour nursing/medical supervision, completion of medical treatment, and end-of-life care. Issues pertaining to the need for advance care planning and palliative care are particularly important for HIV/AIDS residents (see also Chapter 21).

END-OF-LIFE CARE

LTCFs play an important role in the care of people nearing the end of life. In 1993, 20% of U.S. deaths occurred in nursing homes. By 2040, this proportion is expected to rise to 40% (22). Optimizing care near the end of life for LTCF residents goes beyond advance care planning and advance directives. Effective symptom management, maximization of functional capacity, and assistance with issues pertaining to life closure are additional important services that must be offered consistently as part of a system that achieves good care for those nearing the end of life.

Over the past few years, the health-care profession has recognized the need to improve the quality of care for people near the end of life, but consensus about how to accomplish this has not yet been achieved. Those living with serious chronic illness near the end of life are likely to follow one of three trajectories: (i) a relatively brief period of severe functional decline at the end of life (typical of cancer), (ii) long-term disability with periodic exacerbations and unpredictable timing of death (as in congestive heart failure and chronic obstructive pulmonary disease), or (iii) slow dwindling course to death with significant self-care deficits (usually from extreme frailty or dementia). These trajectories shed light on possible care systems that would serve residents' needs better (23).

A number of studies have identified effective communication and pain management as shortcomings in the care of dying persons. Bereaved family members are generally satisfied with life-sustaining treatment decisions but voice concerns about failures in communication and pain control. Nursing home care has received the smallest proportion of positive comments, including mention of poorly trained or inattentive staff and remoteness of physicians. Families recommend that care could be improved through better communication, greater access to physicians' time, and better pain management.

LTCF residents near the end of life are focused on the quality of living rather than dying. They have concerns with day-to-day life, difficulty chewing and swallowing, better pain relief and sense of control, strengthening relationships with loved ones, importance of religious activities, giving care to others, and appreciation of respectful and prompt care (24).

INFECTION CONTROL PRACTICES

The LTCF staff plays an important role in infection control through the use of precautions and routines (see chapters on these topics). From an ethics standpoint, these are measures that carry little risk or burden to the staff and are effective in enhancing infection control. Hand washing is perhaps the most obvious low-risk strategy, yet marked shortcomings in the use of hand washing and gloves continue to exist in LTCFs. Hand-washing practices vary considerably across hospital wards and type of worker, and lack of good hand washing appears to be associated with understaffing (25).

A common ethical dilemma is the question of whether a sick employee should be working. Prohibiting a staff member with a contagious illness from working with residents follows from the ethical concept of utility that strives to maximize good outcomes while minimizing harm. Institutional staffing shortfalls or the staff member's reluctance to take a sick day may compete with this value.

Another ethical quandary is presented when staff members fail to get influenza vaccines. The medical director should work with infection control professionals and other members of the IDT to create an institutional ethic of good infection control practices, supported by strong educational programs for staff, and effective employee health services.

The management of residents colonized with antibiotic-resistant organisms has come to represent a significant challenge for practitioners in LTCF settings. Contact isolation of a resident colonized with a resistant organism curtails that resident's freedom in order to protect the rights of other residents to be free from harm, particularly posthospital residents in subacute settings. Adverse effects of contact isolation include less frequent care and negative psychological consequences. More needs to be learned about the risks to residents and to develop antibiotic resistance precautions that are effective, inexpensive, and achievable in LTCFs. The IDT may address the psychological problems that the isolated resident experiences and develop strategies to avoid unnecessary complications of isolation procedures. For example, the IDT might permit a resident to wash his face and hands, don freshly laundered clothes, and walk in the halls to physical therapy at the end of the day.

COST CONCERNS

The financing incentives in LTCFs create a number of ethical dilemmas for facilities and practitioners. Every treatment option has a cost that must be factored into the process of clinical decision-making. Financial incentives to accept residents with complex medical needs exist with some facilities. Some payors encourage transfer of the acutely ill resident to the hospital, and others reward the LTCF and the practitioner for treating the acutely ill resident in the LTCF. The high cost of antibiotics, such as vancomycin, may create significant dilemmas. In some cases, for cost reasons, residents may not be able to return to the LTCFs they consider home. Significant variation exists in prescribing and the cost of antimicrobials among LTCFs, and formularies and guidelines are increasingly in use to standardize prescribing practices.

RESEARCH ISSUES

Research is an important avenue to improve treatment and prevent infectious disease in LTCF residents. There are multiple facets of ethical obligation in the LTCF research endeavor. Guidelines for ethical investigations have been put forth (26). The Ethics Committee of the American Geriatrics Society has outlined guidelines for appropriateness of the informed consent process for patients with dementia who are research subjects (27). The interest of the individual resident may be at times in opposition to the interest of the population within the facility. A mandate to do no harm and protect confidentiality exists for both the individual and the population. However, the individual resident seeks privacy and autonomy, whereas the concern of the population lies in investigating, reporting, and achieving justice. Infection control activities ought to investigate clusters of adverse outcomes, identify and implement cost-effective interventions, safeguard the health of residents and staff, measure the efficacy of interventions, and avoid conflicts of interest around recommendations of products and equipment. Residents who become subjects for research (or their health-care proxies) must provide informed consent, and they must be assured that their welfare, privacy, and confidentiality will be protected. Staff members should also be protected from harm (taking precedence over staff freedom). Although basic standards of research ethics are not usually reported in nursing home research, the instructions of a journal for the author or other features of peer review can affect the quality of reporting research ethics. Well-written policies on the protection of cognitively impaired research subjects are an important way that research institutions can demonstrate that serious attention is paid to the rights and welfare of cognitively impaired residents.

THE FUTURE

LTCFs are likely to continue to be places where functionally dependent persons receive medical and personal care, either episodically or as a final place of residence towards the end of life. The ethical issues interwoven into this environment are powerful determinants of the outcomes that LTCF residents experience. An articulation of a vision for the future guides

Table 2 Promises to Those with Advanced Stages of Serious Illness

Good medical treatment—you will have the best of medical treatment, aiming to
  prevent exacerbation, improve function and survival, and ensure comfort
Never overwhelmed by symptoms—you will never have to endure overwhelming
  pain, shortness of breath, or other symptoms
Continuity, coordination, and comprehensiveness—your care will be continuous,
  comprehensive, and coordinated
Well prepared, no surprises—you and your family will be prepared for everything
  that is likely to happen in the course of your illness
Customized care, reflecting your preferences—your wishes will be sought and
  respected, and followed whenever possible
Use of patient and family resources (financial, emotional, and practical)—we will
  help you and your family consider your personal and financial resources, and we
  will respect your choices about the use of those resources
Make the best of every day—we will do all we can to see that you and your family
  have the opportunity to make the best of every day

Source: From Ref. 28.

practitioners and others to achieve the best possible quality of life and care
for LTCF residents (Table 2) (28).

SUGGESTED READING

American Geriatrics Society Ethics Committee position statement: making treatment
  decisions for incapacitated elderly patients without advance directives. (Accessed
  January 1998 at http://www.americangeriatrics.org/products/positionpapers/
  treatdec.shtml.).
American Geriatrics Society Ethics Committee position statement: measuring quality
  of care for nursing home residents—considering unintended consequences.
  (Accessed November 2002 at http://www.americangeriatrics.org/products/
  positionpapers/unintended_conseq.shtml.).
Mueller PS, Hook CC, Fleming KC. Ethical issues in geriatrics: a guide for clinicians.
  Mayo Clin Proc 2004; 79:554–562.
Snyder L, Leffler C, for the Ethics and Human Rights Committee, American College
  of Physicians. Ethics Manual. 5th ed. Ann Intern Med 2005; 142:560–582.

REFERENCES

1. Mueller PS, Hook CC, Fleming KC. Ethical issues in geriatrics: a guide for
   clinicians. Mayo Clin Proc 2004; 79:554–562.
2. Olson MD. The heart still beats, but the brain doesn't answer. Perception and
   experience of old-age dementia in the Milwaukee Hmong community. Theoret
   Bioethics 1999; 20:85–95.
3. Gurwitz JH, Field TS, Judge J, et al. The incidence of adverse drug events in two
   large academic long-term care facilities. Am J Med 2005; 118:251–258.

4. Stelfox HT, Bates DW, Redelmeier DA. Safety of patients isolated for infection control. JAMA 2003; 290:1899–1905.
5. Quill TE, Brody H. Physician recommendations and patient autonomy: finding a balance between physician power and patient choice. Ann Intern Med 1996; 125:763–769.
6. Cantor MD, Pearlman RA. Advance care planning in long-term care facilities. J Am Med Dir Assoc 2003; 4:101–108.
7. Lynn J, Goldstein N. Advance care planning for fatal chronic illness: avoiding commonplace errors and unwanted suffering. Ann Intern Med 2003; 138:812–818.
8. Vaughn G, Kiyasu E, McCormick WC. Advance directive preferences among subpopulations of Asian nursing home residents in the Pacific Northwest. J Am Geriatr Soc 2000; 48:554–557.
9. van der Steen JT, Ooms ME, Ader HJ, Ribbe MW, van der Wal G. Withholding antibiotic treatment in pneumonia patients with dementia. Arch Intern Med 2002; 162:1753–1760.
10. Gillick M, Berkman S, Cullen L. A patient-centered approach to advance medical planning in the nursing home. J Am Geriatr Soc 1999; 47:227–230.
11. Liao Y, McGee DL, Cao G, Cooper RS. Quality of the last year of life of older adults: 1986 vs 1993. JAMA 2000; 283:512–518.
12. Mozley CG, Huxley P, Sutcliffe C, et al. "Not knowing where I am doesn't mean I don't know what I like": cognitive impairment and quality of life responses in elderly people. Int J Geriatr Psychiatry 1999; 14:776–783.
13. Cosgrove SE, Fishman NO, Talbot TR. Strategies for use of a limited influenza vaccine supply. JAMA 2005; 293:229–232.
14. Bradley E, Walker L, Blechner B, Wetle T. Assessing capacity to participate in discussions of advance directives in nursing homes: findings from a study of the Patient Self Determination Act. J Am Geriatr Soc 1997; 45:79–83.
15. Mezel M, Teresi J, Ramsey G, Mitty E, Bobrowitz T. Decision-making capacity to execute a health care proxy: development and testing of guidelines. J Am Geriatr Soc 2000; 48:179–187.
16. Berger JT, Majerovitz D. Stability of preferences for treatment among nursing home residents. Gerontologist 1998; 38:217–223.
17. Saliba D, Kington R, Buchanan J, et al. Appropriateness of the decision to transfer nursing facility residents to the hospital. J Am Geriatr Soc 2000; 48:154–163.
18. Fried TR, Mor V. Frailty and hospitalization of long-term stay nursing home residents. J Am Geriatr Soc 1997; 45:265–269.
19. Fried TR, Gillick MR, Lipsitz LA. Short-term functional outcomes of long-term care residents with pneumonia treated with and without hospital transfer. J Am Geriatr Soc 1997; 45:302–306.
20. Donohue SJ. Lower limb amputation: some ethical considerations. Br J Nurs 1997; 6:1311–1314.
21. Van der Steen JT, Muller MT, Ooms ME, van der Wal G, Ribbe MW. Decisions to treat or not to treat pneumonia in demented psychogeriatric nursing home patients: development of a guideline. J Med Ethics 2000; 26:114–120.
22. Brock DB, Foley DJ. Demography and epidemiology of dying in the U.S. with emphasis on deaths of older persons. Hosp J 1998; 13:49–60.

23. Lynn J. Serving patients who may die soon and their families. JAMA 2001; 285:925–932.
24. Singer PA, Martin DK, Kelner M. Quality end-of-life care: patients' perspectives. JAMA 1999; 281:163–168.
25. Pittet D, Mourouga P, Perneger TV. The Members of the Infection Control Program. Compliance with hand washing in a teaching hospital. Ann Intern Med 1999; 130:126–130.
26. Sachs GA, Rhymes J, Cassel CK. Biomedical and behavioral research in nursing homes: Guidelines for ethical investigations. J Am Geriatr Soc 1993; 41:771–777.
27. American Geriatrics Society Ethics Committee. Informed consent for research on human subjects with dementia. J Am Geriatr Soc 1998; 46:1308–1310.
28. Lynn J, Schuster JL, Kabcenell A. Improving Care for the End of Life: a Sourcebook for Health Care Managers and Clinicians. New York: Oxford University Press, 2000.

8

Clinical Manifestations of Infections

Dean C. Norman

*Department of Medicine, David Geffen School of Medicine
at UCLA, and Veterans Affairs Greater Los Angeles Healthcare System,
Los Angeles, California, U.S.A.*

Megan Bernadette Wong

University of California–Los Angeles, Los Angeles, California, U.S.A.

KEY POINTS

1. Atypical presentation, variability of diagnostic testing, and other factors common to frail patients residing in LTCFs may lead to increased morbidity and mortality from infectious diseases by causing delays in diagnosis and therapy.
2. Fever, the "cardinal sign" of infection, may be blunted or absent in infected older persons.
3. Baseline temperatures are lower in older persons as are peak temperature responses to infection; thus, new criteria have been developed for determination of a clinically significant fever in this population.
4. The mechanism for the blunted fever response to infection observed in many infected older persons may be due to changes with age in both afferent and efferent pathways for fever production.
5. Fever in older persons is usually due to a serious viral or bacterial infection and warrants clinical evaluation.

INTRODUCTION

Infectious diseases are a leading cause of morbidity and mortality in the frail nursing home population and are also a leading cause of transfer from a long-term care facility (LTCF) to an acute care facility. Higher morbidity and mortality rates in older patients result in part because of diminished physiologic reserves and altered host defenses brought on by aging and comorbidities. This problem is magnified in the long-term care setting population because of debility due to chronic disease. Elderly patients in long-term care institutions are typically prescribed multiple medications, which coupled with changes in pharmacology of drugs, including antibiotics, increase the risk for adverse drug interactions. As mentioned above, nursing home residents with infections are frequently transferred to acute care hospitals, and their hospitalization may be complicated by nosocomial infection and iatrogenic illness. In recent years, colonization and infection by antimicrobial-resistant pathogens and antibiotic-associated infections, such as *Clostridium difficile*, occur commonly both in the acute care hospital and in LTCFs. Once hospitalized, the elderly are more likely to undergo invasive procedures and are more likely to suffer complications from a given procedure. Only prevention and control of infectious diseases, including addressing the problem of antibiotic resistance as well as rapid diagnosis and the timely initiation of appropriate empiric antimicrobial therapy, will reduce the impact of infectious diseases on the long-term care population. Unfortunately, atypical presentation and variability of diagnostic testing and other factors may lead to increased morbidity and mortality from infection by causing delays in diagnosis and therapy in a population that can least afford diagnostic and treatment delays.

Fortunately, the differential diagnosis of important infectious diseases in residents of LTCFs is somewhat limited. Respiratory infections (including pneumonia), urinary tract, soft tissue infections, and gastrointestinal infections make up the majority of acute infections in this patient population (1). Although the types of infections may be limited, the microbial etiology of infections in the aged is more diverse when compared with the younger population. In general, a variety of pathogens may account for a given infection. For example, pneumonia in the young is usually due to a relatively few pathogens, such as *Streptococcus pneumoniae* and *Mycoplasma pneumoniae*. Urinary tract infection in the young is usually caused by *Escherichia coli*. However, in the old a variety of pathogens are possible for both of these common infections. A small but significant number of cases of community-acquired pneumonia in the elderly are caused by gram-negative bacilli, and a higher percentage of lower respiratory tract infections in nursing homes are caused by gram-negative bacilli and mixed flora (2–6). Similarly, urinary tract infection in the elderly in both the community and extended care setting may be caused by any one of several species of gram-negative and gram-positive bacteria. Chronic indwelling bladder catheter-associated infections are typically polymicrobial. The diverse microbial etiology of urinary tract infections in the elderly necessitates obtaining urine cultures prior to initiation of antibiotic therapy for symptomatic urinary tract infection in the elderly.

ATYPICAL PRESENTATIONS OF INFECTION

Once an infection develops, the cornerstone of successful treatment is timely diagnosis and the rapid initiation of empirical antimicrobial therapy. Nonclassical presentations of acute illnesses occur frequently in the frail elderly and acute infections are no exception. In the nursing home, infectious diseases provide unique diagnostic challenges because of atypical presentations, the frequent presence of cognitive impairment, and often a lack of timely laboratory data. The clinician caring for residents of LTCFs should be aware that virtually any acute change in functional status may herald the onset of a serious infectious disease. These include but are not limited to lethargy, anorexia, falls, focal neurologic signs, and delirium (Table 1). Changes in mental status from baseline are commonly seen even when the infection does not involve the central nervous system. Common infections may present without classical symptoms: pneumonia may develop without cough, purulent sputum, fever or chest pain, and the only sign alerting the clinician may be tachypnea (7,8); meningitis may occur without a stiff neck; and symptomatic urinary tract infection may at times present solely as a decline in cognitive function but without dysuria, urgency, or frequency. The presentation of illness may not be in proportion to severity of the underlying infection; a large percentage of elderly women presenting

Table 1 Clinical Features of Infection in Older Persons

Nonspecifc signs indicating possible infection
  Falls
  Anorexia
  Any acute change in cognition (e.g., delirium, agitation)
  Lethargy
  Hypotension
  Change in baseline body temperature
Atypical features of common infections and bacteremia
  Pneumonia: may occur without cough, sputum production, chest pain, fever; tachypnea may be sole presenting sign
  Urinary tract infection: may occur without dysuria, frequency, flank pain, fever
  Meningitis: may occur without stiff neck
  Septic arthritis: may occur without obvious inflammation of joints
  Bacteremia: may occur without fever; tachypnea, confusion, hypotension common

with symptoms and signs of pylenephritis indistinguishable from those of younger women will be bacteremic, which is not the case for younger women (9). Moreover, costovertebral angle tenderness may not be present in older persons with pylenephritis (10). Localizing peritoneal findings may be delayed in cases of severe intra-abdominal infection (11,12).

FEVER

Diminished Fever Response and Its Pathogenesis

Studies of specific infections in older adults including pneumonia (8,13,14), bacteremia (15,16), endocarditis (17–19), nosocomial febrile illness (20), meningitis (21), and intra-abdominal infection (22) confirm that fever, the hallmark of invasive microbial infection, may be blunted or absent in up to a third of infected elderly patients (23–25). In one study of 320 hospitalized patients, the magnitude of the fever response to infection was reduced with increasing age (26). The absence of this cardinal sign of infection has implications beyond confounding clinical diagnosis. First, an absent or blunted fever response to infection is a poor prognostic sign, as demonstrated in a study of several hundred patients with bacteremia and fungemia (27). The results of this study confirmed that those patients responding to bacteremia or fungemia with a robust fever response were more likely to survive. This older study's conclusion is now well established for many infectious diseases and applies to both the young and the old. Second, although the prognostic significance of the febrile response to infection in humans is clear, it is less well established that fever is an essential adaptive mechanism that augments host defenses. There is strong supporting evidence that fever is an important host defense for a variety of organisms (28). Cold-blooded animals, such as certain species of lizards and fish, move to warmer environments in order to raise body temperatures in response to infection, and laboratory experiments confirm that fever is an important host defense in these animals (29,30). In fact, enhanced resistance to infection appears to occur with increased body temperature in a variety of mammalian animal models (31). Thus, based on these animal data, fever is potentially an important host defense in humans. The effect of fever on host defenses is independent of a direct effect of elevated body temperature on bacterial replication. The exceptions are that physiologically achievable temperature elevations may inhibit bacterial growth directly of *Treponema pallidum*, the gonococcus and certain strains of pneumococci. The mechanism by which fever enhances immune response appears to be multifactorial and minimally involves elevating cytokine production and activity (interleukins 1 and 6, tumor necrosis factor, and interferon). These cytokines, which are called pyrogenic cytokines (previously known as endogenous pyrogens), may have many effects on the cellular components of the immune response. One effect is to facilitate adherence of leukocytes to endothelial cells and leukocyte migration to extravascular areas of infection.

The mechanism by which a significant number of infected older adults fail to mount a febrile response is not known. Potential mechanisms have been proposed based on the current understanding of the pathogenesis of fever. The role of cytokines as potential endogenous mediators of fever has been established (31,32). Bacterial products, such as lipopolysaccharide, bind to toll-like receptors present on immune, endothelial, and epithelial cells and induce these cells to produce endogenous pyrogens, including interleukin 1, tumor necrosis factor, interleukin 6, and interferon-alpha. These pyrogens that are produced either locally at the site of infection and enter the circulation or locally by macrophages adhering to endothelium in circumventricular organs of the brain then act on the anterior hypothalamus resulting in a biochemical cascade including the release of prostaglandin E2. This cascade raises the central nervous system "thermostat" (31). This results in shivering, vasoconstriction, and various behavioral responses, all of which elevates the core body temperature, which then becomes the new baseline. When the infection resolves, the thermostat is reset to baseline and sweating and temperature lowering behaviors occur, thus returning body temperature to normal. It is possible that these pathways could be affected by aging and it has been established that thermoregulation in the elderly appears to be impaired to some degree. This is evidenced by the increased morbidity and mortality in older persons from heat stroke and hypothermia.

Recently, the role of cytokines in the pathogenesis of the early fever response has been challenged. This is in part because endotoxin-challenged animal models develop fever before peripheral macrophages can produce cytokines. It is now postulated that endotoxin may act directly on the vascular endothelium of the anterior hypothalamus or by activating the complement cascade to stimulate prostaglandin E2 by macrophages, which in turn may enter the central nervous system or by exciting hepatic vagal afferents that signal the preoptic area of the hypothalamus (33,34).

A variety of endogenous pyrogens result in a lower fever response in older compared with younger mice (35–37). Intracerebroventricular injection of interleukin 1 showed similar immediate fever responses between young and old rats, suggesting an inability of peripheral endogenous mediators to reach the central nervous system rather than an unresponsiveness of the central nervous system (38). Diminished production of pyrogenic cytokines with age in various rodent models has also been demonstrated (39). Additional rodent experiments have suggested that changes in thermogenic brown fat may play a role in the blunted fever response of aging (40). Thus, reduced production and response to pyrogenic cytokines may be important in the pathogenesis of the blunted febrile response to infection observed in the elderly. Given the most recent data, one must consider that aging may affect toll-like receptors, endogenous pyrogen production, and any of the efferent pathways involved in the fever response.

Baseline Temperatures in Nursing Home Residents and Significance of Fever

The normal and febrile body temperature for older adults has been thoroughly reviewed (25). Studies have demonstrated that baseline temperature was decreased in a nursing home patient population (41,42). It was also found that baseline body temperature and diurnal variation as measured by electronic thermometry was reduced in frail nursing home residents (42). Mean baseline morning rectal temperature was 98.6°F (37°C) in 22 patients in whom oral temperatures could not be easily obtained. The mean oral temperature of 85 additional residents was 97.4°F (36.3°C). Diurnal variation was only 0.6°F (0.3°C) for rectal temperatures and 0.4°F (0.2°C) for oral temperatures. In another study, similar findings were shown in 50 randomly selected nursing home residents with a mean oral baseline temperature of 97.4°F (36.3°C) (41). A further review of this group found 69 infections in 26 of these residents with the mean maximum temperature reaching 101.3°F (38.5°C). In nearly half of these infections the temperature did not reach 101°F. Yet, a majority of these residents significantly increased their temperature over baseline by at least 2.4°F (1.3°C). Lowering the criterion for fever to 100°F (37.8°C) or greater raised the sensitivity to 70% for predicting infection with a specificity of 90%. These findings led to the recommendation by the Practice Guidelines Committee of the Infectious Diseases Society of America that a clinical evaluation for an infection be performed for nursing home residents with (i) a single oral temperature exceeding 100°F (37.8°C), (ii) persistent oral temperature exceeding 99°F (37.2°C), (iii) persistent rectal temperature of 99.5°F (37.5°C) or greater, or (iv) two or more readings of greater than 2°F (1.1°C) over baseline regardless of site of measurement (43). The chance of an infection is further increased if obvious symptoms and signs of infection exist or if there is any change in functional status accompanying the temperature changes. It should be remembered that in some cases a significant decrease in temperature might indicate a serious infection complicated by bacteremia.

Elderly residents of LTCFs who do mount a normal febrile response to infection as defined by 101°F (38.3°C) orally can be expected to have a serious or life-threatening infection. This conclusion is extrapolated from a classic study of 1200 ambulatory care patients (44) and two other confirmatory studies (45,46). In contrast to the young in whom fevers tended to be associated with benign viral infections, these studies demonstrated that the elderly, in particular the old patients who presented with this magnitude of temperature elevation, did have a serious life-threatening infection.

Fever of Unknown Origin

Infection is the leading etiology of fever of unknown origin in the elderly, followed by such connective tissue, diseases as temporal arteritis. A lesser number of cases are due to malignancy (47–50). Many of these underlying conditions are treatable and unless advance directives preclude an extensive evaluation, an underlying cause should be sought.

CONCLUSION

Infections in nursing home residents may manifest with atypical clinical features, which may delay diagnosis and treatment. Fever, the hallmark of infection, may be absent or blunted in 20% to 30% of elderly persons with serious infections. In contrast, the presence of a fever in the geriatric patient is more likely to be associated with a serious viral or bacterial infection compared with younger patients.

SUGGESTED READING

Bentley DW, Bradley S, High K, Schoenbaum S, Taler, G, Yoshikawa TT. Evaluation of fever and infection in long-term care facilities. Clin Infect Dis 2000; 31:640–653.

Blatteis CM, Li S, Li Z, Feleder C, Perkik CF. Cytokines, PGE2 and endotoxic fever: a re-assessment. Prostaglandins Other Lipid Mediat 2005; 76:1–18.

El-Solh AA, Sikka P, Ramadan F, Davies J. Etiology of pneumonia in the very elderly. Am J Respir Crit Care Med 2001; 163:645–651.

Norman DC. Fever in the elderly. Clin Infect Dis 2000; 31:148–151.

Tal S, Guller V, Gurevich A, Levi S. Fever of unknown origin in the elderly. J Int Med 2002:295–304.

REFERENCES

1. Bradley SF. Infections and infection control in the long-term care setting. In: Yoshikawa TT, Norman DC, eds. Infectious Disease in the Aging. A Clinical Handbook. Totowa: Humana Press, 2001:245–256.
2. Marrie TJ. Pneumonia in the long-term-care facility. Infect Control Hosp Epidemiol 2003; 23:159–164.
3. Medina-Walpole AM, Katz PR. Nursing home-acquired pneumonia. J Am Geriatr Soc 1999, 47:1005–1015.
4. Furman CD, Rayner AV, Tobin EP. Pneumonia in older residents of long-term care facilities. Am Fam Physician 2004; 70:1495–1500.
5. El-Solh AA, Sikka P, Ramadan F, Davies J. Etiology of pneumonia in the very elderly. Am J Respir Crit Care Med 2001; 163:645–651.
6. El-Solh AA, Pietrantoni C, Bhat A, et al. Microbiology of severe aspiration pneumonia in institutionalized elderly. Am J Respir Crit Care Med 2003; 167:1650–1654.

7. Norman DC. Clinical features of infection. In: Yoshikawa TT, Norman DC, eds. Infectious Disease in the Aging. A Clinical Handbook. Totowa: Humana Press, 2001:13–17.

8. Metlay J, Schulz R, Li YH, et al. Influence of age on symptoms at presentation in patients with community-acquired pneumonia. Arch Intern Med 1997; 157:1453–1459.

9. Gleckman RA, Bradley PJ, Roth RM, Hibert DM. Bacteremic urosepsis. A phenomenon unique to elderly women. J Urol 1985; 133:174–175.

10. Estathiou SP, Pefanis AV, Tsioulos DI, et al. Acute pyelonephritis in adults: prediction of mortality and failure of treatment. Arch Intern Med 2003; 163: 1206–1212.

11. Norman DC, Yoshikawa TT. Intraabdominal infection: diagnosis and treatment in the elderly patient. Gerontology 1984; 30:327–338.

12. Campbell, Wilson SE. Intraabdominal infections. In: Yoshikawa TT, Norman DC, eds. Infectious Disease in the Aging. A Clinical Handbook. Totowa: Humana Press, 2001:91–98.

13. Bentley DW. Bacterial pneumonia in the elderly: clinical features, diagnosis, etiology and treatment. Gerontology 1984; 30:297–307.

14. Marrie TJ, Haldane EV, Faulkner RS, Durant H, Kwan C. Community-acquired pneumonia requiring hospitalization: Is it different in the elderly? J Am Geriatr Soc 1985; 33:671–680.

15. Gleckman R, Hibert D. Afebrile bacteremia. A phenomenon in geriatric patients. JAMA 1982; 248:1478–1481.

16. Finkelstein M, Petkun WM, Freedman ML, Antopol SC. Pneumococcal bacteremia in adults: age-dependent differences in presentation and outcome. J Am Geriatr Soc 1983; 31:19–27.

17. Terpenning MS, Buggy BO, Kauffman CA. Infective endocarditis: clinical features in young and elderly patients. Am J Med 1987; 83:626–634.

18. Werner GS, Schulz R, Fuchs JB, et al. Infective endocarditis in the elderly in the era of transesophageal echocardiography: clinical features and prognosis compared with younger patients. Am J Med 1996; 100:90–97.

19. Dhawan VK. Infective endocarditis in elderly patients. Clin Infect Dis 2002; 34:806–812.

20. Trivalle C, Chassagne PMD, Bouaniche M, et al. Nosocomial febrile illness in the elderly: frequency, causes, and risk factors. Arch Intern Med 1998; 158:1560–1565.

21. Gorse GJ, Thrupp LD, Nudleman KL, Wyle FA, Hawkins B, Cesario TC. Bacterial meningitis in the elderly. Arch Intern Med 1984; 144:1603–1607.

22. Potts FE IV, Vukov LF. Utility of fever and leukocytosis in acute surgical abdomens in octogenarians and beyond. J Gerontol A Biol Sci Med Sci 1999; 54A:M55–M58.

23. Yoshikawa TT, Norman DC. Fever in the elderly. Infect Med 1998; 15:704–706.

24. Norman DC. Fever and aging. Infect Dis Clin Pract 1998; 7:387–390.

25. Norman DC. Fever in the elderly. Clin Infect Dis 2000; 31:148–151.

26. Roghmann M-C, Warner J, Mackowiak PA. The relationship between age and fever magnitude. Am J Med Sci 2001; 322:68–70.

27. Weinstein MP, Murphy JR, Reller RB, Lichtenstein KA. The clinical significance of positive blood cultures: a comprehensive analysis of 500 episodes of

bacteremia and fungemia II: clinical observations with special reference to factors influencing prognosis. Rev Infect Dis 1983; 5:54–70.

28. Mackowiak PA. Physiological rationale for suppression of fever. Clin Infect Dis 2000; 31(suppl 5):S185–S189.

29. Kluger MJ, Ringler DM, Anver MR. Fever and survival. Science 1975; 188: 166–168.

30. Covert JB, Reynolds WM. Survival value of fever in fish. Nature 1977; 267:43–45.

31. Netea MG, Kullberg BJ, Van der Meer JWM. Circulating cytokines as mediators of fever. Clin Infect Dis 2000; 31:S178–S184.

32. Dinarello CA. Cytokines as endogenous pyrogens. J Infect Dis 1999; 179(suppl 2): S294–S304.

33. Blatteis CM, Li S, Li Z, Feleder C, Perkik CF. Cytokines, PGE2 and endotoxic fever: a re-assessment. Prostaglandins Other Lipid Mediat 2005; 76:1–18.

34. Dinarello CA. Infection, fever, and exogenous and endogenous pyrogens: some concepts have changed. J Endotoxin Res 2004; 10:201–222.

35. Norman DC, Yamamura RH, Yoshikawa TT. Fever response in old and young mice after injection of interleukin. J Gerontol 1988; 43:M80–M85.

36. Miller D, Yoshikawa TT, Castle SC, Norman DC. Effect of age in fever response to recombinant tumor necrosis factor alpha in a murine model. J Gerontol 1991; 46:M176–M179.

37. Miller DJ, Yoshikawa TT, Norman DC. Effect of age on fever response to recombinant interleukin-6 in a murine model. J Gerontol 1995; 50A:M276–M279.

38. Plata-Salamán CR, Peloso E, Satinoff E. Interleukin-1-induced fever in young and old Long–Evans rats. Am J Physiol 1998; 275:R1633–R1638.

39. Bradley SF, Vibhagool A, Kunkel SL, Kauffman CA. Monokine secretion in aging and protein malnutrition. J Leukocyte Biol 1989; 45:510–514.

40. Scarpace PJ, Bender BS, Burst SE. The febrile response of *E. coli* peritonitis in senescent rats. Gerontologist 1990; 30:215A.

41. Castle SC, Norman DC, Yeh M, Yoshikawa TT. Fever response in elderly nursing home residents: are the older truly colder? J Am Geriatr Soc 1981; 39:853–857.

42. Castle SC, Yeh M, Toledo S, Yoshikawa TT, Norman DC. Lowering the temperature criterion improves detection of infections in nursing home residents. Aging Immunol Infect Dis 1993; 4:67–76.

43. Bentley DW, Bradley S, High K, Schoenbaum S, Taler G, Yoshikawa TT. Evaluation of fever and infection in long-term care facilities. Clin Infect Dis 2000; 31:640–653.

44. Keating HJ III, Klimek JJ, Levine DS, Kiernan FJ. Effect of aging on the clinical significance of fever in ambulatory adult patients. J Am Geriatr Soc 1984; 32:282–287.

45. Wasserman M, Levinstein M, Keller E, Lee S, Yoshikawa TT. Utility of fever, white blood cell, and differential count in predicting bacterial infections in the elderly. J Am Geriatr Soc 1989; 37:534–543.

46. Schoeinfeld CN, Hansen KN, Hexter DA, Stearns DA, Kelen GD. Fever in geriatric emergency patients: clinical features associated with serious illness. Ann Emerg Med 1995; 26:18–24.

47. Esposito AL, Gleckman RA. Fever of unknown origin in the elderly. J Am Geriatr Soc 1978; 26:498–505.

48. Berland B, Gleckman RA. Fever of unknown origin in the elderly: a sequential approach to diagnosis. Postgrad Med 1992; 92:197–210.
49. Knockaert DC, Vanneste LJ, Bobbaers HJ. Fever of unknown origin in elderly patients. J Am Geriatr Soc 1993; 41:1187–1192.
50. Tal S, Guller V, Gurevich A, Levi S. Fever of unknown origin in the elderly. J Intern Med 2002:295–304.

9

Establishing an Infection Control Program

Lona Mody

Division of Geriatric Medicine, University of Michigan Medical School, Geriatrics Research, Education, and Clinical Center, Veterans Affairs Ann Arbor Healthcare System, Ann Arbor, Michigan, U.S.A.

KEY POINTS

1. Infections are common in LTCFs and are responsible for significant morbidity and mortality.
2. LTCFs face unique challenges necessitating individualized infection control programs.
3. LTCFs have to comply both with Centers for Medicare and Medicaid and Omnibus Budget Reconciliation Act regulations to establish infection control programs and with Occupational Safety and Health Administration regulations for the protection of residents and staff within the facilities.
4. An infection control practitioner plays a vital role in setting up a comprehensive yet targeted infection control program.
5. Infection control programs should address the following: surveillance for infections and antimicrobial resistance, outbreak investigation and control plan for epidemics, isolation precautions, hand hygiene, staff education, employee and resident health programs, and infection control program for rehabilitation services.

BACKGROUND

Infections in long-term care facilities (LTCFs) increase the mortality and morbidity of residents and generate additional costs for the facilities themselves as well as for hospitals. Every year, approximately 1.6 to 3.8 million infections occur in residents in LTCFs and are responsible for a substantial proportion of resident transfers to acute care hospitals (1). The hazards of hospitalization are numerous and include functional decline, delirium, pressure ulcers, and the potential for adverse events. Nationally, deaths attributable to infections initiated in LTCFs could be as high as 400,000 each year.

Urinary tract, respiratory, and skin and soft tissue infections are the most common endemic infections among LTCF residents. Epidemic infections most commonly reported include gastroenteritis, influenza, and skin infections (1). In addition, LTCF residents are susceptible to antimicrobial-resistant organisms, such as methicillin-resistant *Staphylococcus aureus* (MRSA), vancomycin-resistant enterococci (VRE), cephalosporin and quinolone-resistant gram-negative organisms, and extended spectrum β-lactamase-producing gram-negative organisms (see also Chapters 23 and 24).

The health-care costs of these infections can be immense. The direct costs for antibiotics can range from $38 million to $137 million per year. The costs of hospitalizations resulting from transfer for infection treatment can range from $673 million to $2 billion each year (1). The resulting medical consequences to a patient from loss of function and delirium leading to prolongation of hospital stay and antimicrobial resistance may be enormous, both physically and financially. Thus, infection control is considered to be a vital element in the operation of LTCFs.

This chapter provides an overview of the unique challenges to infection control in LTCFs. It also provides guidelines, resources to establish and sustain efficient infection control programs, and the information on regulations governing infection control practices in LTCFs.

UNIQUE CHALLENGES TO INFECTION CONTROL

Older adults, especially those in LTCFs, have characteristics that create special challenges to implementing an effective infection control program. These include diagnostic uncertainty, time and resource limitations, rapid staff turnover, limited and intermittent physician coverage, increasing acuity of care, and frequent care transitions. These characteristics can be divided into in three categories: host factors, structural factors, and process factors.

Host Factors

LTCF residents are particularly susceptible to infections because of immunosenescence, an increased prevalence of chronic diseases, increasing severity of illness, medications that affect resistance to infection (such as corticosteroids and frequent antibiotic usage), level of debility, impaired mental status (predisposing to aspiration and pressure ulcers), incontinence and resultant indwelling catheter usage, and the institutional environment in which they live (2). Most infections found in these residents are thought to be endogenous in nature and often resulting from the resident's own flora.

LTCF residents may also serve as host reservoirs for certain infectious agents, such as MRSA and VRE. With reduction in the length of hospital stay, the severity of illness among residents of the subacute care nursing unit has increased with resultant inherent rapid transfers to a hospital and increased polypharmacy. All of these factors combined create a vulnerable resident, highly prone to infections and higher disease transmission of resistant pathogens in a closed environment.

Structural Factors

An assessment of the structural factors that affect infection control at an LTCF begins with an evaluation of the facility's capacity to provide care as opposed to an assessment of the process of care, which is an evaluation of the actual delivery of service. Structural factors of concern in implementing an effective infection control program in an LTCF include suboptimal full-time equivalents for registered nurses, nursing aides, and therapists, high staff turnover, changing case mix, and limited availability of information systems.

The number of staff per resident varies considerably among facilities. Hospital-based LTCFs and skilled LTCFs for residents covered by Medicare have almost twice the nursing staff of other community nursing facilities. The relationship between nursing care intensity and health outcomes for LTCF patients has been examined for years, and associations between increased nursing hours per patient and improved health outcomes have been reported (3). For example, registered nurse turnover has been associated with increased risk of infection and a higher risk of hospitalization due to infection in a sample of Maryland LTCFs (4). Potential explanations for these findings may include difficulties in establishing and maintaining effective infection control practices, reduced familiarity between staff and resident to detect minor changes in the resident's health status, and inconsistent supervision and training.

In order to reduce length of acute hospital stay, LTCFs are now accepting sicker patients with higher severity of illness. This change in case mix has led to increased care transitions between hospitals and LTCFs, leading to increased lapses in information exchange. These care transitions also lead to increased risk of transmission of pathogens between the hospital and LTCFs.

Process Factors

Processes of care in LTCFs pertain to actual health-care service delivery. Process factors affecting infection control in LTCFs include variable staff education, availability and utility of diagnostic specimens, use of such quality improvement tools as regional databases, quality indicators, and Minimum Data Sets.

Although the effectiveness of education alone is controversial, the value of education as a part of a comprehensive quality control program has long been recognized in all health-care settings. The importance of staff education is further accentuated by the phenomenal turnover in LTCF personnel. Currently, however, there are no standard guidelines regarding curriculum or frequency for staff education in LTCFs, including in infection control. Nursing aides who are the frontline personnel in recognizing any change in clinical status of LTCF residents may receive little or no formal educational training in various infection control issues, such as hand hygiene, antimicrobial resistance, early symptoms and signs of common infection, and infection control measures to reduce infections related to indwelling devices. LTCFs can overcome these barriers to infection control by scheduling monthly in-services. However, the content, frequency, and attendance at these in-services may vary among facilities.

Diagnostic specimens have limited usefulness in the LTCF population for two reasons: (i) they cannot be or are not obtained, and (ii) if obtained, the results may not be communicated to the appropriate person in a timely fashion, or, in the case of radiological investigations, may not be interpreted accurately. The onsite availability of diagnostic or radiologic services is lacking in many LTCFs. In addition, residents may not be able or willing to cooperate in the collection of valid specimens. Diagnostic tests may thus be infrequently requested, resulting in initiation of therapy without having appropriate clinical information. Alternatively, since the prevalence of bacteriuria in 30% to 50% in LTCFs, obtaining urine specimens without an assessment can also lead to inappropriate prescribing of antimicrobial therapy (see Chapter 12).

REGULATORY ASPECTS OF INFECTION CONTROL

The Centers for Medicare and Medicaid Centers and Omnibus Budget Reconciliation Act (OBRA) regulations require that LTCFs establish prevention and control of infection processes in accordance with the resident populations they serve. Additionally, LTCFs have to comply with Occupational Safety and Health Administration (OSHA) regulations, which address the protection of health-care workers (HCWs) in workplaces, including blood-borne pathogens such as hepatitis B and human immunodeficiency virus. Moreover, facilities have to comply with local and state regulations.

This information can usually be obtained from the state government Web site. Facilities may also choose to comply with the long-term care requirements of voluntary organizations, such as the Joint Commission on Accreditation of Healthcare Organizations.

In summary, application of currently available hospital guidelines to LTCFs may be unrealistic and to some extent inappropriate. In view of the unique infection control challenges that exist in LTCFs, infection control must be simple, focused, and practical as well as recognize the staffing, budget, and care concerns of older adults. Recognizing these challenges, a Canadian consensus group published surveillance definitions for infections in LTCFs (5) and the minimum criteria to initiate antibiotics (6). In addition, the Society for Healthcare Epidemiology (SHEA) has published guidelines on antimicrobial use (7) and an approach to antimicrobial-resistant pathogens (8), *Clostridium difficile* diarrhea and management (9). An approach to infection (10) and fever in LTCFs was recently published (11) (see Appendix B). SHEA and the Association of Professionals in Infection Control (APIC) have also published guidelines that describe the structure and components of infection control in LTCFs (12).

COMPONENTS OF INFECTION CONTROL

Infection Control Program

An effective infection control program includes a method of surveillance for infections and antimicrobial-resistant pathogens, an outbreak control plan for epidemics, isolation and standard precautions, hand hygiene, staff education, an employee health program, a resident health program, policy formation and periodic review with audits, and a policy to communicate reportable diseases to public health authorities (Fig. 1).

Surveillance

Infection surveillance in LTCFs involves collection of data on LTCF-acquired infections and antimicrobial resistance. Surveillance is defined as "ongoing, systematic collection, analysis, and interpretation of health data essential to the planning, implementation, and evaluation of public health practice, closely integrated with timely dissemination of these data to those who need to know" (13). Surveillance can be limited to a particular objective or may be facility-wide. Surveillance is often based on individual patient risk factors, focused on a unit, or based on a particular pathogen or infection type. These varying methods have similar sensitivity and specificity; however, surveillance utilizing laboratory data has the advantage of measuring facility-wide occurrences.

Surveillance can be either passive or active. In passive surveillance, also known as routine surveillance, an infection control professional (ICP)

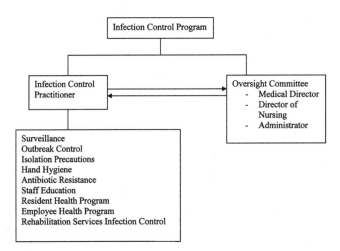

Figure 1 Components of infection control program in long-term facilities.

uses data collected for routine patient care. Although less costly in terms of resources, passive surveillance is inherently biased. It may also under-estimate the magnitude of outcomes measured and delay detection of outbreaks. The feasibility of passive surveillance has been demonstrated and has led to continuing education opportunities. In contrast, active sur-veillance utilizes multiple data sources to detect infections and antimicrobial resistance early. It requires routine infection control professional or practi-tioner (ICP) rounds to detect infections early and may involve patient screening for resistant pathogens. Active surveillance for antimicrobial-resistant pathogens in acute care has created significant debate in recent years regarding its cost effectiveness and clinical utility, although data in LTCFs are lacking. Nonetheless, it may be very useful in detecting certain highly contagious infections such as tuberculosis and influenza.

For surveillance to be conducted correctly, objective and valid defini-tions of infections are crucial. Hospital surveillance definitions are based on the National Nosocomial Infection Surveillance criteria, which depend rather extensively on laboratory investigations. Radiology and microbiol-ogy data are less available, and if available are delayed; therefore, these criteria may not be applicable in LTCF settings. Modified LTCF-specific criteria were developed by a Canadian consensus conference, which took into account the unique limitations of the LTCF setting (5). They have been used widely, although not uniformly (14) (see Appendix A).

Besides using valid surveillance definitions, a facility must have clear goals and aims for setting up a surveillance program. These goals, as with other elements of an infection control program, have to be reviewed periodi-cally to reflect changes in the facility's population, pathogens of interest, and changing antimicrobial resistance patterns. Plans to analyze the data and use of these data to design and implement proven preventive measures must also be made in advance.

The analysis and reporting of infection rates in LTCFs are typically conducted monthly, quarterly, and annually to detect trends. Because the length of stay at an LTCF is long, and each resident is at risk for a prolonged duration, an analysis of absolute numbers of infections can be misleading. Infection rates (preferably reported as infections/1000 resident-days) can be calculated by using resident-days (number of residents × number of days in a month) or average resident census for the surveillance period as the denominator, using the following equation:

$$\frac{\text{Number of new nosocomial infections}}{\text{Number of resident} - \text{Days in the month}} \times 1000$$

For example, if there are 30 infections in a month (30 days) in an LTCF with an average daily census of 300, then the infection rate is

$$\frac{30 \times 1000}{9000} = \frac{3.33 \text{ infections}}{1000 \text{ resident} - \text{days}}$$

These data can then been used to establish endemic baseline rates and to recognize variations from the baseline that could represent an outbreak. Critical to the success of any surveillance program is the feedback of these rates to the nursing staff, physicians, and appropriate quality control and review committees. This information should eventually lead to specific, targeted infection control initiatives and follow-up surveillance to evaluate the success of the changes.

Furthermore, surveillance data can be combined at a regional or a national level, and individual facility rates can be compared with an aggregate of other facilities using visual and simplified statistical methods (Table 1). The success in the reduction of nosocomial infection rates in acute care hospitals that participate in a National Nosocomial Infection Surveillance system has been demonstrated. Although one study has demonstrated the feasibility of using interfacility comparisons among 17 LTCFs, it needs to be studied further at other sites (15).

Outbreak Control

An illness in a community or region is considered an outbreak when it clearly exceeds normal expectancy. The existence of an outbreak is thus always relative to the number of cases that are expected to occur in a specific population in a specific time period.

The main objectives of an outbreak investigation are control and elimination of the source, prevention of new cases, prevention of future outbreaks, research to gain additional knowledge about the infectious agent

Table 1 Summary of Results from Surveillance for Infection from 17 Regional Nursing Homes

Facility	Infection rates[a]							
	Total UTIs[b]	Catheter UTIs[c]	Respiratory	GI	Skin	Bloodstream	Febrile	Total
A	0.61	0.00	2.55	0.12	2.67	0.00	0.00	5.95
B	0.69	3.70	1.56	0.09	1.26	0.00	0.00	3.60
C	0.63	3.70	1.77	0.14	1.12	0.00	0.03	3.69
D	0.66	3.15	1.12	0.03	0.66	0.03	0.00	2.50
E	0.53	5.14	0.23	0.00	0.69	0.00	0.00	1.45
F	0.30	2.92	2.11	0.08	0.83	0.00	0.00	3.31
G	0.40	1.80	1.76	0.09	0.97	0.00	0.00	3.21
H	0.68	4.56	2.02	0.09	0.68	0.02	0.00	3.49
I	0.21	1.33	1.65	0.15	0.72	0.00	0.05	2.78
J	0.27	1.66	1.06	0.64	0.77	0.00	0.00	2.75
K	0.69	4.74	2.36	0.25	1.16	0.04	0.00	4.50
L	2.28	6.90	2.88	0.22	1.54	0.00	0.04	6.96
M	0.00	0.00	1.90	0.38	1.43	0.10	0.10	3.91
N	0.28	7.43	2.24	0.09	0.75	0.00	0.00	3.36
O	0.29	2.99	0.79	0.13	2.30	0.00	0.00	3.51
P	0.67	1.32	2.88	0.15	1.83	0.00	0.04	5.58
Q	0.44	3.04	1.54	0.00	0.83	0.00	0.00	2.81
Mean infection rates[d]	0.57	3.20	1.79	0.16	1.19	0.01	0.01	3.73
SD	0.49	2.12	0.72	0.16	0.60	0.02	0.03	1.36
Total infections	282	130	828	77	520	4	6	1717

[a]Expressed as number of infections per 1000 resident- or device-days.
[b]Catheter-associated and non-catheter-associated UTIs combined.
[c]Catheter-associated UTIs.
[d]Interfacility mean of the number of infections per 1000 resident-days.
Abbreviations: UTIs, urinary tract infections; GI, gastrointestinal; SD, standard deviation.
Source: From Ref. 15.

and its mode of transmission, program evaluation and strategies for improvement, and epidemiological training to conduct outbreak investigations.

It is vital that the ICP know the following: (i) appropriate data collection methods, (ii) how to interpret the data using simple epidemiologic measures, (iii) effective study designs in order to conduct an effective and efficient outbreak investigation, and (iv) effective and appropriate infection control measures. It may also be beneficial for the ICP to have access to a hospital epidemiologist for consultation. These issues are discussed in greater depth in the Chapter 10.

Antibiotic Resistance

Infection and colonization with antimicrobial-resistant pathogens are important concerns in LTCFs and develop primarily due to widespread use of empirical antibiotics, functional impairment, use of indwelling devices, mediocre adherence to hand hygiene among HCWs, and cross-transmission during group activities. An LTCF can reduce infections and colonization with resistant pathogens by emphasizing hand hygiene, developing an antimicrobial utilization program, encouraging evidence-based clinical evaluation and management of infections, and ensuring that the facility has a well-established, individualized infection control program. Guidelines to control MRSA and VRE have been published by SHEA and provide a good base for developing facility-specific policies (8). These issues are discussed in greater depth in Chapters 23 and 24.

Isolation Precautions

The Hospital Infection Control Practice Advisory Committee (HICPAC)/ Centers for Disease Control and Prevention has proposed a two-tiered structure for isolation precautions. In the first tier, HICPAC proposes use of "standard precautions," which have been designed for the care of all patients in hospitals, regardless of their diagnosis, infectious or otherwise. In the second tier are "transmission-based precautions," which have been designed for the care of patients suspected of or known to be infected with epidemiologically important pathogens that have been acquired by physical contact or airborne or droplet transmission (16).

Standard precautions apply to blood, all body fluids, secretions, and excretions regardless of whether they contain visible blood, nonintact skin, and/or mucous membranes. Designed to reduce the risk of transmission of pathogens, both from apparent and ambiguous sources of infection, these precautions include hand hygiene, glove use, masks, eye protection, and gowns, as well as avoiding injuries from sharps. Transmission-based precautions are intended for use with patients who may be infected with highly transmissible or epidemiologically significant pathogens. These include airborne precautions (e.g., for tuberculosis), droplet precautions (e.g., for influenza), and contact precautions (e.g., for *C. difficile*). Although these guidelines were designed for acute care settings, several of them, especially the universal precautions, apply to LTCFs as well. These recommendations have to be adapted to the needs of the facility.

There has been some debate on the role of active surveillance cultures and their impact on isolation policies in acute care hospitals. The SHEA guideline for preventing nosocomial transmission of multi-drug-resistant organisms advocates for aggressive active surveillance cultures (17), whereas the recent draft of HICPAC guidelines call for individual facilities to assess their own needs and conduct surveillance cultures as necessary (16). None of these guidelines specifically address LTCFs and whether there is a role for surveillance cultures in a targeted subgroup of LTCF residents, such as those with indwelling devices or those recently admitted from an acute care hospital. Until there are further data, recommendations put forth by the SHEA long-term care committee on VRE and MRSA should be used when setting up a LTCF isolation and precautions policy.

Hand Hygiene

Contamination of the hands of HCWs has been recognized to play a role in the transmission of pathogenic bacteria to patients since the observations of Holmes, Semmelweis, and others more than 100 years ago. Hand antisepsis remains the most effective and least expensive measure to prevent transmission of nosocomial infections. However, compliance with hand-washing recommendations among HCWs averages only 30% to 50% and improves only modestly following educational interventions. Reasons frequently reported for poor compliance with hand hygiene by HCWs include skin irritation from frequent washing, too little time due to a high workload, and simply forgetting.

The use of waterless, alcohol-based hand rubs as an adjunct to washing with soap and water has become a routine practice by HCWs in many acute care facilities. Introduction of alcohol-based hand rubs has been shown to significantly improve hand hygiene compliance among HCWs in acute care hospitals and to decrease overall nosocomial infection rates and transmission of MRSA infections (18,19). Alcohol-based hand rubs have also been shown to enhance compliance with hand hygiene in the LTCF setting and should be used to complement educational initiatives (20). Although the cost of introducing alcohol-based hand rubs could be a concern of LTCFs, recent data in acute care have shown that total costs of a hand hygiene promotion campaign including alcohol-based rubs corresponded to less than 1% of costs that could be attributed to nosocomial infections (21).

While introducing the alcohol-based hand rub is a prudent, cost-effective measure, several issues should be considered. Alcohol-based hand rubs should not be used if hands are visibly soiled, in which case hand hygiene with antimicrobial soap and water is recommended. Alcohol-based hand rubs can cause dryness of skin; however, recent data on rubs containing emollients have shown to cause significantly less skin irritation and dryness (19). Facilities should be aware that alcohols are flammable. Facilities have reported difficulties in implementing the current hand hygiene guidelines and use of alcohol-based hand rubs due to the fire-safety concerns. Existing national fire codes permit use of alcohol-based hand rub dispensers in patient rooms but cannot be used in egress or exit corridors. Because the state and local fire codes may differ from national codes, facilities should consult with their local fire marshals to ensure that installation of alcohol-based hand rubs are consistent with local fire codes.

Staff Education

Ongoing education is critical in health-care settings due to the plethora of literature published every year, advancement in technology, and regulatory demands. The Joint Commission on Accreditation of Healthcare Organization expects new employee orientation to include the facility's infection control program and the employee's individual responsibility to prevent infections. OSHA also requires training for blood-borne pathogens and tuberculosis for any employee expected to come in contact with potentially infectious agents.

The ICP plays a vital role in meeting these requirements and in educating LTCF personnel on various infection control measures, particularly in view of rapid staff turnover. Informal education during infection control and quality improvement meetings as well as during infection control walking rounds should be complemented with in-services on various topics including hand hygiene, antimicrobial usage and antimicrobial resistance, appropriate and early diagnosis of infections, infection control and prevention measures to prevent these infections, and isolation precautions and policies.

Resident Immunization Program

Adults aged 65 and older should receive pneumococcal vaccination at least once, influenza vaccination every year, and tetanus booster every 10 years. Despite proven effectiveness, compliance with these measures remains dismally low.

A recent study showed that influenza and pneumococcal immunizations are associated with reduced hospitalization rate during influenza seasons (22). In a study describing invasive pneumococcal infection in an LTCF outbreak, the attack rate was 16% in the unvaccinated group and 0% in the vaccinated group (23). Investigators also found that 28 of 361 (7.8%) facilities that responded to their questionnaire did not offer pneumococcal vaccination to their residents. Average influenza and pneumococcal vaccination rates among LTCF residents are 60% and 40%, respectively. In addition to poor documentation, some of the reasons for lower immunization rates cited in the literature include lack of physician emphasis, patient concerns about the side effects of vaccinations, and inability to obtain consent. Adopting a standing-order policy could eliminate delays in immunization due to the consent process.

Employee Health Program

The employee health program mainly concerns employees with potentially communicable diseases, policies for sick leave, immunizations, and OSHA regulations to protect them from blood-borne pathogens. LTCFs must prevent employees with communicable diseases or infected skin lesions from providing direct contact with the residents and prevent employees with infected skin lesions or infectious diarrhea from having direct contact with residents' food. Moreover, when hiring new employees, an initial medical history must be obtained, along with a physical examination and screening for tuberculosis. Infection control education must also be provided.

Policies and measures in LTCFs must be in place to address post-exposure prophylaxis for such infections as HIV and hepatitis B. Varicella vaccine should be given to employees not immune to the virus. Employees are expected to be up to date with their tetanus boosters and to receive influenza vaccinations every year. Not only is the vaccine effective in preventing influenza and reducing absenteeism in HCWs, it has also been associated with a decrease in influenza mortality in patients (24). Annual influenza vaccination campaigns play a central role in deterring and preventing nosocomial transmission of the influenza virus and should be promoted by the ICP and LTCF leadership.

Rehabilitation Services

LTCFs increasingly are responsible for postacute care rehabilitation, including physical therapy, occupational therapy, and wound care with or without hydrotherapy. These therapists, like other clinical staffs, such as nurses and nurses' aides, provide many opportunities for transmission of pathogens between LTCF residents. In an LTCF, physical therapy and occupational therapy can be provided either at the bedside or in a central therapy unit. For bedside therapy, therapists move between different rooms and units and do not routinely wear gloves and gowns. For care at a central therapy unit, residents are transported to an open unit, where hand-washing sinks may not be readily available. Although these therapists have not been implicated in any major outbreaks, hydrotherapy for wounds has been shown to cause outbreaks with resistant pathogens (25).

A detailed infection control program for rehabilitation services should be prepared and should focus on facility design to promote hand hygiene using convenient and easy access to sinks and to promote the use of alcohol-based hand rubs. Patients who are infectious should not be treated at the central facility. Facilities providing hydrotherapy should consider providing the service in a separate room with a separate resident entrance.

INFECTION CONTROL PRACTITIONER

An ICP, usually a staff nurse, is assigned the responsibility of directing infection control activities in a LTCF. The ICP is responsible for implementing, monitoring, and evaluating the infection control program. Due to financial constraints, an ICP usually also functions as an assistant director of nursing or is involved in staff recruitment and education. Whether a full-time ICP is needed usually depends on the number of beds, the acuity level of residents, and the level of care provided at the facility. Nonetheless, for an infection control program to succeed, the ICP should be guaranteed sufficient time and resources to carry out infection control activities. A basic background in infectious disease, microbiology, geriatrics, and educational methods is advisable. The ICP should also be familiar with the federal, state, and local regulations dealing with infection control.

The LTCF leadership should be supportive of the mission and directives of infection control. They should encourage the educational activities proposed by the ICP and should provide the ICP with a computer with Internet access for the current literature and LTCF policies and procedures. Adequate funding for these activities should also be provided. The ICP should have written authority to implement emergency infection control measures.

Additionally, an alliance with and access to an infectious disease epidemiologist should be encouraged. Such collaborations could also provide assistance with outbreak investigations, emergency preparedness in the event of bioterrorism and vaccine shortages, and the use of microbiologic and molecular methods for infection control.

REVIEW COMMITTEE

In the early 1990s, OBRA mandated the formation of a formal infection control committee to evaluate infection rates, implement infection control programs, and review policies and procedures. However, this mandate has been dropped by OBRA at the federal level, although some states may still require them. A small subcommittee or a working group comprised of a physician/medical director, an administrator, and ICP should evaluate the LTCF infection rates on a regular basis and present the data at quality control meetings, review policies and any research in the area, and make decisions to implement infection control changes. This subcommittee can review and analyze the surveillance data, assure that these data are presented to the nursing and physician staff, and approve targeted recommendations to reduce such infections. Records pertaining to these activities and infection data should be kept and filed for future reference.

Principles guiding infection control practices also provide a model for enhancing quality of care and patient safety for other noninfectious adverse outcomes, such as falls, delirium, inappropriate medication usage, and adverse drug events.

RESOURCES FOR INFECTION CONTROL PRACTITIONERS AND SUGGESTED READING

Local APIC chapters provide a network for infection control practitioners to socialize, discuss infection control challenges and practical solutions to overcome them, and provide access to educational resources and services. Infection control practitioners should become members of APIC at both local and national levels to remain up-to-date with practice guidelines, position statements, information technology resources, and changes in policies and regulations.

Society for Healthcare Epidemiology of America (SHEA) and the Association for Professionals in Infection Control (APIC) both have long-term care committees that publish and approve LTCF infection guidelines and publish periodic position papers related to pertinent infection control issues. Their websites have several educational resources for staff education and in-services. In addition, APIC also publishes a quarterly long-term care newsletter.

Glen Mayhall C, ed. Hospital Epidemiology and Infection Control. 3rd ed. Philadelphia, PA: Lippincott Williams & Wilkins.

Selected Internet Websites

Association for Professionals in Infection Control (APIC): http://www.apic.org
Centers for Disease Control and Prevention (CDC): http://www.cdc.gov
Joint Commission on Accreditation of Healthcare Organizations-Infection Control Initiatives: http://www.jcaho.org/accredited+organizations/patient+safety/infection+control/ic+index.htm
Occupational Health and Safety Administration (OSHA): http://www.osha.gov
Society for Healthcare Epidemiology of America (SHEA): http://www.shea-online.org/

REFERENCES

1. Strausbaugh LJ, Joseph CL. The burden of infection in long-term care. Infect Control Hosp Epidemiol 2000; 21:674–679.
2. Nicolle LE. Infection control in long-term care facilities. Clin Infect Dis 2000; 31:752–756.

3. Loeb MB, Craven S, McGeer AJ, et al. Risk factors for resistance to antimicrobial agents among nursing home residents. Am J Epidemiol 2003; 157:40–47.
4. Zimmerman S, Gruber-baldini AL, Hebel JR, Sloane PD, Magaziner J. Nursing home facility risk factors for infection and hospitalization: importance of registered nurse turnover, administration and social factors. J Am Geriatr Soc 2002; 50:1987–1989.
5. McGeer A, Campbell B, Emori TG, et al. Definitions of infection for surveillance in long-term care facilities. Am J Infect Control 1991; 19:1–7.
6. Loeb M, Bentley DW, Bradley S, et al. Development of minimum criteria for the initiation of antibiotics in residents of long-term care facilities: results of a consensus conference. Infect Control Hosp Epidemiol 2001; 22:120–124.
7. Nicolle LE, Bentley D, Garibaldi R, Neuhaus E, Smith P. Antimicrobial use in long-term care facilities. Infect Control Hosp Epidemiol 1996; 17:119–128.
8. Strausbaugh LJ, Crossley KB, Nurse BA, Thrupp LD. Antimicrobial resistance in long-term care facilities. Infect Control Hosp Epidemiol 1996; 17:129–140.
9. Simor AE, Bradley SF, Strausbaugh LJ, Crossley K, Nicolle LE, SHEA Long-Term Care Committee. *Clostridium difficile* in long-term care facility for the elderly. Infect Control Hosp Epidemiol 2002; 23:696–703.
10. Bradley SF. Prevention of influenza in long-term care facilities. Long-term care committee of the Society for Healthcare Epidemiology of America. Infect Control Hosp Epidemiol 1999; 20:629–637.
11. Bentley DW, Bradley S, High K, Schoenbaum S, Taler G, Yoshikawa TT. Practice guideline for evaluation of fever and infection in long-term care facilities. J Am Geriatr Soc 2001; 49:210–222.
12. Smith PW, Rusnak PG. Infection prevention and control in long-term care facility. Infect Control Hosp Epidemiol 1997; 18:831–849.
13. Horan TC, Gaynes RP. Surveillance of nosocomial infections. In: Glen Mayhall C, ed. Hospital Epidemiology and Infection Control. 3rd ed. Philadelphia, PA: Lippincott Williams & Wilkins, 2004:1661–1702.
14. Mody L, Langa KM, Saint S, Bradley SF. Preventing infections in nursing homes: a survey of infection control practices in Southeast Michigan. Am J Infect Control 2005; 33:489–492.
15. Stevenson KB, Moore J, Colwell H, Sleeper B. Standardized infection surveillance in long-term care: interfacility comparisons from a regional cohort of facilities. Infect Control Hosp Epidemiol 2005; 26:231–238.
16. Garner JS, the Hospital Infection Control Practices Advisory Committee. Guideline for isolation precautions in hospitals. Infect Control Hosp Epidemiol 1996; 17:53–80.
17. Muto CA, Jernigan JA, Ostrowsky BE, et al. SHEA guideline for preventing nosocomial transmission of multidrug-resistant strains of *Staphylococcus aureus* and enterococcus. Infect Control Hosp Epidemiol 2003; 24:362–386.
18. Pittet D. Improving adherence to hand hygiene practice: a multidisciplinary approach. Emerg Infect Dis 2001; 7:234–240.
19. Centers for Disease Control and Prevention. Guideline for hand hygiene in health-care settings: recommendations of the Healthcare Infection Control Practices Advisory Committee and the HICPAC/SHEA/APIC/IDSA Hand Hygiene Task Force. MMWR 2002; 51:S3–S40.

20. Mody L, McNeil SA, Sun R, Bradley SE, Kauffman CA. Introduction of a waterless alcohol-based hand rub in a long-term care facility. Infect Control Hosp Epidemiol 2003; 24:165–171.
21. Pittet D, Sax H, Hugonnet S, Harbarth S. Cost implications of successful hand hygiene promotion. Infect Control Hosp Epidemiol 2004; 25:264–266.
22. Kazakova SV, Curtis A, Bratzler D, Nsa W, McKibben L, Shefer A. Impact of pneumococcal and influenza vaccination on the risk of hospitalization among nursing home residents [abstr]. Presented at the Society for Healthcare Epidemiology of America, April 2004.
23. Tan CG, Ostrawski S, Bresnitz EA. A preventable outbreak of pneumococcal pneumonia among unvaccinated nursing home residents in New Jersey during 2001. Infect Control Hosp Epidemiol 2003; 24:848–852.
24. Carman WF, Elder AG, Wallace LA, et al. Effects of influenza vaccination of health-care workers on mortality of elderly people in long-term care: a randomized controlled trial. Lancet 2000; 355:93–97.
25. Embril JM, McLeod JA, AL-Barrak AM, et al. An outbreak of methicillin-resistant *Staphylococcus aureus* on a burn unit: potential role of contaminated hydrotherapy equipment. Burns 2001; 27:681–688.

10

Epidemiologic Investigation of Infectious Disease Outbreaks in Long-Term Care Facilities

Chesley L. Richards, Jr.

*Geriatric Research, Education, and Clinical Center (GRECC),
Atlanta Veterans Affairs Medical Center, and Emory University School of Medicine,
Atlanta, Georgia, U.S.A.*

William R. Jarvis

*Division of Pediatric Infectious Diseases, Emory University
School of Medicine, Atlanta, Georgia, U.S.A.*

KEY POINTS

1. Infectious disease outbreaks are common in long-term care facility residents.
2. Individual risk factors for outbreaks include decreased immunity, malnutrition, chronic disease, functional impairment, multiple medications, and invasive devices.
3. Institutional risk factors for outbreaks include larger size facilities, facility design, group activities, low immunization rates, excessive antimicrobial use, and widespread colonization with antimicrobial-resistant organisms.
4. The key to effective outbreak investigation is a well-coordinated infection control program and plan.
5. The most common outbreaks are viral respiratory infections, foodborne or viral gastroenteritis, and skin infections.

INTRODUCTION

Infectious disease outbreaks in long-term care facilities (LTCFs) are common, can cause serious morbidity and mortality for residents, and can be time-consuming to investigate and control (1). Epidemiologic investigations of these outbreaks can be as complicated as outbreak investigations in hospital settings and yet fewer infection control resources are generally available in LTCFs. Despite these challenges, interdisciplinary infection control programs that include infection control professionals (ICPs), administrators, clinicians (e.g., physicians, nurse practitioners, physician assistants), pharmacists, laboratorians, and nursing staff can prevent many infectious disease outbreaks and successfully control those outbreaks that do occur.

This chapter will review the principles of epidemiologic investigation as they apply to outbreaks in LTCFs, review aspects of selected infectious disease outbreaks, and discuss approaches to their prevention and control. Although LTCFs encompass a broad range of facilities from nursing homes for the elderly to long-term psychiatric facilities, the focus of this chapter is on outbreak investigation in nursing homes for the elderly. Many of the recommendations contained in the chapter, however, can be adapted and used in other LTCF settings.

CHARACTERISTICS OF LONG-TERM CARE FACILITIES

LTCFs are an increasingly important site of medical care and drug prescribing for the elderly. An important distinction between LTCFs and acute care facilities is that LTCFs are residential and persons in LTCFs are generally referred to as "residents" instead of as "patients." Even though medical care is provided to LTCF residents, other aspects of an LTCF resident's life take on greater importance than in acute care facilities. Socialization through group activities, both in and outside the LTCF, promotes good mental health for residents, although these activities may increase the risk of exposure to infectious agents. Group settings for eating and physical therapy, vital to the maintenance of resident independence and functional status, may increase risk for foodborne outbreaks, person-to-person transmission, or exposure to potential fomites, such as physical therapy equipment. Not surprisingly, the management of infectious disease outbreaks in LTCFs is complicated. The availability of clinicians to evaluate febrile residents may be limited and diagnostic studies, including microbiologic cultures, are generally less available than in acute care facilities. Consequently, nursing assistants usually perform the initial resident assessment, and licensed nurses relay important findings to clinicians, usually by telephone. In an effort to improve the evaluation of LTCF residents with fever or suspected infection, recommendations for the minimal evaluation of patients who develop fever in LTCFs were published recently (2). These guidelines specify tasks appropriate for nursing assistants and licensed nurses.

In LTCFs, antimicrobials for the empirical treatment of suspected infection often are prescribed without on-site clinician evaluation or diagnostic testing (1–3). When diagnostic testing is performed, only limited tests are available in most LTCFs. This, together with outsourcing of most laboratory work, may lead to suboptimal timeliness of reporting and, in some situations, inaccurate or misleading results. When residents are acutely ill or diagnostic testing is not available in LTCFs, residents often are transferred to the emergency departments of acute care hospitals. Not surprisingly, evaluation and management of infection accounts for approximately one-quarter of resident transfers from LTCFs to hospitals.

RISK FACTORS FOR OUTBREAKS IN LTCFs

Risk factors for outbreaks include both resident and institutional factors (Table 1). The typical resident in an LTCF is female, >80 years of age, cognitively impaired, and living with several underlying medical conditions. Individual risk factors for infection include immunologic senescence, malnutrition, multiple chronic diseases, medications (e.g., immunosuppressants, central nervous system agents that diminish cough reflex), cognitive deficits that may complicate resident compliance with basic sanitary practices (e.g., hand washing), functional impairments (e.g., fecal and urinary incontinence, immobility, diminished cough reflex), or invasive device use (e.g., urinary catheters, enteral feeding tubes, tracheostomies) (1–3). Institutional factors associated with increased risk for outbreaks are varied. In a study of outbreaks among New York LTCFs, institutional risk

Table 1 Potential Risk Factors for Infectious Disease Outbreaks in Long-Term Care Facilities

Resident level
  Decreased immunity to infection
  Malnutrition
  Chronic disease
  Functional impairment included diminished cough reflex, urinary incontinence, fecal incontinence, immobility
  Medications, especially psychoactive medications that diminish cough reflex and consciousness
  Invasive devices, such as urinary catheters, enteral feeding tubes, tracheostomies, etc.
Institutional level
  Larger size (e.g., larger number of residents)
  Facility design (e.g., single versus multiple resident rooms)
  Group activities, such as meals, physical therapy, recreational activities
  Low immunization rates
  Excessive antimicrobial use
  Widespread colonization of residents with antimicrobial-resistant organisms

factors for respiratory or gastrointestinal infection outbreaks included larger LTCFs (risk ratio 1.71 per 100 bed increase), LTCFs with a single nursing unit, or LTCFs with multiple units but shared staff (4). Risk for outbreaks was lower in LTCFs with paid employee sick leave. Frequent group activities, such as meals, physical therapy, recreational activities, or the common use of shared facilities (e.g., showers or whirlpool baths), increase the risk for outbreaks (1–3). Risk for outbreaks caused by specific pathogens (e.g., influenza, *Streptococcus pneumoniae*) is increased in settings where resident and healthcare worker immunization coverage is low. Finally, widespread excessive antimicrobial use and high rates of colonization with antimicrobial-resistant organisms increase risk of outbreaks from these organisms.

KEY ASPECTS OF INFECTIOUS DISEASE OUTBREAK INVESTIGATION

The epidemiologic investigation of infectious disease outbreaks in LTCFs should be conducted in a systematic fashion. Key components of the investigation are described below and are listed in Table 2.

Infection Control Program and Plan

Unlike hospitals, most LTCFs do not have substantial resources committed to infection control (5). Every infection control program should have an infection control plan outlining personnel, responsibilities, reporting relationships, and surveillance activities (see also Chapter 9). Designating a staff

Table 2 Key Aspects of Outbreak Investigation in Long-Term Care Facilities

Have an infection control plan and program
Ask two important questions
    Is this surveillance artifact?
    Is an epidemiologic investigation needed?
Develop the case definition and line listing
Ascertain cases
Determine person, place, and time
    Host factors (person)
    Geographic assessment (place)
    The epidemic curve (time)
Develop preliminary hypotheses
Evaluate hypotheses
    Cohort and case–control studies
    Observational studies
    Microbiologic studies
Implement intervention(s)
Evaluate impact of intervention(s)

member as the "infection control person" is not sufficient; ideally, a trained, experienced ICP should be responsible for the program, either as a staff member at the facility or on a consulting basis. It is critical for a facility to know who is responsible for conducting surveillance and identifying, investigating, intervening, and reporting an outbreak. Finally, establishing an infection control committee with active participation by the LTCF administrator, medical director, ICP, and nursing staff is important not only for support and guidance during an outbreak but for continued vigilance in optimizing infection control prevention efforts to avoid outbreaks. Several reviews, guidelines, and position statements for infection control in LTCFs have been published previously (3). In addition, guidelines from the Centers for Disease Control and Prevention for many aspects of infection control are available through the Internet (www.cdc.gov/ncidod/hip).

Is This Surveillance Artifact?

An important first question to ask in a potential outbreak situation is whether the "outbreak" actually represents surveillance artifact. Common causes of surveillance artifact include: (i) introduction of new infection definitions or surveillance methods, (ii) a new ICP, nurse, or clinician, (iii) new laboratory tests or populations, or (iv) change in microbial cultures. For example, surveillance data may demonstrate a markedly increased rate of pneumonia in LTCF residents. This increase may represent a true outbreak of bacterial or viral pneumonia requiring infection control intervention. Alternatively, a facility decision to admit more residents at high risk for aspiration (e.g., severe neurological conditions) may increase the rate of pneumonia without representing a true infectious disease outbreak.

Deciding When to Conduct an Investigation

The decision to conduct an epidemiologic investigation is generally driven by three situations: (i) identification of unusual infections or organisms with high potential for morbidity or mortality (e.g., a single case of meningococcal meningitis), (ii) identification of organisms or infections that, though relatively common, have high risk for morbidity, mortality, and transmission to other residents (e.g., influenza, norovirus), or (iii) identification of epidemiologically important organisms (i.e., several cases of methicillin-resistant *Staphylococcus aureus* pneumonia).

First, the definition for what constitutes an outbreak depends on the type of infection and to some extent the facility. If, for example, a single episode of a highly contagious, potentially lethal infection, such as meningococcal meningitis, is identified in an LTCF resident, an epidemiologic investigation and early, aggressive infection control interventions are necessary. In contrast, knowing when to call a cluster of several LTCF residents with acute respiratory infections or gastroenteritis an outbreak is more difficult. Generally, most authorities suggest that when the rate of infections is significantly higher than baseline endemic rates, an epidemic is occurring and an epidemiologic investigation is warranted. This definition depends on two factors. The LTCF should have a surveillance system in place for detecting infections and calculating and comparing infection rates. More important, the LTCF should have a clinical staff member who understands basic principles of infection control and infectious disease epidemiology and is knowledgeable about changes in the LTCF's resident population and infection trends in the facility.

A second important early consideration is whether and when to seek outside assistance to assist in the epidemiologic investigation. If the facility has a trained ICP, the initial investigation for most types of infectious disease outbreaks can be conducted and appropriate infection control interventions instituted by the ICP. If the facility lacks an ICP, then the clinical staff member charged with conducting the epidemiologic investigation may wish to seek assistance from an ICP or health-care epidemiologist, a professional organization, such as the Association of Professionals in Infection Control or the Society for Healthcare Epidemiology in America, a state or local public health agency, or the Centers for Disease Control and Prevention. Although regulations vary from state to state, in general, LTCFs are required to report infectious disease outbreaks to local or state public health agencies.

Case Definition and Line Listing

Although some challenges to conducting an epidemiologic investigation in LTCF are unique, the basic approach to epidemiologic investigation is the same, whether the investigation occurs in a hospital or an LTCF. The initial step in an investigation is usually a case review. When clinical staff or ICPs note increases in rates of infection, an unusual clustering of infections, or infections with unusual agents, all residents thought to fit in the cluster should be reviewed. The easiest tool for this review is a line listing containing demographic, clinical, and exposure information for each patient (Table 3). As early as possible, investigators should develop a tentative case definition. The case definition should include who, what, where, and when— a description of the infectious disease (what) along with three important parameters: person (who), place (where), and time (when). For example, a case definition that could be used in a hypothetical pneumonia outbreak caused by influenza is outlined in Table 4.

If necessary, the initial case definition may be modified during the course of the investigation. For example, the above case definition might need to be changed in several ways: the definition of the respiratory illness might be made more general or specific, employees might be added to the population considered, the time-frame might be broadened or narrowed, and additional wards in LTCF A might be considered. In general, the case

Table 3 Example of a Line Listing—Influenza Outbreak

Case	Age	Sex	Ward/ room	Onset	Cough	Fever	CXR	RA test[a]	Meals	Physical therapy
1	87	M	4A/401	3/01/01	Yes	Yes	+	+	In room	Yes
2	90	F	3A/304	3/02/01	Yes	No	+	+	On ward	Yes
3	99	F	2A/208	3/02/01	Yes	Yes	−	+	Main dining room	Yes
4	80	F	2A/208	3/03/01	Yes	No	−	+	Main dining room	Yes
5	90	M	2B/240	3/05/01	Yes	Yes	+	+	Main dining room	Yes

[a]Rapid antigen test.
Abbreviation: CXR, chest radiograph.

definition should be changed judiciously; each change of the definition will affect the number of cases identified and modify results of comparative studies that are conducted during the course of the investigation. An alternative to changing the case definition completely is to modify the case definition to allow for "definite" and "possible/probable" cases. Using the example above, a "definite" case might be a resident with clinical symptoms and a positive laboratory test for influenza A, whereas a "possible" case might be a resident with clinical symptoms but no or negative laboratory testing. Although difficult, some attempt should also be made to identify the first case patient (e.g., index case), especially if the presumed transmission is person to

Table 4 Example of Case Definition Pneumonia

What (disease)	Respiratory illness with at least 2 of the following symptoms/signs: New or increased cough New or increased sputum production Fever (temperature >38°C) Pleuritic chest pain New or increased shortness of breath Respiratory rate >25 breaths per minute Worsening mental or functional status Positive rapid antigen test or respiratory tract culture for influenza A
Person (population)	Elderly residents
Place	Ward B of LTCF A
Time	Jan 1–Jan 30, 2001

Abbreviation: LTCF, long-term care facility.

person. By designating an index case, assumptions important to the investigation, such as incubation period and duration of the outbreak, can be made. As with the case definition, additional cases found during case ascertainment also may lead to a change in the designated index case.

Case Ascertainment

Case ascertainment should be as comprehensive as possible. Multiple sources of information and data are potentially available. Interviews with nursing staff, including nursing assistants, may be a quick way to ascertain cases; however, because many LTCFs experience rapid staff turnover and chronic understaffing, relying solely on what staff can recall may result in incomplete case ascertainment. Microbiology and radiology reports may be helpful, especially if the case definition includes results of these studies. In addition to chart review, existing infection control surveillance records may be helpful, especially in determining the endemic rate of infection. Because most LTCFs have a single pharmacy provider, antimicrobial prescription data may be a potential source of data to ascertain cases. Finally, medical records for residents transferred to hospitals may be another source for case ascertainment and to evaluate resident outcomes (e.g., death).

Person, Place, and Time

Host Factors (Person)

In addition to clearly defining the persons (or populations) affected by the infectious disease outbreak, investigators should review characteristics of case patients on the line listing to identify specific host factors that may increase risk. The usual risk factors to be considered include intrinsic host factors (i.e., age, sex, race, underlying disease, nutritional status) and extrinsic factors (e.g., urinary catheters, feeding tubes, central vascular catheters, environmental exposures, receipt of medications, personnel exposure, food, or nutritional product received).

Geographic Assessment (Place)

Determining the geographic relationship between cases involved in the outbreak may be difficult and is influenced by a number of interrelated factors. First, determining if the cases occur in a single area of the LTCF is critical. Using a spot map to identify the room of each case is important and usually can be made using a blueprint of the LTCF. Geographic clustering around a single living area may be readily apparent. In contrast, identifying common facilities (e.g., dining rooms, shower/bath facilities) that may be shared by residents from different parts of the LTCF may be both more subtle and, yet, more productive in some outbreak investigations where a geographic pattern is not readily apparent. Finally, if the outbreak is believed to be due to an air- or waterborne organism, reviewing ventilation or plumbing diagrams may be helpful.

The Epidemic Curve (Time)

The epidemic curve is a simple graphical tool using information from the line listing to display the time relationship of cases in the outbreak. Epidemic curves generally display time on the horizontal axis and number of cases on the vertical axis. Epidemic curves have some important features. First, the time axis should be shorter than the presumed incubation period of the infection. Second, the time period should include both the pre-epidemic (e.g., time before the index case) and epidemic periods.

The shape of the epidemic curve is important. If there is an abrupt rise in cases, this is suggestive of a point source for the outbreak (e.g., contaminated product or food). A more prolonged series of cases suggests person-to-person transmission. On some occasions, the epidemic curve may have features of both modes of transmission suggesting that transmission may be occurring by several routes.

Preliminary Hypotheses

Once an initial set of cases is identified, an attempt should be made to generate hypotheses about what may be causing the outbreak. Sometimes, with a distinct cluster in time and space and an obvious source, quick action can be taken. More often, several potential sources and modes of transmission may be suggested by the preliminary data. At a minimum, hypotheses about the potential sources and the potential mode of transmission are needed to properly design comparative studies (described below). Once hypotheses are developed, comparative studies can be designed and used to test the hypotheses with the aim of identifying the most likely causative factors for the outbreak.

Studies

Cohort and Case–Control Studies

There are generally two types of comparative studies used in outbreak investigations to identify risk factors for the outbreak: cohort and case–control studies. In cohort studies, all members of a defined population (i.e., cohort) are evaluated. The data can be collected retrospectively or prospectively. In cohort studies, relative risk, a quantitative measure of the strength of association between the exposure and the risk of developing the adverse condition, can be calculated; this quantifies the strength of association between the presumed exposure and the event. The primary advantage of cohort studies is that the whole population is assessed; bias through the process of selecting controls is not introduced. The primary drawbacks to the cohort design are that the appropriate population may not be defined and cohort studies require significantly more resources to complete, especially if the frequency of cases is low.

In case–control studies, known cases are compared to selected control residents. Selecting appropriate controls may be tricky. It usually is advisable to randomly select controls from the population affected. Confounding may be a concern and can be controlled by using stratification or multivariate analyses. In some case–control studies, cases and controls may be "matched" on a particular characteristic, especially if a particular group of residents appears to be at significantly greater risk (e.g., only females are affected, or only individuals in a particular wing of the LTCF). However, variables on which controls are matched cannot then be analyzed as risk factors. The advantage of case–control studies is that, especially with low-frequency events or outbreaks occurring over a long period of time, the resources needed to collect data (e.g., chart reviews, microbiologic reviews, etc.) will be less than with a cohort study. In case–control studies, odds ratios are calculated and represent approximations of relative risk. Odds ratios indicate whether cases are more likely to have been exposed to a risk factor than controls.

Observational Studies

Often outbreaks may involve suboptimal compliance by health-care workers with facility policies and procedures (i.e., hand hygiene, food preparation, sanitation). Observational studies where ICPs actually observe compliance with these procedures may be an important part of the overall epidemiologic investigation. Before observation, infection control personnel should review policies and procedures with administrative personnel and identify changes or modifications that have occurred. The actual observations should occur for short periods (i.e., one hour) on all shifts and in locations where both case and noncase patients reside, especially if within a facility there are areas of high attack rate and other areas with few or no cases. It is important that observers have a clear understanding of what constitutes the indication for a particular procedure and what constitutes failure to comply. For example, in an observational study on hand hygiene, the observer must know if hand hygiene is expected to occur before a patient encounter, before the health-care worker leaves the patient room, or before they touch another resident or patient-care device.

Microbiologic Studies

In outbreak investigations, microbiologic studies should be based upon epidemiologic findings. In addition to identification of bacteria or viruses from case-patient clinical specimens, several potential microbiologic studies may be considered depending on epidemiologic results. First, in outbreaks where colonization may play an important role (e.g., antimicrobial-resistant bacteria), resident or health-care worker culture surveys may be useful. Important considerations include determining the best methods for culture collection, planning for the number of cultures or site of cultures, laboratory support for rapid processing of specimens, consistency of obtaining specimens, and appropriate record keeping to correctly identify the resident or health-care worker, site of culture, and type of specimen. Environmental cultures only should be considered in situations where the presumed pathogen and the epidemiologic findings suggest an environmental source. Widespread resident, health-care worker, or environmental culturing before the epidemiologic investigation is not recommended and may often lead to erroneous conclusions about the outbreak. Furthermore, such widespread culturing is burdensome on personnel, costly, and, often in the absence of epidemiologic direction, fails to identify the outbreak source.

Implementing Interventions

Once risk factors and potential sources are identified, interventions to terminate the outbreak should be instituted. These interventions must be fully discussed with the LTCF administrator, nursing director, medical director, and health-care staff. Implementation of the interventions is dependent on support and acceptance by the staff. Especially in large, explosive outbreaks, some interventions, such as cohorting infected and colonized residents, institution of facility-wide resident or health-care worker vaccination, or enhanced glove use, may be easily understood and accepted by staff. However, in longer-duration, lower-intensity outbreaks, acceptance may be suboptimal for interventions (e.g., improved compliance with hand hygiene, changes in food preparation policies, etc.) and more focus on education and training may be necessary. In these situations, incorporating ongoing process measurement of the intervention (e.g., observational study of hand hygiene among nursing assistants) with feedback periodically to staff may be helpful in increasing compliance with the intervention.

SELECTED INFECTIOUS DISEASE OUTBREAKS

Selected examples of the more common types of infectious disease outbreaks occurring in LTCFs are presented below. The reader should also refer to other Chapters 13–15, 17–20, 23–27 devoted to specific infections.

Respiratory Tract Infections

Outbreaks of respiratory tract disease in LTCFs are relatively common. In a recent report from five Canadian LTCFs, 16 outbreaks involving 480 of 1313 residents were reported, occurring year-round with no seasonal predilection (6). The most common symptoms among residents during these outbreaks were cough (83%), fever (40%), and coryza (45%), and a minority (15%) of residents developed pneumonia. The most common pathogens included influenza, parainfluenza, or respiratory syncytial viruses; *Legionella* spp.; or *Chlamydia pneumoniae*. Approximately 12% of residents were transferred to hospitals, and 8% died.

Influenza

The most important cause of respiratory tract disease outbreaks in LTCFs is influenza. Outbreaks of influenza A or B usually occur from early October to April but may sometimes extend into summer. Of the 20,000 deaths from influenza each year, 90% occur in persons aged ≥65 years. Primary risk factors are lack of influenza vaccination among residents and health-care workers. Ventilation and architectural issues may also play a role. In a report of an outbreak of influenza A affecting 68 residents, the LTCF had four separate buildings, one of which was newly constructed (7). Interestingly, the attack rate in the new building was significantly lower than the other buildings. Key differences in the new building included: (1) a ventilation system that did not recirculate air, (2) more public space per resident, and (3) no office space in the building serving the entire facility. Even widespread use of immunization, the cornerstone of influenza prevention, may be insufficient to prevent some LTCF outbreaks. Especially in older residents, influenza vaccine effectiveness may be diminished, increasing the risk for influenza outbreaks. These failures may be secondary to poor immunologic response to the vaccine in this elderly population. In an LTCF with high rates (>85%) of resident influenza vaccination, outbreaks involving 172 residents were reported despite a match between the vaccine strain and outbreak strain (8). When antiviral prophylaxis or treatment failures occur, the presence of an antiviral-resistant influenza strain should be considered (9). In addition, clinicians in LTCFs should pay particular attention to public health reports on circulating influenza strains, especially in light of the emergence of avian influenza strains in Asia.

Other Respiratory Viruses

In addition to influenza, infections with parainfluenza virus, respiratory syncytial virus, adenoviruses, and rhinoviruses can cause respiratory tract disease in LTCF residents (see also Chapter 13). Parainfluenza virus type 3 was associated with an outbreak of respiratory disease on a 50-bed nursing unit of a large Wisconsin LTCF. The attack rate was 50% and resulted in 16% mortality within nine days of symptom onset (10). In contrast, a study of 30-day mortality suggested that noninfluenza viruses have lower mortality than influenza viruses with mortality ranging from 6.1% (influenza B) and 5.4% (influenza A) to virtually nil for respiratory respiratory syncytial virus (RSV) and rhinoviruses (11). The key observations from reports on respiratory tract outbreaks are that early identification of the infectious agents, institution of appropriate treatment or prophylaxis, and aggressive use of infection precautions, especially isolation of residents and improved health-care worker compliance with hand-hygiene recommendations, are critical to minimize serious morbidity and deaths.

Streptococcus pneumoniae

Although not a common cause of outbreaks in LTCFs, *S. pneumoniae* is the most common pathogen identified in endemic respiratory tract disease in LTCF residents, is an important cause of invasive disease, and is increasingly resistant to antimicrobials. In a review of 26 *S. pneumoniae* outbreaks since 1990, the majority occurred in elderly patients in LTCFs or hospitals (12). The most common serotypes identified in these outbreaks were 23F, 14, and 4, all of which are included in current formulations of the pneumococcal vaccine. Outbreaks of *S. pneumoniae* pneumonia and bacteremia in Oklahoma, Massachusetts, Maryland, and, more recently, New Jersey were associated with low pneumococcal vaccination rates (13). Despite some skepticism regarding the efficacy of pneumococcal vaccine, these outbreaks reinforce the need for aggressive pneumococcal vaccination programs and policies in LTCFs (14).

Legionnaire's Disease

Legionnaire's disease, caused by *Legionella pneumophila*, remains an important consideration during respiratory tract disease outbreaks. Outbreaks in both LTCFs and hospitals are generally associated with contaminated water systems. *L. pneumophila* may persist in health-care facility water systems despite the use of various interventions (15). In order to identify these outbreaks earlier, clinicians and ICPs should maintain a high index of suspicion for Legionnaire's disease and obtain the proper laboratory support for microbiologic testing to identify *L. pneumophila*.

Gastrointestinal Infections

Outbreaks of gastroenteritis and diarrhea in LTCFs are common and commonly include *Escherichia coli*, *Salmonella* spp., or enteric viruses. The usual mode of transmission for these outbreaks is foodborne or person-to-person transmission. In a 250-bed LTCF in Tennessee, 14% of residents developed gastroenteritis due to *Salmonella hadar* (16). Among the 244 health-care workers, the attack rate was 27% in laundry workers, whereas only 3% in nursing staff and 4% in kitchen staff. Although the index case was probably a member of the kitchen staff, the high attack rate among the laundry staff was probably secondary to inconsistent use of gloves and lack of protective clothing while handling of increased volumes of soiled linen during the outbreak. More recently, outbreaks of fluoroquinolone-resistant *Salmonella* have been reported in LTCFs (17). In an Australian LTCF, 25 residents developed gastroenteritis caused by *Clostridium perfringens* due to contamination of pureed food (18).

Apparently, once the food was liquefied, it was not reheated and subsequently became contaminated. Consequently, the authors recommended that pureed food be reheated to 70°C to inactivate potential contaminating pathogens before consumption. An outbreak of campylobacteriosis occurred in a Connecticut senior center due to contaminated sweet potatoes and raw meat used during a special meal at the center (e.g., Hawaiian luau) (19).

Outbreaks due to enteric viruses occur frequently in LTCFs. In Virginia LTCFs during one year, caliciviruses were responsible for eight different reported outbreaks (20). In a Maryland LTCF with 121 residents, 51% of residents and 47% of the staff developed gastroenteritis due to a calicivirus over a four-month period (21). The index case in the outbreak was a nurse who continued to work for two additional days after becoming ill. The outbreak illustrates the need to exclude ill employees in a timely fashion by providing sick leave and not expecting staff to take annual or vacation leave for illnesses. In a norovirus outbreak in an LTCF, the majority (57%) of residents developed acute gastoenteritis following exposure to an ill LTCF resident, the index case (22). In the residents, prominent symptoms included vomiting (90%), diarrhea (70%), and fever (12%). Four residents required hospitalization, and three died. Many health-care workers (35%) also developed gastroenteritis. Based on molecular typing, the outbreak appeared to occur among debilitated residents and the nurses caring for them implied that the outbreak was propagated through LTCF staff rather than ambulatory residents. Cohorting of ill patients and strict adherence to infection control practices, such as hand hygiene, glove use, and barrier precautions, stopped the outbreak.

Skin Infections

Previous LTCF skin infection outbreaks include *Streptococcus pyogenes*-associated cellulitis, *Pseudomonas aeruginosa* associated with a contaminated whirlpool bath, group A *Streptococcus* or antimicrobial-resistant organisms causing infections of pressure ulcers. Most of these outbreaks are caused by poor infection control practices resulting in transmission of the causative agents. For example, a recent outbreak due to group A *Streptococcus* in LTCF residents was terminated through improved hand hygiene (23). Scabies is an important parasitic skin infection that not infrequently causes outbreaks in LTCFs. Transmission of scabies may occur by contact with mite-contaminated inanimate objects (e.g., bed linens) or direct person-to-person contact. Outbreaks of scabies in three Norwegian LTCF lasted for five months and involved 27 patients or health-care workers (24). Initial treatments with permethrin were not successful; however, benzyl benzoate was effective. Ultimately, more than 600 residents and staff were treated. A key observation from these outbreaks was the need for simultaneous treatment of residents and staff and disinfection of bedding, clothing, and the environment. As with other outbreaks, early identification is optimal for management of scabies outbreaks and may occasionally require dermatological consultation or skin biopsy for diagnosis (see also Chapter 17).

Infections with Antimicrobial-Resistant Organisms

Antimicrobial-resistant pathogen outbreaks affect the elderly in both hospitals and LTCFs (3). Important antimicrobial-resistant pathogens include methicillin-resistant *S. aureus*; multiply resistant gram-negative bacilli, such as *E. coli, Acinetobacter, Enterobacter,* or *P. aeruginosa*; or vancomycin-resistant enterococcus. Widespread colonization of residents in LTCFs with antimicrobial-resistant organisms provides a potential reservoir for subsequent transmission and outbreaks. In Chicago, a citywide outbreak of multidrug-resistant *Klebsiella pneumoniae* and *E. coli* demonstrated that LTCFs were important reservoirs for antimicrobial-resistant organisms (25). Furthermore, in a single Chicago skilled nursing facility, 43% of residents were colonized with at least one antimicrobial-resistant organism (26) (see also Chapters 23–25).

CONCLUSIONS

Infectious disease outbreaks in LTCFs are an important public health concern, can result in serious illnesses and death in LTCF residents, and can be disruptive to LTCF staff. The major patient risk factors include chronic illnesses, incontinence, and poor respiratory function. These risk factors may not be amenable to interventions. However, institutions can attempt to prevent outbreaks by ensuring that residents receive appropriate immunizations, promote judicious use of antimicrobials, and ensure that the LTCF has a well-staffed and organized infection control program. Once infectious disease outbreaks occur, epidemiologic investigation of the outbreak should proceed quickly. The key components of the investigation should include developing a case definition, compiling a line listing of known case patients, conducting additional case ascertainment, constructing an epidemic curve and geographic plots, and developing working hypotheses as to the source, mode of transmission, and possible organisms. The types of studies (e.g., case–control, cohort, observational, microbiologic) performed will depend on the available resources. Interventions to terminate the outbreak should be consistent with epidemiologic findings and be effectively communicated to administrators, staff, and public health officials.

Over the next several decades, the population of elderly LTCF residents will dramatically increase; resources for infection control programs and outbreak prevention in LTCF will be an important investment toward improving the quality of care in this increasingly important health-care setting.

SUGGESTED READING

Bentley DW, Bradley S, High K, Schoenbaum S, Taler G, Yoshikawa TT. Practice guidelines for evaluation of fever and infection in long-term care facilities. Clin Infect Dis 2000; 31:640–653.

Nicolle LE. Infection control in long-term care facilities. Clin Infect Dis 2000; 31:752–756.

Strausbaugh LJ, Sukumar SR, Joseph CL. Infectious disease outbreaks in nursing homes: an unappreciated hazard for frail elderly persons. Clin Infect Dis 2003; 36:870–876.

REFERENCES

1. Strausbaugh LJ, Sukumar SR, Joseph CL. Infectious disease outbreaks in nursing homes: an unappreciated hazard for frail elderly persons. Clin Infect Dis 2003; 36:870–876.
2. Bentley DW, Bradley S, High K, Schoenbaum S, Taler G, Yoshikawa TT. Practice guidelines for evaluation of fever and infection in long-term care facilities. Clin Infect Dis 2000; 1:640–653.
3. Nicolle LE. Infection control in long-term care facilities. Clin Infect Dis 2000; 31:752–756.
4. Li J, Birkhead GS, Strogatz DS, Coles FB. Impact of institution size, staffing patterns, and infection control practices on communicable disease outbreaks in New York state nursing homes. Am J Epidemiol 1996; 143:1042–1049.
5. Goldrick BA. Infection control programs in skilled nursing long-term care facilities: an assessment, 1995. Am J Infect Control 1999; 27:4–9.
6. Loeb M, McGeer A, McArthur M, Peeling RW, Petric M, Simor AE. Surveillance for outbreaks of respiratory tract infections in nursing homes. Can Med Assoc J 2000; 162:1133–1137.
7. Drinka PJ, Krause P, Schilling M, Miller BA, Shult P, Gravenstein S. Report of an outbreak: nursing home architecture and influenza-A attack rates. J Am Geriatr Soc 1996; 44:910–913.
8. Ohmit SE, Arden NH, Monto AS. Effectiveness of inactivated influenza vaccine among nursing home residents during an influenza type A (H3N2) epidemic. J Am Geriatr Soc 1999; 47:165–171.
9. Schilling M, Gravenstein S, Drinka P, et al. Emergence and transmission of amantadine-resistance influenza A in a nursing home. J Am Geriatr Soc 2004; 52:2069–2073.
10. Faulks JT, Drinka PJ, Shult P. A serious outbreak of parainfluenza type 3 on a nursing unit. J Am Geriatr Soc 2000; 48:1216–1218.
11. Drinka PJ, Gravenstein S, Langer E, Krause P, Shult P. Mortality following isolation of various respiratory viruses in nursing home residents. Infect Control Hosp Epidemiol 1999; 20:812–815.
12. Gleich S, Morad Y, Echague R, et al. *Streptococcus pneumoniae* serotype 4 outbreak in a home for the aged: report and review of recent outbreaks. Infect Control Hosp Epidemiol 2000; 21:711–717.

13. Tan CG, Ostrawski S, Bresnitz EA. A preventable outbreak of pneumococcal pneumonia among unvaccinated nursing home residents in New Jersey during 2001. Infect Control Hosp Epidemiol 2003; 24:848–852.
14. Loeb M, Stevenson KB. SHEA Long-Term-Care Committee. Pneumococcal immunization in older adults: implications for the long-term-care setting. Infect Control Hosp Epidemiol 2004; 25:985–994.
15. Fiore AE, Nuorti JP, Levine OS, et al. Epidemic Legionnaires' disease two decades later: old sources, new diagnostic methods. Clin Infect Dis 1998; 26:426–433.
16. Standaert SM, Hutcheson RH, Schaffner W. Nosocomial transmission of salmonella gastronenteritis to laundry workers. Infect Control Hosp Epidemiol 1994; 15:22–26.
17. Olsen SJ, DeBess EE, McGivern TE, et al. A nosocomial outbreak of fluoroquinolone-resistant salmonella infection. N Engl J Med 2001; 344: 1572–1579.
18. Tallis G, Ng S, Ferreira C, Tan A, Griffith J. A nursing home outbreak of *Clostridium perfringens* associated with pureed food. Aust N Z J Public Health 1999; 23:421–423.
19. Winquist AG, Roome A, Mshar R, Fiorentino T, Mshar P, Hadler J. Outbreak of campylobacteriosis at a senior center. J Am Geriatr Soc 2001; 49:304–307.
20. Jiang X, Turf E, Hu J, et al. Outbreaks of gastroenteritis in elderly nursing homes and retirement facilities associated with human caliciviruses. J Med Virol 1996; 50:335–341.
21. Rodriguez EM, Parrott C, Rolka H, Monroe SS, Dwyer DM. An outbreak of viral gastroenteritis in a nursing home: importance of excluding ill employees. Infect Control Hosp Epidemiol 1996; 17:587–592.
22. Marx A, Shay DK, Noel JS, et al. An outbreak of acute gastroenteritis in a geriatric long-term care facility: combined application of epidemiological and molecular diagnostic methods. Infect Control Hosp Epidemiol 1999; 20:306–311.
23. Greene CM, Van Beneden CA, Javadi M, et al. Cluster of deaths from group A *Streptococcus* in a long-term care facility—Georgia, 2001. Am J Infect Control 2005; 33:108–113.
24. Andersen BM, Haugen H, Rasch M, Heldal HA, Tageson A. Outbreak of scabies in Norwegian nursing homes and home care patients: control and prevention. J Hosp Infect 2000; 45:160–164.
25. Wiener J, Quinn JP, Bradford PA, et al. Multiple antibiotic-resistant *Klebsiella* and *Escherichia coli* in nursing homes. JAMA 1999; 281:517–523.
26. Trick WE, Kuehnert MJ, Quirk SB, et al. Regional dissemination of vancoymcin-resistant enterococci resulting from interfacility transfer of colonized patients. J Infect Dis 1999; 180:391–396.

11

An Approach to Antimicrobial Therapy

Jay P. Rho

*Inpatient Pharmacy, Kaiser Foundation Hospital Los Angeles,
and School of Pharmacy, University of Southern California,
Los Angeles, California, U.S.A.*

KEY POINTS

1. Recognition of age-related physiologic, pharmacokinetic, and pharmacodynamic changes will enhance the appropriate selection and dosing of antimicrobial agents.
2. Promoting optimal use of antimicrobials in LTCFs requires diligent antimicrobial utilization review.
3. A high percentage of adverse drug events are generally considered preventable.
4. . Diminished clearance of antimicrobials in the geriatric patient is primarily associated with the decline in renal excretion.
5. Vast majority of common bacterial infections in LTCF residents can be successfully treated with an oral antibiotic, avoiding the need to initiate invasive parenteral therapy.

GENERAL ISSUES OF ANTIMICROBIAL THERAPY

Clinical Relevance

The overall approach to medication management in the long-term care setting remains an important topic of practical and clinical significance for clinicians. The number of residents receiving care in nursing homes in the United States on any given day has increased by 27% over the years from 1.28 million in 1977 to 1.63 million in 1999 (see also Chapter 1). The percentage of residents aged 65 years and older has also increased during this time span from 13% of residents were under 65 years of age in 1977 to less than 10% of residents in 1999 (1). Traditionally, clinicians have hospitalized long-term care residents following the diagnosis of an infection. More recently, treatment of the long-term care resident occurs within the long-term care facility (LTCF). The availability of well-tolerated and effective oral and intramuscular antimicrobial agents (e.g., fluoroquinolones and ceftriaxone) has provided greater options in therapeutic management in the LTCF. The availability of newer and more potent medications is certainly not without risks. In one study, 40% of long-term care residents were prescribed drugs that were thought to be inappropriate by a panel of geriatricians and geropharmacologists (2). The average number of medications used by residents in LTCFs was reported as 7.2 in a Los Angeles study (2) and 8.1 in a Boston study (3). Antimicrobial agents are among the most commonly prescribed drugs in LTCFs except for gastrointestinal drugs, analgesics, and psychoactive medications (3). Antimicrobial usage may seem disproportionately low compared with the 1.5 million infections observed in the long-term care setting annually (4), but indiscriminate prescribing of antimicrobial agents with lack of adequate documentation of infection, potential adverse drugs reactions, and emergence of antimicrobial resistance are major concerns (5). Clinicians must thus exercise caution in their approach to antimicrobial prescriptions: vulnerable populations, for example frail elderly persons residing in LTCFs, need particular consideration because of the additional increased morbidity and mortality associated with age-related decline in immune function, debility, and comorbid illnesses (diabetes mellitus, cerebrovascular accidents, alcoholism, malnutrition, etc.). There should be a rational approach to antimicrobial prescribing in residents of LTCFs, with focus on age-related physiologic, pharmacokinetic, and pharmacodynamic changes that can affect the selection and dosing of such chemotherapeutic agents.

Assessment of Antimicrobial Use in LTCFs

Data evaluating the appropriateness of the therapeutic utility of antimicrobial agents in LTCFs suggest that a substantial proportion of antibiotic treatments are often initiated in the absence of important diagnostic information, such as the presence of fever, leukocytosis, or culture information (6–8). One study surveying 42 nursing homes and 11 affiliated intermediate care facilities suggested that systemic antibiotics were initiated in 62.4% of cases with inadequate initial diagnostic evaluation (9). Another study that included 3899 residents from 52 nursing homes indicated that 22% of all antibiotics prescribed were unnecessary, that is, viral upper respiratory infection and asymptomatic bacteriuria (7). A similar study that focused on the usage pattern of a specific antibiotic, ciprofloxacin, in a long-term care setting found that only 25% of orders for that agent were appropriate and 23% were prescribed for inappropriate indications; 49% were considered inappropriate because of more effective and/or less expensive available alternatives (10). One study demonstrated that antibiotic prescribing for 282 elderly residents of an LTCF who received an antibiotic for a presumed urinary tract infection was inappropriate in 40% of cases; 222 (78.7%) cases, however, showed clinical improvement (11). Using a medication appropriateness index (12) to measure appropriateness of antibiotic prescribing, 113 antibiotic orders (39.7%) were considered inappropriate. The three antibiotics most often inappropriately prescribed were ciprofloxacin (too expensive), trimethoprim–sulfamethoxazole (TMP–SMX) (incorrect duration), and nitrofurantoin (improper dosage). In addition, inappropriate prescribing accounted for an additional $560 per day in treatment costs.

OPTIMIZING THE USE OF ANTIMICROBIAL AGENTS IN THE LTCF

The optimal use of antimicrobials in LTCFs remains problematic largely because of a delay in the diagnosis and initiation of appropriate treatment of infections. Typical manifestations of infection, such as fever, may be absent or blunted in many elderly patients with serious or life-threatening infections (13,14). Limited availability of laboratory and radiological data may, in addition, preclude a precise diagnosis. General principles for initiating antimicrobial therapy are described in Table 1.

Minimum Criteria for Initiation of Antimicrobial Agents

Minimum criteria for initiating systemic antibiotics for bacterial infections have been proposed by a consensus group of physicians, geriatricians, microbiologists, and epidemiologists (Appendix C) (15). These criteria were developed to provide guidelines for the appropriate initiation of empirical antibiotics in clinically stable LTCF residents; critically ill patients with sepsis or sepsis syndrome necessitating transfer to an acute care facility were not included. Empirical regimens for common infections found in LTCF residents, such as skin and soft-tissue infections, respiratory infections, and urinary infections, as well as fever of unknown origin, are outlined in Table 2. Other potential infections, such as intravenous catheter-related infections or infections of mucous membranes and conjunctivae, topical antibiotic use, use of antiviral and antifungal agents, prophylactic antibiotics; and chronic suppressive antibiotics were not addressed. Prospective assessment of these guidelines for appropriate antibiotic use has not been analyzed.

Table 1 Approach to Antimicrobial Prescribing in LTCFs

Not all clinical or functional changes in LTCF residents should be attributed
  to infections
Antibiotics should be administered only when there is potential clinical benefit.
  For example, studies have clearly shown that both men and women residing
  in LTCFs derive no benefit from treatment of asymptomatic bacteriuria
Chronic suppressive therapy with antibiotics or antimicrobial chemoprophylaxis
  should be restricted unless there is a documented evidence of clinical efficacy
  and therapeutic benefit
Continuation of antibiotic therapy beyond standard recommended periods should
  be discouraged. For example, catheter-related urosepsis should be treated until
  clinical sepsis is improved but should not be continued in an attempt to
  maintain sterile urine
In circumstances in which a specific pathogen is isolated and antibiotic sensitivity
  studies are available, the initial broad-spectrum antibiotic should be changed to
  a more narrow-spectrum agent, if the organism is susceptible to such an agent

Abbreviation: LTCF, long-term care facility.

Empirical Antimicrobial Therapy

An empirical antimicrobial regimen should be directed against the most
likely pathogens and able to achieve the desired therapeutic concentrations
at the suspected site of infection. The choice of a specific empirical antimicrobial regimen should be based on the severity of the patient's illness, the
nature of underlying diseases, prior exposures to antimicrobials, and history
of drug allergies. The Society of Healthcare Epidemiology of America has
published a position paper on antimicrobial use in LTCFs that provides
recommendations for empirical antimicrobial therapy for the most frequent
types of infections in nursing home residents, including upper and lower
respiratory tract infections, urinary tract infections, skin and soft-tissue
infections, diarrhea, and fever of unknown origin (Table 2) (16). (Please
refer to Chapters 12–22 on specific infections. Treatment recommendations
may vary from these suggestions.)

The common cold, pharyngitis, and sinus infections are the most frequent infections of the upper respiratory tract. Because the vast majority of
upper respiratory tract infections are viral in etiology, empirical antimicrobial
therapy is seldom indicated. However, if a throat culture or a reliable streptococcal screening test documents the presence of group A streptococci, penicillin
would be the drug of choice. For acute bacterial sinusitis, first-line therapy
includes any of the following antibiotics: trimethoprim–sulfamethoxazole,
amoxicillin, and cefuroxime axetil. The selection of amoxicillin–clavulanic
acid for acute bacterial sinusitis should be reserved for patients who
respond poorly to treatment with one of the first-line antibiotics (16).

Table 2 Empirical Antimicrobial Therapy for Common Infections[a]

Clinical syndrome	Empiric antimicrobial
Upper respiratory infection	
Coryza/common cold	None
Pharyngitis	None; treat only if group A *Streptococcus*
Sinus infection	TMP–SMX + amoxicillin, cefuroxime axetil, macrolide; second line: amoxicillin–clavulanic acid, quinolone
Lower respiratory infection	
Acute bronchitis	Most cases viral, no antibiotics indicated
Acute exacerbation of chronic bronchitis	Amoxicillin, TMP–SMX, doxycycline
Pneumonia	TMP–SMX, amoxicillin, cefuroxime axetil, macrolide, doxycycline; second line: amoxicillin–clavulanic acid, quinolone, clindamycin (aspiration pneumonia)
Urinary tract infection	TMP–SMX, quinolone, aminoglycoside (parenteral)
Skin/soft tissue	
Cellulitis	Cephalexin; second line: dicloxacillin, clindamycin, amoxicillin–clavulanic acid
Infected pressure ulcer[b]	Metronidazole or clindamycin and TMP–SMX or quinolone: amoxicillin–clavulanic acid
Candidiasis	Topical antifungal
Diarrhea	
Clostridium difficile	Metronidazole
Salmonella, Shigella	TMP–SMX, quinolone
Escherichia coli O157:H7	None

[a]Please refer to Chapters 12–22 on specific infections for treatment recommendations, which may differ from these recommendations because of clinician preference or more than one therapeutic option.
[b]May require surgical debridement; if severe systemic symptoms, initial parenteral therapy should be considered.
Abbreviation: TMP–SMX, trimethoprim–sulfamethoxazole.
Source: From Ref. 15.

Antimicrobial Utilization Review

Promoting the optimal use of antimicrobials in LTCFs requires diligent antimicrobial utilization review. Surveillance and control activities are the major foci of these programs. Antimicrobial utilization is logically within the purview of the infection control program. Infection control programs traditionally have advocated education, isolation techniques, and hand washing to control nosocomial infections; however, they now are beginning to address problems of antimicrobial use. A recent survey found that more than one-half of LTCFs had an antimicrobial utilization program (17).

Adverse Drug Events

Approximately 350,000 adverse drug events, 20,000 of which are fatal, occur each year among the 1.5 million residents of LTCFs in the United States (18). Studies that have evaluated the patterns and quality of medication prescribing in nursing homes (18,19) have found antimicrobials to be among the most frequently implicated drugs in causing adverse drug events. In a study of 18 community-based nursing homes located in eastern Massachusetts encompassing 28,839 nursing home resident-months, 546 adverse drug events (1.89 per 100 resident-months) and 188 potential adverse drug events (0.65 per 100 resident-months) were identified (18). Overall, 51% of the adverse drug events were judged to be preventable, including 171 (72%) of the 238 fatal, life-threatening, or serious events and 105 (34%) of the 308 significant events. Antibiotics were associated with 36% of nonpreventable adverse drug events, but fewer than 5% of the adverse drug events were considered preventable. The majority of adverse drug events associated with antibiotics were rashes and confirmed *Clostridium difficile* diarrhea.

Clinicians should be aware that adverse drug events occur more frequently in frail elderly, and, therefore, a systematic examination of adverse events to identify risk factors should be undertaken. Markers of adverse drug event risk include the absolute drug numbers taken by an individual patient. There is an exponential relationship between the number of concurrently used medications and the likelihood of an adverse drug event (20).

Certain drug classes are more commonly implicated in adverse drug events. Although cardiovascular drugs, nonsteroidal anti-inflammatory agents, and psychotropic drugs, by virtue of their frequency of use, are the most commonly implicated drug classes, antimicrobial agents are still commonly associated with adverse drug events in the elderly population.

Cost of Inappropriate Use of Antimicrobial Agents

The consequences of inappropriate use (or overuse and misuse) of anti-infective agents and resultant financial implications include exposing patients to the potential risk of adverse drug reactions, selection of resistant bacteria, and high rates of nosocomial infections—all of which will increase health-care costs (21,22). The total cost of inappropriate prescribing of antimicrobials can be grossly estimated. These agents are among the most costly of all drugs prescribed in the United States, accounting for sales between $3 and $4 billion (22). If a quarter of all prescriptions for anti-infective agents are considered inappropriate for various reasons, this could account for an additional annual cost to the health-care system of $1 billion. Further, the increased costs of treating adverse drug reactions, infections, and their complications resulting from drug resistance also have to be considered. Because the geriatric population is becoming the highest user of health-care services and the largest consumers of drugs, it is essential that a rational approach to prescribing drugs for the elderly, including antimicrobial agents, be emphasized.

DRUG FACTORS TO CONSIDER IN PRESCRIBING ANTIMICROBIAL THERAPY

Once an antimicrobial agent is selected on the basis of known or anticipated activity against the pathogen(s), the goal of therapy is to deliver that drug to the site of infection in concentrations sufficient to inhibit or kill the organism(s). Most serious infections require antibiotic concentrations to exceed the minimum inhibitory concentration of the infecting organism at the site of infection. Some drugs, such as aminoglycosides and fluoroquinolones, exhibit concentration-dependent antimicrobial effects, with high drug concentrations exerting more rapid bactericidal action and longer postantibiotic effects (PAE) than lower concentrations. The elderly undergo age-related physiologic changes that directly influence the disposition and efficacy of various antimicrobial agents (23). The progressive decrease in the ability of vital organ systems of the elderly to maintain homeostasis can lead to alterations in drug clearance and drug receptor sensitivity.

Pharmacokinetics

Pharmacokinetics describes the fundamental mechanics of drug movement through the body over time, including factors that describe the absorption, distribution, metabolism, and elimination, or the overall fate of a drug in vivo (24). A summary of age-related physiological changes is shown in Table 3 (24,25).

Absorption

Age-related changes in the gastrointestinal tract may influence drug absorption. A decrease in gastric acid secretion and an increase in gastric pH are associated with the aging process. The absorption of antimicrobials that are dependent on increased acidity (e.g., sulfonamides, ketoconazole) may be decreased, whereas drugs that are degraded in an acidic environment will have greater bioavailability. The significance of these changes is generally minimal and rarely affects dosing requirements.

Distribution

Age-related changes that can affect the distribution of drugs include changes in body composition and cardiac output. In the elderly, the ratio of body fat to total body water is increased compared with younger individuals. A decrease in lean body mass, coupled with a decrease in total body water, is associated with a decreased volume of distribution for water-soluble drugs. Thus, with older adults, antimicrobials that are distributed primarily

Table 3 Physiological Changes Associated with Aging

Pharmacokinetic parameter	Physiological change with aging
Absorption	↑ Gastric emptying
	↓ Gastric acidity
	↓ Gastrointestinal motility
	↓ Absorptive surface
Distribution	↓ Lean body mass
	↑ Body fat
	↓ Serum albumin
	↑ α1-acid glycoprotein
Elimination	↑↓ Enzyme activity
	↓ Hepatic (liver) blood flow
	↓ Renal (kidney) blood flow
	↓ Glomerular filtration rate
	↓ Tubular secretion

Key: ↓, decrease activity or function; ↑, increase activity or function; ↑↓, may increase or decrease activity or function.

in body water or lean mass may have higher blood concentrations than in younger adults, which can lead to potential toxicity (e.g., aminoglycosides). Conversely, in the elderly, lipid-soluble drugs have a greater body fat distribution, which may reduce blood concentrations and lead to potential subtherapeutic blood concentrations.

Metabolism

Age appears to have no significant effect on the functional activity of various cytochrome P450 isoenzymes, either in terms of in vitro protein content, immunohistochemical content, or in vivo enzyme activity for older patients, as compared with younger patients.

Clearance

Age-related changes in renal function are probably the most significant contributors to alteration in drug clearance. Reduction in kidney mass, renal blood flow, and the subsequent number of functioning nephrons, glomerular filtration rate, and the rate of tubular secretion accounts for the decreased renal excretory capacity observed with aging (24,25). Diminishing renal function and lack of compensatory increases in nonrenal clearance in elderly patients have been associated with prolongation of the serum half-lives of beta-lactams, aminoglycosides, glycopeptides, sulfonamides, and fluoroquinolones. The primary route of clearance for selected antimicrobial agents is listed in Table 4.

Table 4   Routes of Antimicrobial Clearance

Drug	Primary route of clearance
Penicillins	
Ampicillin	Tubular secretion
Ampicillin/sulbactam	Tubular secretion
Methicillin	Tubular secretion
Nafcillin	Hepatic/biliary excretion/renal
Oxacillin	Hepatic/biliary excretion/renal
Penicillin G	Tubular secretion
Piperacillin	Tubular secretion/hepatic
Ticarcillin	Tubular secretion
Cephalosporins	
Cefazolin	Tubular secretion
Cephapirin	Tubular secretion
Cefotetan	Tubular secretion
Cefoxitin	Tubular secretion
Cefuroxime	Tubular secretion
Cefoperazone	Biliary excretion
Cefotaxime	Hepatic/tubular secretion
Ceftazidime	Tubular secretion
Ceftizoxime	Tubular secretion
Ceftriaxone	Renal/hepatic
Carbapenems	
Ertapenem	Tubular excretion
Imipenem/cilastatin	Tubular excretion
Meropenem	Tubular excretion
Monobactams	
Aztreonam	Glomerular filtration and tubular secretion
Quinolones	
Ciprofloxacin	Hepatic/tubular secretion
Ofloxacin	Tubular secretion
Lomefloxacin	Tubular secretion
Levofloxacin	Hepatic/tubular secretion
Moxifloxacin	Hepatic
Gatifloxacin	Hepatic/tubular secretion
Tetracyclines	
Doxycycline	Hepatic
Minocycline	Hepatic
Tetracycline	Glomerular filtration
Macrolides	
Azithromycin	Hepatic
Clarithromycin	Hepatic/renal
Erythromycin	Hepatic
Vancomycin	Glomerular filtration
Aminoglycosides	Glomerular filtration

Tissue Penetration

Some drugs, such as aminoglycosides, macrolides, and fluoroquinolones, bind extensively to certain tissue components. Intracellular accumulation of aminoglycoside is slow, however, because of its poor membrane permeability. Intracellular aminoglycoside concentrations tend to be low after initial drug exposure but are high after more sustained exposure and multiple dosing. However, the drug is microbiologically inactive in an acidic environment, such as in the phagolysosome. Indeed, the high intracellular aminoglycoside concentrations achieved in the renal cortex after multiple doses may be the cause of their nephrotoxicity.

Pharmacodynamics

Pharmacodynamics refers to the action of drugs or the biological effects resulting from the interaction of a drug and its receptor site. Pharmacodynamics describes the antimicrobial effect at the site of infection as well as toxic effects in relation to the concentrations of the antimicrobial drug during the course of drug therapy.

For drugs with concentration-dependent bacterial activity, such as aminoglycosides and fluoroquinolones, the rate and extent of bactericidal action increase with increasing drug concentrations above the minimum bactericidal concentration (MBC) up to a point of maximum effect, usually 5 to 10 times the MBC. In addition, the duration of the PAE is concentration-dependent with these drugs, and thus longer PAEs are induced by higher drug concentrations.

In contrast, the bactericidal activity of most beta-lactam antibiotics against gram-negative bacilli is relatively slow and continues as long as the concentrations are in excess of the MBC. It does not increase as the drug concentration is increased, that is the bactericidal action of beta-lactams is time-dependent and not concentration-dependent. For time-dependent agents that exhibit little to no postantibiotic intervals—such as extended-spectrum beta-lactams effective against most gram-negative bacilli—multiple, small, frequent doses or continuous intravenous infusion produces similar or superior bactericidal effects compared with infrequently administered larger doses.

Drug Interactions

Drug interactions constitute an often predicable and avoidable cause of adverse drug events. It has been well documented that the potential for drug–drug interactions increases with both age and with the number of medications prescribed (26–28). One report suggests that the potential for an interaction reaches 100% once the number of drugs used reaches eight (29). The mechanisms of adverse drug interactions are varied, but the inhibition or induction of drug metabolism is considered of highest importance.

Oxidative metabolism by cytochrome p450 enzymes is a primary method of drug metabolism. The purpose of drug metabolism is to make drugs more water-soluble so that they can be more easily excreted from the body. Drug interactions involving the cytochrome p450 system are common and generally result from either enzyme inhibition or induction. Enzyme inhibition generally involves competition with another drug for enzyme binding sites and usually begins with the first dose of the inhibitor. Duration of inhibition corresponds to the half-lives of the respective drugs. Inhibitors and inducers of the hepatic monoxygenase system include the following antimicrobial agents: fluconazole, miconazole, ketoconazole, erythromycin, clarithromycin, sulfonamides, and fluoroquinolones (30).

POTENTIALLY USEFUL AND SAFE ANTIMICROBIAL AGENTS FOR LTCF RESIDENTS

The vast majority of common bacterial illnesses in LTCF residents responded promptly to broad-spectrum oral antibiotics, but parenteral therapy is occasionally necessary for more severe infections. Some LTCFs have the capacity to provide parenteral therapies. There are antibiotics that may be administered via the intramuscular route, for example select third-generation cephalosporins, such as ceftriaxone, that, when administered intramuscularly, demonstrate similar efficacy compared with the intravenous injection. In addition, several antibiotics, such as quinolones, have oral formulations that achieve systemic concentrations comparable to a parenteral route (31). Such advances should mitigate the need for transfer of LTCF residents to an acute care facility for mild to moderate or uncomplicated infections (32).

Aminoglycosides

Aminoglycosides in the elderly must be prescribed with caution because of the well-documented risks of enhanced ototoxicity and nephrotoxicity associated with these agents and the availability of safer and less toxic drugs with comparable spectra (i.e., cephalosporins, monobactams, carbapenems, beta-lactam/beta-lactamase inhibitor combination antibiotics, and quinolones). However, these agents are rapidly bactericidal against staphylococci and gram-negative aerobic bacteria, including *Pseudomonas* sp., and often provide synergy with other agents (e.g., beta-lactams) for treatment of serious or life-threatening infections, such as enterococcal endocarditis (33). Renal impairment (generally reversible) and ototoxicity (generally irreversible) are the two most common and important potential adverse effects of these antibiotics (34). Because plasma half-life is increased in patients with decreased renal function (most common in elderly persons), the dose should be reduced on the basis of the creatinine clearance. Nephrotoxicity is less likely with once-daily dosing compared with the conventional every eight-hour dosing and is usually reversible (35). However, nephrotoxicity may lead to high serum levels of aminoglycosides, which can cause irreversible ototoxicity. Risk of ototoxicity increases with age and is highest in patients with preexisting hearing deficiencies. Thus, aminoglycoside use in older LTCF residents should be reserved for those with serious or life-threatening infections that require hospitalization and are caused by pathogens susceptible to aminoglycosides (36).

Beta-Lactams

Select beta-lactam antibiotics (penicillins, cephalosporins, carbapenems, monobactams, and beta-lactamase inhibitors) may be useful in the management of infections in LTCFs because of their broad spectrum, favorable pharmacokinetics, and favorable safety profiles. These would include parenteral cefotetan, cefriaxone, cefoperazone, and cefipime, as well as oral agents, such as penicillin, dicloxacillin, amoxicillin, amoxicillin–clavulanate, cephalexin, cefuroxime axetil, and cefixime (36).

Macrolides

Erythromycin, clarithromycin, and azithromycin have a limited role in the management of infections in the elderly in general. Clarithromycin and azithromycin have more favorable dosing regimens, improved antimicrobial activity, and lower gastrointestinal intolerance compared with erythromycin. These agents are moderately active against most strains of streptococci, methicillin-sensitive *Staphylococcus aureus*, anaerobes, *Moraxella catarrhalis, Haemophilus influenzae, Legionella, Mycoplasma pneumoniae*, and *Chlamydia pneumoniae*, as well as such atypical mycobacteria as *Mycobacterium avium* complex. Limited data are available regarding pharmacokinetics of these newer macrolides in elderly persons; decrease in drug clearance has been attributed to reduced renal clearance. The indications for the newer macrolides in elderly LTCF residents are no different from that for the general population. Although macrolides have been recommended in community-acquired pneumonia, it is unclear whether these agents are indicated in LTCF residents with such infections (37) (see also Chapter 14).

Ketolides

Telithromycin is the first Food and Drug Administration–approved member of a new class of antimicrobials called the ketolides. Telithromycin is similar in chemical structure to the macrolides, including the same basic 14-member lactone structure as erythromycin. Telithromycin differs in chemical structure from macrolides in the replacement of the cladinose ring with a ketone group at position 3 and the addition of an 11–12 cyclic carbamate. These chemical modifications enhance telithromycin's spectrum of activity while maintaining the acid stability of the newer macrolides (38).

Telitromycin is active against common community-acquired respiratory pathogens, including penicillin or macrolide-resistant strains of *S. pneumoniae*. Telitromycin is also active against the atypical, intracellular pathogens *M. pneumoniae*, and *Legionella pneumophila*. Telithromycin has poor activity against other gram-negative bacilli, including Enterobacteriaceae and *Pseudomonas aeruginosa* (39).

Clindamycin

This agent is commonly used for anaerobic and staphylococcal infections and for life-threatening group A beta-hemolytic streptococcal infections (streptococcal toxic shock syndrome, necrotizing fasciitis), the latter necessitating acute care facility transfer. Residents of LTCFs are particularly susceptible to antibiotic-associated colitis caused by *C. difficile*; clindamycin use is a relatively common association. The drug has utility in the LTCF for treating mild to moderate infections, such as skin and soft-tissue infections, including infected pressure ulcers, oral and dental infections, and respiratory tract infections caused by susceptible bacteria.

Fluoroquinolones

The fluoroquinolones are a group of synthetic antibiotics that have a broad spectrum of antimicrobial activity, good absorption from the gastrointestinal tract, a unique mechanism of action (inhibition of bacterial topoisomerases), favorable pharmacokinetic properties, and a good safety profile (40).

As a group, the fluoroquinolones have excellent in vitro activity against a wide range of gram-positive bacteria and many gram-negative bacteria, such as Enterobacteriaceae and *Aeromonas, Brucella, Camphylobacter, Haemophilus, Legionella, Moraxella, Neisseria,* and *Vibrio*. These agents are active against *P. aeruginosa* but are significantly less active against other pseudomonal species, including *P. capacia* and *P. fluorescens*. Ciprofloxacin is the most active quinolone against *P. aeruginosa*. The newer generation fluoroquinolones have activity against gram-positive bacteria, including *S. pneumoniae* and staphylococcal species, i.e., methicillin-sensitive *S. aureus* and coagulase-negative species. The fluoroquinolones have less activity against streptococcal species and enterococci.

These agents in general have very poor activity against anaerobes and *Nocardia* organisms. Ciprofloxacin and ofloxacin are active against many species of *Mycobacterium*, including *M. tuberculosis, M. kansasii, M. fortuitum,* and *M. xenopi*. Ciprofloxacin initially was introduced to North America in 1987. Since its release, it has been widely used in LTCFs (31). These agents are used because they allow the convenience of oral therapy with an agent with good bioavailability, are easily administered by one- or twice-daily dosing, are perceived to be safe, and have wide spectrum of activity. In the elderly, quinolones are useful in the treatment of complicated urinary tract infections, bacterial prostatitis, skin and soft-tissue infections, pneumonia, malignant external otitis, and bacterial diarrhea caused by susceptible pathogens (31). The newer generation fluoroquinolones (e.g., levofloxacin, gatifloxacin, moxifloxacin) with improved gram-positive (including *S. pneumoniae*) activity over that of the older agents in this class are now considered agents of choice for the treatment of community-acquired pneumonia in adults, including the elderly (41). Adverse effects of quinolones in the elderly occur in 5% to 15% of cases, including gastrointestinal (nausea, vomiting, diarrhea) and central nervous system (dizziness, headache, insomnia) effects. Associated drug interactions with other medications include decreased theophylline clearance associated with increased serum levels of ciprofloxacin, but not norfloxacin or levofloxacin, and multivalent ions (e.g., calcium, iron, aluminum) contained in foods or drugs that significantly reduce absorption of quinolones from the upper gastrointestinal tract. With the intense quinolone use in many LTCFs, quinolone resistance of organisms has increased. Resistance via mutations in the genes encoding topoisomerase II and IV along with increased drug efflux is common in clinical isolates. Quinolone resistance [methicillin-resistant *S. aureus* (MRSA), *Enterococcus faecalis*, *S. pneumoniae*, and *P. aeruginosa*] complicates management of infections by requiring parenteral therapy with other antibiotics for organisms resistant to these oral agents, as well as increasing the burden of resistant organisms (42). Hence, the appropriate use of quinolones in LTCFs must be periodically assessed.

Trimethoprim–Sulfamethoxazole

This antibiotic is commonly prescribed in the elderly, for urinary tract infections, chronic bacterial prostatitis, lower respiratory tract infections, and bacterial diarrhea caused by susceptible pathogens. Data are limited on the pharmacokinetics of this drug in elderly persons (43). Oral drug absorption does not appear to be affected by age. Renal clearance of trimethoprim is decreased in older persons. The recommended doses for use in the elderly are comparable to those prescribed in younger persons; with renal impairment and a creatinine clearance of less than 30 mL/min but greater than 15 mL/min, the dosage is reduced by half. The drug should be avoided if the creatinine clearance is less than 15 mL/min.

Miscellaneous Antibiotics

Other antibiotics that could be prescribed in residents of LTCFs and deserve brief mention include vancomycin, quinupristin + dalfopristin (Synercid®), linezolid (Zyvox®), daptomycin (Cubicin®), and metronidazole. Vancomycin is a glycopeptide antibiotic used primarily for gram-positive bacterial infections. It is highly active against staphylococci (including MRSA) and streptococci (including vancomycin-sensitive enterococci). In the elderly, studies have indicated that reduced clearance of vancomycin is a consequence of reduced systemic and renal clearance as well as enhanced tissue binding of the drug. Lower parenteral doses are recommended for the frail elderly, and the dose should be adjusted according to the serum peak and trough levels as well as the creatinine clearance (44). The side effect profile in the elderly is no different from that in the general population.

Quinupristin–dalfopristin, which is a streptogramin, is indicated in adults, including the elderly, for the treatment of serious and life-threatening or bacteremic infection with vancomycin-resistant enterococci and complicated skin and skin structure infection with methicillin-sensitive *S. aureus* and *Streptococcus pyogenes* (45). The pharmacokinetics of this agent are similar to that in younger adults.

Linezolid, an oxazolidinone, is active against infections caused by sensitive gram-positive bacteria, as well as MRSA and vancomycin-resistant enterococci (46). This agent's availability, both in parenteral and oral formulations, as well as its relatively safe profile, is particularly advantageous in management of infections caused by such gram-positive-resistant organisms commonly encountered in elderly LTCF residents.

Daptomycin is a cyclic lipopeptide indicated for the treatment of complicated skin and skin structure infections caused by susceptible gram-positive organisms such as *Staphylococcus* (including MRSA) and *Streptococcus* (47). Daptomycin should not be used in the treatment of pneumonia. Because daptomycin is eliminated primarily by renal excretion, patients with creatinine clearance less than 30 mL/min should receive a reduced dosage. No dosage adjustment is necessary in geriatric patients with normal renal function (48).

Antituberculous Agents

Because most tuberculosis cases in the elderly are caused by isoniazid-sensitive and rifampin-sensitive *M. tuberculosis*, the primary drugs for the treatment of active tuberculosis disease in this age group are isoniazid and rifampin. Isoniazid also should be used for the treatment of latent tuberculosis infection when the appropriate indications are present (see Chapter 15).

Antifungal Agents

Similar to younger adults, the commonly prescribed systemic antifungal agents in the elderly include amphotericin B, fluconazole, itraconazole, and voraconazole. Because of potential toxicity of amphotericin B to renal function in the elderly, this agent must be used with caution. Fluconazole, because of its relative safety and efficacy and excellent bioavailability when administered by parenteral and oral routes, is prescribed more often in aging individuals. Itraconazole and voraconazole, available by parenteral and oral formulations, are acceptable alternatives, when indicated (see also Chapter 26).

Antiviral Agents

The antiviral agent commonly prescribed in the elderly includes amantadine, rimantadine, acyclovir, valacyclovir, and famciclovir. Amantadine and rimantadine are recommended for influenza A infection within 48 hours of illness onset in the ambulatory elderly to reduce the duration and severity of illness: in institutionalized elderly, these drugs are recommended for prophylaxis during an influenza A outbreak within the institution. Both drugs are continued for a minimum of two weeks or until approximately one week after the end of the outbreak. However, recent data indicate an increasing incidence of influenza A resistant to amantadine and rimantadine, which may limit the clinical utility of these two agents. The neurominidase inhibitors, zanamivir and oseltamivir, are available for use in influenza A and B infections; efficacy and safety in elderly patients have not been extensively studied. The neuraminidase inhibitors oseltamivir phosphate (Tamiflu®) and zanamivir (Relenza®) are used for the symptomatic treatment of uncomplicated acute illness caused by influenza A and B virus in adults who have been symptomatic for no longer than two days. Dosage adjustments based solely on age are not necessary for geriatric patients older than 65 years of age. Oseltamivir may be used as an adjunct agent along with the annual influenza virus vaccine for the prophylaxis of influenza A or B virus infection in adults. The safety and efficacy of zanamivir for the prophylaxis of influenza virus infection remains to be established (49,50) (see Chapter 13).

Acyclovir, valacyclovir, and famiciclovir are effective agents for the treatment of herpes simplex and herpes zoster infection. Pain from herpes zoster and chronic pain (postherpetic neuralgia) may be relatively diminished by administering these agents within the first 72 hours of the onset of illness (see also Chapter 17).

SUGGESTED READING

Nicolle LE, Bentley DW, Garibaldi R, Neuhaus EG, Smith PW. The SHEA Long-Term Care Committee. Antimicrobial use in long-term-care facilities. Infect Control Hosp Epidemiol 2000; 21:537–545.

Rajagopalan S, Yoshikawa TT. Antimicrobial therapy in the elderly. Med Clin North Am 2001; 85:133–147.

Reese RE, Betts RF. Antibiotic use. In: Betts RF, Chapman SW, Penn RL, eds. Reese and Betts. A Practical Approach to Infectious Diseases. 5th ed. Lippincott: Williams & Wilkins, 2003:969–1148.

REFERENCES

1. Decker FH. Nursing Homes, 1977–99: What Has Changed, What Has Not? Hyattsville, MD: National Center for Health Statistics, 2005.
2. Beers MH, Ouslander JG, Finegold SF, et al. Inappropriate medication prescribing in skilled-nursing facilities. Ann Intern Med 1992; 117:684–689.

3. Avorn J, Gurwitz JH. Drug use in the nursing home. Ann Intern Med 1995; 123:195–204.
4. Haley RW, Culver DH, White JW. The nationwide nosocomial infection rate: a new need for vital statistics. Am J Epidemiol 1985; 121:159.
5. Yoshikawa TT. VRE, MRSA, PRP, and DRGNB in LTCF: lessons to be learned from the alphabet. J Am Geriatr Soc 1998; 46:241–243.
6. Katz PR, Beam TR Jr., Brand F, Boyce K. Antibiotic use in the nursing home physician practice patterns. Arch Intern Med 1990; 150:1464–1468.
7. Warren JW, Palumbo FB, Fitterman L, Speedie SM. Incidence and characteristics of antibiotic use and aged nursing home patients. J Am Geriatr Soc 1991; 39:963–972.
8. Lee YL, Thrupp LD, Friis RH. Nosocomial infection and antibiotic utilization in geriatric patients: a pilot prospective surveillance program in skilled nursing facilities. Gerontology 1992; 38:223–232.
9. Zimmer JG, Bentley DW, Valenti WM, Watson NM. Systemic antibiotic use in nursing homes: a quality assessment. J Am Geriatr Soc 1986; 34:703–710.
10. Pickering TD, Gurwitz JH, Zalenznik D, Noonan JP, Avorn J. The appropriateness of oral fluoroquinolone-prescribing in the long-term care setting. J Am Geriatr Soc 1994; 42:28–32.
11. Miller SW, Warnock R, Marshall LL. Appropriateness of antibiotic prescribing for urinary tract infections in long-term care facilities. Consult Pharm 1991; 14:157–177.
12. Hanlon JT, Schmader KE, Samsa GP. A method for assessing drug therapy appropriate. J Clin Epidemiol 1992; 45:1045–1051.
13. Norman DC. Fever and aging. Infect Dis Clin Pract 1998; 7:387–390.
14. Yoshikawa TT, Norman DC. Fever in the elderly. Infect Med 1998; 15:704–706.
15. Loeb M, Bentley DW, Bradley S, et al. Development of minimum criteria for the initiation of antibiotics in residents of long-term-care facilities: results of a consensus conference. Infect Control Hosp Epidemiol 2001; 22:120–124.
16. Nicolle LE, Bentley DW, Garibaldi R, Neuhaus EG, Smith PW, the SHEA Long-Term Care Committee. Antimicrobial use in long-term-care facilities. Infect Control Hosp Epidemiol 2000; 21:537–545.
17. Crossley K, Henry K, Irvine P, Willenbring K. Antibiotic use in nursing homes: prevalence, cost, and utilization review. Bull N Y Acad Med 1987; 63:510–518.
18. Gurwitz JH, Field TS, Avorn J, et al. Incidence and preventability of adverse drug events in nursing homes. Am J Med 2000; 109:87–94.
19. Gurwitz JH, Sanchez-Cross MT, Eckler MA, Matulis J. The epidemiology of adverse and unexpected events in the long-term care setting. J Am Geriatr Soc 1994; 42:33–38.
20. Atkin PA, Shenfield GM. Medication-related adverse reactions and the elderly: a literature review. Adverse Drug React Toxicol Rev 1995; 14:175–191.
21. Rho JP, Yoshikawa TT. The cost of inappropriate use of anti-infective agents in older patients. Drugs Aging 1995; 6:263–267.
22. Mylotte JM. Antimicrobial prescribing in long-term care facilities: prospective evaluation of potential antimicrobial use and cost indicators. Am J Infect Control 1999; 27:10–19.
23. Myers BR, Wilkinson P. Clinical pharmacokinetics of antimicrobial drugs in the elderly: implications for selection and dosage. Clin Pharmacokinet 1989; 17:385–395.

24. Kimirons MT, Crome P. Clinical pharmacokinetic considerations in the elderly: an update. Clin Pharmacokinet 1997; 33:302–312.
25. Bennett W. Geriatric pharmacokinetics and the kidney. Am J Kidney Dis 1990:283–288.
26. Hall MRP. Drug interactions in the elderly. Gerontology 1982; 28(suppl 1):18–24.
27. Reidenberg M. Drug interactions and the elderly. J Am Geriatr Soc 1982; 30(suppl):S67–S68.
28. Hussar DA. Drug interactions in the older patient. Geriatrics 1988; 43:20–30.
29. Sloan RW. Drug interactions. Am Fam Physician 1983; 27:229–238.
30. Seymour RM, Routledge PA. Important drug–drug interactions in the elderly. Drugs Aging 1998; 12:485–494.
31. Guay DRP. Quinolones. In: Yoshikawa TT, Norman DC, eds. Antimicrobial Therapy in the Elderly Patient. New York: Marcel Dekker Inc., 1994:237–310.
32. Ernest ME, Ernest EJ. Effectively treating common infection in residents of long-term care facilities. Pharmacotherapy 1999; 19:1026–1035.
33. Bonza E, Munoz P. Monotherapy versus combination therapy for bacterial infections. Med Clin North Am 2000; 84:1357–1389.
34. Zaske DE. Aminoglycosides. In: Yoshikawa TT, Norman DC, eds. Antimicrobial Therapy in the Elderly Patient. New York: Marcel Dekker Inc., 1994:183–235.
35. Dew RB III, Susla GM. Once-daily aminoglycoside treatment. Infect Dis Clin Pract 1996; 5:12–24.
36. Rajagopalan S, Yoshikawa TT. Antimicrobial therapy in the elderly. Med Clin North Am 2001; 85:133–147.
37. Naughton DJ, Mylotte JM. Treatment guidelines for nursing-home acquired pneumonia based in community practice. J Am Geriatr Soc 2000; 48:82–88.
38. Javala J, Kataja J, Seppala H, Houvinen P. In vitro activities of the novel ketolide telithromycin against erythromycin-resistant *Streptococcus* species. Antimicrob Agents Chemother 2001; 45:789–793.
39. Felmingham D. Microbiological profile of telithromycin, the first ketolide antimicrobial. Clin Microb Infect 2001; 7(suppl 3):S2–S10.
40. Owens RC Jr., Ambrose PG. Clinical use of fluoroquinolones. Med Clin North Am 2000; 84:1447–1469.
41. Marrie TJ. Community-acquired pneumonia in the elderly. Clin Infect Dis 2000; 31:1066–1078.
42. Strausbaugh LJ, Crossley KB, Nurse BA, Thrupp LD. The SHEA Long-Term Care Committee. Antimicrobial resistance in long-care facilities. Infect Control Hosp Epidemiol 1996; 17:129–140.
43. Williams L, Bender BS. Trimethoprim–sulfamethoxazole. In: Yoshikawa TT, Norman DC, eds. Antimicrobial Therapy in the Elderly Patient. New York: Marcel Dekker Inc., 1994:169–181.
44. Yoshikawa TT. Antimicrobial therapy for the elderly patient. J Am Geriatr Soc 1990; 38:1353–1372.
45. Nichols RL, Graham DR, Barriere SL, the Synercid Skin and Skin Structure Infection Group. Treatment of hospitalized patients with complicated gram-positive skin and skin structure infections: two randomized, multicenter studies of quinupristin/dalfopristin versus cefazolin, oxacillin or vancomycin. J Antimicrob Chemother 1999; 44:263–273.

46. Chien JW, Kucia ML, Salata RA. Use of linezolid, an oxazolidinone, in the treatment of multidrug-resistant gram-positive bacterial infections. Clin Infect Dis 2000; 30:146–151.
47. Akins RL, Rybak MJ. In vitro activities of daptomycin, arbekacin, vancomycin, and gentamicin alone and/or in combination against glycopeptide intermediate-resistant *Staphylococcus aureus* in an infection model. Antimicrob Agents Chemother 2000; 44(7):1925–1929.
48. Product Information: Cubicin®, daptomycin for injection. Lexington, MA: Cubist Pharmaceuticals, 2003.
49. Product Information: Tamiflu®, oseltamivir. Nutley NJ: Roche Pharmaceuticals, 2001.
50. Product Information: Relenza®, zanamivir for inhalation. Research Triangle Park, NC: GlaxoSmithKline, 2003.

12

Urinary Tract Infection

Lindsay E. Nicolle

Departments of Internal Medicine and Medical Microbiology,
University of Manitoba, Winnipeg,
Manitoba, Canada

KEY POINTS

1. The prevalence of asymptomatic bacteriuria is high in long-term care facilities, reaching 50% in women and 35% to 40% in men.

2. The diagnosis of symptomatic urinary infection in long-term care facilities is frequently problematic. With the high prevalence of bacteriuria, a positive urine culture has low predictive value. Chronic genitourinary symptoms, difficulties in communication, and aging-associated changes compromise evaluation of clinical symptoms and signs.

3. Treatment of symptomatic urinary infection for noncatheterized patients should be initiated if acute symptoms referable to the genitourinary tract are present.

4. Residents with long-term indwelling catheters are always bacteriuric and have increased morbidity from urinary infection compared with bacteriuric noncatheterized residents.

5. Selection of antimicrobial therapy for symptomatic urinary infection is similar for long-term care facility and younger populations. The potential impact of antimicrobial pressure on institutional and patient antimicrobial resistance should be considered in antimicrobial selection.

INTRODUCTION

Urinary tract infection is the most common infection that occurs in elderly residents of long-term care facilities (LTCFs). It is the most frequent source of bacteremia and a common reason for transfer of residents to acute care facilities. Urinary infection is also one of the most common indications for antimicrobial therapy in these facilities, but much of the antimicrobial use for urinary infection in LTCFs is inappropriate (1). Thus, an understanding of urinary infection in residents of LTCFs is important for optimal resident care and to promote appropriate antimicrobial use in this setting.

The term urinary tract infection simply means the presence of a microbial pathogen within the normally sterile urinary tract. However, it is generally used in the context of isolation of organisms in the urine at a quantitative level, which excludes contamination. Urinary infection may be asymptomatic, also called asymptomatic bacteriuria, when microorganisms are present in the urinary tract, but there are no symptoms or signs referable to urinary infection in the host. Individuals with asymptomatic infection usually have evidence for an inflammatory or immune host response in the urinary tract. The term "colonization" is sometimes used, rather than asymptomatic bacteriuria. However, this term has no clinical relevance and is not used in this chapter.

An important group of individuals with urinary infection in LTCFs are those with bladder drainage by a chronic indwelling catheter. The epidemiology of infection, including morbidity, differs for residents with chronic catheters from elderly individuals with urinary infection without long-term indwelling catheters. Thus, patients in LTCFs with chronic indwelling catheters are considered as a distinct group. Observations should be considered relevant only for residents without indwelling catheters, unless stated otherwise.

EPIDEMIOLOGY AND CLINICAL RELEVANCE

Prevalence and Incidence

The prevalence of urinary infection in elderly residents of LTCFs is high (Table 1). Approximately 30% to 50% of women have positive urine cultures at any time. The prevalence in men is only slightly lower, at 20% to 40%. This reported prevalence is consistent in reports from different institutions and countries.

The incidence of both symptomatic and asymptomatic urinary infection is also high in these populations. Prospective studies of nursing home-acquired infections identify symptomatic urinary infection as the first or second most frequent infection, but with a wide range of incidence varying from 0 to 2.28 infections per 1000 resident days. However, the definitions used for symptomatic urinary infection lack specificity and may overestimate the occurrence of symptomatic infection. Studies that use more restrictive definitions report rates of symptomatic infection of 0.6 per 1000 resident

Table 1 Prevalence of Urinary Infection in Long-Term Care Facility Populations

	Female		Male	
Population (reference)	Number	Positive (%)	Number	Positive (%)
Nursing home, United States (2); incontinent, mean age 85 yr	158	57	56	25
Nursing home, Greece (3); mean age 78 yr	231	27	121	19
Institutionalized elderly, Sweden (4); mean age 84.6 yr	178	26	89	16
Veterans, Canada (5); mean age 80 yr			59	37
Long-term care, Canada (6); mean age 83 yr	101	53		
Nursing home, United States (7); mean age 83 yr	160	18–33		

days (8), or 0.5 per 1000 resident days for infection with fever (9). Symptomatic infection in women is reported to occur at a rate of 1.41 per 1000 resident days when inclusive criteria are used, but only 0.22/1000 resident days with more restrictive criteria, which require genitourinary symptoms (6). In men, 1.37 infections per 1000 resident days are reported with inclusive criteria and only 0.38 infections per 1000 resident days with more restrictive criteria (5).

Asymptomatic bacteriuria has also been characterized by the "turnover" of bacteriuria described by repeated prevalence surveys in the same population. One study reported (3) an initial prevalence of bacteriuria of 19% for men and 27% of women in a Greek home for the aged. At one year, 11% of men and 23% of women with initially negative urine cultures had developed positive cultures; 22% and 27% with initially positive urine cultures had become negative. Another study (7) reported an initial prevalence of bacteriuria of 25% in women, with 8% of residents with negative urine cultures becoming positive every six months and 31% of residents with initial positive urine cultures becoming negative. Another study (10) reported an initial prevalence of bacteriuria of 15% in a group of elderly women resident in both community housing and long-term care. The monthly probability of transition from positive to negative cultures was 0.30, and 0.12 from negative to positive. In another study in elderly institutionalized men, 10% of all nonbacteriuric residents became bacteriuric in a three-month period (5). Some residents have persistent bacteriuria, whereas others have acquisition of new organisms or resolution of bacteriuria. Thus, bacteriuria within a nursing home population is dynamic. Factors that contribute to the variation, including antimicrobial use, are not well studied.

Risk Factors

Urinary infection in residents of LTCFs is predictably associated with increased functional impairment (11). Residents with cognitive impairment, or who are incontinent of urine or bowel, are more likely to have bacteriuria. Impaired mobility and more prolonged duration of stay in the LTCF are also associated with bacteriuria in some studies. No association between specific medication use and urinary infection has been reported. Risk factors for symptomatic and asymptomatic infection appear to be similar.

The most important determinant of bacteriuria in the long-term care population appears to be neurologic impairment of bladder emptying. Chronic neurologic diseases, such as Alzheimer's disease, Parkinson's disease, or cerebrovascular disease, are usually accompanied by impaired voiding. These illnesses also frequently lead to institutionalization and are associated with cognitive impairment and incontinence of bladder and bowel. The neurogenic bladder results in incomplete voiding and increased likelihood of ureteral reflux, promoting both acquisition and persistence of infection. Devices used to manage incontinence may also increase the likelihood of urinary infection. Men who use an external condom catheter for incontinence management have twice the incidence of urinary infection, compared with men with incontinence who do not use external condom catheters. Prior indwelling catheter use may lead to acquisition of bacteriuria and prostate infection. Once prostatic infection is established, it frequently cannot be eradicated and may be a source for bacteriuria, causing relapsing symptomatic or asymptomatic infection.

Physiologic aging changes associated with urinary infection in well, community-living elderly populations may also contribute to urinary infection in the nursing home setting. Women with prior genitourinary surgery, or who have cystoceles, are more likely to have recurrent infection. The use of topical vaginal estrogen decreased the occurrence of both symptomatic and asymptomatic infection in some studies in older women, but the extent to which estrogen deficiency independently contributes to urinary infection in this population is not established. Prostatic hypertrophy is a uniform accompaniment of aging in men. This may result in urethral obstruction and urinary retention requiring instrumentation and also promotes turbulent urethral urine flow, which facilitates ascension of organisms into the bladder. Thus, multiple variables contribute to the high frequency of urinary infection in elderly LTCF residents, with the relative importance of potential factors varying with the individual resident.

Microbiology

The diversity of infecting organisms is greater in urinary infection in the LTCF compared with community populations (Table 2). Enterobacteriaceae are the most common organisms isolated from both symptomatic and

Table 2 Summary of Reported Distributions of Infecting Organisms Isolated in Bacteriuria in Nursing Home Residents

Organism	Percent of isolates (%)	
	Men	Women
Escherichia coli	11–12	50–53
Klebsiella spp.	5.9–8.3	15
Enterobacter spp.	1.0–1.7	3.8
Citrobacter spp.	2.5–3.9	0.8
Serratia spp.	6.4	
Proteus mirabilis	18–30	17–25
Providencia stuartii	4.2	
Morganella morganii	2.5	
Providencia spp.	11.8–19	3.8
Pseudomonas aeruginosa	11–19	
Other gram-negative bacteria		19
Enterococcus spp.	0.6–5.0	1.8–4.5
Coagulase negative staphylococci	1.7–11	1.8–4.5
Staphylococcus aureus	0.6–2.5	0.8
Other gram-positive bacteria	0.6–1.7	
Candida spp.	1.0	NS

Abbreviation: NS, not stated.

asymptomatic infection. *Escherichia coli* is most frequent in women, followed by *Proteus mirabilis* or *Klebsiella pneumoniae*. For men, *P. mirabilis* may be most common. Other Enterobacteriaceae isolated include *Citrobacter* spp. and *Serratia* spp. and such urease-producing organisms as *Providencia stuartii* and *Morganella morganii*. *P. stuartii* appears to have a predilection for institutionalized populations.

Pseudomonas aeruginosa and gram-positive organisms including *Enterococcus* spp. and coagulase-negative staphylococci are also common. Group B streptococci and *Staphylococcus aureus* are less frequent but occur in some patients in most reported series. Yeast infection, principally due to *Candida albicans*, may occur but is uncommon. The determinants of candiduria in LTCF residents are not well described, but this may be more common in women with associated vulvovaginal candidiasis, and in diabetic patients. The distribution of organisms isolated from symptomatic infection is similar to that for asymptomatic infection, although coagulase-negative staphylococci are uncommon in symptomatic infection.

Polymicrobial infection is present in 10% to 25% of bacteriuric residents. Men with external condom catheters used for voiding management often have infection with more than one organism. Bacteria isolated from urinary infection in LTCF residents are also characterized by increased antimicrobial resistance. This reflects the intense exposure of antimicrobials in nursing home residents (1), as well as opportunities for transmission of organisms between residents in the institutional setting.

Host Response

Asymptomatic bacteriuria is not simply the presence of bacteria in the bladder (11). At least 50% of women with asymptomatic infection have bacteria localized to the kidneys. Pyuria is also present in over 90% of bacteriuric subjects, but neither the presence nor degree of pyuria correlates with symptomatic infection or adverse outcomes. Increased urinary cytokine levels and increased local urinary or systemic antibodies to the infecting organism are also present in many residents with bacteriuria—further evidence for a host response with asymptomatic infection.

Symptomatic subjects uniformly have pyuria. They also have elevated levels of urinary cytokines and local urinary antibody. With resolution of the symptomatic episode, urinary antibodies may decrease, particularly with *E. coli* infection. In clinical presentations with systemic manifestations, such as fever, an elevated C-reactive protein is usually present, and systemic antibody to the infecting organism increases.

Clinical Impact

The majority of urinary infections in residents of LTCFs are asymptomatic. Persistent asymptomatic bacteriuria has not been associated with negative long-term outcomes, such as renal failure, hypertension, or decreased survival. Where an association between decreased survival and bacteriuria in residents has been observed, bacteriuria is not an independent association of mortality. Despite the very high prevalence of urease-producing organisms, including *P. mirabilis* and *P. stuartii*, renal or bladder stones have not been identified as a significant clinical problem in LTCF residents without chronic indwelling catheters.

Episodes of fever attributed to urinary infection have been reported with a frequency of 1 to 1.5 per 1000 resident days, comprising about one-tenth of episodes of fever of any cause in this population (9). The urinary tract is the most common source of bacteremia in LTCF residents, although most of these bacterimic patients have indwelling urinary catheters. Urinary infection is also a common reason for transfer of LTCF residents for acute hospitalization, but is infrequently a direct cause of death in residents.

Urinary infection is one of the most common indications for antimicrobial prescriptions in LTCFs. From 20% to 60% of systemic antimicrobial courses are given for treatment of urinary infection (1). This intensive use of antimicrobials contributes to the emergence and persistence of antimicrobial resistance in the long-term care setting.

Chronic Indwelling Catheter

From 5% to 10% of residents of LTCFs have voiding managed with a long-term indwelling urethral catheter (12). The daily incidence of new infection for individuals with a chronic indwelling catheter is similar to that reported with short-term catheters, about 3% to 7% per day. Thus, anyone with a catheter in place for more than 30 days, i.e., a chronic indwelling catheter, will be bacteriuric, and at any time the prevalence of bacteriuria in individuals with chronic catheters approaches 100%.

Biofilm formation occurs on the catheter, primarily on the interior surface. This material consists of bacteria, extracellular bacterial substances, and magnesium, calcium, and Tamm-Horsfall protein derived from urine. It may also contain struvite if infection with a urease-producing organism is present. Residents with long-term catheters are infected with a complex bacterial flora with two to five organisms present at any time. *P. mirabilis*, *Providencia* spp., *M. morganii*, and *P. aeruginosa* are the most common organisms isolated, although many other gram-negative and gram-positive organisms also occur. Biofilm contributes to catheter encrustation and obstruction. Bacteria growing in the biofilm are in an environment where they are relatively protected from the effect of host defenses or antimicrobials.

Residents of LTCFs with chronic indwelling catheters experience excess morbidity attributable to urinary infection compared with LTCF residents with bacteriuria without an indwelling catheter (13). Febrile urinary infection is 10 times more frequent in these individuals, and bacteremia, primarily from a urinary source, is 40 times more frequent (14). A chronic indwelling catheter may also cause episodes of hematuria and sepsis due to catheter trauma. Local suppurative complications include paraurethral abscesses, urethritis, epididymoorchitis, or prostatic abscesses. Residents with indwelling catheters have a higher mortality than LTCF residents without chronic indwelling catheters, but this difference is likely attributable to underlying patient differences rather than urinary infection. At autopsy, there is a higher frequency of histologic evidence for renal inflammation consistent with pyelonephritis in residents with a chronic catheter compared with bacteriuric residents without an indwelling catheter (13).

CLINICAL MANIFESTATIONS

Urinary infection is usually asymptomatic. However, symptomatic urinary infection is an important contributor to morbidity in LTCF residents. When symptomatic infection occurs, the clinical presentation may vary across a spectrum of minor lower tract irritative symptoms to severe systemic symptoms and sepsis requiring hospitalization. Potential clinical presentations of symptomatic infection are listed in Table 3. Symptoms and signs may be similar to those recognized in younger populations. For acute lower tract

Table 3 Potential Presentations of Symptomatic Urinary Tract Infection in Residents of Long-Term Care Facilities

---

Symptomatic urinary infection
    Acute cystitis (frequency, dysuria, suprapubic discomfort)
    Acute deterioration in continence
    Acute pyelonephritis (costovertebral angle pain/tenderness; often with fever)
    Fever with hematuria
    Fever with no localizing findings (10% due to urinary infection)
    Epididymoorchitis
Additional presentations with indwelling catheters
    Fever with catheter obstruction
    Acute confusion
    Urethritis
    Paraurethral abscess
    Bladder spasms with bypassing of catheter by urine
Not symptomatic urinary infection
    Chronic genitourinary symptoms
    Cloudy or foul smelling urine
    Clinical deterioration without fever or localizing genitourinary symptoms or signs

---

infection (acute cystitis), frequency, dysuria, urgency, and suprapubic discomfort may occur. Acute pyelonephritis may present with costovertebral angle (CVA) pain and tenderness with or without fever. However, the clinical diagnosis is often not straightforward because of difficulties in communication due to deafness, cognitive impairment or dysarthria, chronic symptoms that interfere with assessment, and attenuation of clinical findings with aging, such as a decreased or absent fever response (15). Sepsis, often with bacteremia, is more frequent with obstruction or trauma to the genitourinary tract. Epididymoorchitis may occur in male residents. Hematuria is seldom due to urinary infection, but episodes of gross hematuria are frequently associated with secondary fever in the presence of infected urine.

Chronic genitourinary symptoms are common in this population. These include chronic incontinence, nocturia, and frequency. A high proportion of residents with chronic genitourinary symptoms have positive urine cultures, but chronic symptoms are not attributable to urinary infection and are not improved by antimicrobial treatment of urinary infection (11). Thus, chronic genitourinary symptoms are not a manifestation of symptomatic urinary infection. However, acute deterioration in symptoms, such as acute deterioration in continence status, may be consistent with acute infection.

Urinary tract infection may also present as fever without localizing findings. However, fever with no apparent source is a potential clinical manifestation of many different infections in elderly institutionalized populations. About 50% of these episodes occur in residents with positive urine cultures, given the expected prevalence of bacteriuria. Only 10% of episodes of fever without localizing findings, however, appear to be of urinary origin (9). Unfortunately, other than the presence of an indwelling catheter, criteria to differentiate urinary from other potential sources of fever when localizing symptoms or signs are not present have not been identified. Clinical deterioration without fever or localizing genitourinary findings is also often attributed to urinary infection because of the finding of a positive urine culture. However, in the absence of fever, urinary infection is unlikely the cause of a nonspecific decline in clinical status.

Chronic Indwelling Catheter

The most common presentation of symptomatic urinary infection in the resident with a chronic indwelling catheter is fever without localizing genitourinary findings (13). When symptoms or signs localized to the genitourinary tract are present, they may include CVA pain or tenderness, suprapubic tenderness, hematuria, or catheter obstruction. Bacteremia may also be present. Lower tract symptoms, such as suprapubic tenderness or bypassing of the catheter caused by bladder spasms, may also occur but are less common. Local suppurative complications including epididymoorchitis, prostatic abscess, paraurethral abscesses, or urethritis occur in men. Bladder or kidney stone formation is a potential long-term complication in residents with infection with such urease-producing organisms as *P. mirabilis* or *P. stuartii*.

DIAGNOSTIC APPROACH

Microbiologic Diagnosis

A diagnosis of urinary infection requires an appropriately collected and transported urine specimen, which is cultured quantitatively (Table 4). For a diagnosis of asymptomatic bacteriuria, two consecutive urine cultures growing $\geq 10^5$ cfu/mL are necessary. A single urine culture meeting these quantitative criteria is sufficient to diagnose symptomatic infection. A lower quantitative count may be consistent with symptomatic infection in some clinical settings, such as individuals receiving diuretics, with renal failure, or infected with selected fastidious organisms. If complete obstruction is present and the infection is proximal to the obstruction, urine cultures may

Table 4 Quantitative Criteria for Diagnosis of Urinary Infection in Residents of Long-Term Care Facilities

Voided specimens	Symptomatic	Asymptomatic
Women	$\geq 10^5$ cfu/mL	$\geq 10^5$ cfu/mL × 2
Men	$\geq 10^5$ cfu/mL	$\geq 10^5$ cfu/mL
Catheter specimen	$\geq 10^2$ cfu/mL	$\geq 10^2$ cfu/mL

be negative. Urine culture will also usually be negative if antimicrobial therapy is initiated prior to obtaining the urine specimen. Lower quantitative counts are consistent with infection for the clinical presentations of acute cystitis in young women but have not been validated for microbiologic diagnosis of urinary infection in the institutionalized elderly. As 10% to 25% of bacteriuric men or women in LTCFs have more than one organism isolated, urine specimens with more than one uropathogen in appropriate quantitative counts should not be dismissed as contamination.

A valid quantitative urine culture is dependent upon a urine specimen collected to minimize contamination with urethral and periurethral flora. For men, a clean-catch specimen collected with voiding can usually be obtained and is seldom contaminated. If a male resident cannot cooperate to provide a voided specimen, collection using a freshly applied clean condom and leg bag may provide a suitable specimen. For women, a clean-catch technique also provides an adequate specimen, but many women cannot cooperate with voiding for specimen collection. The use of pedibags, bedpans, or diapers in collecting urine specimens from women are subject to substantial contamination with organisms and should be avoided. Where a patient is unable to cooperate, and a urine culture is necessary to assist in clinical management, in-and-out urethral catheterization for specimen collection should be performed. Any quantitative count of a potential uropathogen is diagnostic of infection in a urine specimen collected by catheterization. However, this procedure may introduce infection in as many as 5% of catheterizations and should only be used when there is a compelling clinical indication.

Urinalysis

More than 90% of elderly residents of LTCFs with bacteriuria will have pyuria, regardless of whether infection is symptomatic or asymptomatic (11). In addition, 30% of residents without bacteriuria also have pyuria, presumably due to contamination from genital secretions or associated with inflammatory conditions within the genitourinary tract. Thus, pyuria is not specific for bacteriuria and does not differentiate symptomatic from asymptomatic infection. A urinalysis negative for pyuria is helpful, as the absence of pyuria has a high negative predictive value to exclude bacteriuria. The leukocyte esterase dipstick test has been evaluated for identification of pyuria in elderly institutionalized populations. It has a positive predictive value varying from 18% to 75% and a negative predictive value of 75% to 100% for identifying bacteriuria in this setting, and it may be valid as a rapid screening test to exclude urinary infection.

Clinical Diagnosis

The diagnosis of symptomatic urinary infection may be straightforward if a resident presents with a new onset of irritative lower tract symptoms or with clinical findings of acute pyelonephritis. However, a clinical diagnosis of symptomatic infection is frequently problematic because of impaired communication and concomitant chronic symptoms associated with comorbid disease. The fever response is less marked or may be absent (15). Acute changes in chronic symptoms, such as acute deterioration in continence status or increased frequency, however, may support a clinical diagnosis of symptomatic urinary infection.

The bacteriuric resident with clinical deterioration but without localizing genitourinary findings often presents a diagnostic problem. Despite the positive urine culture, urinary infection is seldom the source. One study reported urinary infection as a source in only 11% of patients with clinical deterioration without localizing findings, and all residents with urinary infection also had fever (11). In another study, fever without localizing findings was attributed to urinary infection in only 10% of episodes in bacteriuric residents (9). However, there were no clinical or laboratory parameters to differentiate the 90% of episodes not due to a urinary source from the 10% attributable to urinary infection. Thus, urinary infection is a diagnosis of exclusion for the clinical presentation of fever without localizing findings in residents with a positive urine culture. Practitioners must be aware of the uncertainty in attributing this clinical presentation to urinary infection. A negative urine culture is helpful as it excludes a urinary source, but a positive urinary culture does not confirm symptomatic urinary infection. Clinical management includes careful initial evaluation, avoidance of antibiotics if possible, and ongoing monitoring. A consensus document suggests that antibiotics should be initiated for presumed urinary infection only with presentations of acute dysuria or of fever ($>37.9°C$) with one of new or worsening urgency, frequency, suprapubic pain, gross hematuria, CVA tenderness, or urinary incontinence (16).

The presence of "foul smelling" or cloudy urine is also sometimes identified as symptomatic urinary infection and interpreted as an indication for antimicrobial therapy (11). Cloudy urine may be caused by crystals as well as pyuria. By itself, it is not sufficient to diagnose symptomatic infection or an indication for antimicrobial therapy. An unpleasant urine odor may certainly be associated with urinary infection, likely caused by polyamine production by infecting bacteria. However, not all residents with this problem have urinary infection, and not all residents with urinary infection have an unpleasant odor. This "symptom" is more appropriately addressed through improved continence management rather than antimicrobial treatment.

Chronic Indwelling Catheter

A microbiologic diagnosis of urinary infection in the resident with a chronic indwelling catheter requires a urine specimen collected aseptically from the catheter port or by aspiration through the catheter tubing. Catheters that have been in situ for several days will have biofilm formation, primarily on the inner surface of the catheter. A urine specimen obtained from the catheter or tubing samples the bacteriology of this biofilm rather than bladder urine. Urine specimens collected through a biofilm-laden catheter have a greater number of bacteria isolated in higher quantitative counts (17). When antimicrobial therapy for urinary infection is indicated, the indwelling catheter should be replaced and a urine specimen should be obtained from the newly inserted catheter prior to initiating therapy. This will sample bladder urine rather than the biofilm. Replacement of the catheter is also associated with more rapid defervescence of fever and a lower frequency of symptomatic relapse following therapy (17).

The most common clinical presentation of symptomatic urinary infection in the catheterized patient is fever without localizing findings. From 30% to 50% of such episodes in residents with an indwelling catheter have a urinary source (9). Localizing findings including hematuria, an obstructed catheter, suprapubic tenderness, or CVA pain or tenderness increase the likelihood of urinary tract infection. A consensus document suggests, for catheterized patients, that antimicrobial therapy should be initiated when there are one or more symptoms of fever > 39.9°C, new CVA tenderness, rigors, or new delirium (16).

THERAPEUTIC INTERVENTIONS

Asymptomatic Bacteriuria

Asymptomatic bacteriuria in residents of LTCFs should not be treated. Prospective, randomized comparative trials have repeatedly shown no benefit in morbidity or mortality with antimicrobial treatment of asymptomatic bacteriuria (5,6,18,19). Specifically, there is no decrease in acute episodes of symptomatic urinary infection, no change in chronic genitourinary symptoms, and no decreased mortality with treatment of asymptomatic bacteriuria (Table 5). Some studies, in fact, report a trend towards increased mortality with intensive antimicrobial therapy, given in an attempt to maintain sterile urine (5,6). Treatment of asymptomatic bacteriuria does result in increased adverse effects from antimicrobial therapy, increased cost, and increased reinfection with more resistant organisms. Thus, studies are consistent in reporting no benefit with treatment of asymptomatic bacteriuria, and several harmful outcomes. As treatment of asymptomatic bacteriuria is not beneficial, it follows that routine screening of asymptomatic residents of LTCFs for the presence of asymptomatic bacteriuria is not indicated.

Antimicrobial Treatment

Antimicrobial therapy is certainly indicated for the treatment of symptomatic infection. Many antimicrobials are effective for treatment of urinary

Table 5 Randomized Clinical Trials of Therapy and No Therapy for Management of Asymptomatic Bacteriuria in Long-Term Care Facility Residents

Population (reference)	Number	Follow-up	Outcomes of therapy and no therapy
Men (5)	36	2 yr	Similar symptomatic episodes; similar mortality
Women (6)	50	12 mo	↑ Infection, ↑ adverse effects, ↑ resistance with antimicrobial therapy; similar symptomatic episodes and mortality
Women (18)	358	8.5 yr	No difference in mortality
Women (19)	191	3 days	Treatment had no effect on chronic incontinence
Chronic catheter (20)	35	Mean 29.2 wk	No difference: bacteriuria, fever, catheter obstruction; ↑ resistant bacteria with antimicrobial

infection (Table 6). Selection of a specific agent is directed by the known or presumed susceptibilities of the infecting organism, patient tolerance, evidence of prior efficacy of the antimicrobial in the management of urinary infection, and facility formulary. Antimicrobial selection is not altered based on age alone. In every case, a urine specimen for culture should be obtained prior to instituting antimicrobial therapy. If possible, empirical antimicrobial treatment should be avoided. For individuals with mild symptoms, institution of therapy should be delayed pending results of the urine culture. With more serious clinical presentations, including acute confusion, high fever, or hemodynamic instability, empirical antimicrobial therapy should be initiated. The initial regimen should be reassessed once the urine culture result is available, usually at 48 to 72 hours after start of treatment. By this time, the initial clinical course and response to antimicrobial therapy can also be reviewed.

There are few studies that address the question of the optimal antimicrobial regimen for treatment of symptomatic urinary infection in residents of LTCFs. Thus, the relative efficacy of different antimicrobials and optimal duration of therapy are not known. For oral therapy, trimethoprim/sulfamethoxazole (TMP/SMX) or trimethoprim alone may be preferred as initial therapy (1). A comparative clinical trial of ciprofloxacin and TMP/SMX in 172 women, 50% of whom were residents of nursing homes, reported improved clinical and microbiologic outcomes with ciprofloxacin (21). This difference appeared to be largely attributable to a higher frequency of TMP/SMX-resistant organisms. If resistant organisms are known or anticipated to be causing infection, a fluoroquinolone antimicrobial may be appropriate. For gram-positive infections, amoxicillin is usually

Table 6 Antimicrobials for Treatment of Urinary Tract Infection in Long-Term Care Facilities Residents

Antimicrobial agent	Regimen	
	Oral	Parenteral
Pencillins		
Ampicillin		1–2 g q6 h
Amoxicillin	500 mg t.i.d.	
Amoxicillin/	500 mg t.i.d.	
clavulanic acid		
Piperacillin		3 g q4 h
Piperacillin/		3.375 g q6 h
tazobactam		
Cephalosporins		
Cephalexin	500 mg q.i.d.	
Cefazolin		1.0 g q8 h
Cefuroxime (axetil)	125–250 mg b.i.d.	750 mg q8 h
Cefixime	400 mg o.d.	
Cefotaxime		1.0 g q8–12 h
Ceftriaxone		1.0 g q24 h
Ceftazidime		1.0 g q8 h
Aminoglycosides		
Gentamicin		1–1.5 mg/kg q8 h or 4–5 mg/kg q24 h
Tobramycin		1–1.5 mg/kg q8 h or 4.5 mg/kg q24 h
Amikacin		3–5 mg/kg q8 h or 15 mg/kg q24 h
Flouroquinolones		
Norfloxacin	400 mg b.i.d.	
Ciprofloxacin	250–750 mg b.i.d.	400 mg q12 h
Extended release	500–1000 mg o.d.	
Ofloxacin	200–400 mg b.i.d.	
Levofloxacin	250–500 mg o.d.	500 mg o.d.
Gatifloxacin	400 mg o.d.	400 mg o.d.
Other		
Trimethoprim	100 mg b.i.d.	
Trimethoprim/	160/800 mg b.i.d.	
sulfamethoxazole		
Nitrofurantoin	100 mg q.i.d.	
Monohydrate/	100 mg b.i.d.	
macrocrystal		
Aztreonam		1.0 g q8 h
Meropenem		500 mg q8 h
Ertapenem		1.0 g q24 h
Vancomycin[a]		1.0 g q12 h

[a]Gram-positive infections only.
Abbreviations: o.d., once a day; b.i.d., two times a day; t.i.d., three times a day; q.i.d., four times a day.

preferred. Nitrofurantoin is useful for episodes of lower tract infection. It has limited impact on the normal host flora and is often an effective therapy for vancomycin-resistant enterococci. However, nitrofurantoin is not effective for *P. mirabilis, K. pneumoniae,* or *P. aeruginosa* infection, is not indicated for upper tract infection, and is contraindicated in patients with renal failure.

Although fluoroquinolone antimicrobials have been widely used, and are usually effective, there are increasing reports of fluoroquinolone resistance amongst gram-negative organisms causing urinary and other infections in LTCFs. The most common association with isolation of a fluoroquinolone-resistant organism is prior fluoroquinolone exposure (22). Thus, fluoroquinolones should be avoided if alternate antimicrobials are appropriate. Empirical fluoroquinolone therapy should likely be avoided if a resident has received prior fluoroquinolone therapy in the previous three months. Where possible, these antimicrobials should be reserved for therapy when other oral options are not available, in an effort to limit emergence of resistance to this class.

Where the patient's clinical status or infection with antimicrobial-resistant organisms warrants parenteral therapy, an aminoglycoside antimicrobial, such as gentamicin, is preferred (1). Aminoglycosides may be given either intravenously or intramuscularly. A once-a-day dose regimen is also convenient without increased toxicity (Table 6). When empirical therapy with an aminoglycoside is initiated, the clinical course and infecting organism should be reassessed after 48 to 72 hours to ensure that the aminoglycoside remains optimal therapy and that parenteral therapy is still required. In many cases, the aminoglycoside may be changed to alternate parenteral or oral therapy at this time. If a more prolonged course of aminoglycoside therapy is indicated, then aminoglycoside levels and renal function should be monitored at least twice weekly. Aminoglycoside use limits antimicrobial pressure from extended-spectrum cephalosporins or fluoroquinolones and may delay emergence of extended-spectrum beta-lactamase-producing Enterobacteriaceae or fluoroquinolone-resistant organisms. Aminoglycosides are not an appropriate empirical choice for individuals with renal failure. In this setting, a parenteral flouroquinolone or an extended-spectrum cephalosporin may be preferred.

Duration of Treatment

Few studies are available to define the optimal duration of treatment. For minor lower tract symptoms a seven-day course of therapy is likely adequate. Shorter courses of three to five days for women with cystitis appear less effective for the institutionalized population and are not recommended. More severe clinical presentations with systemic signs should be treated for 10 to 14 days.

For selected patients with unique clinical presentations, longer courses of antimicrobial therapy may be indicated. Men with symptomatic relapsing infection from a prostatic source may require 6 or 12 weeks of treatment. Residents with recurrent episodes of symptomatic infection associated with a genitourinary abnormality which cannot be corrected, such as persistent infection stones, may require prolonged suppressive therapy. The specific antimicrobial is selected on a case-by-case basis. Long-term antimicrobial therapy should always be embarked on cautiously and is indicated for only highly selected patients, as it may promote emergence of resistant organisms.

Chronic Indwelling Catheter

Treatment of asymptomatic bacteriuria in residents with an indwelling catheter is not beneficial. There is early recurrence of bacteriuria following antimicrobial therapy and no decrease in febrile episodes attributable to urinary infection. However, there is an increased frequency of reinfection with bacteria resistant to the antimicrobial used for treatment (20).

For symptomatic infection, the principles of antimicrobial selection in residents with a chronic indwelling catheter are similar to those for residents without indwelling catheters. As previously discussed, the catheter should be changed prior to initiating antimicrobial therapy, to facilitate optimal specimen collection as well as to improve outcomes (17). The optimal duration of antimicrobial therapy for treatment of symptomatic infection in a patient with a chronic indwelling catheter is not known. The continuing presence of the catheter leads to recurrent urinary infection, and antimicrobial therapy promotes reinfection with organisms of increasing resistance. Thus, the duration of antimicrobial therapy should be as short as possible. In residents with a prompt clinical response and rapid defervescence of fever, a seven-day course of therapy should be sufficient, although this treatment duration has not been evaluated in clinical trials.

INFECTION CONTROL MEASURES

General

The goal of infection control measures in the LTCF is to prevent acquisition of infection by residents. The most important interventions are likely optimal hand hygiene and glove use by staff members, appropriate use of aseptic or clean techniques in patient care practices, and effective cleaning of equipment between patients. A particular concern for urinary infection in the LTCF is appropriate cleaning and drying of leg bags prior to reuse for residents managed with a condom or indwelling catheter.

Surveillance for infection identifies the presence and burden of specific clinical problems and, by itself, may contribute to decreasing infection rates by heightening staff awareness of infections. Surveillance should be undertaken to identify rates and risk factors for symptomatic urinary infection, including bacteremia from a urinary source (23). Routine urine cultures are not appropriate, given the high prevalence of bacteriuria and lack of evidence for harm. Any surveillance strategy must have a capacity for early identification of potential outbreaks. Antimicrobial use for urinary infection should also be monitored, together with an assessment of the appropriateness of such use.

Chronic Indwelling Catheters

The urine from individuals with chronic indwelling catheters is a reservoir for resistant organisms within the long-term care setting. Thus, appropriate practices must be followed to limit transmission of organisms on equipment or the hands of staff between these patients. Urine measuring devices should not be shared between patients, and appropriate gloving and hand hygiene practices by staff members performing catheter care should be maintained. Policies governing catheter care in LTCF patients should be developed and updated regularly. These policies should also specify when chronic indwelling catheters should be used and how catheter use should be monitored.

Surveillance of chronic indwelling catheter use should include the prevalence of catheter use, indications for catheter use, and reasons why the catheter cannot be removed in a given individual. As all residents with chronic indwelling catheters are bacteriuric, there is no indication for routine screening for the presence of bacteriuria. However, surveillance for symptomatic urinary infection should be performed, including surveillance for episodes of catheter obstruction or trauma.

PREVENTION

General Measures

The major factors promoting urinary tract infection in elderly residents of LTCFs are associated comorbid diseases leading to impaired voiding. As these are often the same comorbidities that require admission to the LTCF, and in most cases cannot be modified, it is not clear that any interventions can decrease bacteriuria. Optimizing nutrition, mobility, and medical management of comorbid illnesses is desirable, but the impact of any of these on the occurrence of urinary infection is unknown. One clinical study reported that improving nutrition of long-term care residents did not decrease the occurrence of urinary infection.

Specific Measures

Several specific interventions may decrease the occurrence of urinary infection. The use of condom catheters is associated with an increased frequency of infection, so limiting the use of these devices should decrease the occurrence of bacteriuria. Whether this would also decrease the occurrence of symptomatic infection is unknown. However, in many cases, patient care requires the use of these devices, and it is unrealistic to avoid use. For individuals with voiding managed with intermittent catheterization, the frequency of infection is similar using a clean or sterile catheterization technique (24). Hence, clean intermittent catheterization is appropriate and less costly. Increased intake of cranberry juice has been suggested as an approach to decrease infection. However, increased cranberry juice did not decrease the prevalence of bacteriuria or symptomatic infection in a placebo-controlled trial (25). Topical vaginal estrogen therapy decreased episodes of both symptomatic and asymptomatic infection in elderly noninstitutionalized women with a very high frequency of symptomatic infection, but whether there is any role for topical estrogen in the institutionalized elderly is not known. Systemic estrogen therapy did not decrease the frequency of bacteriuria in a group of female nursing home residents (26).

Trauma to the mucosa with bleeding in an infected genitourinary tract is associated with a high risk of bacteremia and sepsis. Prophylactic antimicrobial therapy should be given before any invasive genitourinary procedure undertaken in a bacteriuric resident, as this is effective in preventing these complications.

Chronic Indwelling Catheter

The most effective way to avoid urinary infection associated with a chronic catheter is, of course, not to use the catheter. When a catheter is necessary, the duration of use should be limited to as short a time as clinically necessary. Beyond this, bacteriuria cannot currently be prevented in a patient with a chronic indwelling catheter. Some specific interventions to decrease catheter-associated infection have been evaluated but not found to be effective. Routine daily bladder irrigation with saline does not decrease the incidence of infection, antimicrobial treatment of asymptomatic bacteriuria does not decrease the frequency of asymptomatic or symptomatic infection, and different catheter materials, such as latex or silicone, do not alter the rate of infection (13). Silicone catheters have been reported to have fewer episodes of obstruction and may be useful in patients with frequent blockage. However, these catheters have not been shown to decrease the occurrence of symptomatic infection, and, as they are more costly, are recommended only for selected patients. Other interventions, such as daily periurethral cleaning with soap and water or with a disinfectant or placing disinfectant in the drainage bag, also do not decrease the frequency of bacteriuria in patients with indwelling catheters.

Urinary infection in the individual with a chronic indwelling catheter is, conceptually, a technical issue attributable to biofilm formation and inadequate urinary drainage. Further developments in catheter materials to prevent or delay biofilm formation will be necessary if progress in limiting catheter-acquired infections in residents with chronic indwelling catheters is to occur. Current studies of different drainage devices and catheter materials are continuing and may lead ultimately to meaningful advances. Approaches include intraurethral catheters, new catheter biomaterials, or antimicrobial impregnated catheters. None of these devices, however, have yet been documented to have a benefit for patients.

The focus of current prevention efforts must be to minimize the occurrence of symptomatic episodes. Appropriate catheter care to limit trauma and prompt identification and replacement of an obstructed catheter should prevent some episodes of symptomatic infection. The use of prophylactic antimicrobials prior to an invasive genitourinary procedure will prevent postprocedure sepsis and bacteremia. Prophylactic antimicrobials are not indicated with catheter change, as the frequency of infectious complications with catheter change is low.

SUGGESTED READING

Nicolle LE. SHEA Long-term Care Committee. Urinary tract infections in long-term care facilities. Infect Control Hosp Epidemiol 2001; 22:167–175.

Nicolle LE, Bradley S, Colgan R, Rice JC, Schaeffer A, Hooton TM. IDSA guideline for the diagnosis and treatment of asymptomatic bacteriuria in adults. Clin Infect Dis 2005; 40:643–654.

Saint S, Chenoweth CE. Biofilms and catheter-associated urinary tract infections. Infect Dis Clin North Am 2003; 17:411–422.

REFERENCES

1. Nicolle LE, Bentley D, Garibaldi R, Neuhaus E, Smith P. SHEA Long-term Care Committee. Antimicrobial use in long-term care facilities. Infect Control Hosp Epidemiol 2000; 21:537–545.
2. Ouslander JG, Schapira M, Finegold S, Schneille J. Accuracy of rapid urine screening tests among incontinent nursing home residents with asymptomatic bacteriuria. J Am Geriatr Soc 1995; 43:772–775.
3. Kasviki-Charvati P, Drolette-Kefakis B, Papanayiotou PC, Dontas AS. Turnover of bacteriuria in old age. Age Aging 1982; 11:169–174.
4. Hedin K, Petersson C, Wideback K, Kahlmeter G, Molstad S. Asymptomatic bacteriuria in a population of elderly in municipal institutional care. Scand J Prim Health Care 2002; 20:166–168.
5. Nicolle LE, Bjornson J, Harding GKM, MacDonell JA. Bacteriuria in elderly institutionalized men. N Engl J Med 1983; 309:1420–1425.
6. Nicolle LE, Mayhew WJ, Bryan L. Prospective randomized comparison of therapy and no therapy for asymptomatic bacteriuria in institutionalized elderly women. Am J Med 1987; 83:27–33.

7. Abrutyn E, Mossey J, Levison M, Boscia J, Pitsakis P, Kaye D. Epidemiology of asymptomatic bacteriuria in elderly women. J Am Geriatr Soc 1991; 39:388–393.
8. Stevenson KB, Moore J, Colwell H, Sleeper B. Standardized infection surveillance in long-term care. Interfacility comparisons from a regional cohort of facilities. Infect Control Hosp Epidemiol 2005; 26:231–238.
9. Orr PH, Nicolle LE, Duckworth H, et al. Febrile urinary infection in the institutionalized elderly. Am J Med 1996; 100:71–77.
10. Monane M, Gurwitz JH, Lipsitz LA, Glynn RJ, Choodnovskiy I, Avorn J. Epidemiology and diagnostic aspects of bacteriuria: a longitudinal study in older women. J Am Geriatr Soc 1995; 43:618–622.
11. Nicolle LE. Asymptomatic bacteriuria in the elderly. Infect Dis Clin North Am 1997; 11:647–662.
12. Nicolle LE. The chronic indwelling catheter and urinary infection in LTCF residents. Infect Control Hosp Epidemiol 2001; 22:316–321.
13. Warren JW. Catheter-associated urinary tract infection. Int J Antimicrob Agents 2001; 17:299–303.
14. Rudman D, Hontanosas A, Cohen Z, Mattson DE. Clinical correlates of bacteremia in a Veteran's administration extended care facility. J Am Geriatr Soc 1988; 36:726–732.
15. Bentley DW, Bradley S, High K, Schoenbaum S, Taler G, Yoshikawa TT. Evaluation of fever and infection in long-term care facilities. Clin Infect Dis 2000; 31:640–653.
16. Loeb M, Bentley DW, Bradley S, et al. Development of minimum criteria for the initiation of antibiotics in residents of LTCFs: results of a consensus conference. Infect Control Hosp Epidemiol 2001; 22:120–124.
17. Raz R, Schiller D, Nicolle LE. Does replacement of catheter improve the outcome of patients with a permanent urinary catheter and symptomatic bacteriuria? J Urol 2000; 164:1254–1258.
18. Abrutyn E, Mossey J, Berlin JA, et al. Does asymptomatic bacteriuria predict mortality and does antimicrobial treatment reduce mortality in elderly ambulatory women? Ann Intern Med 1994; 120:827–833.
19. Ouslander JG, Shapira M, Schnelle JF, et al. Does eradication of bacteriuria affect the severity of chronic urinary incontinence in nursing home residents. Ann Intern Med 1995; 122:749–754.
20. Warren JW, Anthony WC, Hoopes JM, Muncie HL Jr. Cephalexin for susceptible bacteriuria in afebrile long-term catheterized patients. JAMA 1982; 248:454–458.
21. Gomolin IH, Siami PF, Reuning-Scherer J, Haverstock DC, Heyd A. Efficacy and safety of ciprofloxacin oral suspension versus trimethoprim–sulfamethoxazole oral suspension for treatment of older women with acute urinary tract infection. J Am Ger Soc 2001; 49:1606–1613.
22. Loeb MB, Craven S, McGeer AJ, et al. Risk factors for resistance to antimicrobial agents among nursing home residents. Am J Epidemiol 2003; 157:40–47.
23. Smith PW, Rusnak PG. Infection prevention and control in the LTCF. Infect Control Hosp Epidemiol 1997; 18:831–849.
24. Duffy LM, Cleary J, Ahern S, et al. Clean, intermittent catheterization: safe, cost-effective bladder management for male residents of VA nursing homes. J Am Geriatr Soc 1995; 43:865–870.

25. Avorn J, Monane M, Gurwitz JH, Glynn RJ, Choodnovsky I, Lipsitz LA. Reduction of bacteriuria and pyuria after ingestion of cranberry juice. JAMA 1994; 271:751–754.
26. Ouslander JG, Greendale GA, Uman G, Lee C, Paul W, Schnelle J. Effects of oral estrogen and progestin on the lower urinary tract among female nursing home residents. J Am Geriatr Soc 2001; 49:803–807.

13

Influenza and Other Respiratory Viruses

Ghinwa Dumyati

Department of Infectious Diseases, University of Rochester School of Medicine and Dentistry, Rochester, New York, U.S.A.

KEY POINTS

1. Respiratory viral infections have a significant impact on elderly nursing home residents, resulting in deconditioning, hospitalization, and death.
2. Influenza is well known to cause explosive outbreaks in nursing homes, but recently RSV emerged as an important pathogen, causing significant morbidity and mortality approaching that of influenza infection.
3. Other viruses, such as parainfluenza, coronavirus, human metapneumovirus, and rhinoviruses, have also been described as pathogens in elderly adults and may also contribute to morbidity and mortality.
4. Infection control measures to prevent the spread of these viruses include yearly vaccination of residents and staff for influenza, a surveillance program for respiratory illnesses, early initiation of isolation, and appropriate use of influenza prophylactic and treatment agents.
5. Establishing a specific viral diagnosis is crucial for institution of specific treatment and isolation. It is difficult to clinically differentiate between the various viral infections; therefore, diagnosis by antigen detection or viral culture is highly desirable.

INTRODUCTION

Viral respiratory infections, although extremely common during childhood, decrease in frequency with increasing age. In general, older adults experience approximately one upper respiratory infection (URI) per year (1). Although the incidence of infection is lower, the morbidity of these respiratory viruses is significantly greater in the elderly compared to the young. The reasons for more severe disease are multifactorial and include an aging lung, the presence of comorbid conditions, and age-related immune dysfunction. In long-term care facilities, the rates of acute respiratory tract infection vary depending on the season studied and the methods used for diagnosis. Several studies estimate the rate of URI to be 1–3 per resident per year. Acute respiratory tract infection was reported at a rate of 6.3/100 person-months in a study conducted during the winter at a 590-bed long-term care facility in Rochester, New York (2). Forty-two percent of these infections were proven to be caused by viruses. The devastating effect of influenza outbreaks is well defined in the nursing home population, but the impact of other viruses is less well known. Respiratory syncytial virus (RSV) infection has emerged as an important pathogen causing significant morbidity and mortality approaching that of influenza infection. Although less data are available, other viruses, such as parainfluenza, coronavirus, human metapneumovirus, and rhinoviruses, have also been described as pathogens in elderly adults and may also contribute to increased mortality. Control of viral respiratory infections in chronic care facilities can be challenging because specific diagnosis is often difficult. Congregate settings, hands-on attention required by staff and residents, and cognitive deficits that hamper disease recognition all contribute to the spread of viruses and the development of outbreaks. In this chapter, the clinical presentation and impact of influenza, RSV, coronavirus, parainfluenza, human metapneumovirus, and rhinovirus infections in residents of long-term care facilities will be reviewed. The mode of transmission and methods for prevention of these viruses will also be discussed.

INFLUENZA

Epidemiology and Clinical Relevance

Viral Characteristics

Influenza virus is well known to cause worldwide pandemic and epidemic disease. Three types exist: A, B, and C, which are classified based on antigenic differences between the internal proteins. Both influenza A and B cause severe disease, whereas type C has been reported to cause milder upper respiratory tract infection. Immunity to influenza infection is both humoral and cell mediated. Protective antibodies are produced against the viral envelope proteins, hemagglutinin (H) and the neuraminidase (N). Repeated infections can occur because of yearly antigenic variations in these envelope proteins. Such variations are due to point mutations in the envelope protein-genes. This process, referred to as "antigenic drift," leads to annual epidemics and is the reason for yearly changes in the components of the influenza vaccine. A major change due to an introduction of a completely new H or N genes, referred to as "antigenic shift," leads to influenza pandemics. Pandemics occur because all members of the community are susceptible to infection by the new strain of influenza virus. Antigenic shift only occurs in influenza A viruses. In recent years, influenza A (H3N2 and H1N1) and influenza B have been cocirculating. H1N1 viruses are uncommon causes of infection in the elderly nursing home resident, possibly because of immunity acquired in younger life (3).

Attack Rate, Morbidity, and Mortality

In the United States, yearly influenza epidemics lead to an excess of 54,000 to 430,000 hospitalizations and an estimated excess death of 20,000 to 36,000. The highest excess mortality and hospitalization rates were observed over the past two decades. This increase is attributed to an aging U.S. population, a rising prevalence of high-risk conditions that predispose to more complicated influenza infection, and the predominance of influenza A (H3N2) infections during 1990–1999 seasons (4,5). The burden of influenza is highest in the elderly population because 80% to 90% of the influenza-related deaths and 65% of influenza-related hospitalizations occur in persons 65 years or older. Death is due to pneumonia or exacerbation of cardiovascular, respiratory, and other underlying diseases. The impact of influenza is worse in the "old old." A patient above the age of 85 years is 36 times more likely to die of influenza compared to one aged 65 to 69 years. The mortality also increases with each high-risk condition, such as cardiovascular diseases, pulmonary diseases, metabolic diseases (such as diabetes), renal dysfunction, anemia, and immunosuppresion. The estimated death rates are 104 and 240 per 100,000 for persons with cardiovascular and chronic pulmonary diseases, respectively. The presence of both pulmonary and cardiovascular diseases results in the highest mortality at 870 per 100,000 deaths (6). In addition to causing excess mortality, influenza infection also causes significant morbidity in the elderly. Approximately 10% of older persons who are hospitalized are discharged to a higher level of care even though many were independent prior to admission. Frail nursing home patients have been noted to have a decline in their functional status after influenza infection.

Influenza is an important pathogen in long-term care facilities because of the propensity to cause explosive outbreaks of severe illness. Attack rates vary between 20% and 40% with a reported mortality of 15% to 30% during influenza A outbreaks and 10% during influenza B outbreaks. Risk factors for outbreaks in long-term care facilities include low resident and staff vaccination rates, larger homes, presence of closed wards, and common dining areas. Other risk factors also include crowding and poor ventilation.

Clinical Manifestations

After an incubation period of approximately one to two days, the classic influenza syndrome is characterized by the abrupt onset of fever, chills, headache, and myalgias, accompanied by respiratory symptoms of sore throat, nonproductive cough, and nasal congestion. Ocular symptoms, such as tearing, burning, and pain with movement of the eyes, help to distinguish influenza from other viral illnesses (3). Elderly and debilitated patients may have a less "classic" picture and present with only high fever, lassitude, or confusion with minimal respiratory symptoms. Fever typically lasts for three days but can persist as long as eight days. In the nursing home population, it is difficult to clinically differentiate influenza from other respiratory viruses, such as RSV, because symptoms overlap and not infrequently viruses co-circulate. However, the presence of fever, systemic and gastrointestinal complaints suggests influenza (Table 1).

Diagnostic Approach

Viral culture from the nasopharynx is the gold standard method for the diagnosis of influenza. Virus may also be recovered from sputum. A nasopharyngeal specimen is obtained by swabbing the nose and the throat separately and combining both swabs in the same viral transport media. Nasal washes are difficult to obtain from elderly, debilitated patients, and nasopharyngeal swabs are preferred. Viral culture is important for epidemiological purposes and is also essential for making decisions regarding the best antiviral treatment and prophylaxis. However, it takes three to five days to identify the virus by culture. Time is critical for controlling outbreaks and instituting appropriate antiviral treatment, and, therefore, rapid diagnostic methods, such as immunofluorescence (IFA) or enzyme immunoassay (EIA), have been developed. These tests detect viral antigens directly

Table 1 Clinical Findings in Elderly Patients with Influenza Virus Versus Respiratory Syncytical Virus Infection

Finding	Influenza (%)	RSV (%)
Upper respiratory symptoms	97	100
Lower respiratory symptoms	66	44
Systemic	84[a]	44
Gastrointestinal	38[a]	0
Temperature above 99°F	90[a]	56

[a]Statistically significant difference.
Abbreviation: RSV, respiratory syncytial virus.
Source: Form Ref. 7.

from respiratory secretions and can be used for influenza A or influenza A and B together. Results can be obtained within an hour. Many tests are available; the most commonly used test is the Directigen Flu (Becton-Dickenson). It can detect influenza A alone or influenza A and B. Other tests available are FLU OIA (Thermo Electron), QuickVue Influenza test (Quidel), XPECT Flu (Remel), Now Influenza (Bimax), SAS influenza, and ZstatFlu (Zyme TX). Both QuickVue Influenza and ZstatFlu are eligible for Clinical Laboratory Improvement Amendment of 1998 and can be used on site (8). The sensitivity of various tests compared to culture as gold standard depends on the quality of the specimen, with better results obtained from nasal washes and swabs compared to pharyngeal specimens alone. The sensitivity varies between 40% and 80%, and the specificity ranges between 85% and 100%. Lower sensitivities have been reported in nursing homes and in elderly and patients with cardiopulmonary conditions hospitalized with influenza (9,10). Other techniques include reverse transcription-polymerase chain reaction (RT-PCR), which although very sensitive is not widely available. PCR is presently expensive and requires specimens to be sent to specialized laboratories. Serology using acute and convalescent sera is not helpful for the acute management of patients but is useful in retrospective analysis of outbreaks.

Therapeutic Interventions and Infection Control

The explosive nature of the influenza outbreaks suggests aerosol transmission. However, this has not been as well documented as for tuberculosis or varicella. A large amount of virus is present in the respiratory secretions of infected persons and is dispersed into the air by sneezing, coughing, and talking. Virus shedding begins approximately 24 hours before onset of symptoms and rapidly increases for the first 24 to 48 hours of illness and then diminishes to low levels for up to 5 to 10 days (3). Higher rates of transmission occur in crowded and confined settings, such as in hospitals, nursing homes, and college dormitories. Transmission may also occur through fomites and contaminated hands. Influenza virus can survive up to 24–48 hours on hard nonporous surfaces and on hands for up to five minutes.

Treatment and Chemoprophylaxis

Two classes of antiviral agents are available for prophylaxis and treatment of influenza infection. The M2 channel inhibitors, amantadine and rimantadine, and the neuraminidase inhibitors, zanamivir and oseltamivir, have both been proven efficacious.

Amantadine and Rimantadine: Amantadine and rimantadine inhibit growth of influenza A viruses only. They act by blocking the M2 channels that span the viral membrane and result in inhibition of viral uncoating from the host cell (3). Amantadine and rimantadine have been licensed for prophylaxis and treatment of influenza A infection.

Efficacy: Both amantadine and rimantadine have similar efficacy in prevention and treatment of influenza A. Most studies that have shown amantadine and rimantadine to be effective in preventing influenza have used challenge experiments in healthy adults or natural infections in the family setting. These drugs prevent 50% of laboratory-documented influenza infections and 70% to 90% of illnesses. Amantadine and rimantadine are also effective in the treatment of uncomplicated influenza. Treatment of healthy adults and children, when started within the first two days of illness, results in a decrease of illness duration by one to two days. One placebo-controlled study, carried out in nursing home patients, showed more rapid reduction in fever and symptoms and less use of antibiotics, antitussives, and antipyretics in rimantadine-treated patients (11). The effectiveness of early therapy of high-risk patients with amantadine and rimantadine in reducing frequency of subsequent complications is unknown. A number of observational studies have shown that both amantadine and rimantadine are effective in controlling nursing homes outbreaks, when prophylaxis and treatment have been started early. However, no randomized, placebo-controlled studies to assess the effectiveness of widespread chemoprophylaxis with rimantadine or amantadine have been carried out.

Dosing: Although amantadine and rimantadine have similar mechanisms of action, they differ in their pharmacokinetics. Amantadine is excreted unmetabolized in the urine. The half-life is two times longer in elderly compared to young adults and further prolonged in patients with impaired renal function. The recommended dose is 100 mg/day in patients above the age of 65; further adjustment is needed for elderly patient with renal insufficiency (12). Rimantadine is metabolized in the liver with 20% excreted by the kidney. Because a dose of 200 mg/day was associated with high plasma levels in elderly nursing home patients, the recommended dose for rimantadine is also 100 mg/day. However, modifications are not needed for renal and liver dysfunction. The recommended doses of amantadine and rimantadine are summarized in Table 2. Treatment duration is three to five days.

Side effects: Amantadine and rimantadine are both known to cause central nervous system (CNS) and gastrointestinal effects, but the CNS side effects are more common with amantadine and have been reported in 33% of cases. The CNS symptoms include nervousness, anxiety, difficulty concentrating, lightheadedness, and seizures. Seizures are more common with amantadine than rimantadine, and, therefore, its use is contraindicated in persons with a seizure history. A 4% to 8% increase in the frequency of falls among nursing home residents has been reported during periods of amantadine prophylaxis. Both drugs cause nausea and anorexia in 1% to 3% of cases. The highest incidence of adverse effects is associated with high plasma levels seen in renal failure and with the use of 200 mg of amantadine. Further

Table 2 Recommended Treatment and Prophylactic Dosage of Antiviral Drugs for Influenza in Nursing Home Patients

Drug	Route	Dose	Dose in renal failure (cr cl <50 mL/min)[a]
Amantadine	Oral (tablet or syrup)	100 mg/day	100 mg every 48–72 hr
Rimantadine	Oral (tablet or syrup)	100 mg/day	100 mg/day
Zanamivir	Oral inhalation (powder)	2 inhalations of 5 mg each, twice a day	No change
Oseltamivir	Oral	75 mg twice a day	75 mg/day

[a]Consult the drug package insert for patients with severe renal insufficiency.
Abbreviation: cr cl, creatinine clearance.

adjustment of amantadine dose, based on creatinine clearance, was better tolerated in a Canadian nursing home (12).

Resistance: Resistance to both those agents occurs rapidly (within two to three days) in one-third of influenza-infected patients receiving these drugs (5). It is therefore recommended that treated patients be isolated from patients receiving prophylaxis. Amantadine- and rimantadine-resistant viruses do not demonstrate increased virulence and they remain sensitive to zanamivir and oseltamivir.

Zanamivir and Oseltamivir: Zanamivir and oseltamivir are neuraminidase inhibitors of both influenza A and B viruses. Neuraminidase is an enzyme that cleaves terminal sialic acid residues from carbohydrate moieties on the surface of host cells and influenza virus envelopes. This process promotes the release of progeny viruses from infected cells, prevents the aggregation of virus, and possibly decreases viral inactivation by respiratory mucus. Inhibition of neuraminidase results in virus aggregation and a decrease in the amount of infectious virus released (3). Both agents have been approved for treatment of influenza A and B infections, but only oseltamivir has been licensed for prophylactic use.

Dosing: Oseltamivir is administered orally and zanamivir by oral inhalation. Zanamivir requires a cooperative patient who can inspire effectively. Zanamivir deposits primarily in the oropharynx and throat, with 20% reaching the lungs. Less than 20% is systemically absorbed. Oseltamivir is excreted unchanged in the urine, and, thus, the dose must be reduced in renal failure. The treatment duration is five days for both drugs. Recommended doses for both medications are summarized in Table 2.

Efficacy: The efficacy of zanamivir and oseltamivir in treatment and prophylaxis of influenza has also been studied primarily in healthy, young adults. Data regarding the efficacy of these drugs in high-risk patients is limited. Both drugs prevent naturally acquired influenza infection by 30–40% and illness by 67–84%. Zanamivir reduced the time to alleviation of influenza illness by one day in all subjects and by three days in those with febrile illness or those treated within 30 hours after the onset of symptoms. In elderly and high-risk subjects, a 2.5-day reduction in symptoms was observed. Nonfebrile patients or patients treated after 30 hours derive little or no benefit. Oseltamivir used in healthy adults showed a reduction in influenza symptoms by 1 to 1.5 days. In some studies, oseltamivir reduced the frequency of such complications as otitis media, sinusitis, bronchitis, and other , infections requiring antibiotics; however, the frequency of pneumonia in these study was too low to assess its effect on lower respiratory complications (13–15). The experience with prophylactic use of zanamivir and oseltamivir in long-term care facilities is limited but encouraging. One small, randomized, unblinded study in a Wisconsin nursing home population compared zanamivir to rimantadine for prophylaxis against influenza A and placebo against influenza B epidemics (16). Zanamivir was given for two weeks, and protection was comparable to rimantadine in influenza A epidemic. No cases of influenza B occurred in residents receiving zanamivir prophylaxis. Another randomized, double-blind, placebo-controlled study of oseltamivir used for six weeks showed a statistically significant decrease of laboratory-confirmed influenza compared to placebo. The protective efficacy was 92%. This protection was in addition to that provided by influenza vaccination (17). An influenza surveillance study in several Michigan nursing homes with a high rate of influenza immunization showed that outbreak control with oseltamivir varied depending on the rapidity of outbreak recognition and extent of antiviral use (e.g., limited to units or floors compared to entire nursing home) (9).

Side effects: Both zanamivir and oseltamivir are better tolerated than amantadine and rimantadine. CNS side effects have been infrequently reported. Zanamivir can reduce FEV1 and peak expiratory flow rates and should be used cautiously in patients with chronic obstructive lung disease. Oseltamivir use is associated with nausea of mild to moderate intensity with rare vomiting. These symptoms are transient and usually occur after the first dose.

Resistance: The emergence of virus resistant to zanamivir and oseltamivir is uncommon. One influenza B strain resistant to zanamivir was isolated from an immunocompromised child (5). In one pediatric study of oseltamivir treatment, 5.5% of posttreatment isolates were found to be resistant (5). There was no clinical deterioration and, unlike resistant viruses recovered during M2 channel blocker treatment, neuraminidase-resistant viruses were less virulent in animal models.

Influenza Control in Long-Term Care Facilities

Infection Control

Recommendations for influenza control in long-term care facilities were recently reviewed by Arden and the recommendations of the Society for Healthcare Epidemiology of America and Centers for Disease Control (CDC) have been published (5,18–20). All emphasize that the best method of influenza control in the nursing home is prevention of infection by yearly immunization of residents and staff. A standing order programs for vaccination are recommended by many authorities, to improve the number of long-term residents receiving vaccination (21). Despite vaccination, nursing home residents continue to become infected with influenza because of suboptimal vaccine response, high frequency of exposure, and ease of transmission of influenza virus in closed, crowded settings. Another contributing factor is failure to immunize staff who are frequently responsible for the introduction of influenza to the nursing home.

The key to controlling outbreaks is to identify cases rapidly so that isolation and treatment can be initiated promptly. To achieve this goal, a surveillance program for influenza-like respiratory illnesses (ILI) should be in place during the influenza season. The CDC defines ILI as a temperature of 37.8°C or greater, accompanied by any symptoms of cough, coryza, or sore throat. However, only 70% of all elderly with influenza will have fever, so some cases will be missed. Another proposed definition includes symptoms of cough, sore throat, nasal congestion, or rhinorrhea with or without fever. None of these definitions, however, have been validated in a large prospective study in nursing homes. Residents exhibiting any of the above symptoms should have a nasopharyngeal swab taken for rapid influenza detection and viral culture. Laboratory documentation of influenza infection is important because other respiratory infections have similar clinical manifestations in the elderly (7). Rapid diagnostic tests are also important for the purpose of early treatment and prophylaxis. Lower attack rates of influenza have been demonstrated in an uncontrolled study in nursing homes that used both rapid influenza tests and culture compared to those that used culture alone.

The CDC recommends that when institutional outbreaks occur, chemoprophylaxis should be administered to all residents regardless of their vaccine status. The definition of an outbreak, however, remains controversial. Most recommend starting chemoprophylaxis when 10% of residents on a ward have ILI and influenza has been documented. Others define an outbreak as two to three cases of ILI occurring within 48 to 72 hours. Once prophylaxis is started it should be continued for two weeks or one week after the last documented case of influenza. Other measures during an outbreak include vaccination and chemoprophylaxis of unvaccinated staff. Chemoprophylaxis should be continued for two weeks after vaccination of staff members when protective antibodies are generated. In epidemics where the vaccine virus does not match the circulating virus strain, staff members should receive chemoprophylaxis only.

The present recommendation is to use either amantadine or rimantadine in influenza A outbreaks. No recommendations have been published regarding the prophylactic use of zanamivir or oseltamivir in nursing homes. Although more expensive, rimantadine is preferable to amantadine for influenza A outbreaks because of fewer side effects. Influenza cases that develop on rimantadine prophylaxis may be treated with oseltamivir because of the possibility of rimantadine-resistant virus. For influenza B outbreaks and patients with seizure disorders, the use of the zanamivir or oseltamivir should be considered. Oseltamivir is preferred because of the ease of administration and at this time it is the only agent approved for prophylaxis.

Another measure to control outbreaks in long-term care facilities is isolation. Because transmission of influenza virus can occur by aerosol and fomites, isolation of ill residents is recommended (19). Patients should be confined to their rooms, and centralized activities should be decentralized or postponed. Health-care workers should wear masks when in close contact with ill residents and should wash their hands after contact (Table 3). The optimal duration of isolation is unclear, but three to five days is reasonable. The effectiveness of these isolation methods has not been proven in long-term care facilities but have been useful in hospital-based outbreaks. Other measures include closing the facility or ward to new admissions, restricting visitors, requesting sick personnel remain home, and restricting personnel from floating to others wards.

Vaccination

The most effective measure to prevent influenza outbreak in nursing homes is annual administration of inactivated trivalent influenza vaccine to both staff and residents. Previous surveys of nursing homes have reported vaccination rates of residents varying between 15% and 100%. Recent surveys in 1998–1999 by the CDC, which included 1017 homes in the United States, have shown an increased rate of nursing home resident vaccination ranging from 79% to 91% with a mean of 83% (18). This is the percentage of vaccination recommended to provide protection by herd immunity. The increase in the vaccination rate of nursing home staff has been less impressive. Low rates of staff vaccination at 7% to 10% have been previously reported during nursing homes outbreaks. More recent surveys report the rates to have increased to 32% to 57% of staff with a mean of 46%. Attempts at increasing staff vaccination is important because studies have shown that immunization of staff in nursing homes is associated with a decrease in the mortality of residents living in long-term facilities, irrespective of their vaccination status. Vaccination of staff is also associated with less frequent nursing home outbreaks (22,23).

In healthy young adults, the inactivated trivalent vaccine has 70% to 90% protective efficacy if there is a good antigenic match between the vaccine strain and the circulating influenza virus. Few prospective studies have been conducted in elderly population. Retrospective case-controlled studies have shown a vaccine protective efficacy of 30% to 40% (24). In elderly living in the community, influenza vaccination is associated with a reduction of hospitalization for cardiac and cerebrovascular disease, pneumonia, or influenza, as well reducing risks of death (25,26). Although protective efficacy is lower in nursing home residents, benefit from vaccination is still derived (27–29). Hospitalization rates are reduced by 50% to 60% and mortality by 80%. Influenza vaccine also reduces the duration of illness. Because the effectiveness of vaccination is lower in individuals over age 65 than younger adults, ways to improve the level of protection against influenza infection are being studied. Use of higher doses of vaccine and adjuvants have been tried with mixed success. Live attenuated virus vaccines generated by genetic reassortment with cold adapted influenza A and B viruses have also been studied in children, young adults, elderly, and high-risk patients. Intranasal trivalent cold adapted vaccine was shown to have more than 90% efficacy in preventing influenza A and B in children and is approved for use in 5 to 49 year-olds, including health-care workers, with no high-risk conditions predisposing to complicated influenza (30). The immune response to cold adapted influenza vaccine in elderly persons has been less than optimal when compared with younger subjects. Studies combining both inactivated and activated vaccines in nursing home residents indicate only modest benefit. Because T-cell function declines with age and is one of the reasons for poor response of elderly patient to influenza vaccination, novel virosomal influenza vaccines inducing both humeral and cellular immunity are undergoing studies. Virosomes are viruslike particles consisting of reconstituted viral envelopes lacking the viral genetic material. Preliminary data in elderly show a more sustained humeral response compared to the inactivated virus vaccine. Cytotoxic responses are still undergoing investigation (31).

RESPIRATORY SYNCYTIAL VIRUS

Epidemiology and Clinical Relevance

RSV is an RNA virus of the paramyxovirus family. Two antigenically distinct groups have been recognized: group A and B. RSV is well known to cause severe disease in infants and young children and causes winter epidemics of bronchitis, bronchiolitis, and pneumonia in temperate climates. Reinfection occurs throughout life because immunity is incomplete. RSV typically causes URI in young healthy adults but is more severe in immunocompromised, frail elderly and in patients with underlying cardiopulmonary diseases (32).

Using U.S. national mortality and viral surveillance data, Thompson estimated that RSV is associated with an annual mean of 10,000 deaths in patients above the age of 65 years (4). RSV accounts for an estimated 2% to 11% of hospitalizations for lower respiratory tract disease in persons over age 65. It also accounts for 2% to 9% of deaths from pneumonia in hospitalized elderly patients, and mortality could be as high as 38% in patients admitted from LTCF (33,34). The highest risk of complications, as in influenza infection, occurs in patients with underlying cardiac or pulmonary diseases (35). Morbidity in the elderly is similar to influenza and results in prolonged hospitalizations averaging two weeks with approximately 9% to 18% requiring intensive care admission and mechanical ventilation. More than 10% of patients experienced functional decline and required a higher level of care at discharge (34).

In long-term care facilities, RSV ranks second to influenza as a cause of respiratory infections. RSV accounts for 5% to 27% of respiratory illnesses in these facilities. Attack rates vary widely, depending on the diagnostic test used, and range between 12% and 89% in outbreak situations and 1% and 40% in prospective studies. The severity of the disease and complications also vary, with pneumonia reported in 0% to 55% of cases and mortality in 0% to 53%. One recent population-based study, to assess the burden of influenza and RSV in LTCF, was conducted over four years and included residents of 381 Tennessee nursing homes. The authors report that the impact of RSV on hospitalization, use of antimicrobials, and mortality was as important as influenza. In high-risk residents, influenza and RSV accounted for 7% of cardiopulmonary hospitalizations and 14% of deaths. RSV accounted for an average of 15 hospitalizations due to cardiopulmonary disease, 76 courses of antibiotic courses, and 17 deaths per 1000 persons. In comparison, influenza was responsible for 28 hospitalizations and 15 deaths per 1000 persons (36).

Clinical Manifestations

Rhinorrhea, cough, sputum production, dyspnea, and wheezing characterize RSV infections (2,37). Fever and constitutional symptoms are seen in approximately half of cases. In nursing home residents or hospitalized elderly patients, the clinical presentation of RSV infection is similar to influenza (34). Both infections cause overlapping of upper and lower respiratory symptoms. Systemic symptoms, such as malaise, myalgias, and chills, are more common with influenza, as are gastrointestinal complaints or fever above 99.0°F. Nasal congestion followed by cough and wheezing are more characteristic of RSV infection (32). Although certain features suggest influenza or RSV, no signs or symptoms are pathognomonic, and, thus, the clinical distinction between the two infections is extremely difficult. In a study of patients above the age of 65 years admitted to the hospital with cardiopulmonary illnesses, the only significant difference in signs and symptoms between RSV and influenza cases was the greater frequency of fever above 38°C, which was reflected in a greater number of blood cultures taken in the influenza A group (Table 2). Because both influenza and RSV infections cause a similar clinical picture, it is important to perform diagnostic tests for both influenza and RSV when a cluster of respiratory infection occurs in long-term care facilities.

Diagnostic Approach

The diagnosis of RSV infection is made by viral culture of respiratory secretions. Because nasal wash is difficult in older persons, a nasopharyngeal swab is an acceptable method for specimen collection. In adults, the sensitivity of culture is poor because the titer of virus shed is low and RSV is thermolabile and does not survive long in transit time. The reported sensitivity of culture in nursing home patients is at best 50% and usually significantly lower (38). More rapid methods to diagnose RSV rely on antigen detection from a nasopharyngeal specimens using IFA or EIA. Although useful in children, these tests are not very sensitive in older persons. Only 1 out of 11 elderly patients with RSV infection proven by culture or serology was positive by IFA, and none tested positive by commercial EIA (38). RT-PCR is a new diagnostic technique that shows much promise for the rapid diagnosis of RSV in elderly patients. The test has been shown to be very sensitive and specific (39). At the present time, however, drawbacks include expense and limited commercial availability. Serology, using a fourfold rise antibody in acute and convalescent specimens, is also useful but not for the immediate diagnosis of RSV infection. Detection of antibody rises by EIA appears to be about twice as sensitive as complement fixation tests.

Therapeutic Interventions

Treatment of RSV infection in the elderly patient is supportive using hydration and oxygenation. Bronchospasm may be treated with bronchodilators and steroids, but they are not of proven benefit. No antiviral treatment has been studied in randomized trials in adults or elderly, but aerosolized ribavirin could be considered in certain situations. The drug is approved for the treatment of severe RSV infection in high-risk infants and is usually given by inhalation for two to five days (40). It has been shown to decrease viral shedding but had no clear effect on symptoms in the treatment of experimentally infected young adults. Case reports using aerosolized ribavirin, mostly in adults, also suggest that its use might be beneficial in selected severe cases. In elderly volunteers with chronic obstructive pulmonary disease, the drug has been found to be safe when given for six or 12 hours per day for four days. If treatment is considered, it should be started within few days of symptom onset. In the hospitalized elderly patient, a high dose of aerosolized ribavirin (60 mg/mL) administered over a short duration of two hours three times per day may be better tolerated than continuous inhalation. This dosing regimen was found to be as effective in children as the recommended 20 mg/mL dose aerosolized over 18 hours (41).

Infection Control

Transmission of RSV is from person to person and requires close contact (within 3 ft), suggesting large droplet or fomite spread. RSV can survive for more than six hours on nonporous environmental surfaces. Natural challenge experiments during nosocomial outbreaks on pediatric wards showed that

RSV spread with 70% efficacy during close contact with infected infants, such as cuddling, and with 30% efficiency when only surfaces in the rooms were touched. Airborne transmission is not seen, and, thus, masks are not recommended. Virus inoculation is usually in the eye or nose, less commonly in the throat. The use of goggles that cover the eyes and nose was associated with a decrease in the rate of nosocomial infections on pediatric wards; however, these devices are not felt to be practical. RSV outbreaks in long-term facilities are less explosive than influenza outbreaks and are characterized by a steady trickle of cases with clustering by building, floor, and hallway. Controlling outbreaks requires early diagnosis, interruption of either hand carriage or self-inoculation of the eyes and nose. Strict hand washing is the most important measure to control the spread of infection. Because compliance with hand washing is frequently poor, some authorities have advocated the additional use of gowns and gloves. Isolating symptomatic patients in their room, cohorting staff, and closing the units to new admissions are other recommended measures (Table 3) (42).

PARAINFLUENZA

Epidemiology and Clinical Relevance

Parainfluenza virus (PIV) is a paramyxovirus. Four serotypes have been identified: types 1 to 4, with type 4 having two subgroups (A and B). The PIV serotypes vary in their clinical presentation and seasonality. Parainfluenza types 1 and 2 are more common in fall and usually alternate years. PIV 1 and 2 primarily cause croup and bronchiolitis in children. Parainfluenza type 3 most frequently infects infants below the age of six months. It occurs year round but usually follows the influenza season in late winter and spring. By the age of five years 59% to 100% of children have been infected (43). Parainfluenza 3 causes relatively severe disease and is second only to RSV as a cause of serious lower respiratory infection in infants and children (43). Like RSV recurrent PIV infections are common throughout life. PIV1 and PIV3 have been most commonly described as the cause of serious infections in elderly. Overall, parainfluenza infections are not as commonly reported in older persons as influenza or RSV and account for approximately 5% to 6% of respiratory illnesses in nursing home residents and elderly in community dwelling. PIV accounts for 2.5% to 3.1% of adult hospitalizations for lower respiratory tract infection (44). Several outbreaks have been described in long-term care facilities, with attack rates varying between 2% and 56% and significant morbidity (45,46). Secondary pneumonia occurred in 0% to 36% and death in 0% to 11% of cases. Close contact with the infected patients resulted in an attack rate of 35% in staff members, compared to 11% in those without resident contact, suggesting the importance of person-to-person transmission.

Table 3 Control of Nursing Home Nosocomial Viral Respiratory Infections

Virus	Influenza	RSV	PIV	Rhinovirus	Coronavirus	Human metapneumovirus
Mode of spread	Close contact, aerosol, ? skin, fomite	Close contact skin, fomite	Close contact skin, fomite	Close contact skin, fomite, ? aerosol	Unknown	Unknown
Control measures						
Hand washing	+	+	+	+	+	+
Gloves	+	+				
Masks	+					
Isolation of ill patients in their room	+	+	+	±		
Cohort staff	+	+	+			
Limiting group activities	+	+	+			
Closing facility or ward to new admissions	+	±	±			
Limit visitors with respiratory illness	+	±	±			

Abbreviations: RSV, respiratory syncytial virus; PIV, parainfluenza virus.
Source: From Ref. 42.

Clinical Manifestations

The incubation period is short, two to six days. Virus can be isolated for up to seven days or longer after onset of illness. In healthy adults, the symptoms of PIV are not distinct from the common cold. Patients typically have nasal discharge, congestion, and sneezing. Cough, generalized malaise, and fever may also occur. The most common symptoms reported from an outbreak of PIV 3 among residents of a nursing home in Canada were rhinorrhea and cough. Some patients also had wheezing, fever, and sore throat. Approximately half of the residents developed lower respiratory symptoms (47).

Diagnostic Approach

The gold standard for PIV diagnosis is viral culture of nasopharyngeal secretions, but identification may take up to one week. It is important to process the culture rapidly and to keep it at 4°C during transport. Rapid tests being developed include direct detection by IFA, which is less sensitive than culture, and RT-PCR, which although sensitive is not widely available. Serologic analysis can establish the diagnosis retrospectively.

Therapeutic Interventions

Treatment of PIV in adults is supportive. A few anecdotal reports on the use of aerosolized ribavirin in lower respiratory infections have been reported in immunocompromised children and adults with severe parainfluenza virus pneumonia. In children, systemic steroids for treatment of croup resulted in lower rate of hospitalization compared to placebo or aerosolized steroids (43). At present, no general recommendations can be made.

Infection Control

The exact mode of PIV transmission is not defined, but the slow transmission suggests a person-to-person spread either through contaminated hands or droplets. The virus can survive at least few hours on environmental surfaces and for a short duration on hands. Therefore, hand washing, disinfecting of environmental surfaces, and case isolation are all important in controlling outbreaks of PIV in institutional settings.

CORONAVIRUS

Epidemiology and Clinical Relevance

Coronaviruses are single stranded RNA viruses. Two subtypes, 229E and OC43, cause human infection. These viruses cause symptoms similar to the common cold. Coronavirus 229E grows in cell culture, but OC43 is more difficult to isolate and requires human embryonic tracheal organ culture. Because of the difficulty with viral isolation, the overall clinical impact of coronaviruses in adults has not been well defined. Longitudinal serologic studies in different populations of children, healthy adults, and army recruits report that coronavirus infection accounts for 4% to 15% of acute respiratory disease per year. The percentage increases to 35% during outbreaks. Infection occurs throughout the year but has peaks in winter and early spring.

Data of the impact of coronavirus infections in nursing homes are limited. One published study that used serology to test for OC43 and 229E infection in patients from 11 nursing homes in England found an 11% infection rate (48). Lower respiratory complications occurred in a quarter of the infected patients. A surveillance study in an adult day care performed over 44 months showed that coronavirus infection accounted for 8% of all respiratory tract infections (49). Infection of the staff members typically preceded infection in the elderly daycare participants.

Clinical Manifestations

The incubation period for coronaviruses is two to four days. Disease is indistinguishable from that of the common cold. In older persons in day care, the infection with coronavirus was associated with nasal congestion, cough, constitutional symptoms, and low-grade fever (49). The subjects recovered without sequelae, but illnesses were prolonged lasting an average of 14 days. Fifty percent of subjects had lower respiratory involvement, as evidenced by sputum production, shortness of breath, wheezing, or rales. No pneumonia or deaths were documented. In hospitalized patients with coronavirus infection, lower respiratory symptoms are common: 83% experience dyspnea, 75% have wheezing, 58% have sputum production. Myalgias, fatigue, and fever are less common when compared to hospitalized patients with influenza. Some patients developed pneumonia (50).

Diagnostic Approach

Outside of research settings, diagnosis of coronavirus infection is rarely made because of difficulty in culturing the virus and because the clinical features are indistinguishable from the common cold. As with other respiratory viruses, RT-PCR shows promise as a useful tool to diagnosis acute coronavirus infections (51). Although serologic assays using complement fixation can be used for retrospective analysis, these tests are also not available for general use.

Therapeutic Interventions

Treatment of coronavirus infections is symptomatic. One report of intranasal interferon in adult experimentally challenged with type 229E showed a reduction severity of the clinical illness; however, no antiviral drugs are currently approved to treat coronavirus infections.

Infection Control

The mode of transmission of coronavirus has not been well studied, and no firm recommendations can be given for infection control. Good hand washing seems most reasonable.

RHINOVIRUS

Epidemiology and Clinical Relevance

Rhinoviruses are the most frequent cause of the common cold and are recovered from approximately one-third of patients in the community with cold symptoms (52). More than 100 serotypes have been identified accounting for the recurrence of infection throughout life. In temperate climates, rhinovirus infections tend to peak in fall and spring, although they do occur sporadically in winter. Rhinovirus infection is also common in older adults when specifically tested for using sensitive diagnostic techniques, such as RT-PCR. Rhinovirus accounted for 24% of respiratory illnesses in subjects over age 60 living in the community in a study from the United Kingdom (53). In frail older persons attending senior day care program, rhinoviruses were the cause of 7% of respiratory illnesses (49). Both studies show that in the older population the infection is more severe than in younger adults, with symptoms lasting for 14 to 16 days. Frail elderly with underlying heart and lung problems have more severe disease, in some cases leading to hospitalization (50).

Two outbreaks of rhinovirus infection in a long-term facility are reported (54,55). A high rate of lower respiratory symptoms was noted. In one of the outbreak involving 56 residents with a 100% attack rate, 27% of the residents had radiologic evidence of pneumonia, and 21% died. Of note, several of the health-care workers were affected and might have played a significant role in transmission. Overall, rhinoviruses generally do not result in the significant morbidity observed with influenza or RSV infection (2,35).

Clinical Manifestations

The clinical symptoms of rhinovirus illness can be quite variable in the elderly patient ranging from trivial sniffles to cough and dyspnea (49,54). Nasal congestion and scratchy throat characterize most illnesses. Fever, cough, dyspnea, and constitutional symptoms may also be observed and are more common in the elderly patients than in young adults. Again, the infection cannot be clinically differentiated from other viruses causing respiratory infections.

Diagnostic Approach

Both viral culture and RT-PCR may be used for diagnosis.

Therapeutic Interventions

Treatment is usually symptomatic with oral decongestant, antihistamine, and nonsteroidal anti-inflammatory medications. Pleconaril, an antiviral agent with activity against picornaviruses, has been shown to be of value in decreasing symptoms of rhinovirus infection in young healthy adults, but no data are available in the elderly. Studies using interferon alpha 2 with ipratropium applied topically in the nose with naproxen orally have also shown modest benefit for symptom relief. Further studies are needed before any of these therapies can be recommended.

Infection Control

Rhinoviruses are transmitted by contact with infected secretions, which are spread from hand to hand, followed by autoinoculation of nasal or conjunctival mucosa. Virus may also be transmitted from contaminated surfaces. Aerosol transmission has also been documented under experimental conditions but is not felt to be the primary mechanism of spread in nosocomial settings. Hand washing and avoidance of hand-to-nose or-eye contact are important infection control measures. Containing infected secretions by using tissues and covering the mouth during coughing are encouraged. The use of masks to prevent the spread of infection has not been studied.

HUMAN METAPNEUMOVIRUS

Epidemiology and Clinical Relevance

Human metapneumovirus is a newly discovered respiratory pathogen isolated in the Netherlands from young children with respiratory tract disease (56). The virus is a member of the Paramyxoviridae family and is composed of two groups (group A and B). Few seroprevalence studies indicate that virtually all children are infected by the age of five years (56). Reinfection occurs throughout life, possibly due to loss of protective antibodies or due to reinfection by different genotypes. In temperate zones, most cases are reported in late March and early April, frequently overlapping with RSV season. The virus is often recovered with other pathogens, such as influenza, RSV, or streptococcus pneumonia. It is unclear if coinfection leads to a more severe disease (57–59). Similar to influenza and RSV, metapneumovirus illness is more severe in elderly and in adult patients with underlying cardiopulmonary disease, immunocompromise, or neurologic disease (59,60). Disease has been reported in patient residing in long-term care, but no outbreaks have yet been described.

Clinical Manifestations

The incubation is not well defined, but from a nosocomial pediatric outbreak it is estimated to be five to six days (57). The virus causes lower respiratory disease in children, mostly bronchiolitis, with or without pneumonia, otitis media, laryngitis, or pharyngitis. In adult, the illness is difficult to differentiate from an influenza-like illness or cold. Adults complain of congestion, hoarseness, productive cough, and rhinorrhea. Fever and sore throat are less common. In the older adult population, the virus causes lower respiratory disease with dyspnea, wheezing, and in some cases pneumonia. Illness is more prolonged, lasting between 10 and 17 days (61,62). Many patients with an underlying cardiopulmonary disease or who are immunocompromised are hospitalized and some require intensive care unit (ICU) stay (60). Death has also been reported (61).

Diagnostic Approach

The virus grows very slowly in cell culture, and it takes up to 10 to 14 days after inoculation for the development of cytopathogenic effect. Diagnosis of acute disease will therefore have to rely on rapid testing, and presently the diagnostic method of choice is RT-PCR. Serologic testing requires a fourfold rise in antibody level and will not be useful in the diagnosis of an acute infection.

Infection Control

The mode of transmission has not been studied but is probably similar to RSV.

SUGGESTED READING

Falsey AR, Erdman D, Anderson LJ, Walsh EE. Human metapneumovirus infections in young and elderly adults. J Infect Dis 2003; 187:785–790.

Falsey AR, Walsh EE. Respiratory syncytial virus infection in elderly adults. Drugs Aging 2005; 22:577–587.

Falsey AR, Walsh EE, Hayden FG. Rhinovirus and coronavirus infection-associated hospitalizations among older adults. J Infect Dis 2002; 185:1338–1341.

Walsh EE, Cox C, Falsey AR. Clinical features of influenza A virus infection in older hospitalized persons. J Am Geriatr Soc 2002; 50:1498–1503.

Wright PF. Parainfluenza viruses. In: Mandell GL, Bennett JE, Dolin R, eds. Principles and Practices of Infectious Disease. Philadelphia: Elsevier Churchill Livingstone, 2005:1998–2003.

REFERENCES

1. Nicholson KG, Kent J, Hammersley V, et al. Acute viral infections of upper respiratory tract in elderly people living in the community; comparative, prospective, population based study of disease burden. Br Med J 1997; 315: 1060–1064.
2. Falsey AR, Treanor JJ, Betts RF, et al. Viral respiratory infections in the institutionalized elderly: clinical and epidemiologic findings. J Am Geriatr Soc 1992; 40:115–119.

3. Treanor, John J. Influenza virus. In: Mandell GL, Bennett JE, Dolin R, eds. Principles and Practice of Infectious Diseases. Philadelphia: Elsevier, Churchill Livingstone, 2005:2060–2085.
4. Thompson WW, Shay DK, Weintraub E, et al. Mortality associated with influenza and respiratory syncytial virus in the United States. J Am Med Assoc 2003; 289:179–186.
5. Centers for Disease Control and Prevention. Prevention and control of influenza: recommendations of the Advisory Committee of Immunization Practices (ACIP). MMWR 2005; 54:1–41.
6. Barker WH, Mullooly JP. Pneumonia and influenza deaths during epidemics— implications for prevention. Arch Intern Med 1982; 142:85–89.
7. Wald TG, Miller BA, Shult P, et al. Can respiratory syncytial virus and influenza A be distinguished clinically in institutionalized older persons? J Am Geriatr Soc 1995; 43:170–174.
8. Center for Disease Control. Lab diagnosis—role of laboratory diagnosis. (Accessed on 7–22–05 at http://www.cdc.gov/flu/professionals/labdiagnosis. htm 7–13–2005.).
9. Monto AS, Rotthoff J, Teich E, et al. Detection and control of influenza outbreaks in well-vaccinated nursing home populations. Clin Infect Dis 2004; 39:459–464.
10. Walsh EE, Cox C, Falsey A. Clinical features of influenza A virus infection in older hospitalized Persons. JAGS 2002; 50:1498–1503.
11. Betts RF, Treanor J, Braman P, et al. Antiviral agents to prevent or treat influenza in the elderly. J Respir Dis 1987; 8(suppl):S56–S59.
12. Kolbe F, Sitar DS, Papioannou A, et al. An amantadine hydrochloride dosing program adjusted for renal function during an influenza outbreak in elderly institutionalized patients. Can J Clin Pharmacol 2003; 10:119–122.
13. Monto AS, Fleming DM, Henry D, et al. Efficacy and safety of the neuraminidase inhibitor zanamivir in the treatment of influenza A and B virus infections. J Infect Dis 1999; 180:254–261.
14. The MIST Study Group. Randomised trial of efficacy and safety of inhaled zanamivir in treatment of influenza A and B virus infections. Lancet 1998; 352(9144):1877–1881.
15. Treanor JJ, Hayden FG, Vrooman PS, et al. Efficacy and safety of the oral neuraminidase inhibitor oseltamivir in treating acute influenza (a randomized controlled trial). JAMA 2000; 283(8):1016–1024.
16. Schilling M, Povinelli L, Krause P, et al. Efficacy of zanamivir for chemoprophylaxis of nursing home influenza outbreaks. Vaccine 1998; 16:1771–1774.
17. Munoz FM, Galasso GJ, Gwaltney JR, et al. Current research on influenza and other respiratory viruses: II international symposium. Antiviral Res 2001; 46:91–124.
18. Arden NH. Control of influenza in the long-term-care facility: a review of established approaches and newer options. Infect Control Hosp Epidemiol 2000; 21(1):59–64.
19. Bradley SF. Long-Term-Care Committee of the Society for Healthcare Epidemiology of America. Prevention of influenza in long-term-care facilities. Infect Control Hosp Epidemiol 1999; 20(9):629–637.
20. Gravenstein S, Davidson HE. Current strategies for management of influenza in the elderly population. Clin Infect Dis 2002; 35:729–737.

21. Advisory Committee on Immunization Practices. Use of standing orders programs to increase adult vaccination rates. MMWR 2005; 49(RR01):15–26.
22. Carman WF, Elder AG, Wallace LA, et al. Effects of influenza vaccination of health-care workers on mortality of elderly people in long-term care: a randomised controlled trial. Lancet 2000; 335:93–97.
23. Potter J, Stott DJ, Roberts MA, et al. Influenza vaccination of health care workers in long-term-care hospitals reduces the mortality of elderly patients. J Infect Dis 1997; 175:1–6.
24. Gross PA, Hermogenes AW, Sacks HS, et al. The efficacy of influenza vaccine in elderly persons—a meta-analysis and review of the literature. Ann Intern Med 1995; 123:518–527.
25. Nichol KL. The efficacy, effectiveness and cost-effectiveness of inactivated influenza vaccines. Vaccine 2003; 21:1769–1775.
26. Nichol KL, Nordin J, Mullooly J, et al. Influenza vaccination and reduction in hospitalizations for cardiac disease and stroke among the elderly. NEJM 2003; 348:1322–1332.
27. Voordouw BC, van der Linden PD, Simonian S, et al. Influenza vaccination in community-dwelling elderly: impact on mortality and influenza-associated morbidity. Arch Intern Med 2003; 163:1089–1094.
28. Nordin J, Mullooly J, Poblete S, et al. Influenza vaccine effectiveness in preventing hospitalizations and deaths in persons 65 years or older in Minnesota, New York, and Oregon: data from 3 health plans. J Infect Dis 2001; 184:665–670.
29. Monto AS, Hornbuckle K, Ohmit SE. Influenza vaccine effectiveness among elderly nursing home residents: a cohort study. Am J Epidemiol 2001; 154:155–160.
30. Belshe RB, Mendelman PM, Treanor J, et al. The efficacy of live attenuated, cold-adapted, trivalent, intranasal influenza virus vaccine in children. NEJM 1998; 338(20):1405–1412.
31. de Bruijn IA, Nauta J, Cramer WCM, et al. Clinical experience with inactivated, virosomal influenza vaccine. Vaccine 2005; 35:S39–S54.
32. Falsey AR, Walsh EE. Respiratory syncytial virus infection in elderly adults. Drugs Aging 2005; 22:577–587.
33. Han LL, Alexander JP, Anderson LJ. Respiratory syncytial virus pneumonia among the elderly: an assessment of disease burden. J Infect Dis 1999; 179:25–30.
34. Falsey AR, Hennessey PA, Formica MA, et al. Respiratory syncytial virus infection in elderly and high-risk adults. N Engl J Med 2005; 352:1749–1759.
35. Walsh EE, Falsey AR, Hennessey PA. Respiratory syncytial virus and other infections in persons with chronic cardiopulmonary disease. Am J Respir Crit Care Med 1999; 160:791–795.
36. Ellis SE, Coffey CS, Mitchel EF, et al. Influenza and respiratory syncytial virus-associated morbidity and mortality in the nursing home population. J Am Geriatr Soc 2003; 51:761–767.
37. Falsey AR, McCann RM, Hall WJ, et al. Acute respiratory tract infection in daycare centers for older persons. J Am Geriatr Soc 1995; 43:30–36.
38. Falsey AR, McCann RM, Hall WJ, et al. Evaluation of four methods for the diagnosis of respiratory syncytial virus infection in older adults. J Am Geriatr Soc 1996; 44:71–73.

39. Walsh EE, Falsey AR, Swinburne IA, et al. Reverse transcription polymerase chain reaction (RT-PCR) for diagnosis of respiratory syncytial virus infection in adults: use of a single-tube "hanging droplet" nested PCR. J Med Virol 2001; 63:259–263.

40. Hall CB, McCarthy CA. Respiratory syncytial virus. In: Mandell GL, Bennett JE, Dolin R, eds. Principles and Practices of Infectious Disease. Philadelphia: Elsevier Churchill Livingstone, 2004:2008–2026.

41. Englund JA, Piedra PA, Ahn Y-M, et al. High-dose, short-duration ribavirin aerosol therapy compared with standard ribavirin therapy in children with suspected respiratory syncytial virus infection. J Pediatr 1994; 125:635–641.

42. Graman PS, Hall CB. Epidemiology and control of nosocomial viral infections. Infect Dis Clin North Am 1989; 3(4):815–841.

43. Wright PF. Parainfluenza viruses. In: Mandell GL, Bennett JE, Dolin R, eds. Principles and Practice of Infectious Diseases. Philadelphia: Elsevier, Churchill, Livingstone, 2005:1998–2003.

44. Marx A, Gary HE, Martston BJ et al. Parainfluenza virus infection among adults hospitalized for lower respiratory tract infection. Clin Infect Dis 1999; 29(1):134–140.

45. Public Health Laboratory Service Communicable Disease Surveillance Centre. Parainfluenza infections in the elderly 1976–82. Br Med J 1983; 287:1619.

46. Anonymous Epidemiologic Notes and Reports. Parainfluenza outbreaks in extended care facilities—United States. MMWR 1978; 27:475–476.

47. Loeb M, McGeer A, McArthur M, et al. Surveillance for outbreaks of respiratory tract infections in nursing homes. Can Med Assoc J 2000; 162(8):1133–1137.

48. Nicholson KG, Baker DJ, Farquhar A, et al. Acute upper respiratory tract viral illness and influenza immunization in homes for the elderly. Epidemiol Infect 1990; 105:609–618.

49. Falsey AR, McCann RM, Hall WJ, et al. The "common cold" in frail older persons: impact of rhinovirus and coronavirus in a senior daycare center. J Am Geriatr Soc 1997; 45:706–711.

50. Falsey AR, Walsh EE, Hayden FG. Rhinovirus and coronavirus infection-associated hospitalizations among older adults. J Infect Dis 2002; 185:1338–1341.

51. Glezen PW, Greenberg SB, Atmar RL, et al. Impact of respiratory virus infections on persons with chronic underlying conditions. JAMA 2000; 283:499–505.

52. Monto A, Bryan ER, Ohmit S. Rhinovirus infections in Tecumseh, Michigan: frequency of illness and number of serotypes. J Infect Dis 1987; 156:43–49.

53. Nicholson KG, Kent J, Hammersley V, et al. Risk factors for lower respiratory complications of rhinovirus infections in elderly people living in the community: prospective cohort study. Br Med J 1996; 313:1119–1123.

54. Wald TG, Shult P, Krause P, et al. A rhinovirus outbreak among residents of a long-term care facility. Ann Intern Med 1995; 123:588–593.

55. Louie JK, Yagi S, Nelson FA, et al. Rhinovirus outbreak in a long term care facility for elderly persons associated with unusually high mortality. Clin Infect Dis 2005; 41:265.

56. van den Hoogen BG, DeJong JC, Groen J, et al. A newly discovered human pneumovirus isolated from young children with respiratory tract disease. Nature Med 2001; 7:719–724.

57. Falsey AR. Human metapneumovirus. In: Mandell GL, Bennett JE, Dolin R, eds. Principles and Practice of Infectious Diseases. Philadelphia: Elsevier, Churchill, Livingstone, 2005:2026–2031.
58. Lazar I, Weibel C, Dziura J, et al. Human metapneumovirus and severity of respiratory syncytial disease. Emerg Infect Dis 2004; 10:1318–1320.
59. Hamelin ME, Abed Y, Boivin G. Human metapneumovirus: a new player among respiratory viruses. Clin Infect Dis 2004; 38:983–990.
60. Hamelin ME, Cote S, Laforge J, et al. Human metapneumovirus infection in adults with community-acquired pneumonia and exacerbation of chronic obstructive pulmonary disease. Clin Infect Dis 2005; 41:498–502.
61. Falsey AR, Erdman D, Anderson LJ, et al. Human metapneumovirus infections in young and elderly adults. J Infect Dis 2003; 187:785–790.
62. Boivin G, Abed Y, Pelletier G, et al. Virological features and clinical manifestations associated with human metapneumovirus: a new paramyxovirus responsible for acute respiratory-tract infections in all age groups. J Infect Dis 2002; 186:1330–1334.

14

Pneumonia and Bronchitis

Joseph M. Mylotte

*Department of Medicine, School of Medicine and Biomedical Sciences,
State University of New York, Buffalo, New York, U.S.A.*

KEY POINTS

1. Pneumonia is associated with the highest mortality of any infection in nursing home residents.
2. Most residents with pneumonia will have at least one respiratory symptom or sign (cough, tachypnea, localized findings on chest exam, or hypoxemia) to suggest the diagnosis.
3. Most residents (>75%) with pneumonia can be treated in the nursing home, as there is no evidence that hospitalization impacts significantly on outcome.
4. A quinolone alone is effective therapy for most episodes of pneumonia treated in the nursing home or hospital.
5. Bronchitis in nursing home residents is usually viral in etiology and does not require antibacterial therapy.

NURSING HOME–ASSOCIATED PNEUMONIA

Pneumonia is the second most common cause of infection among residents in nursing homes and is associated with the highest mortality of any infection occurring in this setting (1). In addition, pneumonia is a common reason for transfer from the nursing home to the hospital (1). This section reviews the literature on nursing home–associated pneumonia (NHAP) and has a particular focus on the management and prevention of this infection.

Epidemiology and Clinical Relevance

Incidence

The reported incidence of NHAP has ranged from 0.3 to 2.5 episodes per 1000 resident care days (1). The variation in incidence may be related to several factors, including differences in incidence over time, study design, number of facilities evaluated, intensity of surveillance, or facility affiliation (veterans affairs vs. community). Two studies carried out more than 10 years apart found rates of NHAP of 1 episode per 1000 resident care days (2) and 0.7 episodes per 1000 resident care days (3). Therefore, it would appear reasonable to assume that the incidence of NHAP in most facilities is 1 episode per 1000 resident care days per month. In 1997, of 623,718 episodes of pneumonia among those ≥65 years of age admitted to nonfederal hospitals in the United States, 4.3% occurred in nursing home residents (4).

Risk Factors for NHAP

Independent predictors of NHAP have included poor functional status (5,6), presence of a nasogastric tube (5), swallowing difficulties (3,6,7), an unusual event defined as confusion, agitation, falls, or wandering (6), chronic lung disease (8), tracheostomy (8), increasing age (5), male sex (5), and inadequate oral care (7). In one study (3) influenza vaccination was associated with a significantly lower risk for NHAP. In summary, it is the debilitated and poorly functional nursing home resident, especially those at high risk for aspiration, who are most likely to develop pneumonia.

Pathogenesis

Most episodes of NHAP are due to aspiration of oropharyngeal flora into the lung and failure of host defense mechanisms to eliminate aspirated bacteria (1). One study (9) recently reviewed new insights into the pathogenesis of aspiration among the elderly. The so-called silent aspiration of oropharyngeal flora is said to be an important risk factor for community-acquired pneumonia (CAP) in the elderly (10). Diseases of the central nervous system, such as stroke, are complicated frequently by pneumonia, especially those with dysphagia (11). Basal ganglia infarcts are associated with an especially high risk for pneumonia, compared with those with infarcts involving the cerebral hemispheres (12). Infarcts of the basal ganglia may reduce production of neurotransmitter in the sensory components of the glossopharyngeal and vagal nerves, which results in impaired swallowing and cough reflexes (9).

Although less common according to many authors, acute aspiration of gastric contents as a cause of "pneumonia" in nursing home residents is well described (13). The chemical inflammatory response that results in the lung after gastric content aspiration may lead to symptoms and signs identical to bacterial pneumonia (14). However, the distinction between bacterial pneumonia and gastric content aspiration can be difficult, especially if the aspiration is not witnessed (14). One study (13) found that 69 (27%) of 257 patients in one nursing home had 98 aspiration events during an intensive eight-month observation period. Seventy percent of aspiration episodes were associated with fever and tachypnea, and among 53 chest X-rays obtained after an aspiration, 37 (70%) had a new infiltrate. In a multivariate analysis, a hyperextended neck (elevation of the chin above the horizontal plane with resistance to efforts to return the chin to a normal position), malnutrition, benzodiazepine use, contractures, and use of feeding tubes were independent risk factors for aspiration. Whether or not residents with gastric content aspiration and associated abnormal chest radiographs require antimicrobial therapy remains unclear. Recent studies, using specific definitions of an aspiration event (witnessed, unwitnessed, and suspected), have suggested that aspiration pneumonitis may be more common in nursing home residents presenting as "pneumonia" than previously recognized (15,16).

Etiology

The etiology of NHAP has been the subject of debate for some time, especially regarding the importance of aerobic gram-negative bacilli as causative agents of this infection. When strict criteria were utilized to evaluate sputum specimens (>25 polymorphonuclear leukocytes and <10 epithelial cells per 100-power field) among patients with NHAP, isolation of gram-negative bacilli ranged from 0% to 12%, compared with 9% to 55% when less strict or no criteria were utilized (1). Overall, *Streptococcus pneumoniae* is the most common bacterial pathogen isolated among nursing home residents with pneumonia, followed by nontypeable *Haemophilus influenzae*, and *Moraxella catarrhalis* (1). Atypical organisms, such as *Legionella*, *Chlamydia pneumoniae*, and *Mycoplasma*, have rarely been identified in the small group of studies in which these pathogens were carefully sought (1). The role of viruses as a cause of NHAP has not been adequately studied.

Mortality

Mortality of NHAP treated in the hospital setting has tended to be higher than that treated in the nursing home setting. For residents admitted to the hospital mortality has ranged from 13% to 41%, compared with 7% to 19% among those treated only in the nursing home (1). This variation in mortality is related to differences in definition of mortality, in study design (one facility vs. a population of residents from multiple homes), and in facility affiliation (Veterans Affairs facilities vs. community nursing homes).

One study (17) compared processes of care, clinical characteristics, and crude hospital mortality in elderly Medicare recipients with pneumonia from the community or nursing home admitted to 34 hospitals in Connecticut in 1996–1997. There was no difference in the level of various processes of care achieved between the two groups. However, those with NHAP had a significantly higher crude hospital mortality compared with those with community-acquired pneumonia.

Risk Factors for Mortality

Pre-pneumonia functional status (low, medium, or high dependence) has been identified as an important predictor of mortality due to NHAP in several studies (1). Other factors found to be predictive of mortality related to NHAP include dementia (18), increased respiratory rate (18,19), increased pulse (18), change in mental status (18), witnessed aspiration (20), sedative prescription (20), and comorbidity score (20). In a study in one Veterans Affairs long-term care facility, residents with an episode of pneumonia had a significant risk of death that persisted for up to two years following the episode, compared with age- and dependency-matched controls (20). One study (21) found that improved survival was associated with achieving a higher level of compliance with process of care criteria after controlling for severity of pneumonia.

Physicians have difficulty in accurately assessing severity of CAP (22), and this is true for NHAP as well (23). To address this problem, one group of investigators (22) derived and validated a model for measuring severity of CAP, which has also been validated in NHAP (23). However, the model has limited usefulness in the nursing home setting because it requires laboratory testing that is infrequently done. Other investigators (18) derived a simplified severity of NHAP model that did not require laboratory tests and has the potential to be used by staff in the nursing home. In the derivation cohort, this model defined a low-risk mortality group (≤10% 30-day mortality) and a high-risk mortality group (>35% 30-day mortality). Others (24) have developed a model for predicting mortality in nursing home residents with lower respiratory tract infection (pneumonia or bronchitis), but their model requires laboratory testing and measurements not commonly available in this setting (e.g., body mass index) and may not be practical for clinical use.

Clinical Manifestations

The dogma has been that nursing home residents have an "atypical" presentation, meaning that respiratory symptoms (cough, shortness of breath, pleuritic chest pain, chills) and signs (fever, tachypnea, rales on chest examination) occur less frequently than among age-matched community-dwelling elderly or younger people (1). In a recent study of 378 episodes of NHAP occurring among residents of 11 nursing homes, the findings were: fever, 70%; respiratory rate >30 per minute, 23%; pulse >125 per minute, 6%; cough, 61%; and altered mental status, 38% (18). One study (25) found that nonspecific symptoms (e.g., generalized weakness, loss of appetite, falls, delirium, and new or worsening incontinence) were more common presentations of pneumonia in the elderly compared with those <65 years of age; however, this difference was the result of a confounding effect of dementia in the elderly group. A study focusing on characteristics associated with radiographic pneumonia in nursing home residents found that at least one lower respiratory symptom (cough, sputum production, or pleuritic chest pain) was present in >90% of episodes, but none of these were useful as predictors of pneumonia compared with a respiratory rate ≥30 breaths per minute or the presence of localized crackles on lung auscultation (26). In a case control study, a single oxygen saturation of <94% breathing room air had a positive predictive value of 95% for pneumonia in nursing home residents (27). As part of an evidence-based guideline for the management of NHAP, investigators developed criteria for the diagnosis of "probable" pneumonia. A modification of these criteria is provided in Table 1 (20).

Diagnostic Approach

An expert panel has developed a practice guideline for evaluation of fever and infection in nursing homes Appendix B (29). This guideline clearly acknowledges the problem of obtaining adequate specimens for culture in the nursing home setting. Table 2 lists the panel's recommendations regarding the diagnostic studies in nursing home residents with clinically suspected pneumonia. Consideration should also be given to an assessment of the hydration status of the resident with pneumonia, e.g., blood urea nitrogen determination. Blood cultures should not be done routinely in the diagnostic evaluation of NHAP because the yield is exceedingly low (18).

The bedside assessment of residents by nursing staff is a critical component in diagnosing infections because onsite evaluation by physicians is infrequent (29). Therefore, nursing staff education regarding proper evaluation of residents with suspected infection is an important issue. The diagnostic criteria for pneumonia listed in Table 2 should be considered a starting point for evaluating residents for this infection and should be part

Table 1 Bedside Criteria for the Diagnosis of Suspected Pneumonia in Nursing Home Residents

Pneumonia should be considered a possible diagnosis if two or more of the following symptoms or signs are present:
    New onset of cough with or without sputum production
    Fever (rectal temperature ≥100° F)
    Complaints of shortness of breath
    Respiratory rate ≥25 breaths per minute
    Heart rate ≥100 beats per minute
    Hypoxemia (oxygen saturation <94% breathing room air)
    Acute change in cognitive or functional status
    Localized congestion (rales/ronchi) on chest auscultation

Source: From Ref. 28.

Table 2 Diagnostic Studies for Nursing Home Residents with Suspected Pneumonia[a]

Pulse oximetry to identify hypoxemia (hypoxemia is defined as an oxygen
  saturation <94% breathing room air)
Chest radiograph
Complete blood count with differential
Blood urea nitrogen to assess hydration status

[a]Blood cultures are not recommended in those managed in the nursing home because the yield is low; sputum for Gram stain and culture is not recommended because of the difficulty in obtaining an adequate expectorated specimen, and suctioned specimens are not recommended due to discomfort of the procedure with little if any benefit overall.
Source: From Ref. 29.

of a written protocol for the overall evaluation of infection in the nursing home. Written protocols would tend to reduce variability in the assessment of residents with suspected infection and assist physicians in making management decisions.

Therapeutic Interventions

Once the diagnosis of NHAP is suspected or established and there are no advance directives to the contrary, there are four major decisions to consider in addition to the actual choice of a specific antibacterial agent: (1) location of treatment—nursing home or hospital; (2) initial route—oral versus parenteral—of a treatment for those treated in the nursing home; (3) timing of switch to an oral agent in those given parenteral therapy in the nursing home or hospital; and (4) duration of treatment (30).

Treatment Location

In recent studies, 63% to 78% of NHAP episodes were treated in the nursing home (1). For the majority of residents with NHAP, who usually have mild to moderate infection, treatment in the nursing home is preferable because hospitalization is associated with complications, including loss of functional status, development of pressure ulcers, delirium, and infection. However, because the treatment of pneumonia is expensive and reimbursement may not cover the cost in the nursing home there may be a financial incentive to transfer residents to the hospital for treatment, because nursing homes do not pay for hospital costs (31). One study (31) found that nursing home ownership (for profit vs. not for profit) and payer source strongly influenced rates of hospitalization. Another study (32) found that, after controlling for severity of illness and probability of hospitalization, hospitalization had no impact on mortality of NHAP and was threefold more expensive than treatment in the nursing home. In a separate study, these authors found that residents with a do-not-resuscitate order before development of pneumonia were significantly less likely to be hospitalized for treatment of pneumonia (33). This suggested to the authors that the do-not-resuscitate order functioned as an unstated proxy for limiting care in the absence of explicit discussions about such limitations with family or a surrogate. In addition, other factors may be important in the decision to hospitalize a resident with pneumonia, including a resident's or proxy's preference, time when decompensation occurs (hospitalization may be more likely if decompensation occurs at night or on weekends), or severity of the clinical manifestations [delirium with inability to maintain oral intake, hypotension, severe hypoxemia, high respiratory rate (>30 breaths per minute), tachycardia]. Taking all these factors into consideration, plus the benefits/risks of hospitalization of nursing home residents with NHAP, the goal should be to treat in the nursing home as often as possible.

Initial Route of Treatment in the Nursing Home Setting

Parenteral antibiotics (usually given by intramuscular injection) have been prescribed for 16% to 44% of episodes of NHAP initially treated in the nursing home (1). One study reported no significant difference in mortality between those treated initially with an oral agent or an intramuscular agent in the nursing home and was unable to define factors predictive of prescribing parenteral therapy initially for NHAP in the nursing home setting (30). The inability to identify factors associated with prescribing initial parenteral therapy for NHAP may explain the wide variation in the use of this approach in published studies, and this requires further evaluation.

Timing of Switch to Oral Therapy

Timing of the switch to oral therapy is dependent upon reaching clinical stability (improvement in symptoms and signs, afebrile for 16 hours, no other acute life-threatening complications, and ability to take oral medications) (34). One study specifically addressed the issue of timing of switch to oral therapy among residents with NHAP. In this study (30), 75% of residents who were prescribed an intramuscular antibiotic received this therapy for three days or less, whereas in the hospital the median duration of intravenous antibiotic therapy was five days and 75% were treated for seven days. Thus, it is recommended to assess residents treated in the nursing home for clinical stability and switch to an oral agent beginning on day 2 of therapy and for those initially treated in the hospital on day 3 of therapy (23).

Duration of Treatment

Duration of treatment of NHAP has not been evaluated in randomized clinical trials. One study (30) has retrospectively assessed duration of therapy of NHAP. For episodes treated initially in the nursing home, there was no significant difference in mean duration of therapy between those treated with an oral agent only (9.4 days) and those with a parenteral agent followed by an oral agent (9.0 days; $P = 0.42$). The 75th percentile for duration of therapy was 10 days for those treated in the nursing home. Thus, 7 to 10 days of therapy appeared to be the standard approach to treating NHAP in the facility (30). For episodes treated initially in the hospital, the 75th percentile for total duration of treatment (intravenous plus oral) was 14 days.

Choice of Antimicrobial Agent

In early 2000, the first guideline specifically for NHAP was published and was based on community practice (30). In this guideline, a wide range of oral agents was recommended for treatment in the nursing home, because there was no clear consensus among practicing physicians. Likewise in the hospital setting, several different regimens were recommended. Noteworthy is that a macrolide was not recommended for NHAP for three reasons: gastrointestinal side effects, the issue of increasing macrolide resistance among *S. pneumoniae*, and rare episodes due to atypical pathogens. Subsequently, the Canadian Infectious Diseases Society published a CAP treatment guideline (35) that included specific recommendations for NHAP. This guideline recommended an oral "respiratory" quinolone (levofloxacin, gatifloxacin, or moxifloxacin) alone or amoxicillin/clavulanate plus a macrolide as the first choice for treatment of NHAP in the nursing home, and for treatment in the hospital a respiratory quinolone alone was the first choice, and the second choice was a second- or third-generation cephalosporin plus a macrolide. In 2003, the Infectious Diseases Society of America updated a prior guideline and made recommendations for treatment of NHAP that were similar to the Canadian guideline (36). More recently, the American Thoracic Society and the Infectious Diseases Society of America have collaborated on a guideline for hospital-acquired, ventilator-associated, and health-care-associated pneumonia (37). In this guideline, NHAP is included in the health-care-associated pneumonia group. The rationale for this grouping appears to be the results of invasive diagnostic testing in the small group of residents with pneumonia who are intubated and in whom *Staphylococcus aureus* and enteric gram-negative bacilli were the most commonly isolated pathogens. However, as the authors of the guideline point out, there are few data about the bacteriology of health-care-associated pneumonia in those who are not mechanically ventilated and this includes more than 90% of episodes of NHAP. Therefore, the appropriateness of recommending antibiotic treatment of NHAP based on the findings of a small group of residents who are severely ill with pneumonia is unclear.

The author's recommendations for empirical regimens for treatment of NHAP in the nursing home or hospital are listed in Table 3 and are similar to the 2003 Infectious Diseases Society guideline (36), except a macrolide is not recommended. The most logical and simple approach is to use a respiratory quinolone (levofloxacin, gatifloxacin, or moxifloxacin) as initial

Table 3 Management of Nursing Home–Acquired Pneumonia

Hospitalization decision (assumes that there is no "do-not-hospitalize" request from the resident or surrogate)

Most residents can be treated in the nursing home if they can take medications and fluids enterally (either by swallowing or by tube feeding)

Hospitalization should be considered if there is:

Hypotension

Significant hypoxemia that persists despite maximum oxygen supplementation in the nursing home or respiratory rate >30 breaths/min

Significant alteration in mental status

Temperature >103°F that does not respond to an antipyretic

Tachycardia (>120 beats per minute) that is persistent with or without hypotension

Empirical antimicrobial treatment in the nursing home[a]

Decide on the route of administration—oral or parenteral (intramuscular). Consider the intramuscular route if the resident is unable to take oral medications and there is no alternative enteral route available

Oral regimens:

Quinolone—

Gatifloxacin 400 mg PO daily

Levofloxacin 250–500 mg PO daily

Moxifloxacin 400 mg PO daily

Amoxicillin/clavulanate (Augmentin) 875 mg PO BID

Cefuroxime axetil (Ceftin) 500 mg PO BID

Parenteral regimens: ceftriaxone 500–1000 mg IM daily or cefotaxime 500 mg IM BID

If a parenteral regimen is used initially, evaluate the resident for clinical stability beginning on day 2 to identify the time to switch to an oral regimen. Clinical stability is defined as improvement in symptoms and signs, afebrile for 16 hr, no evidence of other organ compromise, and able to take oral medication

Duration of treatment does not need to exceed 7 days in most patients

Empirical antimicrobial treatment in the hospital[a]

Parenteral regimens:

Gatifloxacin 400 mg IV daily

Levofloxacin 250–500 mg IV daily

Moxifloxacin 400 mg IV daily

or

Ceftriaxone 500–1000 mg IV daily

Cefotaxime 500 mg IV q12h

Cefuroxime 750 mg IV q8h

or

Ampicillin/sulbactam 1.5 g IV q6–8 hr

Timing of switch to an oral regimen should be determined by achievement of clinical stability as defined above. Once it is determined that the resident can be switched to an oral regimen, there is no need to continue hospitalization unless there are extenuating circumstances.

(Continued)

Table 3   Management of Nursing Home–Acquired Pneumonia (*Continued*)

Oral regimens: same as for treatment in the nursing home
Duration of therapy does not need to exceed 10 days but should be no longer than
  14 days

[a]In the 2003 Infectious Diseases Society of America Community-Acquired Pneumonia guideline
(36), amoxicillin–clavulanate plus a macrolide is listed as an alternative to a quinolone alone for
empirical treatment in the nursing home. Likewise for empirical treatment of the hospitalized
resident with pneumonia, the guideline recommends an "advanced" macrolide (azithromycin
or clarithromycin) plus a beta-lactam as an alternative to a quinolone alone. In the recommendations in this table a macrolide-containing regimen is not listed because pathogens, such as
Chlamydia pneumoniae, *Mycoplasma pneumoniae*, and *Legionella pneumophila*, rarely cause
pneumonia in nursing home residents.
Abbreviations: PO, per os (oral); BID, two times a day; IM, intramuscular; IV, intravenous.

therapy. The respiratory quinolones provide excellent antimicrobial activity
agent for the common bacterial pathogens causing NHAP, can be administered as a once-a-day treatment, and has a low side-effect profile. Although
concerns about the development of quinolone resistance among pneumococci are appropriate, this caveat does not apply to the treatment of true
bacterial infection. It is the unnecessary use of quinolones and macrolides
in the treatment of viral upper respiratory tract infection in the community
and nursing home settings that is increasing the resistance to these agents
among pneumococci.

Withholding Antibiotic Therapy for NHAP in Nursing Home Residents with Advanced Dementia

Nursing home residents with advanced dementia are at risk of pneumonia,
and it is often the cause of death in these individuals (1) (see also Chapter 7).
Severity of dementia is an independent predictor of both short- (one week;
28% mortality) and long-term (three months; 50% mortality) mortality
in NHAP, after adjusting for multiple confounding factors, including
antibiotic therapy (38). Given this high mortality in the late stages of dementia, the benefit of aggressive therapy with antibiotics, intravenous hydration,
etc., has been questioned (39). One study (40) found that care for nursing
home residents with lower respiratory tract infection and dementia was more
aggressive in the United States than care for residents in the Netherlands,
regardless of the severity of dementia (40). In the Netherlands, it has been
reported that antibiotic treatment is withheld in 23% of nursing home
residents with pneumonia and severe dementia (41). This difference in management of NHAP in the severely demented nursing home resident reflects
differences in attitudes by physicians and families about the use of aggressive
interventions in this group of people as well as the fact that in the Netherlands, unlike the United States, the physician ultimately is responsible for

decision-making in consultation with family (40). A concern in withholding antibiotic therapy in NHAP is the degree of suffering that may occur compared with when treatment is prescribed. One study (42) found that those dying of pneumonia (with or without treatment) suffered more than those dying of other causes, but there was no difference in level of suffering in those dying with pneumonia with or without antibiotic therapy (40). This report emphasized optimal care of NHAP including "prudent consideration of curative treatment, treatment to relieve discomfort, and supportive treatment in view of expected and desirable outcomes."

Managing Volume Depletion

A factor that has got little attention in the management of NHAP is the state of hydration of the resident with this infection. Fever and the accompanying tachypnea observed with NHAP can lead to considerable insensible water loss. In addition, oral intake of liquids may be substantially decreased with any infection including pneumonia (40). Therefore, it is important to assess the hydration status of each resident with NHAP. However, the bedside evaluation of hydration status of the nursing home resident is not particularly useful in identifying those with dehydration. An objective assessment of hydration status of the resident with pneumonia should be done, e.g., by measuring the serum blood urea nitrogen. The management of volume depletion related to NHAP in the nursing home setting is also difficult, especially if the resident has decreased mentation. Ineffective hydration of the resident with pneumonia in the nursing home may be one explanation for treatment failure that leads to hospitalization, but this has not been adequately studied. Because intravenous hydration is usually not an option in the nursing home setting, alternative methods, such as clysis (43), deserve further study.

Summary Management of NHAP

Due to the adverse effects of hospitalization on functional status and the lack of improvement in outcome with hospitalization for treatment of NHAP except possibly in immediate mortality among the severely ill, most residents with pneumonia should be treated in the nursing home. Route (oral or parenteral) of initial treatment in the nursing home should be determined after considering the severity of pneumonia, ability to take oral medications, mental status, and state of hydration. If intramuscular antibiotic treatment is utilized, switching to the oral route should be done as soon as clinical stability has been achieved, especially if the resident can take oral medications. Total duration of treatment of NHAP in the nursing home setting rarely needs to exceed seven days. If initial treatment of NHAP takes place in the hospital, duration of treatment should not exceed 10 days usually; on the day treatment is switched to an oral agent the resident should usually be discharged back to the nursing home to complete therapy unless there are complicating factors. Treatment of discomforting symptoms, such as shortness of breath, excessive secretions, etc., should be considered an important part of the management of pneumonia.

Prevention

Vaccination

The burden of pneumococcal disease in terms of incidence and mortality falls on the elderly (44). As a result pneumococcal vaccination is recommended for persons age 65 and older (45) (see also Chapter 22). However, the efficacy of pneumococcal vaccine in preventing pneumonia in the elderly has been the subject of considerable debate due to the lack of prospective, randomized controlled trials (46). Despite this limitation, vaccination of all elderly people is recommended because the vaccine is safe, inexpensive, and cost effective (45). The elderly appear to respond with a significant antibody response to pneumococcal vaccine in most but not all studies (47). However, antibody levels appear to decline rapidly in the elderly beginning as early as three years after vaccination (47), and this supports periodic revaccination of the elderly nursing home resident to attempt to maintain effective serum antibody levels. Revaccination of the elderly with the 23-valent vaccine appears to be safe (48). The Centers for Disease Control and Prevention's Advisory Committee on Immunization Practices has recommended only a onetime revaccination after five or more years for those 65 years or older if vaccinated before age 65 (45). Based on published retrospective studies of efficacy of pneumococcal vaccine and evidence of safety of revaccination (47), this writer recommends that after initial vaccination of the nursing home resident vaccination should be repeated every five years thereafter.

The morbidity and mortality of influenza virus infection is greatest among the elderly (49). Efficacy of influenza vaccine in the elderly in preventing acute influenza is probably no greater than 40%, and as a result outbreaks continue to occur in nursing homes despite high rates of resident vaccination (49). However, the value of influenza vaccination in the elderly lies in the reduction in the complications related to this infection. Vaccination among the elderly in nursing homes can decrease hospitalizations by 50% to 60% and decreases mortality as much as 80% (49). One study found that influenza vaccination significantly reduced the risk of developing NHAP (3). Based on these findings, influenza vaccine is strongly recommended for all nursing home residents each year unless there is some contraindication.

Oral Hygiene

Some investigators hypothesized that poor oral hygiene in nursing home residents increases the rate of colonization of dental plaque and oral mucosa by potential respiratory pathogens (50). Because aspiration of oropharyngeal flora into the lung is the major route of pathogenesis of NHAP, colonization of dental plaque and oral mucosa may represent a reservoir of potential pathogens that can reach the lung. Therefore, it follows that maintaining good oral hygiene in nursing home residents has the potential benefit of reducing colonization with respiratory pathogens, thereby decreasing the occurrence of NHAP. Recent studies have found evidence that lack of oral hygiene is associated with pneumonia in nursing home residents (7,51). A study in Japanese nursing homes demonstrated that residents randomized to an intensive oral care regimen had a significantly lower rate of pneumonia than did residents following a standard oral care regimen (52). Further investigation of the link between oral hygiene and development of NHAP is warranted, as well as studies of practical methods to improve oral hygiene in nursing home residents.

Controlling Gastroesophageal Reflux

Gastroesophageal reflux is common in the elderly and aspiration of material from the stomach can damage the trachea. The supine position and nasogastric tubes also promote gastric content aspiration. The simplest approach to managing gastroesophageal reflux is to elevate the head of the bed and minimize the use of nasogastric tubes. There is no evidence presently that decreasing reflux reduces the risk of gastric content aspiration or NHAP.

Pharmacologic Interventions

A group of investigators recently reviewed the literature on interventions to prevent pneumonia among the elderly (52). They quote anecdotal studies published as letters to the editor that suggest that therapy with angiotensin converting enzyme inhibitors, which increase the sensitivity of the cough reflex and improve the swallowing reflex in elderly prone to aspiration, or amantadine, which may improve swallowing by releasing dopamine, is associated with a decreased risk of pneumonia. Although these observations are provocative, none of these interventions can be recommended at this time because these studies have not been published in complete form. Efforts should also be made to minimize the use of sedative hypnotics and narcotic analgesics that may suppress the cough reflex.

Feeding Tubes and Gastric Content Aspiration

One of the primary reasons for the use of feeding tubes has been to attempt to reduce the risk of aspiration among residents with dysphagia (53). However, there is now ample evidence that feeding tubes do not prevent aspiration in residents with dementia (54). There is also no evidence that tube feeding improves quality of life or prolongs survival of nursing home residents with advanced dementia (54). Several authors (53,54) have concluded that there is a limited role for tube feeding among residents with dysphagia, and advanced dementia and their use should be discouraged.

BRONCHITIS

Epidemiology and Clinical Relevance

A prospective study of infections in one nursing home over a three-year period (1984–1987) found that the incidence of bronchitis was one episode per 1000 resident care days (2). In another prospective study in five nursing homes in Toronto, Ontario, Canada, between 1993 and 1996, the incidence of bronchitis was 0.5 episodes per 1000 resident care days, and the cumulative incidence after three years was 24% (3). Univariate predictors of bronchitis were increasing age, immobility, and female sex, whereas influenza and pneumococcal vaccinations were associated with a decreased risk of bronchitis. In the multivariate analysis, only increasing age (in deciles) and immobility were predictors of bronchitis and influenza vaccine was protective (3).

The study also specifically addressed the microbial etiology of bronchitis in nursing home residents. Nasopharyngeal swab cultures and paired acute and convalescent sera were used to identify the etiology of both pneumonia and bronchitis in the study population. These authors did not specifically separate the etiology of pneumonia from that of bronchitis. Of 272 episodes of pneumonia and bronchitis, 166 had nasopharyngeal swabs of which 60 (36%) grew respiratory viruses [influenza A and B ($N = 18$), parainfluenza ($N = 40$), and respiratory syncytial virus ($N = 2$)]. In only 15 episodes a bacterial etiology was identified, of which the most common organisms were *H. influenzae* ($N = 3$), *S. aureus* ($N = 3$), and *C. pneumoniae* ($N = 3$). These results suggest that respiratory viruses are the most common cause of bronchitis among nursing home residents.

Clinical Manifestations

The manifestations of bronchitis in nursing home residents have not been carefully delineated in any specific study. One study provided a reasonable definition of bronchitis as follows: one or more of the following must have been present, including cough, pleuritic chest pain, fever $\geq 100°$ F, or purulent sputum plus no auscultatory findings of pneumonia (rales, rhonci, or dullness to percussion) or a chest radiograph without evidence of pneumonia (2).

Diagnostic Approach

The guideline for evaluation of fever and infection in nursing homes Appendix B (29) does not specifically address the issue of the diagnosis of bronchitis. However, symptoms and signs of pneumonia and bronchitis overlap considerably. Therefore, the presence of symptoms and signs of lower respiratory tract infection should prompt an evaluation for pneumonia as previously outlined in the section on NHAP using the guideline (29). Those who have no evidence of pneumonia on chest radiograph or with no findings on auscultation of chest should be considered to have bronchitis.

Because most episodes of bronchitis in nursing home residents have a viral etiology (5), there is no value to obtaining sputum for bacterial culture.

Therapeutic Interventions

There are no studies specifically addressing the antimicrobial treatment of bronchitis in nursing home residents. However, because most of these infections are caused by viruses, treatment with antibacterial agents is usually not indicated. This recommendation is consistent with a recent review of the treatment of uncomplicated acute bronchitis in healthy adults (55). Supportive measures, such as antipyretics and antitussives, should be prescribed.

Infection Control Measures and Prevention

Infection control measures related to bronchitis are a function of the mechanisms of spread of respiratory viruses for the most part. Prevention relates to the use of influenza vaccine (see also Chapter 9)

SUGGESTED READING

Bentley DW, Bradley S, High K, Schoenbaum S, Taler G, Yoshikawa TT. Practice guideline for evaluation of fever and infection in long-term care facilities. Clin Infect Dis 2000; 31:640–653.

Marik PE. Aspiration pneumonitis and aspiration pneumonia. N Engl J Med 2001; 344:665–671.

Mylotte JM. Nursing home-acquired pneumonia. Clin Infect Dis 2002; 35:1205–1211.

van der Steen JT, Kruse RL, Ooms ME, et al. Treatment of nursing home residents with dementia and lower respiratory tract infection in the United States and the Netherlands: an ocean apart. J Am Geriatr Soc 2004; 52:691–699.

Watson L, Wilson BJ, Waugh N. Pneumococcal polysaccharide vaccine: a systemic review of clinical effectiveness in adults. Vaccine 2002; 20:2166–2173.

REFERENCES

1. Mylotte JM. Nursing home-acquired pneumonia. Clin Infect Dis 2002; 35: 1205–1211.
2. Jackson MM, Fierer J, Barrett-Connor E, et al. Intensive surveillance for infections in a three-year study of nursing home patients. Am J Epidemiol 1992; 135: 685–696.
3. Loeb M, McGeer A, McArthur M, Walter S, Simor AE. Risk factors for pneumonia and other lower respiratory tract infections in elderly residents of long-term care facilities. Arch Intern Med 1999; 159:2058–2064.
4. Kaplan V, Angus DC, Griffin MF, Clermont G, Scott Watson R, Linde-Zwirble WT. Hospitalized community-acquired pneumonia in the elderly. Age- and sex-related patterns of care and outcome in the United States. Am J Respir Crit Care Med 2002; 165:766–772.

5. Alvarez S, Shell CG, Woolley TW, Berk SL, Smith JK. Nosocomial infections in long-term care. J Gerontol 1988; 43:M9–M17.
6. Harkness GA, Bentley DW, Roghman RJ. Risk factors for nosocomial pneumonia in the elderly. Am J Med 1990; 18:151–159.
7. Quagliarello V, Ginter S, Han L, Van Ness P, Allore H, Tinetti M. Modifiable risk factors for nursing home-acquired pneumonia. Clin Infect Dis 2005; 40:1–6.
8. Magaziner J, Tenney JH, DeForge B, Hebel JR, Muncie HL Jr., Warren JW. Prevalence and characteristics of nursing home-acquired infections in the aged. J Am Geriatr Soc 1991; 39:1071–1078.
9. Yamaya M, Yanai M, Ohrui T, Arai H, Sasaki H. Interventions to prevent pneumonia among older adults. J Am Geriatr Soc 2001; 49:85–90.
10. Kikuchi R, Watabe N, Konno T, Mishina N, Sekizawa K, Sasaki H. High incidence of silent aspiration in elderly patients with community-acquired pneumonia. Am J Respir Crit Care Med 1994; 150:251–253.
11. Horner J, Massey EW, Riski JE, Lathrop DL, Chase KN. Aspiration following stroke: clinical correlates and outcome. Neurology 1988; 38:1359–1362.
12. Nakagawa T, Sekizawa K, Arai H, Kikuchi R, Manabe K, Sasaki H. Incidence of pneumonia in elderly patients with basal ganglia infarction. Arch Intern Med 1997; 157:321–324.
13. Pick N, McDonald A, Bennett NN, et al. Pulmonary aspiration in a long-term care setting: clinical and laboratory observations and an analysis of risk factors. J Am Geriatr Soc 1996; 44:763–768.
14. Marik PE. Aspiration pneumonitis and aspiration pneumonia. N Engl J Med 2001; 344:665–671.
15. Mylotte JM, Goodnough S, Naughton BJ. Pneumonia versus aspiration pneumonitis in nursing home residents: diagnosis and management. J Am Geriatr Soc 2003; 51:17–23.
16. Mylotte JM, Goodnough S, Gould M. Pneumonia versus aspiration pneumonitis in nursing home residents: prospective application of a clinical algorithm. J Am Geriatr Soc 2005; 53:755–761.
17. Meehan TP, Chua-Reyes JM, Tate J, et al. Process of care performance, patient characteristics, and outcomes in elderly patients hospitalized with community-acquired or nursing home-acquired pneumonia. Chest 2000; 117:1378–1385.
18. Naughton BJ, Mylotte JM, Tayara A. Outcome of nursing home-acquired pneumonia: derivation and application of a practical model to predict 30 day mortality. J Am Geriatr Soc 2000; 48:1292–1299.
19. Mehr DR, Foxman B, Colombo R. Risk factors for mortality from lower respiratory infections in nursing homes. J Fam Pract 1992; 34:585–591.
20. Vergis EN, Brennen C, Wagener M, Muder RR. Pneumonia in long-term care. A prospective case-control study of risk factors and impact on survival. Arch Intern Med 2001; 161:2378–2381.
21. Hutt E, Frederickson EB, Ecord M, Kramer AM. Processes of care predict survival following nursing home-acquired pneumonia. JCOM 2002; 9:249–256.
22. Fine MJ, Auble TE, Yealy DM, et al. A prediction rule to identify low-risk patients with community-acquired pneumonia. N Engl J Med 1997; 336:243–250.
23. Mylotte JM, Naughton B, Saludades C, Maszarovics Z. Validation and application of the pneumonia prognosis index to nursing home residents with pneumonia. J Am Geriatr Soc 1998; 46:1538–1544.

24. Mehr DR, Binder EF, Kruse RL, et al. Predicting mortality in nursing home residents with lower respiratory tract infection. JAMA 2001; 286:2427–2436.
25. Johnson JC, Jayadevappa R, Baccash PD, Taylor L. Nonspecific presentation of pneumonia in hospitalized older people: age effect or dementia? J Am Geriatr Soc 2000; 48:1316–1320.
26. Mehr DR, Binder EF, Kruse RL, Zweig SC, Madsen RW, D'Agostino RB. Clinical findings associated with radiographic pneumonia in nursing home residents. J Fam Pract 2001; 50:931–937.
27. Kaye KS, Stalam M, Shershen WE, Kaye D. Utility of pulse oximetry in diagnosing pneumonia in nursing home residents. Am J Med Sci 2002; 324: 237–242.
28. Hutt E, Kramer AM. Evidence-based guidelines for management of nursing home-acquired pneumonia. J Fam Pract 2002; 51:709–716.
29. Bentley DW, Bradley S, High K, Schoenbaum S, Taler G, Yoshikawa TT. Practice guideline for evaluation of fever and infection in long-term care facilities. Clin Infect Dis 2000; 31:640–653.
30. Naughton BJ, Mylotte JM. Treatment guideline for nursing home-acquired pneumonia based on community practice. J Am Geriatr Soc 2000; 48:82–88.
31. Konetzka RT, Spector W, Shaffer T. Effects of nursing home ownership type and resident payer source on hospitalization for suspected pneumonia. Med Care 2004; 42:1001–1008.
32. Kruse RL, Mehr DR, Boles KE, et al. Does hospitalization impact survival after lower respiratory tract infection in nursing home residents? Med Care 2004; 42:860–870.
33. Zweig SC, Kruse RL, Binder EF, Szafara KL, Mehr DR. Effect of do-not-resuscitate orders on hospitalization of nursing home residents evaluated for lower respiratory infections. J Am Geriatr Soc 2004; 52:51–58.
34. Halm EA, Fine MJ, Marrie TJ, et al. Time to clinical stability in patients hospitalized with community-acquired pneumonia: implications for practice guidelines. JAMA 1998; 279:1452–1457.
35. Mandell LA, Marrie TJ, Grossman RF, Chow AW, Hyland RH. Canadian guidelines for the initial management of community-acquired pneumonia: an evidence-based update by the Canadian Infectious Diseases Society and the Canadian Thoracic Society. Clin Infect Dis 2000; 31:383–421.
36. Mandell LA, Bartlett JG, Dowell SF, et al. Update of practice guidelines for the management of community-acquired pneumonia in immunocompetent adults. Clin Infect Dis 2003; 37:1405–1433.
37. Niederman MS, Craven DE. Guidelines for the management of adults with hospital-acquired, ventilator-associated, and healthcare-associated pneumonia. Am J Crit Care Med 2005; 171:388–416.
38. van der Steen JT, Ooms ME, Mehr DR, van der Wal G, Ribbe MW. Severe dementia and adverse outcomes of nursing home-acquired pneumonia: evidence for mediation by functional and pathophysiological decline. J Am Geriatr Soc 2002; 50:439–448.
39. Morrison RS, Siu AL. Survival in end-stage dementia following acute illness. JAMA 2000; 284:47–52.
40. van der Steen JT, Kruse RL, Ooms ME, et al. Treatment of nursing home residents with dementia and lower respiratory tract infection in the United States and the Netherlands: an ocean apart. J Am Geriatr Soc 2004; 52:691–699.

41. van der Steen JT, Ooms ME, Ader HJ, Ribbe MW, van der Wal G. Withholding antibiotic treatment in pneumonia patients with dementia. A quantitative observational study. Arch Intern Med 2002; 162:1753–1760.
42. van der Steen JT, Ooms ME, van der Wal G, Ribbe MW. Pneumonia: the demented patient's best friend? Discomfort after starting or withholding antibiotic treatment. J Am Geriatr Soc 2002; 50:1681–1688.
43. Dasgupta M, Binns MA, Rochon PA. Subcutaneous fluid infusion in a long-term care setting. J Am Geriatr Soc 2000; 48:795–799.
44. Fedson DS, Anthony J, Scott G. The burden of pneumococcal disease among adults in developed and developing countries: what is known and what is not known. Vaccine 1999; 17:S11–S18.
45. Centers for Disease Control and Prevention. Prevention of pneumococcal disease. Morb Mortal Wkly Rep 1997; 46(RR-8):1–24.
46. Watson L, Wilson BJ, Waugh N. Pneumococcal polysaccharide vaccine: a systemic review of clinical effectiveness in adults. Vaccine 2002; 20:2166–2173.
47. Artz AS, Ershler WB, Longo DL. Pneumococcal vaccination and revaccination of older adults. Clin Microbiol Rev 2003; 16:308–318.
48. Torling J, Hedlund J, Konradsen HB, Ortqvist A. Revaccination with the 23-valent pneumococcal polysaccharide vaccine in middle-aged and elderly persons previously treated for pneumonia. Vaccine 2003; 22:96–103.
49. Bradley SF. Prevention of influenza in long-term care facilities. Infect Control Hosp Epidemiol 1999; 20:629–637.
50. Scannapieco FA, Mylotte JM. Relationships between periodontal disease and bacterial pneumonia. J Periodontol 1996; 67:1114–1122.
51. Terpenning MS, Taylor GW, Lopatin DE, Kerr CK, Dominguez BL, Loesche WJ. Aspiration pneumonia: dental and oral risk factors in an older veteran population. J Am Geriatr Soc 2001; 49:557–563.
52. Yoneyama T, Yoshida M, Ohrui T, et al. Oral care reduces pneumonia in older patients in nursing homes. J Am Geriatr Soc 2002; 50:430–433.
53. Gillick M. Rethinking the role of tube feeding in patients with advanced dementia. N Engl J Med 2000; 342:206–210.
54. Finucane TE, Christmas C, Travis K. Tube feeding in patients with advanced dementia. A review of the evidence. JAMA 1999; 282:1365–1370.
55. Gonzales R, Sande MA. Uncomplicated acute bronchitis. Ann Intern Med 2000; 133:981–991.

15

Tuberculosis

Shobita Rajagopalan

Division of Infectious Disease, Department of Internal Medicine, Charles R. Drew University of Medicine and Science, and Martin Luther King, Jr.–Charles R. Drew Medical Center, Los Angeles, California, U.S.A.

KEY POINTS

1. In industrialized nations including the United States, the geriatric population constitutes one of the largest reservoirs of *Mtb* infection.
2. The well-documented, airborne, highly infectious mode of transmission of *Mtb* puts individuals who reside in congregate settings, such as older residents of LTCFs, at an increased risk of TB.
3. The variable and atypical clinical manifestations of TB in aging individuals can delay diagnosis and treatment, resulting in increased morbidity and mortality in this age group.
4. All LTCFs must develop and maintain appropriate TB prevention and control strategies to ensure protection of its residents and staff against this highly communicable disease.
5. Current published recommendations by the Advisory Committee for Elimination of TB in conjunction with the CDC staff and public health consultants are available to guide such TB control efforts.

INTRODUCTION

In industrialized nations, including the United States, the geriatric population constitutes one of the largest reservoirs of *Mycobacterium tuberculosis* (*Mtb*) infection (1,2). Tuberculosis (TB) case rates in the United States are highest for this age group compared with other age categories (3). The well-documented, airborne, highly infectious mode of transmission of *Mtb* puts individuals who reside in congregate settings, such as older residents of long-term care facilities (LTCFs), at an increased risk for TB. Such vulnerable elderly individuals are both at risk for reactivation of latent TB as well as acquisition of new TB infection in comparison with community-dwelling elderly (4). The prevention and control of TB in these facilities therefore must be strongly emphasized (4–7). The variable and atypical clinical manifestations of TB in aging persons can delay diagnosis and treatment, resulting in increased morbidity and mortality in this age group; this treatable infection may be discovered as a postmortem finding.

The Institute of Medicine report, *Ending Neglect: The Elimination of TB in the U.S.,* sponsored by the Centers for Disease Control and Prevention (CDC) reaffirms the commitment to the goal of elimination TB in the United States by the year 2010, defined as case rates of less than one case per million population per year (8). The focus of such intensive TB control efforts on all high-risk populations, including the institutionalized elderly, must be made a priority (9,10). This chapter reviews the epidemiology, pathogenesis, and clinical features of TB in aging adults and provides updated recommendations for diagnosis, treatment, prevention of transmission, and infection control strategies in health-care settings including elderly residents of LTCFs.

EPIDEMIOLOGY AND CLINICAL SIGNIFICANCE

Although a cure for TB was developed more than 50 years ago, this infectious disease continues to kill between 2 and 3 million people every year. The World Health Organization estimates that, if uncontrolled, 36 million people will die of TB by the year 2020 (11). Eight million people develop active TB every year, nearly 98% of who live in the developing world (12).

In the United States, TB occurs with disproportionate frequency among the elderly (13,14). In 2002, 21% of the TB cases occurred in persons age 65 years and older, even though this group accounted for approximately 12% of the population. The incidence among persons 65+ years was 8.8 per 100,000 in 2002, whereas the incidence for all ages combined was 5.2 per 100,000 (15). In a CDC-sponsored study of 15,379 routinely reported cases in 29 states conducted in 1984–1985, the incidence of TB was estimated at 39.2 cases per 100,000 persons among nursing home (NH) residents, compared with 21.5 cases per 100,000 for elderly living in the community (15). Published data have clearly demonstrated the heightened efficiency of TB transmission within congregate settings, such as prisons, nursing facilities [nursing homes (NHs)], chronic care facilities, and homeless shelters; the awareness about TB infection and disease in the institutionalized elderly has thus been stimulated (4–6,14). The aggregate TB incidence rate for residents of NH's is 1.8 times higher than the rate seen in elderly persons living in the community (16,17). In several studies of patients entering NHs, the percentage of tuberculin skin test (TST) reactors was 10% to 40% (14,18,19). Generally, the risk that a recent converter will develop clinically active TB is highest in the first two years after conversion and then declines (20). However, in TST reactors over the age of 70 years, the case rate of active TB among known reactors may increase greatly (21) The most prevalent risk factors in the nursing home for development of active tuberculosis were diabetes mellitus (42%), being more than 10% below ideal body weight (41.5%), and alcohol abuse (13%) (19). After two-step testing, 60% to 90% of patients entering NHs are TST negative and are, therefore, nonimmune to new infection, although 5% to 10% of nonreactors to tuberculin may be anergic. These patients are at a risk of infection if exposed and of progression to clinically active TB if not then treated. Nonreactors are vulnerable even though many of them may have been TST-positive previously.

PATHOGENESIS

The following is a concise summary of the well-integrated disease mechanisms relevant to the natural history and clinical course of TB in aging adults (22–24). Inhaled tubercle bacilli are engulfed by alveolar macrophages and transported to regional lymph nodes. Infected macrophages and circulating monocytes secrete proteolytic enzymes, generating an exudative lesion. Activated mononuclear phagocytes stimulate granuloma formation with subsequent activation of T lymphocytes, which ultimately triggers the onset of cell-mediated immune and delayed-type hypersensitivity responses, which clinically correlates with a positive dermal reactivity to standard-dose tuberculin antigen. As the major component of the immune system affected by senescence is the T-cell-mediated response, dermal reactivity to tuberculin must be interpreted cautiously [reviewed further in Section, "Diagnosis" (22)]. The characteristic Ghon complex that subsequently develops consists of organized collections of epithelioid cells, lymphocytes, and capillaries. Tubercle bacilli are confined and their growth restrained within caseous necrosis and surrounding fibrosis with ultimate healing. Reactivation (secondary or postprimary) TB is associated with granuloma liquefaction and rupture into the bronchoalveolar and vascular systems, which promotes widespread microbial dissemination.

Approximately 90% of active TB cases (TB disease) in the elderly are the result of reactivation of primary infection (19). TB without overt clinical manifestations and evidenced by positive dermal reactivity to tuberculin (TB infection; latent TB) may occur in 30% to 50% of aging individuals. Rarely, previously infected older persons may eventually eliminate the viable tubercle bacilli and revert to a tuberculin-negative state and a "naïve" immunologic status; these individuals are at risk for new infection (reinfection) with *Mtb*. Thus, older persons potentially at risk for TB include individuals never exposed to *Mtb*, those with latent and dormant primary infection that may reactivate, and others who are no longer infected and at risk of reinfection.

Because animal model studies have clearly documented the association between age-related decline in T-cell responses and the enhanced risk of infections by intracellular pathogens including *Mtb*, immunosenescence or immune dysregulation is likely to play a role in the relapse of dormant infection in the elderly. However, other factors, including age-associated diseases (e.g., malignancy, diabetes mellitus), poor nutrition, immunosuppression, chronic renal failure, and chronic institutionalization, contribute to this increased risk for TB in the elderly.

CLINICAL MANIFESTATIONS

Clinical manifestation of TB disease in the elderly can be relatively atypical. Active tuberculous lung involvement occurs in approximately 75% of elderly persons. In elderly persons infected with *Mtb*, the classic clinical feature of pulmonary TB, that is, cough, hemoptysis, fever, night sweats, and weight loss, may be absent (25). In addition, disseminated or miliary TB, tuberculous meningitis, skeletal and genitourinary TB increase in frequency with advancing age (26–31). TB in this population may present clinically with decline in functional status (e.g., activities of daily living), chronic fatigue, cognitive impairment, anorexia, weight loss, or unexplained low-grade fever. Unrecognized TB must thus be in the differential diagnosis of prolonged, unexplained, nonspecific symptoms and signs in an elderly individual.

DIAGNOSIS

The TST skin has long been one of the traditional methods available for TB screening. A false-negative reaction to tuberculin increases with age, partly because of anergy (32) and the "booster phenomenon" of skin test reactivity to antigen (33). All older persons who receive a tuberculin skin test (using five tuberculin units of Tween-stabilized tuberculin, and results read in 48–72 hours) should thus be retested within two weeks of a negative response (induration of less than 10 mm) to identify potentially false-negative reactors (34). A positive booster effect, and therefore a positive tuberculin reaction, is a skin test induration of 10 mm or more (with an increase of 6 mm or more over the first skin test reaction). This "two-step testing" is now a standard of practice recommended by the American Geriatrics Society for aging adults.

The whole-blood interferon gamma release assay, QuantiFERON®TB Gold test (QFTG) (Cellestis Limited, Carnegie, Victoria, Australia), is a Food and Drug Administration–approved in vitro cytokine-based assay for cell-mediated immune reactivity to *Mtb* and might be used instead of TST in TB screening programs for health-care workers (HCW). This interferon gamma release assay is an example of a blood assay for *Mtb* (BAMT) (35).

QFTG measures cell-mediated immune responses to peptides representative of two *Mtb* proteins that are not present in any (bacille Calmette-Gue'rin) BCG vaccine strain and are absent from the majority of nontuberculosis mycobacteria. This assay was approved by Food and Drug Administration in 2005 and is an available option for detecting *M. tuberculosis* infection. CDC recommendations for the United States on QFT and QFTG have been published.

Because 75% of all TB cases in the elderly occur in the respiratory tract, chest radiography is warranted following documentation of a positive tuberculin skin test after the initial placement (or by the booster effect or by conversion) or if the patient has clinical manifestations suggestive of TB. The majority of pulmonary TB cases in aging patients are attributed to reactivation disease; 10% to 20% of cases occur as a result of primary infection or reinfection. Clinicians must interpret radiographic diagnoses of TB in older patients judiciously, because the infection in the lung fields can often be atypical (36). All patients with pulmonary symptoms, radiographic changes compatible with TB, or both who have not been treated with anti-TB therapy should have sputum examination for *Mtb* by smear and culture. Elderly persons unable to produce sputum may be evaluated for a flexible fiberoptic bronchoscopy to obtain bronchial washings and bronchial biopsy to confirm the diagnosis. Because most LTCFs do not have the capacity to isolate residents suspected of having TB disease, these persons often merit transfer to an appropriate acute or subacute care facility for respiratory isolation and sputa collection.

For suspected pulmonary TB, three fresh consecutive morning sputum specimens are recommended for routine mycobacteriologic studies that include an initial smear and culture for *Mtb* (37). Rapid techniques that use radiometric systems, specific DNA probes, and the polymerase chain reaction help supplement routine mycobacterial culture methods that require up to six weeks for the growth of *Mtb* (38). The rapid diagnosis of TB is particularly important in the high-risk elderly population, as well as human immunodeficiency virus (HIV)-infected persons, other immunocompromised hosts, and patients with multiple drug-resistant TB. Histological examination of tissue from various sites, such as the liver, lymph nodes, bone marrow, pleura, or synovium that show the characteristic caseous necrosis with granuloma formation, is also useful for the diagnosis of TB disease.

TREATMENT

Treatment of TB Infection

Recently published recommendations for targeted skin testing and the treatment of latent TB infection (LTBI) based on TST induration criteria are shown in Tables 1 and 2 (39). Drug therapy for latent TB (based on tuberculin skin test reactivity) considerably decreases the risk of progression of TB infection

Table 1   Skin Test Criteria for Positive Tuberculin Reaction (mm Induration)[a]

$\geq 5\,mm^a$

   HIV-positive persons

   Recent contacts of person(s) with infectious tuberculosis

   Persons with chest radiographs consistent with tuberculosis (e.g., fibrotic changes)

   Patients with organ transplants and other immunosuppressed hosts receiving the
     equivalent of >15 mg/day prednisone for >1 month

$\geq 10\,mm^a$

   Recent arrivals (<5 yr) from high-prevalence countries

   Injection drug users

   Residents and employees of high-risk congregate settings: prisons, jails, nursing
     homes, other health-care facilities, residential facilities for AIDS patients, and
     homeless shelters

   Mycobacteriology laboratory personnel

   High-risk clinical conditions: silicosis; gastrectomy; jejunoileal bypass; $\geq 10\%$
     below ideal body weight; chronic renal failure; diabetes mellitus; hematological
     malignancies (e.g., lymphomas, leukemias); other specific malignancies (carcinoma
     of the head or neck, and lung) (alcoholics are also considered high risk)

$\geq 15\,mm^b$

   Persons with no risk factors for TB

[a]Chemoprophylaxis recommended for all high-risk persons, regardless of age.
[b]Persons considered otherwise low risk regardless of age: ≥ 15 mm induration is positive.
Abbreviations: HIV, human immunodeficiency virus; AIDS, acquired immunodeficiency syndrome.
Source: From Ref. 39.

to TB disease. Because the LTBI treatment recommendations address adults
in general, targeted skin testing and treatment of high-risk populations can
be applied to the elderly. The isoniazid (INH) daily regimen for nine months
has recently replaced the previously recommended six-month schedule for
treatment of LTBI. In instances of known exposure to drug-resistant organisms, alternative preventive therapy regimens may be recommended. In
addition, because recent reports in 2001 of fatal and severe hepatitis are
associated with the two-month rifampin (RIF) and pyrazinamide (PZA) or
rifampin-pyrazinamide (RZ), persons being considered for treatment with
RZ should be informed about the potential hepatotoxicity and screened
for liver disease or adverse effects from INH. To reduce the risk of liver
injury associated with RZ therapy, the American Thoracic Society and
CDC, with the endorsement of the Infectious Diseases Society of America,
have prepared recommendations that supercede previous guidelines (40).

TB Disease

Because of the relatively high proportion of adult patients with TB caused
by organisms that are resistant to INH, TB treatment recommendations
have been modified as shown in Table 3 (41). Four drugs are necessary in

(*Text continues on page 243.*)

Table 2 Revised Drug Regimens for Treatment of Latent Tuberculosis Infection in Adults (Including the Elderly)

Drug	Interval and duration	Comments	Ratings HIV-negative	(Evidence) HIV-infected
Isoniazid	Daily for 9 mo**	In HIV-infected persons, isoniazid may be administered concurrently with nucleoside reverse transcriptase inhibitors, protease inhibitors, or non-nucleoside reverse transcriptase inhibitors	A (II)	A (II)
	Twice weekly for 9 mo**	Directly observed therapy must be used with twice-weekly dosing	B (II)	B (II)
	Daily for 6 mo	Not indicated for HIV-infected persons, those with fibrotic lesions on chest radiographs, or children.	B (I)	C (I)
Rifampin	Twice weekly for 6 mo	Directly observed therapy must be used with twice-weekly dosing	B (II)	C (I)
	Daily for 4 mo	Used for persons who are contacts of patients with isoniazid-resistant, rifampin-susceptible TB	B (II)	B (III)
		In HIV-infected persons, most protease inhibitors or delavirdine should not be administered concurrently with rifampin. Rifabutin with appropriate dose adjustments can be used with protease inhibitors (saquinavir should be augmented with ritonavir) and non-nucleoside reverse transcriptase inhibitors (except delavirdine).		

(Continued)

Table 2 Revised Drug Regimens for Treatment of Latent Tuberculosis Infection in Adults (Including the Elderly) (*Continued*)

Drug	Interval and duration	Comments	Ratings HIV-negative	(Evidence) HIV-infected
		Clinicians should consult Web-based updates for the latest specific recommendations		
Rifampin plus pyrazinamide	Daily for 2 mo	Pyrazinamide generally should not be offered for treatment of LTBI for HIV-infected or HIV-negative persons	D (II)	D (II)
	Twice weekly for 2–3 mo		D (III)	D (III)

Strength of the recommendation: A, both strong evidence of efficacy and substantial clinical benefit support recommendation for use, should always be offered; B, moderate evidence for efficacy or strong evidence for efficacy but only limited clinical benefit supports recommendation for use, should generally be offered; C, evidence for efficacy is insufficient to support a recommendation for or against use, or evidence for efficacy might not outweigh adverse consequences (e.g., drug toxicity, drug interactions) or cost of the treatment or alternative approaches, optional; D, moderate evidence for lack of efficacy or for adverse outcome supports a recommendation against use, should generally not be offered; E, good evidence for lack of efficacy or for adverse outcome support a recommendation against use, should never be offered.

Quality of evidence supporting the recommendation: I, evidence from at least one properly randomized controlled trial; II, evidence from at least one well-designed clinical trial without randomization for cohort or case-controlled analytic studies (preferably from more that one center), from multiple time-series studies, or from dramatic results form uncontrolled experiments; III, evidence from opinions of respected authorities based on clinical experience, descriptive studies, or reports of expert committees.

Note: The substitution of rifapentine for rifampin not recommended as rifapentine's safety and effectiveness not established for LTBI.

Abbreviation: LTBI, latent tuberculosis infection.

Source: From Refs. 39, 40.

Table 3 Drug Treatment Regimens of Tuberculosis

Initial phase			Regimen	Continuation phase			
Regimen	Drugs	Intervals and doses[a] (minimal duration)		Drugs	Interval and doses[a,b] (minimal duration)	Range of total doses (minimal duration)	Rating[c] (evidence)[d] HIV
1	INH, RIF, PZA, EMB	7 day/wk for 56 doses (8 wk) or 5 day/wk for 40 doses (8 wk)	1a	INH/RIF	7 day/wk for 126 doses (18 wk) or 5 day/wk for 90 doses (18 wk)[e]	182–130 (26 wk)	A(I)
			1b	INH/RIF	Twice weekly for 36 doses (18 wk)	92–76 (26 wk)	A(I)
			1c[f]	INH/RPT	Once weekly for 18 doses (18 wk)	44–58 (26 wk)	B(I)
2	INH, RIF, PZA, EMB	7 day/wk for 14 doses (2 wk), then twice weekly for 12 doses (6 wk) or 5 day/wk for 10 doses (2 wk), then twice weekly for 12 doses (6 wk)	2a	INH/RIF	Twice weekly for 36 doses (18 wk)	62–58 (26 wk)	A(II)
			2b[f]	INH/RPT	Once weekly for 18 doses (18 wk)	44–40 (26 wk)	B(I)
3	INH, RIF, PZA, EMB	3 times weekly for 24 doses (8 wk)	3a	INH/RIF	3 times weekly for 54 doses (18 wk)	78 (26 wk)	B(I)

(Continued)

Table 3 Drug Treatment Regimens of Tuberculosis (*Continued*)

Initial phase			Continuation phase			
Regimen	Drugs	Intervals and doses[a] (minimal duration)	Regimen	Drugs	Interval and doses[a,b] (minimal duration)	Range of total doses (minimal duration)	Rating[c] (evidence)[d] HIV
4	INH, RIF, EMB	7 day/wk for 56 doses (8 wk) or 5 day/wk for 40 doses (8 wk)	4a	INH/RIF	7 day/wk for 217 doses (31 wk) or 5 day/wk for 155 doses (31 wk)[e]	273–195 (39 wk)	C(I)
			4b	INH/RIF	Twice weekly for 62 doses (31 wk)	118–102 (39 wk)	C(I)

[a]When directly observed therapy (DOT) is used, drugs may be given 5 days/week and the necessary number of doses adjusted accordingly. Although there are no studies compare five with seven daily doses, extensive experience indicates this would be an effective practice.

[b]Patients with cavitation on initial chest radiograph and positive cultures at completion of two months of therapy should receive a seven-month [31 wk; either 217 doses (daily) or 62 doses (twice weekly)] continuation phase.

[c]*Definitions of evidence ratings*: A, preferred; B, acceptable alternative; C, when A and B cannot be given; E, should never be given.

[d]*Definitions of evidence ratings*: I, randomized clinical trial; II, data from clinical trials that were not randomized or were conducted in other populations; III, expert opinion.

[e]Five-day-a-week administration is always given by DOT. Rating for 5 day/wk regimens is AIII.

[f]Options 1c and 2b should be used only in HIV-negative patients who have negative sputum smears at the time of completion of two months of therapy and who do not have cavitation on initial chest radiograph (see text). For patients started on this regimen and found to have a positive culture from the two-month specimen, treatment should be extended an extra three months.

x Not recommended for HIV-infected patients with CD4 cell counts <100 cells/μL.

Abbreviations: EMB, ethambutol; INH, isoniazid; PZA, pyrazinamide; RIF, rifampin; RPT, rifapentine.

Source: From Refs. 38, 41.

the initial intensive phase of treatment, for the six-month regimen to be maximally effective. Thus, in most circumstances, the treatment regimen for all adults with previously untreated TB should consist of a two-month initial phase of INH, RIF, PZA, and ethambutol (EMB) (Table 1, Regimens 1–3). When drug susceptibility test results are known and the organisms are found to be fully susceptible, EMB need not be included. If PZA cannot be included in the initial phase of treatment, or if the isolate is resistant to PZA alone (an unusual circumstance), the initial phase should consist of INH, RIF, and EMB given daily for two months (Regimen 4). EMB should be included in the initial phase of Regimen 4 until drug susceptibility is determined. The continuation phase of treatment is given for either four or seven months. The four-month continuation phase should be used in the large majority of patients. The seven-month continuation phase is recommended only for three groups: patients with cavitary pulmonary TB caused by drug-susceptible organisms, patients whose sputum culture obtained at the time of completion of two months of treatment is positive, and patients whose initial phase of treatment did not include PZA. The continuation phase may be given daily (Regimens 1a and 4a), two times weekly by directly observed therapy (DOT) (Regimens 1b, 2a, and 4b), or three times weekly by DOT (Regimen 3a).

Most cases of active TB in the elderly result from reactivation of a latent infection. Presumably, these persons acquired the infecting organism before the effective antituberculous chemotherapy was available. Hence, unless the older patient is from a high-prevalence country with *Mtb* drug resistance, had received prior inadequate *Mtb* chemotherapy, or had acquired the infection from a known multiple drug-resistant TB contact, most TB cases in the elderly will be highly susceptible to INH and RIF. Thus, in areas where INH resistance is 4% or less, or if the population in question has a low risk for drug resistance, such as most older persons, the empirical four-drug regimen may not be necessary. The more intensive, shorter duration antituberculous drug regimens can attempt to minimize treatment noncompliance and development of drug resistance, particularly when administered by DOT; however, the potential for drug toxicity often limits their use in older patients.

Monitoring of Drug Therapy

Elderly persons are at a greater risk for hepatic toxicity from INH, but this risk is low in frequency and mild. It is recommended that clinical assessments as well as baseline liver function test be performed before the initiation of INH. Periodic laboratory monitoring seems a prudent practice, particularly in the frail elderly who may not be able to communicate warning symptoms of drug toxicities. A rise in serum aminotransferase (SGOT) level to five times above normal or clinical evidence of hepatitis necessitates the prompt discontinuation of INH (as well as other hepatotoxic agents); these drugs may subsequently be resumed at lower doses and gradually increased to full doses as tolerated. Relapse with drug rechallenge will require trial of an alternative regimen.

PREVENTION

Recently published recommendations for targeted skin testing and the treatment of latent TB infection based on TST induration criteria are shown in Tables 2 and 3 (40,41).

Ideally the TB infection control program in health-care settings (including LTCFs) should consist of three types of control measures; administrative actions (i.e., prompt detection of suspected cases, isolation of infectious patients, and prompt institution of appropriate treatment), engineering controls (negative-pressure ventilation rooms, high-efficiency particulate air filtration, and ultraviolet germicidal irradiation), and personal respiratory protection requirements (masks). The setting should have: (i) a written protocol for the early identification of patients with symptoms or signs of TB disease, and (ii) procedures for referring these patients to a setting where they can be evaluated and managed. Patients with suspected or confirmed infectious TB disease should not stay in LTCFs unless adequate administrative and environmental controls and a respiratory protection program are in place. Persons with TB disease who are determined to be noninfectious can remain in the LTCF and do not need to be in an AII room (formerly called negative pressure isolation room with negative pressure, an air flow rate of 6–12 air changes per hour, and direct exhaust of air from the room to the outside of the building or recirculation of air through a high-efficiency particulate air filter).

While instituting such infection control measures in elderly TB patients, clinicians should be aware of the presence of concomitant chronic conditions and functional disabilities that often require more assistance and care, as well as the importance of minimizing prolonged isolation.

INFECTION CONTROL

In this section, the diagnostic approach, therapeutic interventions, and prevention within the context of TB infection control are reviewed. All LTCFs should develop and maintain appropriate TB prevention and control strategies to ensure protection of its residents and staff against this highly communicable disease. Current published recommendations by the Advisory Committee for Elimination of TB in conjunction with the CDC staff and public health consultants are available to guide such TB control efforts (10). In large facilities, an infection control committee is usually responsible for the TB prevention and control program; in the system that has more than one facility providing long-term care to the elderly, a qualified individual should evaluate the overall infection control implementation at all the facilities. The four principal aspects of effective TB infection control in LTCFs include surveillance, containment, assessment, and education.

Surveillance

Identification and reporting all cases of TB infection and TB disease in the facility among all residents and staff is referred to as surveillance. When an infectious case is documented, additional cases and new infections, as indicated by skin test conversion (described in section, "Diagnosis") should be identified with the help of the state of local health department, and appropriate therapy should be instituted (30–32). The surveillance process is outlined as follows:

- All new residents on admission and all employees should receive a two-step tuberculin test. (In the context of BAMT screening, HCWs should receive only one baseline test preferably within 10 days of starting employment.)
- All individuals with a reaction of 10 mm or more of induration should have a follow-up chest radiograph to identify current or past tuberculous lung involvement. (HCWs with positive baseline BAMT results should be referred for a medical and diagnostic evaluation to exclude TB disease and then treatment for LTBI should be considered in accordance with CDC guidelines. Persons with a positive BAMT result do not need to be tested again for surveillance. For HCWs who have indeterminate test results, providers should consult the responsible laboratorian for advice on interpreting the result and making additional decisions.)
- Skin-test–negative employees or volunteers having contact (of 10 or more hours per week) with patients should periodically have repeat skin tests, the frequency depending on the risk of TB infection at that facility.
- Follow-up skin test should be performed for tuberculin-negative persons after any suspected exposure to a documented case of active TB.
- HIV testing should be recommended for all staff and patients with TB infection or disease.
- Staff members suspected of having TB disease should be relieved of their work responsibilities until the diagnosis is either excluded or they are considered noninfectious as a result of effective antituberculous therapy.

Containment

Containment ensures that transmission of TB infection is effectively halted. Persons for whom treatment of TB infection or TB disease is indicated should complete the recommended course of treatment under direct observation (see section, "Treatment"). Appropriate respiratory isolation and ventilation control measures should be applied in pulmonary TB disease cases. As previously indicated, the vast majority of LTCFs do not have the ability to initiate isolation ventilation control measures. Residents of such LTCFs who are suspected of having TB disease will most likely require transfer to an acute care facility or a facility with the capacity to manage TB cases. Confirmed or suspected infectious TB cases in LTCFs do not require isolation precautions provided the following conditions are met: three consecutive concentrated sputum smears are negative, and chemotherapy is begun promptly at the time of confirmation or suspicion or diagnosis.

Assessment

Assessment refers to monitoring and evaluation of the surveillance and containment activities throughout each facility. A record-keeping system is necessary to track and assess the status of persons with TB infection and disease. Such a system should also generate data needed to assess the overall effectiveness of the TB control efforts. State and local health departments should provide support in updating policies and record-keeping systems for TB control in LTCFs in addition to expert TB medical consultation when needed. A health department representative should also be designated to provide epidemiological and management assistance to such facilities. State health departments are responsible for maintaining an updated TB registry for all persons with TB infection or disease (including LTCFs) within their jurisdiction. The health department staff should annually review the following information for each LTCF, comparing it with previous data and data from similar LTCFs:

- percentage of residents and staff with positive tuberculin skin test within the facility,
- percentage of tuberculin skin test conversion,
- description of treatment and supervision,
- percentage of persons who have successfully completed recommended therapy (goal is >95%),
- number of persons reporting drug intolerance or adverse effects,
- number of persons unable to compete therapy and the reason for therapy discontinuation.

Education

Providing information and imparting skills to LTCF residents, families, visitors, and employees to ensure understanding and cooperation with surveillance, containment, and assessment recommendations are all part of education. Staff from the LTCF, with the assistance of the local health department's designee, can counsel residents, families, and visitors. Reading materials, pamphlets, videotaped demonstration, and Internet access to the

World Health Organization, National Institutes of Health, CDC, and other recommended Web sites may also provide useful tools for TB education. The LTCF staff must have frequent in-service training sessions regarding TB infection control. Because of varying levels of education, differences in cultural background, and potential language barriers, the teaching sessions should be conducted by individuals experienced in educating diverse groups. Finally, quality assurance audits should be linked to such educational efforts with continuous feedback to staff to ensure the required impact.

SUGGESTED READING

American Thoracic Society. Targeted skin testing and treatment of latent tuberculosis infection. Am J Respir Crit Care Med 2000; 161:S221–S247.
Centers for Disease Control and Prevention. Guidelines for preventing the transmission of *Mycobacterium tuberculosis* in health-care settings. Morb Mortal Wkly Rep 2005; 54(RR17):1–141.
Rajagopalan S. Tuberculosis in the elderly: a global health problem. Clin Infect Dis 2001; 33:1034–1039.

REFERENCES

1. Davies PD. Tuberculosis in the elderly: an international perspective. Clin Geriatr 1997; 5:15–26.
2. Rajagopalan S. Tuberculosis in the elderly: a global health problem. Clin Infect Dis 2001; 33:1034–1039.
3. Centers for Disease Control and Prevention Facts Sheets, 1999. Tuberculosis cases and case rates per 100,000 population by age group: United States, 1989–1999.
4. Stead WW. Tuberculosis among elderly persons, as observed among nursing home residents. Int J Tuber Lung Dis 1998; (suppl 1):S64–S70.
5. Stead W, Lofgren J, Warren E, Thomas C. Tuberculosis as an endemic and nosocomial infection among the elderly in nursing homes. N Engl J Med 1985; 312:1783–1787.
6. Stead WW. Special problems in tuberculosis. Tuberculosis in the elderly and in residential homes, correctional facilities, long-term care hospitals, mental hospitals, shelters for the homeless, and jails. Clin Chest Med 1989; 10:397–405.
7. Centers for Disease Control and Prevention. Prevention and control of tuberculosis in facilities providing long-term care to the elderly. Recommendations of the Advisory Committee for Elimination of Tuberculosis. Morb Mortal Wkly Rep 1990; 39/RR-10:7–20.
8. Institute of Medicine (U.S.) Committee on the Elimination of Tuberculosis in the United States. In: Geiter L, ed. Ending Neglect: the Elimination of Tuberculosis in the United States. Washington, D.C.: National Academy Press, 2000:1–269.
9. Ijaz K, Dillara JA, Yang Z, Cave MD, Bates JH. Unrecognized tuberculosis in a nursing home causing death with spread of tuberculosis to the community. J Am Geriatr Soc 2002; 50:1213–1217.

10. Centers for Disease Control and Prevention. Guidelines for preventing the transmission of *Mycobacterium tuberculosis* in health-care settings. Morb Mortal Wkly Rep 2005; 54(RR17):1–141.
11. WHO. The World Health Report. Making a Difference. Vol. 3. Geneva: World Health Organization, 1999:310–320.
12. Fact sheet Bureau of Oceans and International Environmental and Scientific Affairs. Washington, D.C. (Accessed March 18, 2003, at http://www.state.gov/g/oes/rls/fs/2003/18798.htm.)
13. Reichman, LB, O'Day R. Tuberculosis infection in a large urban population. Am Rev Respir Des 1978; 117:705–712.
14. Narain J, Lofgren J, Warren E, Stead WW. Epidemic tuberculosis in a nursing home: a retrospective cohort study. J Am Geriatr Soc 1985; 33:258–263.
15. CDC. Progress towards tuberculosis elimination in low-incidence areas of the United States: recommendations of the Advisory Council for the Elimination of Tuberculosis. Morb Mortal Wkly Rep 2002; 51:1–16.
16. Schultz M, Hernandez JM, Hernandez NE, Sanchez RO. Onset to tuberculosis disease: new converters in long-term care settings. Am J Alzheimers Dis Other Dementias 2001; 16:313–318.
17. Hutton MD, Cauthen GM, Bloch AB. Results of a 29-state survey of tuberculosis in nursing homes and correctional facilities. Public Health Rep 1993; 108:305–314.
18. Welty C, Burstin S, Muspratt S, Tager IB. Epidemiology of tuberculous infection in a chronic care population. Am Rev Respir Dis 1985; 132:133–136.
19. Vega Torres RA, Conde JG, Diaz M. Prevalence of tuberculin reactivity and risk factors for the development of active tuberculosis upon admission to a nursing home. P R Health Sci J 1996; 15:275–277.
20. Powell KE, Farer LS. The rising age of the tuberculosis patient: a sign of success and failure. J Infect Dis 1980; 142:946–948.
21. Stead W, Lofgren JP. Does the risk of tuberculosis increase in old age? J Infect Dis 1983; 147:951–955.
22. Bloom BR. Tuberculosis Pathogenesis, Protection and Control. Immune Mechanisms of Protection. Washington, D.C.: American Society for Microbiology Press, 1994:389–415.
23. Lurie MB. Studies on the mechanism of immunity in tuberculosis. The fate of tubercle bacilli ingested by mononuclear phagocytes derived from normal and immunized animals. J Exp Med 1942; 129:247.
24. Dannenberg AM. Pathogenesis of tuberculosis; native and acquired resistance in animals and humans. In: Leive L, Schlessinger D, eds. Microbiology 1984. Washington, D.C.: American Society for Microbiology, 1984:344–354.
25. Yoshikawa TT. Tuberculosis in aging adults. J Am Geriatr Soc 1992; 40:178–187.
26. Perez-Guzman C, Vargas MH, Torres-Cruz A, Villarreal-Velarde H. Does aging modify pulmonary tuberculosis? A meta analytical review. Chest 1999; 116:961–967.
27. Mert A, Bilir M, Tabak F. Miliary tuberculosis: clinical manifestations, diagnosis and outcome in 38 adults. Respirol 2001; 6:217–224.
28. Kalita J, Misra UK. Tuberculous meningitis with pulmonary miliary tuberculosis: a clinicoradiological study. Neurol India 2004; 52:194–196.

29. Shah AH, Joshi SV, Dhar HL. Tuberculosis of bones and joints. Antiseptic 2001; 98:385–387.
30. Malaviya A. Arthritis associated with tuberculosis. Best Pract Res Clin Rheumatol 2003; 17:319–343.
31. Lenk S, Schroeder J. Genitourinary tuberculosis. Curr Opin Urol 2001; 11:93–98.
32. Nash DR, Douglass JE. Anergy in active pulmonary tuberculosis. A comparison between positive and negative reactors and an evaluation of 5TU and 250TU skin test doses. Chest 1980; 77:32–35.
33. Thompson NJ, Glassroth JL, Snider DE Jr., Farer LS. The booster phenomenon in serial tuberculin screening. Am Rev Respir Dis 1979; 119:587–597.
34. Rosenberg T, Manfreda J, Hershfield ES. Two-step tuberculin testing staff and residents of a nursing home. Am Rev Respir Dis 1993; 148:1537–1540.
35. Centers for Disease Control and Prevention. Guidelines for Using the Quanti-FERON®-TB Gold test for detecting *Mycobacterium tuberculosis* infection, United States. Morb Mortal Wkly Rep 2005; 54(RR15):49–55.
36. Morris CDW. The radiography, haematology and bronchoscopy of pulmonary tuberculosis in the aged. QJ Med 1989; 71:529–536.
37. American Thoracic Society. Diagnostic standards and classification of tuberculosis in adults and children. Am J Resp Crit Care Med 2000; 161:1376–1395.
38. Centers for Disease Control and Prevention. Nucleic acid amplification tests for tuberculosis. Morb Mortal Wkly Rep 1996; 45:950–952.
39. American Thoracic Society. Targeted skin testing and treatment of latent tuberculosis infection. Am J Respir Crit Care Med 2000; 161:S221–S247.
40. Centers for Disease Control and Prevention. MMWR update: fatal and severe liver injuries associated with rifampin and pyrazinamide for latent tuberculosis infection, and revisions in American Thoracic Society/CDC recommendations–United States, 2001. Morb Mortal Wkly Rep 2001; 50(34):733–735.
41. CDC-ATS-IDSA. Treatment of tuberculosis. Morb Mortal Wkly Rep 2003; 52(RR11):1–77.

16

Infected Pressure Ulcers

Steven C. Reynolds and Anthony W. Chow
*Division of Infectious Diseases, Department of Medicine, University of
British Columbia, and Vancouver Hospital Health Sciences Center,
Vancouver, British Columbia, Canada*

KEY POINTS

1. Infected pressure ulcers have a powerful negative impact on the morbidity, mortality, and quality of life of residents in LTCFs. The majority of pressure ulcers can be prevented.
2. Multiple modalities are needed to effectively treat infected pressure ulcers, including mitigation of precipitating factors, appropriate wound care and dressing, debridement (if needed), and proper antibiotic therapy.
3. Infected pressure ulcers often have a polymicrobial etiology. Microbiological specimens may be misleading in superficial wounds and chronic wounds, and, therefore, caution is needed when interpreting culture results.
4. Antibiotic selection is based on a careful consideration of patient and microbiological factors. Broad coverage directed at both facultative and obligate anaerobes is generally required when treating infected pressure ulcers. The presence of MRSA requires careful assessment to distinguish between colonization versus infection and to establish the need for specific antistaphylococcal therapy.
5. There are important infection control issues associated with infected pressure ulcers.

EPIDEMIOLOGY AND CLINICAL RELEVANCE

Definition

Pressure ulcers are defined by the Agency for Healthcare Research and Quality (AHRQ; previously called Agency for Health Care Policy and Research) as lesions caused by prolonged exposure to pressure leading to tissue damage. They represent areas of necrosis due to compression of soft tissues between bony prominences and external surfaces. This damage can be relatively minor or can lead to massive necrosis involving deep tissues that can cause significant morbidity and mortality.

Incidence and Prevalence

The incidence and prevalence of pressure ulcers are quite variable, depending on the patient population being studied and the inclusion criteria. There are several systems for classifying pressure ulcers. The National Pressure Ulcer Advisory Panel classifies pressure ulcers as follows (Fig. 1) (2):

- *Stage I*: Nonblanchable erythema of intact skin.
- *Stage II*: Partial-thickness skin loss involving the epidermis or dermis; lesion presents as an abrasion, blister, or superficial ulcer.

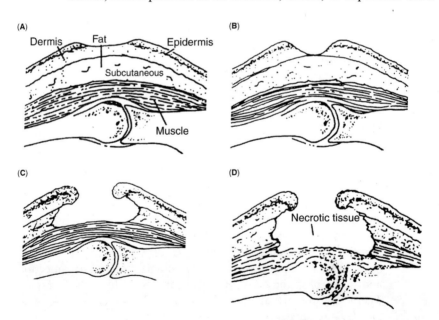

Figure 1 The National Pressure Ulcer Advisory Panel Classification of pressure ulcers. (**A**) Stage I, nonblanchable erythema of intact skin; (**B**) Stage II, partial-thickness skin loss involving the epidermis or dermis; (**C**) Stage III, full-thickness skin loss that may extend to but not through the fascia; (**D**) Stage IV, full-thickness skin loss involving deeper structures beyond the fascia. *Source*: From Ref. 1.

- *Stage III*: Full-thickness skin loss that may extend to but not through the fascia; the ulcer may be undermined.
- *Stage IV*: Full-thickness skin loss involving deeper structures, such as muscle, bone, or joint structures.

Most studies assessing the epidemiology of pressure ulcers include those ulcers that are Stage II and higher. Using this definition, the prevalence of pressure ulcers in nursing homes ranges from 1.2% to 11.3% (3,4). When Stage I ulcers are included, the prevalence rises to between 4% and 29.7% (4). Seventeen percent of patients admitted to nursing homes have Stage II or higher pressure ulcers on arrival. Among these, 81% come from an acute care hospital, 12% from home, and 7% from another nursing home. The incidence of pressure ulcers in patients admitted to nursing homes without pressure ulcers on arrival is 13% in one year, and 21% by two years (4).

Risk Factors

Not all nursing home patients are at equal risk of developing pressure ulcers. Risk factors can be classified as intrinsic or extrinsic (5). Limited mobility and poor nutrition are the strongest intrinsic predictors of pressure ulcer formation. Other factors, such as incontinence, increased age, diabetes mellitus, white race, abnormal skin, male gender, increased temperature, and decreased blood pressure, have also been implicated in at least one multivariate analysis but have not been associated in all studies (Table 1). The extrinsic risk factors for pressure ulcer development are pressure, friction, shear stress, and moisture; of these the most important is pressure.

Pressure

The highest capillary pressure is 32 mmHg (Fig. 2). Pressures above this lead to transudation, which increases interstitial pressure causing edema, ischemia, and autolysis. If the pressure is removed soon enough, reperfusion can occur, and irreversible damage is prevented. If pressure is sustained, necrosis occurs. There is an inverse relationship between the degree of pressure and the time required for irreversible tissue damage (Fig. 3) (7). Several studies indicate that the critical period of applied pressure, before irreversible tissue damage is likely to occur, is within one to two hours. A patient lying on a hospital mattress can generate pressures of 40 to 75 mmHg over bony prominences, particularly over the sacrum, greater trochanters, ischial tuberosities, dorsal spine, and the heels. This degree of pressure is sufficient to compromise the microcirculation, and these bony prominences correspond to the locations where pressure ulcers are most commonly identified clinically (Fig. 4). A patient sitting can generate pressures of 300 mmHg over the ischial tuberosities. Pressure is highest at

Table 1 Risk Factors Associated with Pressure Ulcers

	Studies reporting univariate associations	Studies reporting multivariate associations
Mobility or functional limitation	6	3
Incontinence	5	1
Nutritional factors	4	4
Altered consciousness or impaired cognition	3	0
Increased age	2	1
Diabetes mellitus	2	1
White race	2	1
Skin abnormalities	1	1
Stroke	1	1
Contractures	1	0
Male gender	1	1
Increased body temperature	1	1
Decreased blood pressure	1	1

Source: From Ref. 3.

the bone/muscle interface, and fat and muscle are more susceptible to pressure-related damage than skin. Thus, the superficial damage visible to the caregiver often underestimates the actual degree of destruction in deeper tissue layers (Fig. 5).

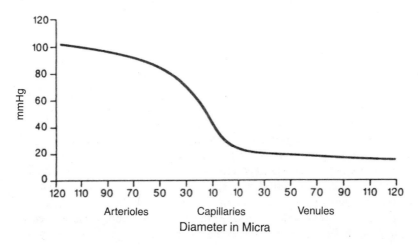

Figure 2 Pressure in various components of the tissue microcirculation. *Source*: From Ref. 6.

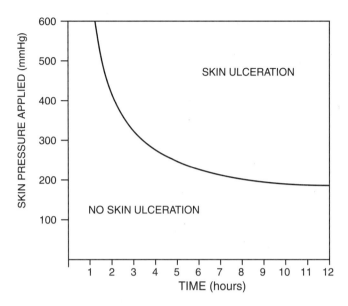

Figure 3 Inverse relationship of pressure to time in the production of pressure ulcers. *Source*: From Ref. 6.

Friction

Friction occurs when two opposing surfaces move across each other. In this case, it is the skin rubbing across sheets when a patient is dragged into a new position. This leads to damage at the surface and can compromise the skin barrier and lead to early ulceration (7).

Shearing Stress

Shearing stress results from the sliding and relative displacement of adjacent structures. This occurs from patients being positioned with the head of the bed up, or from being pulled up the bed. These forces cause vessels to be crimped, increasing ischemia in surrounding tissues. Superficial tissues remain in place due to friction so that damage is exclusively in deep tissues. Therefore, the ulcers produced are often extremely undermined and much worse than external inspection would suggest.

Moisture

Moisture as from urinary or fecal incontinence can increase the risk of pressure ulcers by fivefold. It can also be a source of bacterial contamination.

Other Factors

The National Pressure Ulcer Long-Term Care Study assessed 1524 long-term care residents over a 12-week period (8). Of the total sample, 443 (29.1%) developed new pressure ulcers. Variables predictive for ulcer development

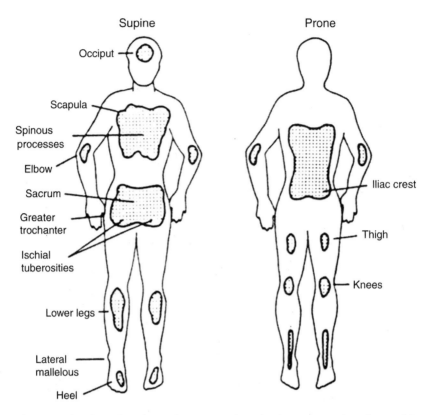

Figure 4 Common locations of pressure ulcers in the prone and supine positions, corresponding to areas of the skin surfaces (*stippled*) where pressures equal to or greater than mean capillary pressure are exerted. *Source*: From Ref. 7.

included a high initially assessed risk score, previous pressure ulcer, significant weight loss, oral problems with eating, requirement for urinary catheterization, and the use of pressure management systems. Protective variables included status as a new resident, nutritional supplements, and use of disposable briefs. Diminishing nursing resources and associated factors had a powerful negative impact on the risk of developing pressure ulcers. Nursing resources were considered to be compromised if a registered nurse was unable to spend more than 15 minutes per day with each resident, if a certified nursing assistant had less than two hours available per resident per day, and if the licensed practical nurse turnover rate was greater than 25%.

Infection

The epidemiology of infection in pressure ulcers has not been well described. One study demonstrated that infected pressure ulcers were the most common

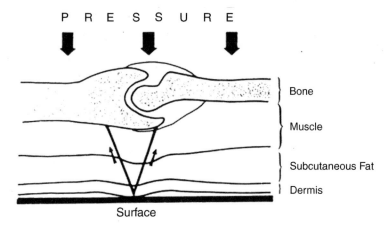

Figure 5 Pressure on any bony prominence is transmitted through the intervening tissues to the skin surface in a three-dimensional cone-shaped gradient, with the greatest pressure over a wide surface of bone and diminishing pressure toward the skin surface. *Source*: From Ref. 7.

infectious problem in nursing homes, occurring in 6% of the 532 patients studied (9). The percentage of patients with pressure ulcers was not provided in this study. Another study prospectively followed 16 long-term care patients with pressure ulcers for 2184 days. One was infected at enrollment, and three developed infections during follow-up, for an incidence of 1.4 infections per 1000 patient-ulcer days (10).

The consequences of pressure ulcers are multiplied when they become infected (11). Superficial infection delays wound healing and prolongs pain and discomfort. Infections can also invade deeper tissues and cause more serious complications, such as osteomyelitis (17–26% of patients with nonhealing pressure ulcers) and bacteremia (3.5 per 10,000 hospital discharges), and are associated with an in-hospital mortality rate of 51% (12). Pressure ulcers also have important implications for infection control and prevention measures in long-term care facilities (LTCFs) (discussed later in this chapter). Finally, there are significant costs associated with pressure ulcers. In one study, the mean cost per ulcer in a midwest LTCF in 1996 was $2731 (13). Nearly 80% of this cost came from the 4% of patients who required hospitalization. In another study, the mean cost for 20 patients with pelvic osteomyelitis associated with pressure ulcers treated between 1994 and 1999 was $59,600 (14).

PATHOGENESIS OF INFECTED PRESSURE ULCERS

Many organisms in chronic wounds, such as infected pressure ulcers, do not live in planktonic suspension but exist in organized complex communities called biofilms (15). Biofilms are formed by populations of organisms that are encased in a secreted extracellular polysaccharide matrix that protects the organisms and facilitates many of the functions necessary for the survival of the individual microorganism and the larger biofilm community.

Biofilms are formed when organisms are able to attach to a solid surface in an environment that is hospitable and rife with nutrients. Subsequently, a microcolony forms, which, given the right circumstances, eventually may mature into a complex biofilm community. The extracellular polysaccharide matrix provides a microenvironment with an intricate structure complete with water channels that allow transport of nutrients and waste. Organisms within biofilms utilize these water channels for the dispersion of intercellular signaling proteins, which can influence the overall growth patterns of the community. The best studied aspect of this biofilm behavior is the "quorum sensing" ability of these microorganisms to alter their phenotypic expression and growth patterns in response to the environment (e.g., adopting a more sessile growth pattern and a slower metabolic rate in response to less hospitable conditions). Biofilms also provide a physical barrier to toxic environmental components, such as the host immune system or antibiotics. It has been well documented that microorganisms in biofilms are 50 to 1000 times more resistant to conventional antibiotics than planktonic bacteria (16). Furthermore, failure to eradicate biofilm-associated bacteria is not due to inadequate antibiotic penetration into biofilms but likely due to a diminished antimicrobial effect of conventional antibiotics on bacteria in the biofilm environment (17).

Understanding this microbiological defense mechanism is important in our management strategy of chronic wounds. Organisms respond very differently to therapeutic interventions when they have access to the resources and defense mechanisms that a biofilm can provide. A chronic wound can provide nutrients and a relatively hospitable environment for microbial growth and biofilm formation. Biofilms help to explain the ubiquity and tenacity of microbial colonization of chronic wounds. Additionally, the ability to manipulate biofilms may result in more effective wound management. For example, wound debridement may physically remove the biofilm glycoprotein matrix and afford greater efficacy by host immune mechanisms and antibiotics on planktonic bacteria. There is some evidence that erythromycin has an inhibitory effect on biofilm formation and that other macrolides are able to induce phagocytic penetration into biofilms (18). Unsaturated lactoferrin may prevent bacterial biofilm development by scavenging free iron (19).

CLINICAL MANIFESTATIONS

Superficial infections will generally manifest with erythema, warmth, and tenderness. Purulent discharge, foul odor, and crepitus may also be seen. Due to advancing age and comorbid conditions, systemic signs, such as fever and leukocytosis, may be minimal or absent even in patients with grossly infected ulcers, and local signs of inflammation may not be readily apparent. Superficial infections can delay wound healing. This can occasionally be the only clue to the presence of infection, reflecting the presence of more than 10^6 microorganisms per gram of tissue (20).

A more serious complication of infection in pressure ulcers is osteomyelitis. This may manifest as a nonhealing wound with systemic toxicity, or it may be suspected on the basis of clinical or radiological findings and should always be considered in LTCF patients with fever, leukocytosis, or other signs of sepsis. Many patients will have few or no signs of infection other than a nonhealing wound (21).

Bacteremia and sepsis, which are usually secondary to deep ulcers and osteomyelitis, is the most feared complication of infected pressure ulcers. Mortality rates among patients with sepsis may approximate 50% (22). Patients usually present with signs of systemic toxicity, such as fever, chills, confusion, and hypotension.

DIAGNOSTIC APPROACH

Appropriate management of pressure ulcers requires careful clinical assessment, microbiological evaluation, imaging studies, and histopathologic confirmation of the extent of infection by deep tissue biopsies.

Clinical Assessment

Diagnosis of pressure ulcers begins with identifying the patients at risk and careful examination for the earliest stages of pressure ulcer formation. The established pressure ulcer is usually easily recognized on the basis of its typical location and the clinical setting. A developing ulcer is often irregular in shape, whereas chronic ulcers tend to have regular edges with a thick fibrous ring below the surface. Because of the pressure gradient phenomenon (Fig. 5), a very small surface defect commonly overlies a large undermining lesion. Whereas the physical examination is critical to identify and locate pressure ulcers as an occult source of sepsis, it is less helpful in determining the extent of soft tissue infection underlying the pressure ulcer or whether there is contiguous osteomyelitis. In one study, the clinical examination was accurate in the diagnosis of histopathologically confirmed underlying osteomyelitis in only 56% of 36 patients, with a sensitivity of 33% and a specificity of 60% (21). Some authors have suggested that the presence of nonhealing ulcers is more likely associated with underlying osteomyelitis, but this association was not substantiated in other studies. Even the presence of exposed bone does not necessarily indicate the presence of osteomyelitis because histopathologically confirmed osteomyelitis was present in only 14% of patients with exposed bone (21).

Microbiologic Evaluation

A critical concept in chronic wounds is that there is a continuum of bacteria–host interactions ranging from contamination to septicemia and that infection must be distinguished from contamination or colonization (Fig. 6) (23). Contamination is defined as the existence of nonreplicative organisms within the wound, whereas colonization is characterized by the replication of microorganisms adherent to a wound in the absence of tissue damage. By definition, colonization does not impede wound healing. The intermediate step between colonization and an invasive infection is encompassed by the term "critical colonization." This is defined as a local infection that impedes wound healing but does not spread beyond the borders of the wound (24). This stage may be difficult to identify by physical examination alone; although the wound bed and granulation tissue may appear unhealthy, other signs of local infection are absent. Transition between the various stages of host–bacteria interactions in wounds is determined by several factors, including the number of bacteria per gram of tissue, virulence of the organism in question, and the ability of the host to mount an appropriate immunological response.

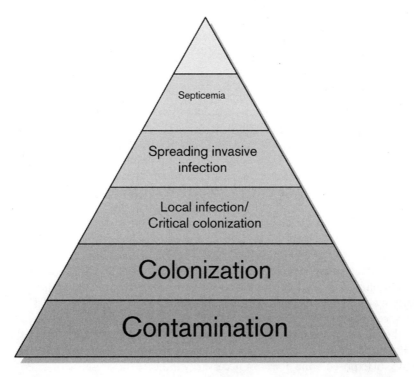

Figure 6 Pyramid schema of bacterial activity in chronic wounds. *Source*: From Ref. 15.

All pressure ulcers will become colonized by skin organisms. Thus, the challenge of microbiologic evaluation is to be able to distinguish between isolates that are more likely to be associated with invasive infection (high virulence) rather than mere colonization (low virulence). Organisms isolated from blood cultures or from deep tissue biopsy bypassing the open wound generally carry higher significance than those isolated from superficial swab cultures of the pressure ulcer. One study (25) assessed the relative value of superficial swabs, needle aspiration, and deep tissue biopsy for the microbiologic evaluation of 72 pressure ulcers in patients over the age of 60. Swabs were taken using saline-moistened gauze in the ulcer bed. Aspirates were obtained by introducing a 22-gauge needle through disinfected intact skin and aspirating briskly while moving the needle in several directions. Deep tissue biopsies were obtained using sharp, sterile scalpels. Ninety-seven percent of cultures obtained from surface swabs were positive, compared with 43% of aspirates and 63% of biopsies. It was concluded that the aspiration method was unreliable, as it underestimated the number of isolates compared with deep tissue biopsies. In addition, correlation between the species of bacteria found on deep biopsy compared with aspirates and swabs was poor. Another study (26) also assessed the reliability of needle aspiration compared with deep tissue biopsy in 32 patients with clinically infected pressure ulcers. Their aspiration technique involved instilling 1 mL of sterile saline into the wound margin and massaging the area before aspiration. Compared with deep tissue biopsy, the irrigation-aspiration technique had a sensitivity of 93% and specificity of 97%. A median of 4.5 bacterial species was recovered per ulcer by this method. However, aspirated samples from noninfected ulcers have also been shown to contain bacteria in 30% of cases, with the majority being usual skin contaminants.

In another study of 23 consecutive patients, the bacteriology of pressure ulcers was examined using both aerobic and anaerobic techniques (27). Specimens were obtained by needle aspiration, surgical drainage, or cotton swab. An average of four isolates per patient (three aerobes and one anaerobe) were recovered. Although five times as many aerobes as anaerobes were isolated from the ulcers, twice as many anaerobes as aerobes were recovered from blood among 19 bacteremic patients. The most common aerobic isolates from the ulcers included *Proteus mirabilis*, group D enterococci, *Escherichia coli*, staphylococci, and *Pseudomonas* species. Anaerobic isolates included *Peptostreptococcus* species, *Bacteroides fragilis*, and *Clostridium perfringens*. Among 19 (79%) patients with documented bacteremia, the predominant blood isolates were *B. fragilis* (11 patients), *Peptostreptococcus* (seven patients), *P. mirabilis* (four patients), and *S. aureus* (three patients). In 10 (41%) patients, bacteremia was polymicrobial. Thus, blood cultures are clearly very important in the initial microbiologic assessment of all patients with suspected infection associated with pressure ulcers.

Culture results must be interpreted with caution in cases of osteomyelitis. In a study of 36 patients with nonhealing pressure ulcers, 17% had histopathologic evidence of chronic osteomyelitis, based on specimens obtained by needle biopsy through a debrided area of the ulcer (21). Bone cultures were positive in all samples showing osteomyelitis but also in 73% of cases without histopathologic evidence of osteomyelitis. The number of different organisms and the use of quantitative cultures also were not predictive of the presence of osteomyelitis. Even in cases where pure growth of the same organism was found in both the swab and bone cultures, there was sometimes no histopathologic evidence of osteomyelitis. Criticisms of this study are that there could have been sampling errors in bone biopsy (it is not as sensitive as ostectomy), so true cases could have been missed. Follow-up information regarding those patients with multiple pure cultures who were not treated as osteomyelitis was not reported. If these patients improved without specific antimicrobial therapy, it would have been stronger evidence that bone cultures obtained through debrided wounds were not predictive of osteomyelitis.

The data regarding culture results from pressure ulcers can be summarized as follows. First, superficial swab cultures are not useful and generally reflect colonization rather than infection. Second, needle aspirates are difficult to interpret and should either not be used or be used with great caution. An exception might be the irrigation-aspiration technique, which demonstrated high sensitivity and specificity compared with deep tissue biopsy results for draining pressure ulcers (26). Third, the culture results themselves, even from bone or other deep tissue biopsies, should not be used as the sole criterion for evidence of osteomyelitis without additional clinical or histopathologic evidence of infection. Because bacterial colonization is an almost universal phenomenon, culture results must be interpreted in the light of clinical data, and histopathological evidence of infection should be sought before the decision to initiate antimicrobial therapy is made.

Imaging Studies

Radiologic studies can play a valuable role in the investigation of infection in pressure ulcers, usually by determining the existence of osteomyelitis and in delineating the extent of the ulcer. The different modalities include plain radiography, computer-assisted tomography (CT), magnetic resonance imaging (MRI), and radionuclide scintigraphy.

Plain Radiography

Plain films are useful for demonstrating the extent of bony damage, but it can take up to 14 days before evidence is visible radiographically. In cases of osteomyelitis due to pressure ulcers, interpretation of plain films may be difficult. Even noninfected ulcers can show periosteal reactive changes and heterotopic new bone formation. Furthermore, lytic bony lesions do not develop very often (21). Because of these difficulties, plain radiographs have limited value in both confirming and excluding the diagnosis of osteomyelitis in cases of pressure ulcers, and routine use of plain films for this purpose is not recommended.

The sinogram may be of value in the patient requiring surgical debridement, because this study will frequently allow the surgeon to delineate the necessary extent of the surgical procedure. Sinography may also yield unexpected findings, such as excessive depth of the sinus tract, extension into neighboring joints, and abscess formation. The role of sinography in assessing pressure ulcers has probably diminished with the wide availability of CT scanning.

Computer-Assisted Tomography

CT scans can be useful for the detection of early osseous erosion and to document the presence of sequestrum or gas formation but is generally less sensitive than either MRI or radionuclide scintigraphy for the diagnosis of bone infections (28). Furthermore, it is often impossible to distinguish between osteomyelitis and pressure-induced osseous changes confined to fat and muscle tissue (29). CTs may be more useful in defining the size of the ulcer, the presence of fistulas, and possible joint involvement.

Magnetic Resonance Imaging

MRI has a sensitivity of 98% and specificity of 89% in the detection of osteomyelitis among patients with spinal cord injuries. MRI provides excellent resolution in defining the extent of local tissue destruction in deep musculoskeletal infections. However, there is less information on the true value of MRI for the detection of osteomyelitis in older patients with infected pressure ulcers.

Radionuclide Scintigraphy

Three-phase technetium-99m (Tc-99m) diphosphate bone scans and indium- or gallium-labeled white blood cell scans are currently the most sensitive and specific imaging modalities for the detection of osteomyelitis in patients with diabetic foot ulcers and other musculoskeletal infections (28). However, these techniques have not been adequately studied in patients with pressure ulcers.

In summary, the clinical examination will indicate the presence of superficial infections but is not useful for the diagnosis of underlying osteomyelitis. Microbiological data, if obtained from deep biopsy or aspiration, are useful for directing antimicrobial therapy after the clinical diagnosis of infection is made. On its own, the presence of bacteria even from deep cultures is not sufficient to diagnose infection. Among the radiographic investigations, CT and MRI may be of some value, but there is currently insufficient data to recommend their general use. Scintigraphy, when used with different tests in combination, can be useful. Bone scans have good negative-predictive value, and white blood cell scans have good positive-predictive value. The bone biopsy for histopathologic diagnosis remains the gold standard for confirmation of osteomyelitis and should be used in cases of uncertainty.

THERAPEUTIC INTERVENTIONS

The goals of treating infected pressure ulcers are to resolve the infection and to aid in wound healing. Therapy should be directed by a multidisciplinary approach drawing from the expertise in nursing, medicine, surgery, and physical rehabilitation. Implementation of the appropriate therapy requires an understanding of the risk factors and the pathophysiology leading to pressure ulcer formation.

Reducing Intrinsic Risk Factors for Pressure Ulcers

Although most intrinsic risk factors for the development of pressure ulcers discussed earlier are, for the most part, not amenable to intervention, it may be possible to reduce some risks by paying attention to underlying comorbid conditions. For example, both congestive heart failure and diabetes mellitus have been shown to interfere with wound healing in patients with pressure ulcers within the intensive care unit. It seems reasonable to extrapolate these findings to LTCF residents and to strive at improving patients' general medical condition. Part of good general medical care is the optimization of a patient's nutritional status. There is convincing evidence that poor nutrition is a risk factor for pressure ulcer development. Conversely, there are also data demonstrating that patients who receive higher dietary protein diets show improved wound healing compared with those with an inadequate diet. This is independent of effects on serum albumin and other markers of nutritional status. The effects of caloric supplementation and enteral feeding are controversial. It seems intuitive that if patients who are receiving more protein demonstrate better healing, then caloric supplementation or tube feeding (in those unable to feed themselves) will also lead to improved healing. However, this has yet to be demonstrated. There are two reasons why caloric supplementation has not been shown to be helpful. First, malnutrition can mean that either patients are underfed or they are cachectic from underlying diseases. Caloric supplementation would be expected to help the underfed but not those with cachexia. The second problem is that tube feeding has its own risks. The patient may become less mobile because of tube feeding or may be tied down to prevent self-extubation. Tube feeding may also increase the risk of aspiration pneumonia. These possibilities can all worsen a patient's condition and may delay wound healing. In addition to caloric and protein malnutrition, attention has been focused on zinc and vitamin C supplements. Patients deficient in these nutrients heal poorly, but supplementation in nondeficient patients has not been proven beneficial. In general, patients with pressure ulcers should receive protein and calories appropriate for those under stress. Tube feeding should not be instituted solely for the treatment of pressure ulcers.

Reducing Extrinsic Risk Factors for Pressure Ulcers

Attention should also be paid to the extrinsic risk factors for pressure ulcer formation. Pressure relief is the cornerstone of pressure ulcer therapy. There are a number of devices for the reduction of pressure (Fig. 7). They can be classified into static and dynamic devices. Static devices, such as foam- or fluid-filled products, maintain constant pressure when the patient is not moving but disperse it over a greater area than standard bed mattresses. These devices are appropriate for patients who can assume different positions without bearing weight on the ulcer and without compressing the support material too much. For patients who cannot avoid weight bearing

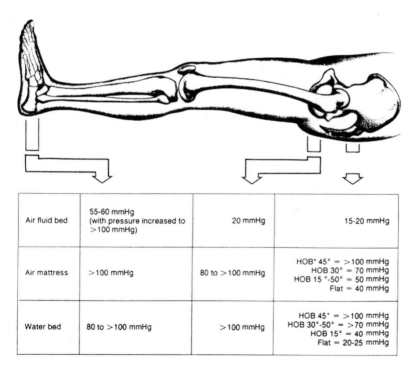

Air fluid bed	55-60 mmHg (with pressure increased to >100 mmHg)	20 mmHg	15-20 mmHg
Air mattress	>100 mmHg	80 to >100 mmHg	HOB˙ 45° = >100 mmHg HOB 30° = 70 mmHg HOB 15 °-50° = 50 mmHg Flat = 40 mmHg
Water bed	80 to >100 mmHg	>100 mmHg	HOB 45˙ = >100 mmHg HOB 30°-50° = >70 mmHg HOB 15° = 40 mmHg Flat = 20-25 mmHg

Figure 7 Degree of pressure reduction, in mmHg, by pressure-relieving devices on varying anatomical locations. *Abbreviation*: HOB, head of bed. *Source*: From Ref. 30.

on the ulcer or who do not show evidence of healing, a dynamic device may be more suitable. Dynamic devices change their support by alternating currents of air to redistribute pressure against the body. Examples are low air-loss beds and air-fluidized beds. Low air-loss systems maintain pressure using a constant air supply moving through a mattress of semipermeable fabric that allows some of the air to escape. Air-fluidized systems contain tiny silicone-coated beads suspended in strong currents of air. Manufacturers of these various dynamic devices claim that contact pressure is less than 10 mmHg. However, evidence supporting the use of any of these devices is relatively scant. Most authorities recommend use of dynamic beds for extensive Stages III–IV pressure ulcers and for ulcers that fail to heal with standard therapy.

Local Wound Care

Local wound care is another fundamental part of pressure ulcer therapy. The important aspects of local care include debridement, wound dressings, negative pressure wound therapy (NPWT), other adjunctive measures, and surgery.

Debridement

Debridement of necrotic tissue is required for optimal healing to occur. The reasons for this are not entirely clear but may be due to decreased bacterial contamination and physical removal of biofilms, resulting in a reduction of chronic inflammation and improved tissue granulation. There are a number of techniques for debriding wounds. Sharp debridement can be performed at the bedside or in the operating room. It is recommended in cases of thick eschars or in infected wounds. It should be remembered that wound debridement can lead to transient bacteremia; systemic antimicrobial prophylaxis should be considered especially in patients with prosthetic devices or those at risk for endocarditis. Mechanical debridement using saline-soaked gauze and irrigation with a 35 mL syringe and 19-gauge needle (this achieves a pressure of approximately 8 psi—enough to remove dead tissue and bacteria but not enough to damage viable tissue) are another possibility. The traditional wet-to-dry dressing can damage viable tissue and should only be used in wounds with large amounts of necrotic tissue. Occlusive dressings, such as hydrocolloids, hydrogels, and foams, allow tissue fluid full of phagocytes and their enzymatic products to accumulate, leading to autolytic debridement. There are also a number of enzymatic products available, that may be of use in noninfected pressure ulcers.

Wound Dressings

Dressings help to protect viable tissue, promote healing, and reduce contamination. A general rule is that dressings should keep the wound bed moist and the surrounding intact skin dry. Saline-soaked gauze has historically been used for pressure ulcer dressing. In superficial wounds, this can lead to excess maceration of intact skin and can impede wound healing if allowed to dry. Synthetic dressings are divided into films, hydrocolloids, foams, hydrogels, and alginates. Films are thin semipermeable membranes appropriate for use in minimally draining Stage II wounds. Hydrocolloids are adherent absorbent dressings useful for moderately draining wounds. Foams are similar but are nonadherent and need a secondary dressing. Hydrogels desiccate more easily than other dressings and are not ideal for pressure ulcers. Alginates are highly absorbable dressings derived from seaweed; they should be used in heavily draining wounds. Synthetic dressings should be avoided in cases of active infection, draining sinus tracts, and exposed bone or tendon.

Negative Pressure Wound Therapy

NPWT is being increasingly used in the treatment of complex ulcers and surgical wounds (31). NPWT uses a foam pad, which has gentle suction applied via tubing, placed into the wound and covered with a semiocclusive, vapor-permeable dressing. The goal is to provide an optimal moist environment for wound healing. NPWT is based on the theory that the wound is drawn closer by the negative pressure and stagnant interstitial fluid is drawn out of the wound. Studies suggest a concomitant increase in local blood flow, which has been attributed to decreased tissue edema. This results in enhanced formation of granulation tissue. There have been multiple case series and a limited number of small randomized controlled trials studying NPWT with somewhat mixed results, although they generally show some improvement in the formation of granulation tissue and chronic wound healing. NPWT is considered best suited for Stage III or IV ulcers or wounds. In particular, wounds and ulcers with poor granulation tissue, relatively large size, and a heavy exudate may derive the most benefit from NPWT. Contraindications include untreated osteomyelitis, local malignancy, nonenteric or unexplored fistulas, necrotic tissue with eschar present, and placement over exposed vessels or organs.

Other Adjunctive Measures

Some authors have advocated topical antibiotics or antiseptics to decrease bacterial contamination and promote healing. The evidence that they show benefit, however, is rather scant. Silver sulfadiazine has been shown to be of no added benefit when compared with its vehicle alone. Thus, the benefit seen in earlier studies might have been derived from the vehicle creams keeping the wound moist rather than the antimicrobial constituents. Antibiotics and antiseptics have also been shown to be toxic to fibroblasts in vitro, and there is a concern with selection of resistant organisms. Topical antimicrobials, therefore, should not be used unless there are new data supporting their beneficial effects in the future. Adjunctive therapies, such as electrical stimulation, hyperbaric oxygenation, ultrasound, and growth factors, continue to be investigated, but clinical data are rather limited at this time. The use of electrical stimulation in particular looks promising and may become a more important treatment modality in the future.

Surgery

Surgery is the treatment of choice for difficult Stages III and IV pressure ulcers. It performs the tasks of debriding necrotic tissue, contouring bony prominences to decrease subsequent pressure loads, and closure of the ulcer by myocutaneous flaps that fill the defect and provide adequate blood supply. Surgery should be reserved for those patients who will gain an improvement in their quality of life from resolution of their pressure ulcer.

Antimicrobial Therapy

Treatment of infectious complications in pressure ulcers depends on both medical and surgical interventions. For the reasons mentioned above, topical antimicrobial therapy should be avoided. Systemic antibiotics have a role both in prophylaxis and treatment. Systemic antibiotics should also be used for patients with serious infections of the pressure ulcer, including those with spreading cellulitis, associated osteomyelitis, or bacteremia.

The choice of antibiotics is based on an understanding of the polymicrobial etiology of infected pressure ulcers and the need to cover for high-virulence microorganisms, both aerobic and anaerobic. There are no trials assessing the superiority of one antibiotic regimen over another. Cultures from deep aspirates can be used to guide the choice of agents and broaden the antibiotic coverage. However, because cultures from aspirates do not correlate well with tissue biopsy results, antibiotics should not be narrowed to treat only those organisms found in aspirate cultures. There are a variety of antimicrobial options for treating infected pressure ulcers (Table 2). Monotherapy with broad-spectrum β-lactam/β-lactamase inhibitor combinations, carbapenems, or later-generation fluoroquinolones are all appropriate choices. Tigecycline has broad-spectrum activity against both aerobic and anaerobic bacteria associated with necrotizing skin and soft tissue infections, including both gram-positive and gram-negative bacteria. It's role in the treatment of infected pressure ulcers in LTCF residents remains to be determined. Monotherapy with extended-spectrum cephalosporins should be avoided due to the emergence of extended-spectrum β-lactamase–producing microorganisms. Combination therapies, such as with a cephalosporin or fluoroquinolone for aerobic coverage plus clindamycin or metronidazole for anaerobes, may also be suitable. The addition of vancomycin may be needed if infection with resistant organisms such as methicillin-resistant *Staphylococcus aureus* (MRSA) is strongly suspected. Due to poor tissue perfusion in infected pressure ulcers, antibiotic therapy should be administered by

Table 2 Antibiotic Regimens for Infected Pressure Ulcers

Regimens	Recommended dose schedule
Monotherapy	
Ticarcillin–clavulanate	2–4 g q4–6 hr IV
Piperacillin–tazobactam	2–4 g q6–8 hr IV
Imipenem	0.5–1 g q6–8 hr IV
Meropenem	0.5–1 g q6–8 hr IV
Ertapenem	1 g IV q24
Cefipime	2 g IV q8
Gatifloxacin	400 mg QD IV or PO
Moxifloxacin	400 mg QD IV or PO
Tigecycline	50–100 mg q12 h IV
Combination therapy	
Clindamycin or metronidazole, plus	450–600 mg q6–8 hr IV or 450 mg qid PO
one of the following:	500 mg q6–8 hr IV or 500 mg tid PO
Ciprofloxacin (with clindamycin only)	200–400 mg q12 hr IV or 500 mg bid PO
Ofloxacin	200–400 mg q12–24 hr IV or
	400 mg bid PO
Levofloxacin	500–750 mg QD IV or PO
Amoxicillin–clavulanate	500/125 mg tid PO
Ceftriaxone	1 g IV q24
Ceftizoxime	1–2 g IV q6–8 hr
Cefotaxime	1 g IV q8
Treatment of MRSA infection	
Vancomycin	0.5 g q6–8 IV or 1–1.5 g IV q12–24
Quinupristin/dalfopristin (Synercid®)	7.5 mg/kg q8–12 hr IV
Oxazolidinone (Linezolid®)	600 mg q12 hr IV
Daptomycin	4 mg/kg q24 IV

Abbreviations: IV, intravenous; QD, day; PO, oral; qid, four times a day; tid, three times a day; bid, two times a day; MRSA, methicillin-resistant *Staphylococcus aureus*.

the intravenous route particularly as initial empirical therapy in patients with signs of sepsis.

When choosing antibiotics for an infected pressure ulcer, there are several factors to consider besides the culture results and in vitro susceptibility data, including bioavailability, dosing requirements, delivery methods, and adverse effects. For example, cephalosporin use has been associated with an observed institutional increase in resistant organisms, specifically vancomycin-resistant enterococci (VRE). In LTCFs, the risk of *Clostridium difficile*-associated diarrhea is particularly problematic. All elderly patients should be carefully monitored when any antibiotics are initiated, particularly with clindamycin and the cephalosporins. Linezolid has a tendency to cause peripheral neuropathies when used for longer than two weeks. Carbapenems and fluoroquinolones are known to lower seizure thresholds.

This is not an exhaustive list, and careful consideration of comorbid conditions and their impact on antimicrobial efficacy and side effects must be undertaken when deciding upon antimicrobial therapy.

The method of drug delivery is a limiting factor in patients with poor intravenous access. Empirical antibiotic combinations, such as clindamycin plus ciprofloxacin, which have excellent oral bioavailability and good tissue penetration, are a reasonable alternative in a nonseptic patient who has good digestive tract function. The later-generation fluoroquinolones, such as gatifloxacin and moxifloxacin, are being investigated as intravenous or oral alternatives for the treatment of soft tissue infections. They hold a great deal of promise due to their broad spectrum, including antianaerobic activity, and excellent oral bioavailability. Additionally, multiple dosing regimens, which cause a significant nursing burden, may be avoided. Both the newer fluoroquinolones and ertapenem require only a single daily dose.

INFECTION CONTROL MEASURES

The goals of infection control in regard to pressure ulcers are to reduce colonization and prevent infection; to reduce the spread of pathogenic organisms to other patients, staff, or the environment; and to prevent selection of resistant organisms. In 1994, the Agency for Health Care Policy and Research (now called AHRQ) included six infection control recommendations in their treatment guidelines for pressure ulcers (32). One of these recommendations pertains to the care of wounds at home and will not be discussed further. Of the recommendations for hospitalized patients, four are designed to reduce contamination of the wound and one aims to reduce the spread of pathogens. Each of these recommendations was given a grade C for strength of evidence, indicating expert opinion rather than solid data from clinical trials.

AHRQ Recommendations to Reduce Contamination of Pressure Ulcers

Recommendation 1: Sterile Instruments Should Be Used to Debride Pressure Ulcers

The use of sterile technique to debride wounds is entirely sensible. The act of sharp debridement changes the physiology of the wound, which renders it more susceptible to infection. Thus, the use of sterile technique to reduce the bacterial burden in the wound is indicated in this instance. The fact that newly debrided wounds may be more susceptible to infection after exposure to smaller numbers of bacteria makes the other AHRQ recommendations for preventing contamination more difficult to apply to the general population. Newly debrided wounds and older wounds may require different precautions, a possibility that remains to be tested.

Recommendation 2: Clean Dressings May Be Used
Instead of Sterile Dressings

Sterile dressings have not been shown to lead to less contamination than clean dressings. The AHRQ, therefore, recommends that as long as clean dressings remain dry and free from heavy contamination, they are still suitable for use. The problem is that one cannot be assured that they are entirely free from any contamination, and in one study as high as 20% of "sterile" dressings yielded a few colonies of bacteria immediately upon opening the package (33). The rate of contamination increases if the dressings are saturated while placed on their wrappings over a nonsterile surface (a common practice used to avoid using another container in which to saturate the gauze).

Recommendation 3: Health-Care Workers Should Use Clean
Gloves for Each Patient, and When Treating Multiple Ulcers
on the Same Patient the Most Contaminated Ulcer Should
Be Treated Last; They Should Also Wash Their Hands
Between Patients

This recommendation is based on the same argument as using sterile dressings. Again, it seems prudent to use sterile gloves with newly debrided pressure ulcers, although clean gloves likely are sufficient for the care of older ulcers. A trial to assess bacterial loads, incidence of clinical infection, and impact on wound healing for pressure ulcers dressed with clean or sterile gloves would be a useful contribution to the field. In general, hand washing and the appropriate use of gloves remains an area in which there is room for improvement. The role of hand washing in preventing nosocomial infections cannot be overstated and should continue to be emphasized.

Recommendation 4: Ulcers Should Be Protected
from Sources of Contamination Such as Feces

This recommendation to protect pressure ulcers from fecal or other contamination also seems intuitively reasonable. Delayed wound healing in patients with fecal incontinence has been shown. Unfortunately, it can be difficult to protect the wound entirely, but every effort to do so should be made.

AHRQ Recommendation to Prevent Spread of Pathogenic Organisms from Pressure Ulcers

Recommendation 1

Follow body substance isolation precautions or an equivalent system when treating pressure ulcers. Body substance isolation has six components applicable to pressure ulcers:

1. Wear gloves for contact with body fluids.
2. Change gloves and wash hands between patients.

3. Wash hands after any type of patient contact.
4. Wear additional barrier, such as gowns, masks, or goggles, when body fluids may come in contact with the clothing or skin.
5. Place soiled reusable items in securely sealed containers.
6. Place needles into designated sharps containers.

These recommendations apply to all patients and should also be followed in the management of patient with pressure ulcers. Wound dressing changes can lead to aerosolization of bacteria that can persist for up to 30 minutes. Thus, masks and gowns should by worn when changing wounds heavily contaminated with resistant or highly virulent bacteria. This may be less of a problem with hydrocolloid as opposed to gauze dressings. The use of whirlpools to debride wounds can also be an infection control hazard. Both pseudomonas and staphylococci have been recovered even from regularly disinfected and serviced whirlpools in nursing homes. Whether the benefit of whirlpools outweighs the infection control risks remains to be seen.

Increasingly, MRSA and VRE are being isolated in LTCFs (see also Chapters 23 and 24). Antimicrobial use is an important evolutionary pressure for selecting these resistant strains. Improved use of antimicrobial agents, therefore, is critically important for preventing or slowing the spread of these organisms. There are a number of studies examining antibiotic use in nursing homes, although no specific information exists regarding antibiotic utilization patterns and infection or contamination of pressure ulcers with resistant microorganisms. It has been estimated that 30% to 50% of long-term care residents will receive at least one course of systemic antimicrobial therapy in any given year. Telephone orders with no evidence that a physician ever saw the patient might account for half of these antibiotic prescriptions in LTCFs. It is recommended that clinical information regarding indications for antimicrobial therapy should be charted for each patient prescribed antibiotics and that institutions should include antimicrobial utilization monitoring in their infection control program. The empirical use of vancomycin in LTCFs with high rates of MRSA carriage and infection is a particular concern because this practice also leads to an increased prevalence of VRE. Every effort should be made to distinguish colonization from clinical infection before any specific antimicrobial therapy is initiated.

PREVENTION

The cornerstones to prevention are identifying patients at risk, improving general health, minimizing external forces, and implementing educational programs to inform caregivers about pressure ulcers. Several prediction tools have been developed to identify patients at risk for developing pressure ulcers. The most widely used are the Braden scale and the Norton scale, both of which have been validated clinically (34). The Braden scale is composed of six broad clinical categories: sensory perception, moisture, activity, mobility, nutrition, and friction and shear; the Norton scale is composed of five broad clinical categories: physical condition, mental state, activity, mobility, and incontinence. Risk assessment should be performed on admission to an institution and at periodic intervals. In addition to assessing the patient's risk of pressure ulcer development, the skin should be examined on a daily basis for signs of breakdown so that further preventative measures can be undertaken.

The key to preventing pressure ulcers is in alleviating pressure-related tissue damage. This can be achieved by proper positioning of the patient or by the use of devices to relieve pressure. Frequent turning to relieve prolonged weight bearing on bony prominences is also important. A two-hour repositioning schedule is considered the minimum interval for patients at risk, and patients who are wheelchair dependent should shift their weight every 15 minutes.

Friction, shear, and moisture are the other extrinsic forces that play a role in pressure ulcer pathogenesis. Friction should be avoided by not dragging a patient across a surface. Instead, a sheet that the patient is lying on should be used to move the patient in the bed. Friction can also be avoided by the use of sheepskins or boots or synthetic dressings. Minimizing the angle of the head of the bed can reduce shear, as can the use of undersheets to move patients. Moisture is usually due to incontinence, which should be treated if reversible. If not controllable, moisture should be detected and removed as soon as possible, and the use of absorbent underpads or briefs should be considered. Barrier creams may also be helpful.

Education is another key to preventing pressure ulcers and should be directed at both the patients and caregivers. The educational program should include information regarding the risk factors of pressure ulcers, skin assessment and staging techniques, pressure relief strategies and devices, wound healing, and infection control. The effects of educational programs have not been extensively studied, but there are some evidences that they reduce pressure ulcer incidence.

Using a comprehensive prevention strategy, one study (35) demonstrated a significant reduction in the incidence of pressure ulcers in two separate LTCFs (from 13.2% to 1.7% per month and from 15% to 3.5% per month, respectively). The average monthly cost of prevention for high-risk residents in this study was $519.73 (plus a one-time cost of $277 for mattress and chair overlays). More than half ($277.15) of the monthly costs were due to labor; the most expensive item cost was for support surfaces. These findings indicate that preventative strategies can be cost-effective, particularly if they are based on risk stratification.

SUGGESTED READING

Edwards R, Harding KG. Bacteria and wound healing. Curr Opin Infect Dis 2004;
    17:91–96.
Gupta S, ed. Guidelines for managing pressure ulcers with negative pressure wound
    therapy. Adv Skin Wound Care 2004; 17(suppl 2):1–16.
Thompson D. A critical review of the literature on pressure ulcer aetiology. J Wound
    Care 2005; 14:87–90.

REFERENCES

1. Shea JD. Pressure ulcers: classification and management. Clin Orthop Rel Res
    1975; 112:81–94.
2. The National Pressure Ulcer Advisory Panel. Pressure ulcers prevalence, cost,
    risk assessment: consensus development conference statement. Decubitus 1989;
    2:24–28.
3. Allman RM. Pressure ulcer prevalence, incidence, risk factors, and impact. Clin
    Geriatr Med 1997; 13:421–437.
4. Brandeis GH, Morris JN, Nash DJ, Lipsitz LA. The epidemiology and natural
    history of pressure ulcers in elderly nursing home residents. JAMA 1990;
    264:2905–2909.
5. Thompson D. A critical review of the literature on pressure ulcer aetiology.
    J Wound Care 2005; 14:87–90.
6. Woolsey RM, McGarry JD. The cause, prevention and treatment of pressure
    sore. Neurol Clin 1991; 9:797–808.
7. Reuler JB, Cooney TG. The pressure sore: pathophysiology and principles of
    management. Ann Intern Med 1981; 94:661–666.
8. Horn SD, Bender SA, Ferguson ML, et al. The National Pressure Ulcer Long-
    term Care study: pressure ulcer development in long-term care residents. J Am
    Geriatr Soc 2004; 52:359–367.
9. Garibaldi RA, Brodine S, Matsumiya S. Infections among patients in nursing
    homes. N Engl J Med 1981; 305:731–735.
10. Nicolle LE, Orr P, Duckworth H, et al. Prospective study of decubitus ulcers in
    two long term care facilities. Can J Infect Control 1994; 9:35–38.
11. Penhallow K. A review of studies that examine the impact of infection on the
    normal wound-healing process. J Wound Care 2005; 14:123–126.
12. Livesley NJ, Chow AW. Infected pressure ulcers in elderly individuals. Clin
    Infect Dis 2002; 35:1390–1396.
13. Xakellis GC, Frantz R. The cost of healing pressure ulcers across multiple health
    care settings. Adv Wound Care 1996; 9:18–22.
14. Hirshberg J, Rees RS, Marchant B, Dean S. Osteomyelitis related to pressure
    ulcers: the cost of neglect. Adv Skin Wound Care 2000; 13:25–29.
15. Edwards R, Harding KG. Bacteria and wound healing. Curr Opin Infect Dis
    2004; 17:91–96.
16. Harrison-Balestra C, Cazzaniga AL, Davis SC, Mertz PM. A wound-isolated
    Pseudomonas aeruginosa grows a biofilm in vitro within 10 hours and is visua-
    lized by light microscopy. Dermatol Surg 2003; 29:631–635.

17. Darouiche RO, Dhir A, Miller AJ, Landon GC, Raad II, Musher DM. Vancomycin penetration into biofilm covering infected prostheses and effect on bacteria. J Infect Dis 1994; 170:720–723.
18. Mitsua Y, Kawai S, Kobayashi H. Influence of macrolides on guanosine diphospho-D-mannose dehydrogenase activity in *Pseudomonas* biofilm. J Infect Chemother 2000; 6:45–50.
19. Singh PK, Parsek MR, Greenberg EP, Welsh MJ. A component of innate immunity prevents bacterial biofilm development. Nature 2002; 417:552–555.
20. Parish LC, Witowski JA. The infected decubitus ulcer. Int J Dermatol 1989; 28:643–647.
21. Darouiche RO, Landon GC, Klima M, Musher DM, Markowski J. Osteomyelitis associated with pressure ulcers. Arch Intern Med 1994; 154:753–758.
22. Galpin JE, Chow AW, Bayer AS, Guze LB. Sepsis associated with decubitus ulcers. Am J Med 1976; 61:346–350.
23. McGuckin M, Goldman R, Bolton L, Salcido R. The clinical relevance of microbiology in acute and chronic wounds. Adv Skin Wound Care 2003; 16:12–23.
24. Schultz GS, Sibbald RG, Falanga V, et al. Wound bed preparation: a systematic approach to wound management. Wound Repair Regen 2003; 11(suppl 1): S1–S28.
25. Rudensky B, Lipschits M, Isaacsohn M, Sonnenblick M. Infected pressure ulcers: comparison of methods for bacterial identification. South Med J 1992; 85:901–903.
26. Ehrenkranz NJ, Alfonso B, Nerenberg D. Irrigation-aspiration for culturing draining decubitus ulcers: correlation of bacteriological findings with a clinical inflammatory scoring index. J Clin Microbiol 1990; 28:2389–2393.
27. Chow AW, Galpin JE, Guze LB. Clindamycin for treatment of sepsis caused by decubitus ulcers. J Infect Dis 1977; 735:565–568.
28. Restrepo CS, Gimenez CR, McCarthy K. Imaging of osteomyelitis and musculoskeletal soft tissue infections: current concepts. Rheum Dis Clin North Am 2003; 29:89–109.
29. Turk EE, Tsokos M, Delling G. Autopsy-based assessment of extent and type of osteomyelitis in advanced-grade sacral decubitus ulcers: a histopathologic study. Arch Pathol Lab Med 2003; 127:1599–1602.
30. Mulder GD, LaPan M. Decubitus ulcers: update on new approaches to treatment. Geriatrics 1998; 43:37–50.
31. Gupta S. Guidelines for managing pressure ulcers with negative pressure wound therapy. Adv Skin Wound Care 2004; 17(suppl 2):1–16.
32. Bergstrom N, Bennett MA, Carlson CE. Treatment of pressure ulcers. Clinical practice guideline. No.15. 1994. (AHCPR publication no.95–0652.) Rockville, MD.
33. Popovich DM, Alexander D, Rittman M, Martorella C, Jackson L. Strikethrough contamination in saturated sterile dressings: a clinical analysis. Clin Nurs Res 1995; 4:195–207.
34. Lyder CH. Pressure ulcer prevention and management. JAMA 2003; 289:223–226.
35. Lyder CH, Shannon R, Empleo-Frazier O, McGeHee D, White C. A comprehensive program to prevent pressure ulcers in long-term care: exploring costs and outcomes. Ostomy Wound Manage 2002; 48:52–62.

17

Herpes Zoster, Cellulitis, and Scabies

Kenneth E. Schmader and Jack Twersky
Center for the Study of Aging and Human Development and Division of Geriatrics, Department of Medicine, Duke University Medical Center, and Geriatric Research, Education, and Clinical Center, Durham Veterans Affairs Medical Center, Durham, North Carolina, U.S.A.

KEY POINTS

1. The main goal of the treatment of herpes zoster in the elderly is the reduction of pain. Early antiviral therapy and analgesics, employing the principles of good pain management, help to achieve this goal.
2. VZV may be transmitted to seronegative, susceptible individuals during the vesicular stage of a herpes zoster rash and cause varicella. Nursing home personnel at risk for varicella include susceptible health-care workers and staff, particularly if they are pregnant or immunocompromised. Susceptible persons should avoid contact with the resident with herpes zoster until the rash has crusted over.
3. Diagnose and treat dermatomycotic infections to prevent new cases of cellulitis.
4. Consider hospital transfer for nursing home residents who have cellulitis due to a drug-resistant organism and other morbidities that would interfere with containment of the organism in the facility, such as dementia or incontinence.

5. Scabies may present atypically in nursing home residents with red nodular, papular, or eczematous lesions that do not itch as opposed to the typical presentation of burrows and excoriations in classical locations on the body (e.g., interdigital spaces) with itching.

6. The first-line scabicide is permethrin cream (5%) applied to all areas of the body from the neck down and washed off after eight to 14 hours. Alternative regimens include lindane applied in a thin layer to all areas of the body from the neck down and thoroughly washed off after eight hours or ivermectin 200 µg/kg orally, repeated in two weeks.

HERPES ZOSTER

Epidemiology and Clinical Relevance

Herpes zoster is a neurocutaneous disease caused by the reactivation of varicella-zoster virus (VZV) from a latent infection of dorsal sensory or cranial nerve ganglia. Nearly all elderly adults in the United States are latently infected with VZV and at risk of zoster. The incidence of zoster increases strikingly with aging. For example, in Boston, investigators reported a zoster incidence of 1.9, 2.3, 3.1, 5.7, and 11.8 per 1000 person-years for the age groups 25 to 34, 35 to 44, 45 to 54, 55 to 64, and 65 to 75+ years, respectively (1). The incidence of zoster in long-term care facilities (LTCFs) is unknown because there are no investigations of zoster in this population. In the general population, the lifetime incidence of zoster is estimated to be 10% to 20% and as high as 50% of a cohort surviving up to age of 85 years. There are approximately 600,000 to 850,000 cases of zoster in the United States each year. Given an incidence of 7 to 11 cases of zoster per 1000 elderly persons per year and approximately 1.5 million elderly nursing home residents in the United States, one may estimate at least 10,500 to 16,500 zoster cases in U.S. nursing homes per year.

Residents of LTCFs are at risk for zoster not only because of aging but also because of immunosuppression from several diseases and/or medications. Patients with HIV infection, lymphomas, leukemias, systemic lupus erythematosus, and immunosuppressive medications are prone to developing zoster and may reside in LTCFs.

The most frequent and feared complication of zoster in the elderly is postherpetic neuralgia (PHN). Like zoster, the prevalence of PHN increases significantly with aging. For example, in a study in Boston (2), outpatients aged 50 years or older had a 14.7-fold higher prevalence of pain 30 days after rash onset, compared with outpatients younger than 50 years old. Most experts now define PHN as any pain 90 to 120 days after rash onset. Defined this way, the prevalence of PHN in older adults in the placebo groups in antiviral trials was about 50%, 90 days from rash onset, and 46%, 120 days from rash onset (3). The prevalence of PHN in LTCFs is unknown because there are no studies of PHN in this population.

Clinical Manifestations

The reactivation and spread of VZV in the affected sensory ganglion and peripheral sensory nerve evokes an intense cellular immune response and neuronal inflammation and destruction. These events elicit a prodrome of pain or discomfort in the affected dermatome before the rash appears. The prodrome masquerades as many other painful conditions in the elderly. The diagnosis may be particularly difficult in residents of LTCFs because of preexisting pain syndromes or cognitive impairment. Clinicians should consider zoster in the differential diagnosis of any acute, unilateral, dermatomal pain syndrome. Clues to prodromal zoster include a description of typical neuropathic pain in a dermatome and very sensitive skin in the affected dermatome. The prodrome usually lasts a few days, although there are case reports of it lasting weeks to months.

The diagnosis becomes apparent when VZV infects cells in the dermis and epidermis and produces the characteristic rash. The zoster rash may "hide" on the back, trunk, or buttocks of some LTCF residents when they are bed bound or cognitively impaired and no one bothers to examine the area. The rash is unilateral, dermatomal, red, maculopapular/vesicular, and most commonly involves the T1 to L2 and V1 dermatomes. Lesions may develop in adjacent dermatomes. Typically, the vesicles crust over in 7 to 10 days. Along with the rash, most patients experience a dermatomal pain syndrome due to acute neuritis. The neuritis is described as burning, deep aching, tingling, itching, or stabbing, and ranges from mild to severe.

Complications of zoster in the elderly include PHN; ocular inflammation with impaired vision in ophthalmic zoster; stroke secondary to granulomatous arteritis of the internal carotid artery in ophthalmic zoster; focal motor paresis in muscles served by nerve roots of the corresponding affected dermatome; disordered balance, hearing and facial paresis in cranial neuritis (Ramsay-Hunt syndrome); meningoencephalitis; and secondary bacterial infection of the rash. However, PHN is the most debilitating aspect of zoster. The PHN patient may suffer from constant pain ("burning, aching, throbbing"), intermittent pain ("stabbing, shooting"), and stimulus-evoked pain like allodynia ("tender"). Allodynia, the experience of pain after a nonpainful stimulus, is a particularly disabling component of the disease. Patients with allodynia suffer from severe pain after the lightest touch of the affected skin by things as trivial as a piece of clothing. These subtypes of pain may produce chronic fatigue, disordered sleep, depression, anorexia, and weight loss, all of which may have serious consequences in LTCF residents. Severe PHN may trigger a series of events that markedly reduce quality of life or that are ultimately fatal in the LTCF resident.

Diagnostic Approach

The clinical diagnosis of zoster is sufficient when an elderly patient presents with the typical dermatomal vesicular rash and pain. Zosteriform herpes simplex is the main consideration in the differential diagnosis, particularly in vesicular rashes on the face or buttocks. Herpes simplex commonly recurs many times and usually does not generate chronic pain. Nonetheless, it may be very difficult to distinguish the two conditions on clinical grounds. Also, like many conditions in geriatrics, zoster may present atypically. The rash may never appear as a diagnostic guide in elderly patients with dermatomal pain alone ("zoster sine herpete"); acute facial palsy, hearing loss, vertigo, and/or dysgeusia (cranial neuritis); and fever, delirium, and meningismus (meningoencephalitis).

Laboratory diagnostic testing is useful for differentiating herpes zoster from herpes simplex, for suspected organ involvement, and for atypical presentations. Immunofluorescence antigen detection of VZV antigens in vesicle fluid is an excellent test because it is rapid (hours), specific, and very sensitive. VZV culture is slower and less sensitive but remains a standard in making the virological diagnosis. Tzanck smears may suggest VZV infection if multinucleated giant cells and intranuclear inclusions are demonstrated in stained vesicle scrapings, but the technique cannot differentiate VZV from herpes simplex virus infections. VZV DNA detection using the polymerase chain reaction is very sensitive and specific and particularly useful for unusual cases or unusual specimens (i.e., only crusts available for testing).

Therapeutic Interventions

The main goal of the treatment of zoster in the elderly is the reduction of pain. Pharmacological approaches to zoster pain include antiviral therapy, anti-inflammatory drugs, and analgesics. With the exception of complicated or severe zoster, these therapies can be delivered in the LTCF.

Antiviral Therapy

Acyclovir, famciclovir, and valacyclovir are guanosine analogues that are phosphorylated by viral thymidine kinase and cellular kinases to a triphosphate form that inhibits VZV DNA polymerase. Randomized controlled trials indicate that oral acyclovir (800 mg five times a day for seven days), famciclovir (500 mg every eight hours for seven days), and valacyclovir (1 g three times a day for seven days) reduce acute pain and the duration of chronic pain in elderly zoster patients with dermatomal zoster who are treated within 72 hours of rash onset (4). It is also reasonable to treat patients with ophthalmic zoster and those forming new vesicles outside of the 72-hour window. Unfortunately, 20% to 30% of treated patients in antiviral trials had pain six months from zoster onset, indicating that treated patients can develop PHN. The most common adverse effects are nausea and/or vomiting, diarrhea, and headache in 8% to 17% of patients. The drugs are excreted via the kidney and must be dose adjusted for renal insufficiency. Any of the three drugs are acceptable agents. A suspension form of acyclovir is available for patient unable to swallow the pill form. Patients with complicated zoster should be transferred to hospital for IV acyclovir therapy. These cases include disseminated zoster, central nervous system infection, visceral infection, and severe ophthalmic zoster in any host and multidermatomal zoster in the immunocompromised host.

Anti-inflammatory Therapy

Corticosteroids, with or without acyclovir, do not prevent PHN. Antiviral therapy and prednisone may accelerate time to uninterrupted sleep and return to daily routines in elderly outpatients with no relative contraindications to corticosteroids, such as hypertension, diabetes mellitus, or osteoporosis. Most LTCF residents have relative contraindications to corticosteroids, and it is unknown as to whether this population would experience these benefits. Corticosteroids may be useful for VZV-induced facial paralysis and cranial polyneuritis to improve motor outcomes and pain. The most common adverse effects in zoster clinical trials were gastrointestinal symptoms (dyspepsia, nausea, vomiting), edema, and granulocytosis.

Analgesics

Clinicians should prescribe analgesics to reduce acute zoster pain regardless of effects on chronic zoster pain. The choice of nonopiate or opiate analgesics depends on the patient's pain severity, underlying conditions, and response to the drug. The principles of excellent pain management, such as scheduled analgesia, use of pain measurements, and close follow-up, should be applied to acute zoster pain management as with any other painful condition. If pain control from antiviral agents and analgesics is inadequate, then regional or local anesthetic nerve blocks should be considered.

Postherpetic Neuralgia

Patients and clinicians have employed a large number of treatments for PHN, but few of these treatments have been carefully evaluated. Recent controlled clinical trials indicate that the topical lidocaine patch 5%, gabapentin, pregabalin, opiates, and tricyclic antidepressants can significantly reduce pain in PHN patients (5). These treatments are considered the first-line agents for the treatment of PHN, but none of these treatments has been evaluated in LTCF residents. Except for the topical lidocaine patch 5%, the starting dose of the above drugs will probably need to be lower and the titration schedule slower than standard recommendations to avoid serious adverse effects in LTCF residents.

Infection Control Measures

VZV may be transmitted to seronegative, susceptible individuals during the vesicular stage of a zoster rash and cause varicella. Most adults and nearly all elderly LTCF residents are latently infected and not at risk for varicella including latently infected immunocompromised patients. Furthermore, there are no controlled studies indicating that exposure of a latently infected individual to zoster causes zoster or varicella. The persons at risk for varicella include susceptible health-care workers and staff, particularly if they are pregnant or immunocompromised.

Direct contact, airborne or droplet nuclei routes may transmit VZV. VZV spreads most efficiently with close contact. The incubation period of varicella is usually between 14 and 16 days with a range of 8–21 days. Although there are no studies of VZV transmission in LTCFs, several studies show that susceptible health-care workers and staff may develop varicella after exposure to zoster in hospital patients. If a susceptible person does develop varicella, they too may transmit the virus to susceptible individuals during the vesicular phase of their rash.

To manage patients with zoster in LTCFs, susceptible persons should avoid contact with the zoster patient until the rash has crusted over. The optimal method to protect susceptible staff in LTCFs is not known. In hospital, the Centers for Disease Control and Prevention (CDC) recommends a private room and contact precautions for immunocompetent hospital patients with dermatomal zoster (6). For immunocompromised patients in hospital with localized zoster or any patient with disseminated zoster, the recommendations are a private room with special ventilation and airborne and contact precautions. These recommendations have to be modified for the more limited resources of LTCFs. Feasible measures include moving the patient to a private room and the use of contact precautions for all zoster patients.

LTCF staff and employees who are exposed to a resident with zoster should have an evaluation of their VZV immune status within one to two days of exposure. An exposure is defined as being in the same room or having face-to-face contact with the zoster patient. Employees with a history of varicella or zoster are considered immune and can return to work. Employees who do not have a prior history of varicella, or who are unsure of their varicella status, should have VZV antibody testing. If the antibody test is positive, they are immune and can return to work. If the are antibody is negative, they may develop varicella in the next 10 to 21 days. These individuals may be candidates for varicella-zoster immune globulin (VZIG). VZIG is recommended for exposed, susceptible individuals who are able to receive VZIG within 72 to 96 hours of exposure and are at risk of significant morbidity from varicella. Adults who are at increased risk and who should receive VZIG include immunocompromised individuals, individuals taking systemic corticosteroids, and pregnant women. The benefit of VZIG for immunocompetent adults is less clear because it may not prevent varicella, but it is generally recommended for any susceptible adult. Alternately, the CDC recommends the varicella vaccine as postexposure prevention, if given within 72 hours of exposure (7). Once exposed, susceptible health-care workers may be infectious in an 8 to 21 days' window post exposure. They probably should not work during this time period. If they develop varicella, they may benefit from acyclovir, particularly if given with within 24 hours of rash onset.

    VZV immunity among health-care workers varies by country of origin. In general, serology studies indicate that less than 10% of persons in temperate climates above 20 years old are susceptible. The percentages are higher in persons who immigrated from countries with tropical climates. Health-care workers in LTCFs should be screened for VZV immunity at the time of their employment by the methods noted above. If the worker reports a history of varicella, the likelihood is very high that the worker is seropositive and, therefore, immune. If the workers report no history of varicella or are unsure and their VZV antibody test is negative, they should receive the varicella vaccine.

Prevention

A recent large ($n = 38,546$) randomized, double-blind, placebo-controlled trial of a high-dose live attenuated VZV vaccine (zoster vaccine) showed that the vaccine markedly reduced morbidity from herpes zoster and PHN among community-dwelling adults ≥ 60 years old (8). A total of 957 confirmed cases of herpes zoster (315 among vaccine recipients and 642 among placebo recipients) and 107 cases of PHN (27 among vaccine recipients and 80 among placebo recipients) were included in the analysis. The zoster vaccine reduced the burden of illness due to herpes zoster by 61.1%, the incidence of PHN by 66.5%, and the incidence of herpes zoster by 51.3%. Reactions at the injection site were more frequent among vaccine recipients but were generally mild. The zoster vaccine probably boosted cell-mediated immunity to VZV, which progressively declines with aging. How these exciting results will extrapolate to LTCF residents is not clear because most study participants were living independently in the community and had no or minimal limitations on their health. The efficacy and safety of the zoster vaccine in frail older adults are not known.

    The varicella vaccine was licensed by the Food and Drug Administration in the United States in 1995 to prevent varicella and is now part of the childhood immunization schedule. It is about 85% to 90% effective in preventing varicella in susceptible children and 75% effective in susceptible adults (7). Zoster can develop in vaccinees but at a much lower rate than zoster after natural varicella. Whether widespread vaccination of children with the vaccine will significantly reduce zoster incidence in the elderly will not be known until the cohorts of vaccinated children become elderly. However, the vaccine virus is highly attenuated and probably less likely to reactivate and cause complications.

CELLULITIS

Epidemiology and Clinical Relevance

Skin and soft tissue infections are the third most common infections in nursing home residents. Cellulitis is defined as a diffuse inflammation of the epidermis, dermis, subcutaneous fat, and/or connective tissue in which a thin watery exudates spreads through the cleavage planes of the interstitial space. Cellulitis is often accompanied by lymphangiitis and lymphadenitis. Surprisingly, there are few high-quality investigations of cellulitis in the nursing home. This chapter will organize data from many sources and make inferences about the impact of cellulitis to nursing home residents.

Skin infections and mortality as a result of skin infections occur at higher rates among elderly patients than among younger patients. The frequency of skin infection appears to be particularly high among nursing home residents who experience skin infections at rates similar to the rates experienced among hospitalized patients. The prevalence of skin and/or soft tissue infections in the nursing home has been reported to be between 1% and 9%, and the incidence is 0.9 to 2.1 per 1000 patient-days (9).

Cellulitis does not usually occur in intact skin. Bacteria are unable to penetrate the keratinized layers of normal skin. The skin's low pH (5.5), the presence of natural antibacterial substances in the sebaceous glands, and circulating immunoglobins all resist local bacterial invasion. Risk factors for cellulitis may be divided into two sets: predisposing factors and portals of entry. A number of conditions have been described as predisposing to the development of cellulitis. In a multivariate analysis, lymphedema, venous insufficiency, leg edema, and being overweight were independently associated with cellulitis. In this study, no association was observed for diabetes mellitus, alcohol, or smoking, all of which were considered risk factors in the past (10). All the positive risk factors noted above cause a disruption in lymphatic flow. Disruption of the local lymphatic drainage system related to saphenous vein harvesting during coronary artery bypass surgery and after hip replacement is a well-described risk factor predisposing to cellulitis and common comorbid conditions among nursing home residents (11). A previous episode of cellulitis, breast cancer with axillary node dissection, cancer of the cervix, uterus, nasopharynx, radical pelvic surgery, lymphedema, nephrotic syndrome, and right-sided congestive heart failure all cause disruption of lymphatic flow and increase the risk of developing cellulitis. Though not described in the literature, patients who have lower extremity amputations commonly develop cellulitis probably due to peripheral vascular disease compounded by disruption of the lymphatic system as a result of the amputation.

A portal of entry is generally recognized in 60% to 100% of cases. The portal may be a surgical site, laceration, wound, pressure ulcer, insect bite, or nonsterile needle (10). Fissured toe webs and intertrigo are particularly important risks for cellulitis in the elderly. Tinea pedis commonly occurs in nursing home residents and predisposes to the development of cellulitis. In one study dermatomycosis was a significant risk factor for cellulitis, as were tinia pedis interdigitalis and tinea pedis plantaris (12). In a study of cellulitis related to saphenous vein harvesting sites, 25 of 31 patients who developed cellulitis had mycologically confirmed tinea pedis in their intertriginous space(s) (11). Another study of elderly patients who developed cellulitis found that 83% had tinea pedis as a predisposing factor (13). Finally, another important portal of entry involves feeding tubes. Superficial infections at the skin entry point to the gastrointestinal tract are reported to occur at a rate of 1% to 4% within 30 days of placement of the gastrostomy tube and 1% to 2% yearly thereafter.

The most likely organism causing cellulitis depends to some extent on the characteristics of the nursing home. Group A hemolytic *Streptococcus* is the most common causative organism. Less commonly *Staphylococcus aureus*, gram-negative bacilli, *Legionella* sp., *Streptococcus pneumoniae*, and *Cryptoccocus* have been reported as a cause of cellulitis. Many nursing homes have residents who are colonized with methicillin-resistant *S. aureus* (MRSA). MRSA is an important pathogen causing cellulitis in these nursing homes. Mucormycosis has been found as the primary organism causing cellulitis patients with diabetes and renal transplant recipients.

Clinical Manifestations

Skin infection runs the gamut from erysipelas to cellulitis to necrotizing fasciitis. These conditions are more common in older adults than younger adults and share common risk factors. They are defined by their level of tissue penetration. Erysipelas is the most superficial infection. It is defined by inflammation of the epidermis and dermis as well as adjacent lymphatics. Erysipelas differs from cellulitis in that lymphatic involvement is prominent (streaking) and that it tends to have margins that are clearly demarcated from uninvolved skin. The initial presentation is a small erythematous lesion, 80% of time in the lower extremity, which is easily overlooked. Facial erysipelas may follow an upper respiratory tract infection. Fever is present in about a fifth of cases and is abrupt in onset, associated with rigors and sometimes with nausea and vomiting. The clinical course is almost always benign. Local complications, such as septic arthritis, skin necrosis, or necrotizing fasciitis, are rare, but recurrence is common.

Necrotizing fasciitis is a deep-seated, life-threatening infection of the subcutaneous tissue that results in progressive destruction of the fascia and fat but may spare the skin. Untreated or unapparent trauma is frequently the initiating event. After 24 hours there may be mild erythema. The infection spreads rapidly. The erythema darkens, changing from red to purple then to blue, and blisters and bullae form that contain clear yellow fluid. By the fourth day there is gangrene. Infection may disseminate in the form of metastatic abscesses and pneumonia.

Cellulitis is a diffuse inflammation of the soft or connective tissue due to infection in which a thin watery exudate spreads through the cleavage planes of interstitial and tissue spaces. Cellulitis is characterized by fever, chills, malaise, and locally ill-defined erythema. The lesion may be brawny, edematous, or indurated (peu d'orange), particularly in the setting of venous insufficiency or chronic lymphatic obstruction, with an advancing elevated margin. The skin is almost always hot, shiny, bright red, and frequently painful to touch. In severe disease associated with less typical organisms, small vesicles and occasionally large bullae may develop. Because predisposing conditions predominate in the lower extremities, e.g., venous insufficiency, peripheral vascular disease, lymphatic obstruction, etc., most cases of cellulitis occur below the waist. Cellulitis has been associated with saphenous vein donor sites for coronary artery bypass grafts and within the flaps of the surgical incision after primary hip replacement. In both circumstances, the cellulitis and erythema may extend along the incision. Among a collection of 31 patients who developed cellulitis after saphenous vein harvesting, all the cases of cellulitis originated at the scar and spread both proximally and circumferentially (11). Symptoms occur generally months after the index surgeries.

As discussed above, the most likely organisms causing cellulitis are group A hemolytic *Streptococcus*, *S. aureus*, gram-negative bacilli, *Legionella* sp., and *Cryptoccocus*. Cellulitis caused by *S. pneumoniae* is particularly virulent. It may be the primary infection or present after a case of pneumonia or otitis media. The cellulitis presents as brawny edema, a violaceous hue, and is more likely to have bullae. Blood stream infections, tissue necrosis, and supporative complications are more likely and surgical intervention is often necessary. Overall mortality can be up to17% in complicated infections.

Diagnostic Approach

The diagnosis of cellulitis in the nursing home is by necessity a clinical diagnosis based on the symptoms and signs described above. Most nursing homes do not have readily available laboratory and imaging resources for complex evaluations. Deep venous thrombosis is the main consideration in the differential diagnosis and should be ruled out when symptoms and signs suggest it. Differentiating cellulitis from deep vein thrombosis can be challenging, which is complicated by the fact that cellulitis and deep venous thrombosis may occur concurrently. Early cases of herpes zoster, osteomyelitis associated with an open wound, necrotizing fasciitis, chronic venous stasis, and eczema may mimic cellulitis.

Because a consideration of the differential diagnosis is critical, a physician, nurse practitioner, or physician assistant needs to see the cellulitis. It is not satisfactory to rely upon a licensed nurse's assessment. Typically a red, hot, and tender area with mild systemic signs, including absent or low-grade fever, is sufficient for initiating therapy for cellulitis. Erysipelas may have a similar presentation and the treatment and risks are similar. Skin and soft tissue cultures are not recommended in typical cases because of low yield (10–25%) and lack of feasibility, because they are not usually available to nursing home providers (14). Skin and soft tissue cultures via fine-needle aspirates may be useful if there is a fluctuant area suggesting an abscess, unusual pathogens are suspected (i.e., immunocompromised host), or initial antimicrobial therapy has been unsuccessful (14). Blood cultures may be positive in about 5% of cases, but the organism is as likely to be a contaminant as it is causative. There are some nursing homes that are attached to hospitals and may have microbiology resources available. In these cases, checking cultures of macerated tissue in the toe webs may be helpful in identifying organisms or more likely ruling out group A *Streptococcus*. When group A *Streptococcus* is not recovered from the toe web space, it is usually not the offending organism (13).

More virulent forms of cellulitis should be treated in the acute care setting. Vesicles, bullae, and high-grade fever would all be indications for transfer to the hospital. In these cases, cultures of the vesicles, bullae, and blood are more likely to yield the pathogen. In cases where necrotizing fasciitis is in the differential diagnosis, a serum test for creatine phosphokinase, magnetic resonance imaging of the lesion, and surgical consultation are indicated.

Therapeutic Interventions

Erysipelas and cellulitis without systemic signs can be treated by an oral first-generation cephalosporin (i.e., cephalexin 500 mg q6h). Clindamycin (150–300 mg q8h), dicloxacillin (250 mg q6h), or amoxicillin (500 mg)–clavulinic acid (one tablet q8h) are reasonable alternatives. The cellulitis associated with gastrostomy tubes is typically mild and may also be treated in this manner.

When cellulitis presents with fever and systemic signs, IV therapy is indicated. Cefazolin (1.0 g IV q8h) or nafcillin (2.0 g IV q4h) are reasonable empirical choices. Cellulitis complicating saphenous vein harvests or hip prosthesis has the same prognosis and should be managed in the same manner as other presentations for cellulitis. When the organism is identified, it is important to individualize the therapy to the inhibitory quotient (IQ), i.e., the ratio of achievable antibiotic concentration to the minimum inhibitory concentration. In one study an IQ greater than 6 was strongly associated with better outcomes in severe bacterial infections (15). Because cellulitis is frequently very challenging to eradicate, using the IQ when possible increases the probability of effectively treating the infection. Treatment with clindamycin and a macrolide theoretically could improve outcomes because of immunomodulary activity of these antibiotics. It has been shown in animal models that these antibiotics inhibit protein synthesis and suppress production of bacterial toxin and penicillin binding proteins. Vancomycin is appropriate for MRSA or suspected MRSA infections.

The experience for treating severe cellulitis is hospital based. There are no studies that investigate outcomes in a long-term care setting or in using oral antibiotic therapy. My experience is that most cellulitis can be managed in the nursing home, but that is with the understanding that the nursing home has the capability of administering IV therapy if necessary, that a physician/physician assistant/nurse practitioner is available to carefully assess the patient's response to treatment, and that licensed nurses are available 24 hours a day and seven days a week to monitor the patient.

Local care of cellulitis includes immobilization, elevation of the extremity, and cool sterile saline dressings to reduce pain. Though application of moist heat is recommended when there are areas of fluctuation suggesting early abscess formation (10), hospitalization for any such complication is recommended. In a retrospective study of 101 cases of cellulitis treated in a hospital, 85 cases treated were well within 10 days of treatment (16).

Infection Control Measures

Outbreaks of cellulitis have been described among nursing home residents with group A *Streptococcus* infections. Transmission was via direct contact between staff and/or other residents. When an outbreak of a bacterial infection due to a specific organism does occur, identification and treatment of carriers are an effective intervention to reducing additional infections (17). The CDC recommends standard precautions for the management of routine skin infections, such as cellulitis. This standard consists of hand washing using a plain nonantimicrobial soap before and after examining the patient with cellulitis. Antimicrobial soaps or a waterless agent are indicated for control of outbreaks or hyperendemic infections. Gloves should be worn when touching skin that is not intact. Hands should be washed before patient contact and after glove removal. Environmental control includes cleaning and disinfecting bed rails, bedside equipment, and other frequently touched surfaces. Environmental interventions may be particularly problematic in a nursing home because of the many personal possessions that frequently clutter the patient's personal space and poor compliance of patients with any regulations due to impaired cognitive function. This is another reason why more complex cases, particularly with open wounds, may be best managed in a hospital setting. Contact isolation is indicated for open bullae with drainage and when treating a resistant organism. Most of these special circumstances are probably more appropriately managed in an acute care facility. If complex patients are managed in the nursing home, they should be placed in a private room or they should share rooms with patients who are infected with the same organism. A gown should be worn if it is anticipated that clothing will have substantial contact with the patient. More aggressive attempts to control infection, such as isolation or limitation of activity, are not justified unless there is evidence that a given resident is a risk to others and barriers will decrease the risk.

The most important infection control measure is good hand washing. It has been well documented that nursing staff and physicians are not compliant with proper hand washing protocols. This is an important problem in nursing homes as well. A study that investigated hand washing in an LTCF found that gloves were worn in 82% of indicated encounters, but they were changed when indicated only 16% of the time. Hands were washed before encounters in 27% of episodes, 0% percent during encounters, and 63% after encounters. The level of training in the staff had no influence on compliance with proper infection control. Physicians, registered nurses, licensed practical nurses, and nurses aides were all equally unlikely to follow proper protocols. To improve hand hygiene among staff, waterless, alcohol-based hand sanitizers and glove boxes should be placed throughout the resident care areas. A problem that is rarely mentioned as a likely hindrance to following appropriate procedures is the damage done to nurses' hands due to the frequent washing. A study that evaluated nurses' hands found that one-quarter had skin damage at the time of the study and 86% had skin damage at some point in time. The damaged hands are more likely to be a reservoir for pathogenic organisms as well as discourage proper hand washing. The alcohol-based, waterless antiseptic agents may decrease the damage to hands and are less time consuming to administer. Together these factors may increase compliance with hand washing.

Prevention

Between 20% and 50% of patients who develop cellulitis have recurrence of the cellulitis (18). Impaired circulation in the arterial, venous, or lymphatic systems and a portal of entry are necessary conditions for the development of cellulitis. Preventive interventions should address these risk factors and specifically target nursing home residents who have had previous episodes of cellulitis. Although there are no studies that address the circulatory risk factors, venous stasis is generally undertreated and compression dressings are an effective nonpharmacologic management strategy.

An important strategy to address portal of entry is the evaluation and management of tinea pedis. Treatment of tinea pedis reduces recurrence of cellulitis. Management strategies include topical antifungal agents, as well as local skin care consisting of warm saline soaks (except in diabetic patients), proper foot hygiene, and avoidance of trauma. Acute infection may be treated with a short course of an oral antifungal agent (griseofulvin, terbinafine, fluconazole, ketoconazole, itraconazole). Macerated web spaces and hyperhydrosis are treated with drying agents, lambs wool, and cotton balls. Chronic tinea infections are treated with antifungal foot powder and disinfectant spray (Lysol®) to shoes once a week (10).

One may consider prophylactic antibiotic therapy in residents who do not comply with preventive measures, but there is no evidence that this strategy is effective in the nursing home. For example, intramuscularly administered injections of benzathine penicillin had no effect on episodes of recurrent cellulitis among subjects with predisposing factors (venous stasis, obesity, leg edema, fracture, diabetes, surgery, lymphedema).

SCABIES

Epidemiology and Clinical Relevance

Scabies is a cutaneous ectoparasitic infestation caused by the mite, *Sarcoptes scabiei* (19). Itching, excoriation, and secondary bacterial infections are the main clinical problems. The clinical manifestations are caused by the adult female mite, which measures about 1/16 inch in length. The body is round without a distinct head, but there are mouth parts at one end of the body and four pairs of legs. Most of the body consists of ovaries and developing eggs. The female mite will copulate with a male mite on the skin, dig through the stratum corneum to the boundary of the stratum granulosum, and create a burrow. The female mite continues to tunnel in the burrow for its life span of about 30 days, increasing its length a few millimeters per day. During this time, it lays a few eggs per day in the burrow. The eggs hatch into larvae. Over a 10- to 14-day period, the larvae move to the skin surface, molt into adults, and begin the reproduction process again.

Scabies is endemic in the most parts of the world. The mite is able to survive outside the human host for a limited time. Live mites can be recovered from the bed, furniture, and floors of nursing homes with recent scabies infestations, but fomites do not appear to be important in the transmission of scabies. Instead, it thrives on humans and requires human infestation to propagate itself. The likelihood of spread is increased with increasing amount and duration of physical contact. Overcrowding, poor hygiene, and institutional settings are associated with epidemics.

Accurate data on the incidence and prevalence of scabies in nursing homes are not available, but the epidemic spread of scabies is well documented in LTCFs. Typically, the mite is introduced into the home by a visitor or newly admitted patient. The infected patient may have an atypical presentation or may be misdiagnosed, so the infection is present for weeks or months. Contact with staff, visitors, and other patients spreads the infection within and outside the home. For example, researchers reported a nursing home outbreak in Norway where the index case had pruritis and rash for several months and was misdiagnosed as eczema (20). The infection spread to 13 patients and six health-care workers before diagnosis and treatment. In another nursing home epidemic, most patients had truncal erythematous papulosquamous lesions and only one patient had an identifiable burrow (21). Only one third of patients had pruritis and two thirds were treated with topical corticosteroids before the correct diagnosis was made.

Clinical Manifestations

The cardinal symptom of scabies is itching. The itching is often nocturnal and varies in severity from mild to severe. Individuals may be infested for weeks or months before itching is noted. On the physical examination, the cardinal sign is the burrow. The burrow appears as a raised, linear tunnel of skin that varies in length from a few mm up to 1 cm. There may be associated erythema, eczematous changes, and excoriations. In immunocompetent patients, the burrows are characteristically distributed in the hands and wrists, especially in the interdigital spaces of the fingers, the palms, the flexor surface of the wrist; the posterior and medial aspects of the elbow; the feet; the anterior axilla; the waist; the buttocks; the penis and scrotum; and the nipple area in women.

The typical itching, appearance, and distribution of lesions in scabies may not be present in nursing home residents (19), who often have coexisting diseases, treatments, and deficient cellular immune responses that mask scabies. The itching and burrows may be minimal or absent. The cutaneous manifestations may be eczema-like lesions, plaques, nodules, or papules. The face and scalp can be infested. In bed-bound residents, the lesions may be found only on the back or sides on skin in contact with bedsheets. A crusted form of scabies ("Norwegian scabies") has been described in nursing home residents. It appears as a marked crusting dermatitis in the hands and feet with thick hyperkeratotic debris. Red scaling plaques on the trunk, neck, and scalp may also develop. This form of scabies is important because the parasite burden is very high and patients are highly contagious. Crusted scabies has also been described in immunosuppressed residents, including those with leukemia and acquired immunodeficiency syndrome.

Left untreated, scabies persists indefinitely and causes several complications. The lesions may become extensive in the setting of poor hygiene. With repeated excoriations, patients experience an eczematous neurodermatitis. Secondary bacterial infection may follow as manifested by impetigo, folliculitis, and cellulitis. If mistreated with topical corticosteroids, the itching and cutaneous signs may be masked for long periods of time. The suppression of symptoms and delay in treatment may result in extensive infestation.

Diagnostic Approach

The differential diagnosis includes any pruritic dermatosis, such as various forms of eczema, atopic dermatitis, contact dermatitis, insect bites, urticaria, vasculitis, and dermatitis herpetiformis. The diagnosis is straightforward when the patient has (1) typical itching, (2) visible burrows in characteristic distributions, (3) a mite demonstrated in the burrow, and (4) resolution of the disease following topical scabicides. The mite can be demonstrated by skin scrapings of burrows. Mineral or microscope immersion oil is placed on a #15 scalpel blade and allowed to flow on the lesions. The lesion is scraped very superficially with the blade in the epidermal layer only, taking care to avoid bleeding. The skin scrapings and oil are transferred to a slide; a cover slip is placed and the specimen is examined under low power for adult mites, larvae, nymphs, eggs, egg casings, or fecal pellets. One may also demonstrate the mite by raising the closed end of the burrow with a needle and looking for the mite with a hand lens, either on the tip of the needle or in the unroofed burrow. Other techniques include epidermal shave biopsies, dermal curettage, videodermatoscopy, a skin swab with adhesive tape, and punch biopsy. Even in highly suspected cases of scabies, it may be surprisingly difficult to find the organism, particularly in excoriated or inflamed areas of skin. To reduce the false-negative rate of these tests, some authorities recommend several slides from nonexcoriated, noninflamed, sites of typical distribution.

The diagnosis is even more difficult in atypical cases in nursing home residents. Nursing home residents may have little or no symptoms of infestation. Itching may be the first clue, but the itching may be ascribed to dry skin or anxiety in nursing home residents. In nursing home residents with unexplained itching, clinicians should perform a careful skin survey for burrows in typical and atypical locations. The lesions may be very sparse in nursing home residents who are bathed regularly. Although bathing will not cure the infestation, it will reduce the number of visible lesions. Lesions other than burrows may be the clue to scabies. These eruptions include persistent reddish pruritic nodules, papular lesions, eczematous lesions, and bullous lesions. The diagnosis should be considered in unexplained, pruritic dermatoses.

Therapeutic Interventions

Scabies can be completely eradicated by prescribing scabicides (22). The recommended regimen by the CDC is permethrin cream (5%) applied to all areas of the body from the neck down and washed off after 8 to 14 hours (23). Permethrin is effective, safe, and well tolerated, but treatment failures can occur in nursing home residents and it is more expensive than lindane. Resistance has not been a problem with permethrin.

Alternative regimens include lindane [gamma benzene hexachloride (1%)] 1 oz of lotion or 30 g of cream applied in a thin layer to all areas of the body from the neck down and thoroughly washed off after eight hours or ivermectin 200 µg/kg orally, repeated in two weeks. Lindane treatment failures and resistance have been reported in the United States. Seizures have been reported in individuals who used lindane after a hot bath or on skin with extensive dermatitis. Ivermectin is an effective, safe, inexpensive, convenient, oral pill for scabies. In the United States, it has not yet been approved for human use by the Food and Drug Administration. In one trial in outpatients, nursing home, and hospitalized patients in Argentina, patients received either a single oral dose of ivermectin (150–200 μg/kg body weight) or topical application of 1% lindane. Treatment was repeated after 15 days if clinical cure had not occurred. At day 15, 14/19 (74%) of group treated with ivermectin were cured compared with 13/24 (54%) of lindane-treated patients. At day 29, 18/19 (95%) of ivermectin patients were cured compared with 23/24 (96%) of lindane-treated patients. Adverse effects were mild, few, and transient (24). Although well tolerated, investigators have not shown that ivermectin is superior to topical treatment. However, it can be useful for scabies outbreaks in nursing homes. In a large group of nursing home patients, topical scabicides may be difficult to apply properly or may be poorly tolerated because of burning or other skin reactions. For crusted (Norwegian) scabies, a single application of permethrin or one dose of ivermectin runs a substantial risk of treatment failure. The CDC notes that combined treatment with a topical scabicide and oral ivermectin or repeated treatments with ivermectin are recommended.

Itching often persists after therapy. If itching persists over one to two weeks, a diagnostic examination should be done again. The differential diagnosis includes hypersensitivity to scabies, cutaneous irritation, contact dermatitis to the scabicide, a recurrence of scabies, an unrelated skin disease, or delusions of parasitosis. Hypersensitivity and contact dermatitis can be treated with topical corticosteroids, provided one is sure that the itching does not represent scabies. Some experts recommend a scabicide retreatment for patients who are symptomatic whether or not live mites are demonstrated, whereas other experts recommend treatment only if live mites are observed. Recurrent scabies requires head-to-toe application of a scabicide or a dose of ivermectin with treatment of all contacts as before. Several relapses raise the issue of resistance, which can be addressed by using a different scabicide.

Infection Control Measures

The CDC recommends contact precautions for patients with scabies. These precautions include gloves upon entering the room, removal of gloves before leaving the room, and washing hands immediately with an antimicrobial agent. A gown is recommended if clothing could have contact with the infested patient. Ideally, the patient should be placed in a private room or cohorted with another patient with scabies. Whether scabies in a nursing home requires a private room is controversial. Skin-to-skin contact should be avoided until after scabicide treatment. The duration of the precautions is 24 hours after the initiation of treatment. Patient transport should be limited during this time.

All staff, relatives, and other patients with prolonged skin to skin contact with the patient should be identified and treated prophylactically with a scabicide whether or not they have symptoms. In addition, close household contacts of employees undergoing treatment should be offered prophylactic treatment. Staff can return to work the day after completing treatment. Staff should remove and decontaminate bedding and clothing by machine washing at 60°C.

Fumigation of Living Areas Is Unnecessary

If clinicians suspect an outbreak of several cases in the institution, it is important to have parasitological diagnostic confirmation, because a full-scale infection control program is costly in time and personnel. When an outbreak is confirmed, the infection control team in the facility should be assembled to manage the epidemic. The entire population at risk—patients, staff, visitors—should be treated. Some time may have passed before the scabies was diagnosed, so many people may have been exposed. Recurrent epidemics of scabies have been reported in nursing homes when all patients were not treated during an outbreak. Furthermore, some exposed staff or patients may have gone to other institutions and need to be treated. It is useful to have an in-service training seminar where everyone is educated about scabies and understands the rational for measures in control program. Staff commonly lacks knowledge about parasite transmission, diagnosis, and clinical manifestations, as well as the methods for confirming the existence of an outbreak.

Prevention

Residents and staff would prefer to prevent an outbreak rather than spend the time and energy on controlling one. Several practices aid prevention. Staff should be educated about scabies and be aware that any nursing home is at risk for infestation. New patients should be screened for scabies in their admission history and physical exam. New employees should be queried for new rashes or pruritis. Any suspect infestations should be evaluated. Clinicians and staff need to have a high index of suspicion for scabies in any case of undiagnosed itching or rash and make an accurate early diagnosis. The index case in many nursing home outbreaks had longstanding scabies that was misdiagnosed. Clinicians need to think about the possibility of scabies and develop competency in skin scraping procedures. In unclear or difficult cases, consultation with dermatology subspecialists is useful. Once a case is identified, employ patient care procedures to end skin-to-skin contact. These procedures include standard precautions with protective gloves and clothing and hand washing. Although simple, many of these steps are difficult to implement in the nursing home because the incidence of scabies is low and the staff and clinicians are occupied with more prevalent problems.

ACKNOWLEDGMENT

This work was supported by the Durham VAMC GRECC and by the Duke Claude D. Pepper Older Americans Independence Center and the National Institute of Allergy and Infectious Diseases (K24-AI-51324–01).

SUGGESTED READING

Bentley DW, Bradley S, High K, Schoebaum S, Taler G, Yoshikawa TT. Practice guideline for evaluation of fever and infection in long-term care facilities. Clin Infect Dis 2000; 31:640–653.

Centers for Disease Control and Prevention. Sexually transmitted diseases treatment guidelines, 2002. Morb Mortal Wkly Rep 2002; 51(RR-6):67–69.

Dubinsky RH, Kabbani H, El-Chami Z, Boutwell C, Ali H. Practice parameter: treatment of postherpetic neuralgia. Neurology 2004; 63:959–965.

Gnann JW Jr., Whitley RJ. Herpes zoster. N Engl J Med 2002; 347:340–346.

Wendel K, Rompalo A. Scabies and pediculosis pubis: an update of treatment regimens and general review. Clin Infect Dis 2002; 35:S146–S151.

REFERENCES

1. Donahue JG, Choo PW, Manson JE, Platt R. The incidence of herpes zoster. Arch Intern Med 1995; 155:1605–1609.
2. Choo PW, Galil K, Donahue JG, Walker AM, Spiegelman D, Platt R. Risk factors for postherpetic neuralgia. Arch Intern Med 1997; 157:1217–1224.
3. Dworkin RH, Schmader KE. The epidemiology and natural history of herpes zoster and postherpetic neuralgia. In: Watson CPN, ed. Herpes Zoster and Postherpetic Neuralgia. Amsterdam: Elsevier, 2001:39–65.
4. Gnann JW Jr., Whitley RJ. Herpes zoster. N Engl J Med 2002; 347:340–346.
5. Dubinsky RH, Kabbani H, El-Chami Z, Boutwell C, Ali H. Practice parameter: treatment of postherpetic neuralgia. Neurology 2004; 63:959–965.
6. Garner JS. Guideline for isolation precautions in hospitals. The Hospital Infection Control Advisory Committee. Infect Control Hosp Epidemiol 1996; 17:53–80.
7. Centers for Disease Control and Prevention. Morb Mort Wkly Rep 1999; 48:RR-6.
8. Oxman MN, Levin MJ, Johnson GR, et al. For the Shingles Prevention Study Group. A vaccine to prevent herpes zoster and postherpetic neuralgia in older adults. N Engl J Med 2005; 352:2271–2284.
9. Nicolle LE. Infection control in long-term care facilities. Clin Infect Dis 2000; 31:752–756.
10. Dupuy A, Benchikhi H, Roujeau JC, et al. Risk factors for erysipelas of the leg (cellulitis): case-control study. BMJ 1999; 318:1591–1594.

11. Karakas M, Baba M, Alsungur VL, et al. Manifestation of cellulitis after saphenous venectomy for coronary bypass surgery. JEADV 2002; 16:438–440.
12. Roujeau JC, Sigurgeirsson B, Korting HC, Kerl H, Paul C. Chronic dermatomycoses of the foot as a risk factor for acute bacterial cellulitis. Dermatology 2004; 209:301–307.
13. Semel JD, Goldin H. Association of athlete's foot with cellulitis of the lower extremities: diagnostic value of bacterial cultures of ipsilateral interdigital space samples. Clin Infect Dis 1996; 23:1162–1164.
14. Bentley DW, Bradley S, High K, Schoebaum S, Taler G, Yoshikawa TT. Practice guideline for evaluation of fever and infection in long-term care facilities. Clin Infect Dis 2000; 31:640–653.
15. Spanu T, Santangelo R, Andreotti F, Cascio GL, Velardi G, Fadda G. Antibiotic therapy for severe bacterial infections: correlation between the inhibitory quotient and outcome. Int J Antimicrob Agents 2004; 23:120–128.
16. Ginsberg MB. Cellulitis: analysis of 101 cases and review of the literature. South Med J 1981; 74:530–533.
17. Greene CM, Van Beneden CA, Javadi M, et al. Cluster of deaths from group A *Streptococcus* in a long-term care facility—Georgia, 2001. Am J Infect Control 2005; 33:108–113.
18. Baddour LM. Cellulitis syndromes: an update. Int J Antimicrob Agents 2000; 14:113–116.
19. Chosidow O. Scabies and pediculosis. Lancet 2000; 355:819–827.
20. Andersen BM, Haugen H, Rasch M, Heldal Haugen A, Tageson A. Outbreak of scabies in Norwegian nursing homes and home care patients: control and prevention. J Hosp Infect 2000; 45:160–164.
21. Wilson MM, Philpott CD, Breer WA. Atypical presentation of scabies among nursing home residents. J Gerontol A Med Sci 2001; 56:M424–M427.
22. Wendel K, Rompalo A. Scabies and pediculosis pubis: an update of treatment regimens and general review. Clin Infect Dis 2002; 35:S146–S151.
23. Centers for Disease Control and Prevention. Sexually transmitted diseases treatment guidelines, 2002. Morb Mortal Wkly Rep 2002; 51(RR-6):67–69.
24. Chouela EN, Abeldano AM, Pellerano G, et al. Equivalent therapeutic efficacy and safety of ivermectin and lindane in the treatment of human scabies. Arch Dermatol 1999; 135:651–655.

18

Infectious Diarrhea

Abbasi J. Akhtar

Divisions of Gastroenterology and Infectious Disease, Department of Internal Medicine, Charles R. Drew University of Medicine and Science, and Martin Luther King, Jr.–Charles R. Drew Medical Center, Los Angeles, California, U.S.A.

Made Sutjita

Division of Infectious Disease, Department of Internal Medicine, Charles R. Drew University of Medicine and Science, and Martin Luther King, Jr.–Charles R. Drew Medical Center, Los Angeles, California, U.S.A.

KEY POINTS

1. Acute infectious diarrhea in the elderly LTCF residents is an important but underappreciated cause of significant morbidity and mortality.
2. Viral infection is the most common cause of infectious diarrhea in LTCF residents. *C. difficile*, *E. coli*, and *Salmonella* spp. are common bacterial causes.
3. Medications, feeding formulas, and various foods or drinks may cause diarrhea in LTCF residents.
4. Prompt diagnosis and definitive treatment along with adequate rehydration with glucose/electrolyte solutions are crucial.
5. Preventive strategies include hand washing, food and water supply safety, infection control measures, and available vaccination against enteric infection.

EPIDEMIOLOGY AND CLINICAL RELEVANCE

Diarrhea is one of the most common gastrointestinal complaints, the second most common cause of death worldwide, and one of the four most common infections in elderly residents of long-term care facilities (LTCFs). Nonspecific diarrhea is the most common type of diarrhea in the United States; however, it is anticipated that an increase in the number of specific infectious causes of diarrhea will be diagnosed with the development of newer diagnostic techniques (1,2).

Physiological protective mechanisms against invasion of pathogenic organisms, such as gastric acidity, forward propulsive gut motility, and normal intestinal flora, may be compromised in the elderly. This may be due to age-related changes or a combination of comorbid conditions and factors such as polypharmacy, decreased antibody formation, and decreased helper T cells and mucosal IgA. Precise implications of immunosenescence on disease acquisition in the elderly are not very clear. However, it appears to increase their susceptibility to infectious diarrhea as compared with younger population (3–6). Moreover, after acquiring a diarrheal disease, elderly patients tolerate it less well and suffer more frequent complications than their younger counterparts with the same disorder.

Infectious diarrhea in LTCF residents may be associated with significant morbidity and mortality, even in developed countries. Mortality from diarrhea is much higher in older LTCF residents, especially in those older than age 75. About one third of all deaths due to diarrheal disease in the United States occur in the elderly residents in LTCFs, probably because of their lack of tolerance to resulting volume depletion with dire complications, such as cardiovascular compromise and organ failure. The hospitalization rate due to diarrheal illness, duration of hospital stay, morbidity, and mortality is significantly higher in older patients in comparison with patients younger than age 50, being highest in those older than age 75 (7,8). Early recognition and prompt treatment of diarrheal disease are, therefore, essential in preventing serious complications of dehydration and electrolyte disturbance that may result in multiple organ system failure and death.

The risk of exposure to pathogens that cause diarrhea is enhanced in LTCF residents, because of shared bathroom and dining facilities, liberal social and physical mixing of residents, and suboptimal infection control measures.

The most common cause of infectious diarrhea in LTCF residents is viral infection. The exact epidemiology of viral diarrhea is difficult to determine because of lack of precise diagnostic measures in many viral illnesses. However, Norwalk virus, Norwalk-like virus, and rotavirus are the most common pathogens (9). Although rotavirus is a recognized cause of childhood diarrhea, it is underappreciated as a cause of diarrhea in older patients (10). Moreover, acute diarrhea may occur as a component of a general viral syndrome caused by such viruses as influenza. Viral diarrhea may occur as a sporadic case or as an outbreak of diarrheal disease in LTCFs. Viral diarrhea is usually a self-limited condition. However, some frail residents may develop complications from dehydration and electrolyte imbalance.

Any microorganism that causes diarrhea in the general population can also cause diarrhea in LTCF residents. However, a definitive laboratory diagnosis of the culprit microorganism is made in no more than half of all patients with diarrhea. Common bacterial causes of diarrhea in LTCFs include *Clostridium difficile, Escherichia coli* (0157:H7, enterotoxigenic, enteropathogenic, and enteroinvasive), *Salmonella* spp., *Shigella* spp., *Campylobacter* spp., *Vibrio cholerae* and other *Vibrio* spp., and *Yersinia enterocolitica* (11). Although common in past, *Salmonella* or *Shigella* organisms are less likely causes of nosocomial diarrhea in hospitalized patients or LTCF residents.

Some cases of acute diarrhea resulting from food poisoning may be caused by *Clostridium perfringens, Bacillus cereus, Staphylococcus aureus,* or *Listeria monocytogenes* (Table 1). Among immune compromised patients with acquired immune deficiency syndrome (AIDS), cancer, chemotherapy, or long-term corticosteroid use, such opportunistic microorganisms as *Mycobacterium avium-intercellulare,* cytomegalovirus, herpes simplex, *Isospora belli, Cryptosporidium, Microsporidium,* and *Cyclospora* should also be considered

Table 1 Etiology of Diarrhea in Long-Term Care Facility Residents

Infectious causes	Noninfectious causes
Viruses	Dietary
Norwalk agent	Hyperosmolar formula
Enteroviruses	Lactose intolerance
Rotavirus	Fructose and sorbitol
Calicivirus	Medications
Bacteria	Antibiotics
Bacillus cereus	Antacids
Clostridium difficile	Laxatives
C. perfringens	Miscellaneous
Campylobacter sp.	Gut disorders
Escherichia coli	Inflammatory bowel disease
Listeria monocytogenes	Ischemic bowel, lymphoma
Salmonella sp.	Celiac disease
Shigella sp.	Systemic diseases
Staphylococcus sp.	Urosepsis
Vibrio sp.	Renal failure
Parasites	Thyrotoxicosis, diabetes mellitus
Giardia lamblia	
Entamoeba histolytica	
Cryptosporidium sp.	
Cyclospora sp.	

in the etiology of infectious diarrhea in addition to common pathogens. The quantity of fecal *Candida* may be increased during antibiotic therapy and diarrhea, due to alteration of intestinal microflora, but there is no persuasive proof to date that *Candida* is a primary cause of antibiotic-associated diarrhea (12).

C. difficile is the most important cause of nosocomial infectious diarrhea in LTCF residents, and because of its spore-forming capacity the organism may persist and cause protracted diarrhea. The incidence of asymptomatic carrier state of *C. difficile* rises from 2% in healthy adults to 9% of LTCF residents; however, antibiotic use and hospitalization may increase the incidence from 16% to as high as 56% (13,14). Tube feeding, prolonged hospitalization (especially in the intensive care units), surgery, chemotherapy, and acid suppression therapy are possible risk factors for *C. difficile* acquisition in elderly patients. Therefore, clinicians should have a low threshold for *C. difficile* testing (15,16).

The clinical spectrum of infection with *C. difficile* may include asymptomatic carrier state, trivial or serious diarrheal disease, toxic megacolon and its complications, fever of undetermined origin, and protein-losing enteropathy. Of note is an uncommon scenario: *C. difficile* infection presenting as acute abdomen with or without preceding diarrhea. Mortality in those patients who develop complications requiring surgery ranges from 38% to 80% (17). *C. difficile* spores may be resistant to commonly used soaps, and stronger chemicals may be required for adequate disinfection; this may be one of possible explanation of recurrent/relapsing cases of *C. difficile*–associated pseudomembranous colitis.

Among the parasitic causes of diarrhea, *Giardia lamblia*, and occasionally *Cryptosporidium* and *Microsporidium*, may be found, although other parasites, such as *Entamoeba histolytica*, may be responsible for some cases in LTCFs depending on underlying disease and exposure.

CLINICAL MANIFESTATIONS

Diarrhea may occur sporadically in one or more residents or as an outbreak in multiple residents. The clinical spectrum of infectious diarrhea may vary from a few loose stools to a potentially life-threatening condition. Most patients in the general population suffering from infectious diarrhea will complain of one or more of the following symptoms: crampy lower abdominal pain, anorexia, nausea, fever, malaise, and watery or bloody diarrhea. However, elderly residents in LTCFs with diarrhea may or may not complain of diarrhea, and thus the condition may escape prompt detection by the nursing or paramedical staff. Sometimes complications resulting from dehydration, such as altered mental status, stroke, myocardial infarction, and renal failure, may prompt the discovery of diarrhea. Infectious diarrhea may or may not be accompanied by fever; occasionally, it may manifest as hypothermia. Severe constipation and fecal impaction may present as overflow diarrhea. *C. difficile*–associated pseudomembranous colitis, which usually is accompanied by low-grade fever and watery diarrhea, may sometimes occur with little or no diarrhea and appear as an acute abdomen and, if unrecognized, may lead to unnecessary surgery, increased morbidity, and even mortality (18).

Bloody diarrhea or blood in stools—usually a sign of infection associated with inflammation, microbial invasion of mucosa, or tissue damage—may occur in *E. coli* 0157-H7, *Yersinia*, *Shigella*, or *Salmonella* infections. This should be differentiated from noninfectious causes of diarrhea, such as inflammatory bowel disease (ulcerative colitis and Crohn's disease), diverticular bleeding, or ischemic colitis (19–21).

An uncommon but clinically important scenario is when elderly persons with underlying inflammatory bowel disease (ulcerative colitis or Crohn's disease) develop infectious diarrhea (22). If the diarrhea episode is mistakenly considered an exacerbation of the underlying inflammatory bowel disease and corticosteroids are administered, catastrophic complications, such as hyperinfection syndrome may develop, leading to significant morbidity and even death.

DIAGNOSTIC APPROACH (FIG. 1)

History

In the evaluation of infectious diarrhea, noninfectious causes of diarrhea must be considered in the differential diagnosis. LTCF residents often consume multiple medications, which may cause diarrhea (Table 2). Likewise, diarrhea can be a manifestation of several systemic diseases, such as diabetes mellitus, hyperthyroidism, or such covert intestinal disorders as inflammatory bowel disease, celiac disease, bacterial overgrowth, and ischemic bowel disease. Attempts should be made to distinguish fecal incontinence, constipation with fecal impaction, and overflow diarrhea from true diarrhea. A careful symptom-specific history should be obtained from the resident, if possible, or from the nursing staff. Thirst and decreased urination may be early symptoms of volume depletion, followed by lethargy and altered level of consciousness, as dehydration progresses. Elderly patients may not volunteer information about diarrhea. This reluctance may be due to embarrassment or lack of understanding. Relevant information includes participation in group gatherings, contact with persons having diarrhea, sharing meals, travel, sexual practices, medication history, in particular antibiotic use within two months, and recent hospitalization. Information about mode of onset of diarrhea (sudden or gradual), sporadic or outbreak in multiple patients, duration of symptoms, character of stools (watery, presence of mucus or blood), and associated symptoms (abdominal pain, nausea, vomiting, tenesmus, fever) is germane for the clinical diagnosis of diarrheal illness. History of recent travel or exposure to a patient or pet

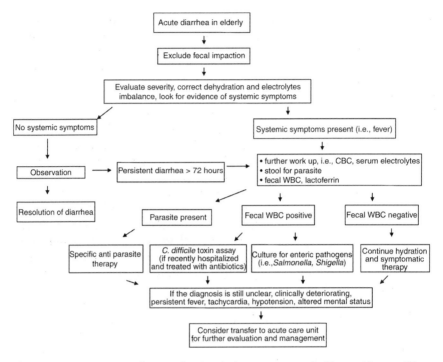

Figure 1 Management of acute diarrhea in long-term care facility residents. *Abbreviations*: CBC, complete blood count; WBC, white blood cells.

with diarrhea, consumption of improperly cooked meat, egg or shellfish, unpasteurized milk or milk products, and juices is also important. Duration of diarrhea may give useful clues to the diagnosis. In general acute diarrhea of less than two weeks duration is more likely to be of infectious origin. In cases of diarrhea due to food poisoning, the incubation period (e.g., *S. aureus, B. cereus,* <6 hours; *C. perfringens,* 6 to 24 hours; *Salmonella, Shigella, Clostridium botulinum,* 16 to 24 hours) may give a clue to the culprit organism (24). In addition, there may be a clue to the etiology of diarrhea in the type of food ingested. Examples include *V. cholera* from eating raw seafood, salmonellosis from improperly cooked eggs and poultry, *E. coli* from improperly cooked meat, and listeriosis from contaminated milk products. *Salmonella, Campylobacter,* and *Yersinia* have been reported to cause diarrheal disease after consumption of raw milk or unpasteurized milk products. Antibiotic-associated diarrhea usually occurs four to seven days after initiation of antibiotic therapy, although it may occur more than a month after stopping the antibiotics.

A careful drug history should be obtained. Besides antibiotic-associated diarrhea and *C. difficile* colitis, many drugs, such as magnesium-containing antacids, may cause diarrhea. Excessive ingestion of sorbitol-containing foods,

Table 2 Some of the Commonly Used Drugs that Can Cause Diarrhea in Older Patients

Cardiovascular medications	Antiarrhythmics: quinidine, procainamide, digoxin Antihypertensives: hydrochlorothiazide, furosemide, angiotensin converting enzyme inhibitors, beta blockers, methyldopa
Gastrointestinal medications	Antacids: magnesium containing antacids, H_2 receptor antagonists, proton pump inhibitors, misoprostol
Pulmonary medications	Theophylline
Cholesterol-lowering agents	Gemfibrozil, lovastatin, fluvastatin
Nervous system medications	Levodopa, lithium, donepezil, haloperidol, selective serotonin reuptake inhibitors, carbamazepine
Medications for infectious diseases	Antibiotics: clindamycin, quinolones, macrolides, tetracyclines, penicillin derivatives, cephalosporins Antivirals: amantadine, interferons, acyclovir, ganciclovir, ribavirin Antiprotozoal agents: tinidazole, metronidazole, trimethoprim and sulfamethoxazole
Antiarthritic medications	Nonsteroidal anti-inflammatory agents, colchicine
Miscellaneous	Laxatives, lactulose, oral hypoglycemic agents, thyroid hormones, ticlopidine, biphosphonates, chemotherapeutic agents, sorbitol-containing medications, ethanol, herbal remedies

Source: Adapted from Ref. 23.

such as grapes, sugar-free candies, etc., may also result in diarrhea, as does milk or milk products ingestion in residents with lactose intolerance. Diarrhea may be a side effect of many medications; therefore, a careful review of all medications (both prescription and nonprescription), including herbal remedies and dietary supplements, is important (Table 2). In residents receiving enteral feeding, the formulation of feeding solution and rate of administration should be carefully reviewed, as rapid administration of hypertonic formulas may cause diarrhea.

Physical Examination

A careful physical examination may help in identifying extraintestinal causes and risk factors for diarrhea. Attempts to identify early clinical evidence of the presence and severity of dehydration and electrolyte disturbance in elderly sick residents with diarrhea are more important than determining the precise etiology of diarrhea. Altered level of consciousness, dry mouth and tongue, sunken eyes, markedly reduced skin turgor over the chest, and >10% loss of body weight suggest significant dehydration. Vital signs, including measurement for orthostatic hypotension and change in body temperature, should be checked. Fever with relative bradycardia and a faint maculopaular rash over the trunk may be a clinical clue to typhoid fever. A gentle digital rectal examination will provide useful information about sphincter weakness caused by neuropathy or muscle injury and presence of hard fecal masses, neoplasms, and blood. Finding of perianal skin tag, fissures, fistulas, and abscesses may be a clue for possible diagnosis of Crohn's disease.

Laboratory Tests

Laboratory tests are expensive and often unnecessary in most cases of self-limiting diarrheal illness. However, a complete blood count (CBC), serum chemistry, and urinalysis (to exclude urinary tract infection presenting as diarrhea) should be obtained in residents with significant diarrhea who appear ill or have rapid decline in function. After consideration of noninfectious causes of diarrhea, stools should be examined for ova, parasites, and fecal leukocytes/fecal lactoferrin. Fecal leukocytes, lactoferrin, and occult blood are markers of bacterial invasion and inflammation of colonic mucosa. Routine stool culture is a low yield test and should only be considered if fever, dysentery, leukocytosis, abdominal pain, and tenderness are present, or in cases of diarrhea outbreaks (25,26). Close collaboration of laboratory staff is essential for rapid and precise diagnosis. If the clinical findings are suggestive of a particular etiological agent, specific laboratory tests, such as special cultures, acid fast stains, the Rotazyme test for rotavirus infection or DNA probes for rapid detection of certain pathogens, may be considered. If confirmed by randomized controlled studies in future, analysis of flatus may become a rapid bedside diagnostic test for infectious diarrhea (27). Unexplained leukocytosis of more than $15,000/mm^3$ may be a potential clue to *C. difficile*-associated diarrhea or colitis; likewise, fever, cramps, and hypoalbuminemia (probably due to protein-losing enteropathy) may act as surrogate markers of *C. difficile* infection or other enteric infectious agents (28).

If the diagnosis is still unclear and the resident is febrile, tachycardic, or hypotensive, transfer to an acute unit should be considered for further evaluation and management. Plain abdominal radiograph and, in some cases, computerized tomography scan may be required to exclude acute abdomen requiring prompt surgical intervention. Sigmoidoscopy may be necessary in some cases. In this scenario, the procedure should be done without any cleansing enemas or oral laxatives, as the cleansing solutions may themselves act as mucosal irritants causing hyperemia and excess mucus that mimic inflammatory changes. In most cases, a limited examination is enough to make a diagnosis. Sigmoidoscopy helps in distinguishing bloody diarrhea from hemorrhoidal bleeding and may also reveal evidence of colonic ischemia or uniformly congested and ulcerated mucosa, suggestive of acute infectious colitis or idiopathic ulcerative colitis. Pseudomembranous colitis can also be diagnosed by sigmoidoscopy (29). However, some cases may have evidence of pseudomembrane formation limited to the right colon and may only be diagnosed by full colonoscopy. Colonoscopy will also facilitate diagnosis of ulcerative colitis, Crohn's disease, and other conditions, such as microscopic colitis, collagenous colitis, and colorectal neoplastic lesions, such as villous adenoma or carcinoma. Colonoscopic biopsies may also assist in the diagnosis of diarrhea due to cytomegalovirus, tuberculosis, amebiasis, and schistosomiasis.

Esophagogastroduodenoscopy (EGD) has a limited role in diagnosis of infectious diarrhea. However, when empirical therapy does not improve symptoms and laboratory tests do not reveal a potential pathogen and diarrhea persists, EGD may be considered. In addition to visual inspection of mucosa, EGD may be helpful in obtaining tissue biopsies for histopathological examination and duodenal aspirate for microbiological examination and cultures, which would assist in the diagnoses of giardiasis, strongyloidiasis, bacterial overgrowth syndrome, etc. EGD and intestinal biopsy may sometimes diagnose less common causes of diarrhea, such as celiac disease, eosinophilic gastroenteritis, and intestinal lymphoma. The decision for an extensive evaluation and therapy should be in accordance with residents' advanced directives or desires of the health-care proxy. However, because diarrhea is often acute, self-limited, and easily treated, care-limiting advance directives may not apply to this condition.

THERAPEUTIC INTERVENTION

A careful history and vigilant physical examination will guide the clinician in proper management of acute infectious diarrhea. Most cases of infectious diarrhea, especially those of viral etiology, are usually self-limiting, and symptomatic supportive therapy with fluid and electrolyte replacement are all that is required. Correction of the primary cause(s) of diarrhea, such as stopping or replacing the culprit medication (30,31), change to isotonic tube-feeding formulas and/or decreasing the rate of infusion, and relief of fecal impaction, may be important therapeutic maneuvers. Initial laboratory studies are more helpful to elucidate the degree of dehydration and electrolyte disorder, rather than to provide organism-specific diagnosis.

Principles of therapy are basically the same irrespective of exact etiology of diarrhea and include adequate hydration and maintaining electrolyte balance. The oral route should be used whenever possible. Oral fluids (water, juices, soups, and electrolyte-containing drinks) should be encouraged as tolerated. To facilitate early recovery, adequate calories should be provided to the extent tolerated. However, milk and milk products, with exception of plain yogurt, should be avoided, at least in the initial phase of diarrheal illness. Any of the commercially available low-osmolarity oral rehydration solutions (ORS) may be used (32). Most of such solutions contain balanced amount of electrolytes and glucose/glucose polymer, such as rice starch, to facilitate fluid absorption by the glucose pathway (33). All elderly patients with acute diarrhea should be assessed frequently, to determine success or failure of ORS therapy and timely intravenous fluid replacement if needed. If the resident shows signs of significant dehydration (poor skin turgor, dry skin, altered level of consciousness, >10% weight loss, hypotension, or orthostasis), then intravenous administration of fluids and electrolyte solutions may be required, and the resident may need a transfer to an acute care facility. Particular care should be exercised in rapid intravenous replacement of fluids and electrolytes, as frail patients may have limited tolerance to fluid overload and can swiftly develop pulmonary edema and electrolyte imbalance due to underlying renal and cardiovascular diseases. ORS as a primary therapy or a supplemental therapy should be considered in all patients who do not have vomiting or altered level of consciousness. Boiled vegetables, starches, plain yogurt may be consumed as tolerated (34).

In general, routine empirical antimicrobial therapy for infectious diarrhea should be avoided because of self-limiting nature of illness and risks of antibiotic therapy. However, antimicrobial therapy should be considered for symptomatic patients with pathogen-specific diarrheal illnesses, such as *C. difficile* colitis, amebiasis, and giardiasis (Table 3). In addition, empirical therapy with fluoroquinolones, such as ciprofloxacin or levofloxacin, may also be considered in patients who manifest evidence of such systemic illness as fever, leukocytosis, and severe diarrhea/dysentery, especially among those at high risk of complications, particularly frail elderly, diabetics, or those who are immunocompromised.

Diarrhea resolves with treatment in most patients with *C. difficile* infection; however, up to 20% of such patients may relapse. Therapeutic strategies for recurrent *C. difficile* infection include repeating the same antibiotics, metronidazole or vancomycin, in tapering doses for several weeks, adding toxin-binding resins, such as cholestyramine and colestipol, and probiotics, such as *Saccharomyces boulardii*, *Lactobacillus GG*; rarely, healthy stool enemas have been tried but are not approved by the Food and Drug Administration. Available data suggest that probiotics may be useful in the management of acute infectious diarrhea; however, further studies are needed before their use can be adopted as standard therapy (35). In general, antidiarrheal medications with antiperistaltic property should be avoided in acute stages of illness because of the risk of developing toxic megacolon. Therefore, the mainstay of therapy should be maintenance of

Table 3 Antibiotic Therapy for Common Pathogens Causing Infectious Diarrhea in the Elderly

Campylobacter jejuni	Azithromycin 500 mg daily for 3 days, or erythromycin 500 mg twice daily for 5 days
Clostridium difficile	Metronidazole 500 mg 3 times daily or vancomycin 125 mg, orally 4 times daily for 10 days
Entamoeba histolytica	Metronidazole 750 mg 3 times daily for 10 days or tinidazole 1 g twice daily for 3 days, followed by either iodoquinol 650 mg orally 3 times daily for 20 days or paramomycin 500 mg 3 times daily for 7 days
Escherichia coli (except 0157-H7)	Ciprofloxacin 500 mg twice daily for 3 days or levofloxacin 500 mg once daily for 3 days
Giardia lamblia	Metronidazole 500 mg 3 times daily for 7 days or tinidazole 2 g single dose
Salmonella typhi/ paratyphi	Ciprofloxacin 500 mg twice daily for 10 days
Shigella	Ciprofloxacin 500 mg twice daily for 3 days, levofloxacin 500 mg once daily for 3 days
Vibrio cholerae	Tetracycline 500 mg 4 times daily for 3 days or doxycycline 300 mg single dose or ciprofloxacin 1 g single dose

fluid and electrolyte balance. Bismuth subsalicylate may be used in some patients who are not toxic; however, vigilance should be exercised for potential drug–drug interaction, salicylate intoxication and bismuth ence-phalopathy, in high-risk elderly patients.

INFECTION CONTROL MEASURES

Whether the case of diarrhea is sporadic or is occurring in an individual resident or in a group of residents in LTCF should be determined. As the mode of transmission of most enteric pathogens is the fecal–oral route, enteric precautions (adequate hand washing with appropriate disinfectant such as chlorhexidine and wearing gloves by visitors and LTCF staff when entering patients' room) should be observed. Diagnosis and prompt treat-ment of the index case, appropriate contact isolation, as well as adequate sterilization of bed linen, towels, and clothing should be implemented with-out delay. Terminal bleaching of rooms after discharge or transfer of the patient is recommended. Appropriate infection control and administrative authorities (e.g., state health departments) should be informed promptly to identify potential outbreaks and to implement effective control measures in a timely manner.

PREVENTION

Food handlers in particular and all staff of LTCF in general should be screened for absence of enteric pathogens, especially after a history of travel to high-risk areas. Food and water supply should be supervised and checked for absence of any possible contamination. Health education should be provided to medical, nursing, and all relevant persons and updates provided periodically. Hand washing and sanitary hygiene should be recommended and strictly observed. Safe food-handling and preparation practices should be emphasized. Vigilance in use of antibiotics in general, and clindamycin and cephalosporins in particular, is an effective prevention measure. Likewise, limiting the use of laxatives and magnesium-containing antacids may also decrease incidence of diarrheal disease in this setting (36). Development of vaccines against enteral pathogens may prevent significant morbidity and mortality from diarrhea in elderly LTCF residents.

SUGGESTED READING

Casburn-Jones AC, Farthing MJ. Management of infectious diarrhoea. Gut 2004; 53:296–305.
Gore JI, Surawicz C. Severe acute diarrhea. Gastroenterol Clin North Am 2003; 32:1249–1267.
Musher DM, Musher BL. Medical progress: contagious acute gastrointestinal infections. N Engl J Med 2004; 351:2417–2427.
Slotwiner-Nie PK, Brandt LJ. Infectious diarrhea in the elderly. Gastroenterol Clin North Am 2001; 30:625–635.

REFERENCES

1. Manatsathit S, Dupont HL, Farthing M, et al. Guideline for the management of acute diarrhea in adults. J Gastroenterol Hepatol 2002; 17:S54–S71.
2. Guerrant RL, Van Gilder T, Steiner TS, et al. Practice guidelines for the management of infectious diarrhea. Clin Infect Dis 2001; 32:331–351.
3. Hall KE. Effect of aging on gastrointestinal function. In: Hazzard WR, Blass JP, Halter JB, Ouslander JG, Tinetti ME, eds. Principles of Geriatric Medicine & Gerontology. New York: The McGraw-Hill Companies, Inc., 2003:593–600.
4. Hall KE. Aging and neural control of the GI tract. II. Neural control of the aging gut: can an old dog learn new tricks? Am J Physiol Gastrointest Liver Physiol 2002; 283:G827–G832.
5. Dharmarajan TS, Pitchumoni CS, Kokkat AJ. The aging gut. Pract Gastroenterol 2001; 25:15–27.

6. Gravenstein S, Fillit HM, Ershler WB. Clinical immunology of aging. In: Tallis RC, Fillit HM, eds. Brocklehurst's Textbook of Geriatric Medicine and Gerontology. London, England: Churchill Livingstone (Elsevier Science Limited), 2003:113–124.
7. Mounts AW, Holman RC, Clarke MJ, Bresee JS, Glass RI. Trends in hospitalization associated with gastroenteritis among adults in the United States. Epidemiol Infect 1999; 123:1–8.
8. Frenzen PD. Mortality due to gastroenteritis of unknown etiology in the United States. J Infect Dis 2003; 187:441–452.
9. Green KY, Belliot G, Taylor JL, et al. A predominant role for Norwalk-like viruses as agents of epidemic gastroenteritis in Maryland nursing homes for the elderly. J Infect Dis 2002; 185:133–146.
10. Anderson EJ, Weber SG. Rotavirus infection in adults. Lancet Infect Dis 2004; 4:91–99.
11. Slotwiner-Nie PK, Brandt LJ. Infectious diarrhea in the elderly. Gastroenterol Clin North Am 2001; 30:625–635.
12. Krause R, Reisinger EC. *Candida* and antibiotic-associated diarrhea. Clin Microbiol Infect 2005; 11:1–2.
13. Simor A, Bradley SF, Strausbaugh LJ, Crossley K, Nicolle LE, SHEA Long-Term Care Committee. *Clostridium difficile* in long-term care facilities for the elderly. Infect Control Hosp Epidemiol 2002; 23:696–703.
14. Gerding DN, Johnson S. Antibiotic-associated colitis/diarrhea. In: Cohen J, Powderly WG, eds. Infectious Diseases. Mosby (Elsevier) New York, 2004: 491–495.
15. Dial S, Alrasadi K, Manoukian C, Huang A, Menzies D. Risk of *Clostridium difficile* diarrhea among hospital inpatients prescribed proton pump inhibitors: cohort and case-control studies. CMAJ 2004; 171:33–38.
16. Starr JM, Martin H, McCoubrey J, Gibson G, Poxton IR. Risk factors for *Clostridium difficile* colonisation and toxin production. Age Ageing 2003; 32:657–660.
17. Dallal RM, Harbrecht BG, Boujoukas AJ, et al. Fulminant *Clostridium difficile*: an underappreciated and increasing cause of death and complications. Ann Surg 2002; 235:363–372.
18. Klipfel AA, Schein M, Fahoum B, Wise L. Acute abdomen and *Clostridium difficile* colitis: still a lethal combination. Digest Surg 2000; 17:160–163.
19. Talan D, Moran GJ, Newdow M, et al. Etiology of bloody diarrhea among patients presenting to United States emergency departments: prevalence of *Escherichia coli* 0157:H7 and other enteropathogens. Clin Infect Dis 2001; 32: 573–580.
20. Brandt LJ. Bloody diarrhea in an elderly patient. Gastroenterology 2005; 128:157–163.
21. Yasuhara H. Acute mesenteric ischemia: the challenge of gastroenterology. Surg Today 2005; 35:185–195.
22. Robertson DJ, Grimm IS. Inflammatory bowel disease in the elderly. Gastroenterol Clin North Am 2001; 30:409–426.
23. Akhtar AJ, Padda M. Fecal incontinence in older patients. J Am Med Dir Assoc 2005; 6:54–60.

24. American Medical Association, American Nurses Association-American Nurses Foundation, Centers for Disease Control and Prevention, et al. Diagnosis and management of foodborne illnesses: a primer for physicians and other health care professionals. MMWR 2004; 553(RR04):1–33.
25. Chan SS, Ng KC, Lam PK, Lyon DJ, Cheung WL, Rainer TH. Predictors of positive stool culture in adult patients with acute infectious diarrhea. J Emerg Med 2002; 23:125–130.
26. Basta SA. Stool cultures for nosocomial diarrhea: money down the drain? Am J Gastroenterol 2002; 97:1054–1056.
27. Probert CS, Jones PR, Ratcliffe NM. A novel method for rapidly diagnosing the causes of diarrhoea. Gut 2004; 53:58–61.
28. Bulusu M, Narayan S, Shetler K, Triadafilopoulos G. Leukocytosis as a harbinger and surrogate marker of *Clostridium difficile* infection in hospitalized patients with diarrhea. Am J Gastroenterol 2000; 95:3137–3141.
29. Johal SS, Hammond J, Solomom K, James PD, Mahida YR. *Clostridium difficile* associated diarrhoea in hospitalized patients: onset in the community and hospital and role of flexible sigmpoidoscopy. Gut 2004; 53:673–677.
30. Scheurlen M. Medication-related diarrhea. MMW Fortschr Med 2003; 145:24–27.
31. Chassany O, Michaux A, Bergmann JF. Drug-induced diarrhoea. Drug Saf 2000; 22:53–72.
32. Murphy C, Hahn S, Volmink J. Reduced osmolarity oral rehydration solution for treating cholera. Cochrane Database Syst Rev 2004; CD003754.
33. Ramakrishna BS, Venkataraman S, Srinivasan P, Dash P, Young GP, Binder HJ. Amylase-resistant starch plus oral rehydration solution for cholera. N Engl J Med 2000; 342:308–313.
34. Adolfsson O, Meydani SN, Russell RM. Yogurt and gut infection. Am J Clin Nutr 2004; 80:245–256.
35. Allen SJ, Okoko B, Martinez E, Gregorio G, Dans LF. Probiotics for treating infectious diarrhoea. Cochrane Database Syst Rev 2004; CD003048.
36. Apisarnthanarak A, Zack JE, Mayfield JL, et al. Effectiveness of environmental and infection control programs to reduce transmission of *Clostridium difficile*. Clin Infect Dis 2004; 39:601–602.

19

Hepatitis in Long-Term Care Facilities

Darrell W. Harrington and Peter V. Barrett

*Department of Medicine, Harbor-UCLA Medical Center,
Torrance, California, U.S.A.*

KEY POINTS

1. Hepatitis A infection, based on serologic evidence, increases in prevalence with age; however, outbreaks of hepatitis A have not been reported in nursing homes.
2. Although hepatitis B infection is relatively uncommon in older persons, small outbreaks have been reported in nursing home residents.
3. HCV is the most frequent cause of acute viral hepatitis in older adults. Chronic infection with this virus does occur in the elderly including complications of cirrhosis and HCC.
4. The prevalence and clinical relevance of hepatitis D, E, and G are unknown or unclear.
5. Health-care workers in LTCFs should be encouraged to be immunized with the hepatitis B vaccine.

INTRODUCTION

Clinical disease in the context of a long-term care facility (LTCF) presents problems for the health-care professional, which differ considerably from those found in the ambulatory setting or in acute care hospitals. This chapter will focus on the acute and chronic forms of the most common types of viral hepatitis encountered in a long-term care setting, as well as on the challenges to infection control that they represent. In general, the comments in this chapter will emphasize the care of older patients, who comprise the greatest number of patients in LTCFs.

Although there are numerous viral agents that may involve the liver, the following discussion will focus on the three major types, hepatitis virus A, B, and C, with additional comments on the less common varieties, hepatitis virus D, E, and G (Table 1). Advances in technology over the past two decades have provided health-care professionals with enormous amounts of new information about the biology and pathogenesis of these viruses, and, as a result, great strides have been made in both the treatment and prevention of disease.

EPIDEMIOLOGY AND CLINICAL RELEVANCE

Hepatitis A Virus

Epidemiology: Hepatitis A virus (HAV) was historically known as "infectious hepatitis." It is prevalent worldwide and is transmitted predominantly by the fecal–oral route through person-to-person contact or by contaminated food or water. Transmission is rarely reported following contact with blood or body fluids other than feces. In countries where HAV is endemic, most of the population becomes exposed in childhood and life-long immunity to the virus is conferred. However, in industrialized societies, improved sanitation has resulted in a decreased frequency of infection and concomitantly has produced a decrease in the proportion of the population that is immune to the virus. In the United States, the highest rates of natural immunity can be found in Native Americans and Hispanics; the rate for Native Americans is greater than 10-fold higher and that for Hispanics greater than twofold higher than for other ethnic groups. During an epidemic, secondary cases of hepatitis A occur two to six weeks following the index case. Infected individuals are most infectious in the late incubation period, a time when they are asymptomatic. Patients are usually no longer contagious by the time jaundice appears. The vast majority of infected individuals recover completely from acute infection. Fulminant hepatitis and death are rare complications, and the virus virtually never persists as a chronic infection.

Groups at risk for HAV infection include household or sexual contacts of infected individuals, international travelers, and persons living in endemic areas; during outbreaks day care center employees or attendees, homosexually active men, and injecting drug users are at risk. However, it should be noted that in nearly one-half of patients with hepatitis A, no known risk factor is identified. It is likely that asymptomatic infections, particularly in children, play an important role. The incidence of hepatitis A varies cyclically, with an interepidemic period of 7 to 10 years. The most recent increase began in 1993 and continued through 1995, with a total of more than 31,000 cases reported in the United States (1). The incidence of hepatitis A also

Table 1 Viral Characteristics and Epidemiology

Viral agent	A	B	C	D	E	G
Type and family	RNA picornavirus	DNA hepadnavirus	RNA flavivirus	Defective RNA virus	RNA calicivirus	RNA flavivirus
Epidemiology						
Incidence	125,000–200,000/yr	140,000–320,000/yr	38,000/yr	Unknown	No reported cases in US	Unknown
Prevalence	Antibodies present in 33% of Americans	1–1.25 million chronically infected	Antibodies present in 1.5% of American	HDV present in 10–20% with chronic HBV	Primarily occurs in developing countries	Estimated antibodies present in 1–2% of Americans
Mode of transmission	Fecal–oral	Blood-borne, sexual, perinatal	Blood-borne, sexual, perinatal	Blood-borne and sexual	Fecal–oral	Blood-borne
Incubation period (day)	15–60	45–160	14–180	42–180	15–60	Unknown
Chronicity	No	15–30%	50–80%	70–80%	No	Yes
Fulminant disease	Uncommon	Common	Rare	Common	No	No
Hepatocellular carcinoma	Unrelated	Strong association	Strong association	Strong association	Unrelated	Unknown
Mortality (%)	<1	1–2	1–2	2–20	1–2	Not significant
Vaccine	Yes	Yes	No	No (vaccinate against HBV)	No	No

Abbreviations: HBV, hepatitis B virus; HDV, hepatitis D virus.
Source: Data compiled from National Notifiable Diseases Surveillance System, Centers for Disease Control and Prevention.

varies regionally, with rates in the West that are two to five times higher than in the rest of the United States.

The prevalence of hepatitis A in the elderly population has been well documented. In population-based surveys, such as the National Health and Nutritional Examination Survey (2,3), the frequency of serologic evidence of past infection increases steadily with age, ranging from 10% in people under five years of age to three quarters of people 50 years and older. This age-associated increase is seen for both males and females and in all racial and ethnic groups. Also noted in this study was an inverse relationship between personal income and the prevalence of anti-HAV antibodies. Studies have shown that closed communities (4) and small food-related outbreaks (5) are potential sites of outbreaks. However, in a recent review, no documented outbreaks of HAV in nursing homes were reported (6). The latter observation is reassuring, but complacency must be avoided because as improved sanitation conditions become widespread, HAV infection will become progressively less frequent in childhood or adolescence, and, as a corollary, the proportion of the adult population that will be susceptible to HAV infection will grow. This is especially important because acute HAV infection is more severe in the aged (7,8).

Diagnosis: The diagnosis of HAV infection is not difficult. Viral cultures are not practical for clinical purposes, but serologic testing can allow the clinician to distinguish between acute infection and remote infections. The detection of HAV IgM immunoglobulins in serum indicates present or recent infection and may persist for several months. There is no chronic infection associated with HAV infection. Antibodies of the IgG class appear after complete resolution of infection and remain throughout life, thus conferring protection from reinfection (Fig. 1). The composition of the virus' antigenic map is preserved throughout the world, and, thus, global protection is conferred by the administration of immune globulin or by vaccination with a vaccine.

Hepatitis B Virus

Epidemiology: Between 140,000 and 320,000 persons become infected with hepatitis B virus (HBV) every year, but more than half remain asymptomatic. As shown in Figure 2, the overall incidence of HBV increased steadily from 1966 to 1985 but has declined more than 60% since that time. Evidence from the Centers for Disease Control and Prevention (CDC) indicates that there are 1.0 to 1.25 million persons in the United States with chronic infection and almost 6000 people will die each year from cirrhosis or hepatocellular carcinoma (HCC) as consequences of the infection. The peak age of infection is 20 to 39 years. Interestingly, the risk of developing symptomatic disease is directly related to age, whereas the risk of persistent infection is inversely related. The incidence of hepatitis B has been decreasing

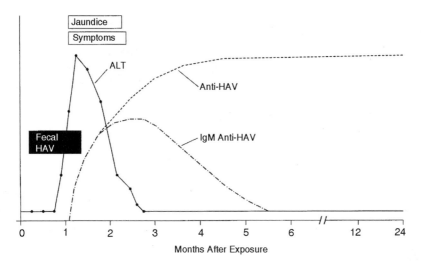

Figure 1 Clinical course of acute viral hepatitis A. *Abbreviations*: HAV, hepatitis A virus. *Source*: From Ref. 9.

in the United States in recent decades, coincident with recognition of the acquired immunodeficiency syndrome (AIDS) epidemic and subsequent decline in high-risk behavior. HBV was known as "serum hepatitis" a generation ago because it was shown to be transmitted to recipients of blood transfusion and serum products; however, it may be transmitted by any

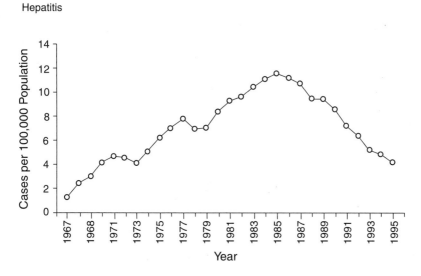

Figure 2 Hepatitis B by year, United States, 1967–1995. *Source*: From Ref. 1.

parenteral route, and it is also transmitted by sexual contact and perinatally. Currently, the most common mode of transmission is high-risk heterosexual contact with an infected individual, followed in frequency by injection drug use and homosexual contact. All of these activities are poorly represented among the elderly population, making acute infection with HBV in the setting of an LTCF unlikely.

The best information about the prevalence of hepatitis B infection in LTCFs and in the elderly may be found in the NHANES II and III surveys (2,3). For persons 65 to 74 years of age, hepatitis B surface antigen (HBsAg) was found less often than in the general population, with a frequency of 0.2% in white subjects and 0.9% in black subjects. A small number of reports have been published describing outbreaks of hepatitis B infection among nursing home residents. These infections were considered to have been spread by sharing bath brushes (10), through sexual contact with an infected nurses aide (11), or through the reuse of nondisposable syringes and shavers (12). Two outbreaks of nosocomial hepatitis B virus infection were reported from nursing homes in Ohio and New York (13). The infections were traced to the use of fingerstick devices, and in both reports personnel failed to restrict the use of the device to individual patients and to discard used parts. Failure to comply with universal precautions and Food and Drug Administration recommendations regarding the use of such devices will provide a continuing risk of exposure to patients requiring multiple percutaneous exposures.

Diagnosis: Two nucleocapsid antigens, hepatitis B core antigen and hepatitis B e-antigen (HBeAg), and a surface marker, HBsAg, are important components of this complex virion. The incubation period is long, ranging from 45 to 160 days (average 120). HBsAg is the first marker detected in serum and appears as early as six weeks after exposure. In acute resolving disease this antigen becomes undetectable six to eight weeks following the resolution of clinical symptoms. HBeAg appears in the serum shortly after HBsAg and is a qualitative marker of viral replication. In the normal host, after HBsAg disappears, antibody to HBsAg becomes detectable in serum and remains detectable indefinitely, conferring immunity to reinfection (Fig. 3). In chronic HBV infection, HBsAg and HBV DNA persist indefinitely in the serum as manifestations of chronic active infection and viral replication.

Hepatitis C Virus

Epidemiology: In the 1980s, hepatitis C virus (HCV) was shown to be the infectious agent responsible for most "non-A, non-B hepatitis" that occurred following transfusion or accidental needlestick. The incubation period for HCV infection has been reported to average six to seven weeks. Although sexual and perinatal transmission occurs, percutaneous exposure to infected blood or transplantation of organs from infectious donors remains the most efficient modes of transmission. However, since the development

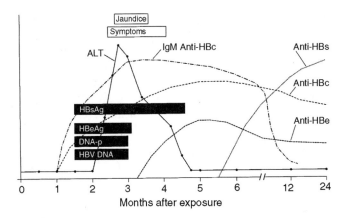

Figure 3 Clinical course of acute viral hepatitis B. *Abbreviations*: HBeAg, hepatitis B e-antigen; HBV, hepatitis B virus. *Source:* From Ref. 9.

of serological markers, such as anti-HCV antibodies, and the institution of mandated testing in 1992, the incidence of transfusion-associated or organ transplant-associated HCV infection has declined rapidly (Fig. 4). In contrast to HBV, HCV circulates at very low titers in infected serum, and this observation may explain why transmission via sexual contact is less common.

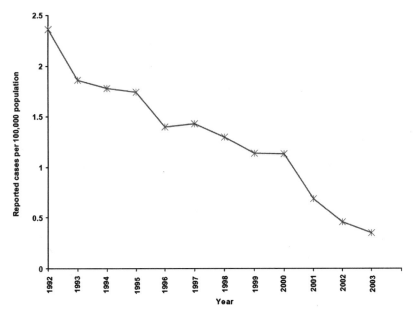

Figure 4 Incidence of reported acute hepatitis C, United States, 1992–2003. *Source*: From Ref. 1.

Although vertical transmission perinatally may occur, there is no evidence to support transmission during breastfeeding. In almost half of HCV sero-positive persons, no definitive risk factor can be identified.

In contrast to both HAV and HBV, the risk of chronic liver disease in patients infected with HCV is extremely high. Three quarters of infected individuals will develop chronic infection and at least one quarter of these will develop cirrhosis (14). Although the prevalence of anti-HCV varies in the U.S. population depending on various risk factors, the interpretation of the results from commonly used screening assays (enzyme immunoassays) is limited by several factors: (i) these assays do not detect anti-HCV in approximately 10% of people infected with HCV; (ii) these assays do not distinguish between acute and chronic or past infection; (iii) in the acute phase of hepatitis C, there may be a prolonged interval between onset of illness and seroconversion; and (iv) in populations with a low prevalence of infection, the rate of false-positive tests for anti-HCV is high.

Hepatitis C virus is the most frequent cause of acute viral hepatitis in older people. In a series of cases of acute viral hepatitis in older patients in the United States, non-A, non-B hepatitis accounted for 74% (15–17). In most studies, the major risk factor for hepatitis C infection in older people is a history of blood transfusion. Because mandatory screening programs have been in effect for less than a decade, the elderly have had a longer period of possible exposure to the virus. Today, rather than infection from blood transmission, the main mode of transmission for this virus is intracommunity from unknown sources (18). Several studies have suggested that the prevalence of anti-HCV in older patients is similar to that of the general population (19–21). In a study evaluating 315 institutionalized elderly people in Italy, anti-HCV was present in 2.2% (19). Conversely, in a recent study of 199 long-term care residents in nursing homes, anti-HCV was present in 4.5% of subjects (22). These results were obtained with screening methodology for anti-HCV that is not as reliable as assays for HCV RNA. In another study of 273 patients in an Israeli geriatric hospital, only five (1.8%) were found to have antibodies to HCV, and HCV RNA was found in only one of those five patients, suggesting a low prevalence in older patients (23). It is also likely that residents of LTCFs will have minimal additional exposure to HCV because of the context of their living arrangements. In a study of 208 elderly subjects living at home compared with 288 elderly subjects living in a nursing home, no difference in the prevalence of anti-HCV was detected (24).

Diagnosis: Hepatitis C is a single-stranded RNA virus similar to flaviviruses and accounts for the majority of non-A, non-B hepatitis. No commercial test is available to detect HCV antigen, but infection with HCV can be detected with antibody to HCV or with testing for HCV RNA. HCV RNA may be detected in infected serum as early as one to two weeks following exposure. Unlike HAV and HBV, antibodies to HCV are detected in the serum of patients during both the acute and chronic phases of infection, and their presence does not confer immunity.

Hepatitis D Virus

Epidemiology: Hepatitis D virus (HDV) has an unusual replication cycle. Infection can be acquired either as a coinfection with HBV or as a superinfection of chronic HBV carriers. People with HBV–HDV coinfection may have more severe acute disease and a higher risk of fulminant hepatitis than those infected with HBV alone. Chronic HBV carriers who acquire HDV superinfection usually contract chronic HDV infection, and in long-term studies of people with HDV superinfection, 70% to 80% had evidence of chronic liver disease with cirrhosis, compared with 15% to 30% of patients with chronic HBV infection alone. The actual incidence of HDV is uncertain because this disease is not reportable in the United States, but the CDC has estimated that there are approximately 7500 infections annually. The prevalence of HDV infection among persons positive for HBsAg is low in the general population (1.4–8.0%) and has been found to be highest in those with repeated percutaneous exposure, such as injection drug users (20–53%) and hemophilia patients (48–80%). Infection with HDV is virtually absent from populations with HBV infection acquired during infancy or childhood. The percutaneous route is the most efficient mode of transmission for HDV infection, but it may also be transmitted through sexual intercourse. No data are available to document the prevalence of HDV infection in the aged, and no outbreaks have been described in LTCFs.

Diagnosis: Testing for HDV infection is rarely indicated. Coinfection is diagnosed by the presence of IgM antibodies to the delta agent (anti-HDV), together with IgM anti-HBc. Tests for IgG anti-HDV are commercially available in the United States, but HDV antigen and HDV RNA are only available in research laboratories.

Hepatitis E Virus

Epidemiology: Hepatitis E virus (HEV) is the major etiologic agent of enterically transmitted non-A, non-B hepatitis worldwide, but in the United States it has been reported primarily in returning travelers. Unlike HAV, which is also transmitted by the fecal–oral route, person-to-person transmission of HEV appears to be uncommon. There is no evidence of chronic infection with this viral subtype. To date, there are no data regarding the prevalence of this infection in nursing home residents in the United States or abroad. However, like hepatitis A, data from endemic areas suggest that the prevalence of anti-HEV antibodies increases with age and probably represents the cumulative chance of being infected by the virus.

Diagnosis: No serologic tests are commercially available in the United States to detect HEV infection.

Hepatitis G Virus

Epidemiology: The hepatitis G virus (HGV) is a newly identified, blood-borne viral agent that often results in chronic infection. As much as 10% of posttransfusion and community-acquired hepatitis that cannot be explained by known types of viral hepatitis may result from HGV. Importantly, HGV infection does not seem to be associated with symptoms or with clinically significant liver disease. The role of HGV in the elderly is not well understood, but in two large series of elderly patients, 11% to 24% were found to have antibodies to HGV, and three individuals were found to be viremic (22,25). In addition, it should be noted that 40% of anti-HGV–positive subjects in one study had evidence of anti-HCV antibodies (25). It appears that in most cases, HGV infection is silent, self-limiting, and clinically unimportant.

Diagnosis: Polymerase chain reaction testing has been used in research studies to detect HGV virus in the serum of infected individuals, but this methodology is not generally available for clinical purposes.

CLINICAL MANIFESTATIONS AND COMPLICATIONS OF VIRAL HEPATITIS

The liver has a great reserve capacity, and the decline in function that usually occurs with aging has little clinical relevance except for altered drug metabolism. Conventional liver function tests, such as serum bilirubin, transaminases, alkaline phosphatase, and gamma glutamyl transpeptidase, do not change with age; therefore, abnormal values should be taken seriously. However, it should be noted that elderly patients often have chronic medical conditions requiring complicated medical regimens, and abnormal liver function tests should be evaluated in the context of symptoms and potential effects of medication.

The clinical manifestations of many diseases have been abundantly described in young and middle-aged subjects, but less is known about the presentation of the same illnesses in the elderly. This is also true regarding viral hepatitis. Generally, the accepted "classic" symptoms and signs are not reliable in the elderly. Furthermore, changes in both immunologic and endocrinologic function, as well as the presence of comorbidities, such as neurologic disease, may have a significant impact on the clinical presentation of disease in the elderly. The elderly population is at risk for all clinical forms and consequences of viral hepatitis including acute hepatitis, chronic active hepatitis, cirrhosis, hepatocellular carcinoma, and even death.

Acute Hepatitis

The most common presenting complaints of acute hepatitis are anorexia, nausea, fatigue, and myalgia, usually developing seven to 14 days before the onset of jaundice. In addition, infected persons may complain of headache, right upper quadrant pain, and arthralgias. These symptoms are virtually identical for all forms of viral hepatitis. In general, elderly patients have milder clinical disease and may present with a simple flulike illness and complain only of malaise or fatigue. Cholestasis rather than hepatocellular inflammation dominates the pathophysiological changes. Clinical recovery and clearance of the virus are usually slower in the aged compared with the younger individual. Jaundice can usually be observed when the bilirubin rises to 3.0 mg/dL or greater and is most easily observed in the sclerae, soft palate, or under the tongue. However, it is important to remember that the absence of jaundice does not exclude the diagnosis of viral hepatitis. These vague symptoms may go unnoticed in the setting of an LTCF, because the prevalence of other comorbidities, such as depression, congestive heart failure, and pulmonary disease, may exist concurrently with the onset of an acute viral infection. Conversely, many elderly with acute infection may be completely asymptomatic. Other physical findings may include hepatomegaly or splenomegaly. The presence of lymphadenopathy or fever should alert the examiner to other viral syndromes or to the possibility of malignancy, such as lymphoproliferative disease. Diagnosis of acute viral hepatitis may be confirmed by the presence of serological markers (Table 2).

One of the most feared complications of acute viral hepatitis is fulminant hepatitis, an illness characterized by rapid prolongation of prothrombin time, hyperbilirubinemia, encephalopathy, and occasionally death. The clinical manifestations of this rare form of acute hepatitis are seen almost

Table 2 Diagnostic Approach to Patients with Acute Viral Hepatitis

		Serological test of patient's serum		
HBsAg	IgM anti-HAV	IgM anti-HBc	Anti-HCV	Diagnostic interpretation
+	−	+	−	Acute hepatitis B
+	−	−	−	Chronic hepatitis B
+	+	−	−	Acute hepatitis A superimposed on chronic B
+	+	+	−	Acute hepatitis A and B
−	+	−	−	Acute hepatitis A
−	+	+	−	Acute hepatitis A and B (HBsAg below detection threshold)
−	−	+	−	Acute hepatitis B (HBsAg below detection threshold)
−	−	−	+	Acute hepatitis C

Abbreviations: HBsAg, hepatitis B surface antigen; HCV, hepatitis C virus.
Source: From Ref. 26.

exclusively in patients infected with HBV, HDV, and HEV and less commonly in HAV and HCV. However, the case fatality rate is disproportionately high in the elderly. Accordingly, the ratio of deaths from hepatitis A to the total number of patients reported increased from 0.07% in the age group 15 to 24 years to 4% in those age 65 and older (8,27). Hepatitis B is the most common viral infection leading to fulminant viral hepatitis and accounts for 35% to 70% of all virus-related cases. In a multivariate analysis of risk factors for fulminant hepatitis, age was an independent predictor of mortality in patients with both HBV and HCV (28,29).

Chronic Hepatitis

Chronic hepatitis is primarily a feature of HBV, HCV, and HDV. Approximately 10% of persons infected with HBV will develop chronic hepatitis, but 80% to 85% of persons infected with HCV and HDV will develop chronic hepatitis. In contrast to the low chronic carrier state in young adults, up to 60% of older people infected with HBV become chronic carriers. The higher frequency of chronicity may be the result of the decline in cellular immunity and decreased viral clearance that have been demonstrated in the older population. Clinical symptoms associated with chronic hepatitis range from patients who are asymptomatic to those with varying degrees of constitutional symptoms (fatigue, anorexia, and nausea), or to cirrhosis and its complications. In addition, it should be noted that up to 25% of persons with chronic infection would be found to have normal aminotransferases.

In older patients with chronic hepatitis B, HBsAg and anti-HBc antibodies can be detected in their serum. However, evidence of active viral replication, such as the presence of HBeAg and/or HBV DNA in the serum, is usually slight or absent (30). It is likely that most hepatitis B carriers in the elderly represent individuals with long-standing infection who acquired their disease many years earlier. Although there is little evidence of viral replication in such patients, they may still be highly infective to others.

Chronic infection with HCV may also occur in the elderly and is a very common sequel to acute infection (30). It is well established that older patients with chronic HCV have significantly higher HCV RNA titers than the younger counterparts (31). This observation may well represent a decreased ability of the immune system in the aged to clear the infection. In addition, it should be noted that genotype 1b is overrepresented in the older population and that patients infected with genotype 1b have higher levels of HCV RNA in the serum compared with those infected by other HCV genotypes (32).

In a study of the natural history of chronic HCV infection in patients with transfusion-associated hepatitis C, it was found that among patients who were 50 years of age or older at the time of transfusion the average time from the transfusion to the development of chronic active hepatitis, cirrhosis, and hepatocellular carcinoma was 10.7, 9.8, and 14.7 years, respectively (33). Among patients who received transfusion before the age of 50, the average time to the development of these diseases was 20.4, 23.6, and 31.5 years, respectively. It is possible that the significantly shorter duration of time from transfusion to symptomatic disease in older subjects may be caused by more rapid progression of disease. Older patients with chronic hepatitis C may present for the first time with complications of cirrhosis or hepatocellular carcinoma.

Whereas histologic stage correlates directly with prognosis in HBV and HDV, it is of little value in the natural history of HCV. Ultimately, morbidity and mortality are associated with the development of end-stage liver disease and cirrhosis.

Hepatocellular Carcinoma

Primary HCC is highly associated with underlying cirrhosis and is over-represented in the elderly, with more than 40% of cases occurring in persons over 70 years. Among the known viral hepatitis agents, only HBV, HDV, and HCV are important in the pathogenesis of HCC. The incidence of HCC associated with hepatitis B and C has been observed to increase with age (34–36).

For example, in a study of Chinese government employees infected with hepatitis B, the incidence of HCC increased from 197 to 927 cases per 100,000 carrier years in age groups 30 to 39 and 60 to 90, respectively (37). The length of time during which an individual has had cirrhosis is an important factor contributing to the development of HCC, thus conferring an increased risk among the elderly. Of note, the mean age of detection of HCC is significantly older in patients with HCV compared with HBV infection, probably because HCV infection is more often acquired later in life than the HBV infection. In addition, HCV is usually associated with more advanced liver disease and cirrhosis at the time of HCC presentation compared with individuals infected with HBV. Prognosis, to a large extent, is dependent on the size of the tumor at the time of diagnosis. Therefore, screening of all patients with known cirrhosis for the development of HCC is recommended. It has been reported that the median survival of HCC in persons aged 65 years and older was 10.5 weeks (38).

THERAPEUTIC INTERVENTIONS

Treatment of Acute Hepatitis

Treatment for acute viral hepatitis remains supportive. Moreover, many older patients will often have mild nonspecific symptoms or may be completely asymptomatic. Acute hepatitis in the elderly only occasionally warrants hospitalization to an acute care facility. Although it is common to prescribe bed rest, forced and prolonged bed rest should be avoided because the associated deconditioning may be difficult to reverse in older patients. Anorexia and nausea may be present, but patients should be encouraged to try to maintain fluid and caloric intake. Drugs that require metabolism by the liver and those with potential for hepatotoxicity should be avoided if possible. Treatment with corticosteroids is not efficacious.

Although clinical trials of interferon in patients with acute HBV and HCV have shown some efficacy, many of these patients recover spontaneously. Accordingly, treatment in the acute phase of infection would unnecessarily expose large numbers of patients to the potentially harmful effects of this drug. Furthermore, observational studies strongly suggest that acute icteric disease resolves spontaneously at a significantly higher rate than silent or asymptomatic acute disease. Therefore, interferon is not recommended for acute, symptomatic hepatitis B or hepatitis C.

Chronic Hepatitis

Both HBV and HCV may have significant chronic infectious stages that lead to profound clinical sequelae, including cirrhosis and hepatocellular carcinoma. Unfortunately, little information about treatment efficacy of the available chemotherapeutic regimens in patients over the age of 60 years has been published. It is likely that they have been excluded from the various clinical studies because of concern about the increased frequency of side effects that may be seen in the elderly population with many drugs. In fact, the National Institutes of Health consensus statement published in 1997 recommends treating patients over age 60 only in the context of a clinical trial (39). Given the growing number of older patients in our society, clinically significant complications from chronic hepatitis will become increasingly common, and the decision to treat or withhold therapy for chronic hepatitis infection must be made while balancing the potential risks and benefits of treatment for an individual patient. All potential candidates for therapy should be referred to a hepatologist.

Patient Selection

The minimal criteria recommended by the National Institutes of Health for candidates who may benefit from interferon-based therapy include the following:

- elevated liver function tests for at least six months;
- the presence of viral genetic material in the serum;
- portal fibrosis or moderate to severe liver inflammation on liver biopsy;
- compensated liver disease.

Table 3 Exclusion Criteria for the Use of Interferon-Based Therapy

Patients with a history of drug or alcohol abuse without abstinence 6 months to a year

History of hepatic encephalopathy, variceal bleeding, ascites, or other signs of hepatic decompensation

History of other causes of chronic hepatitis, including alcoholic liver disease, hemochromatosis, Wilson's disease, alpha-1 antitrypsin deficiency, hepatotoxic drug injury, or autoimmune hepatitis

History of significant cardiovascular disease, such as unstable angina pectoris or congestive heart failure; pulmonary diseases, including chronic obstructive pulmonary disease; uncontrolled diabetes mellitus and other comorbid conditions that would limit treatment

History of previous psychiatric illness, such as severe depression and psychosis

Patients on other antiviral medications

Exclusion criteria are listed in Table 3. The most important factors in assessing the elderly for potential treatment are the patient's motivation and the presence of comorbid disease. A comorbid chronic disease, such as severe chronic obstructive pulmonary disease, coronary artery disease, or malignancy that likely will limit life span, would make treatment for chronic hepatitis a secondary issue. Likewise, patient motivation is critical in dealing with treatment side effects as well as the administration of injections. Age, independent of physiological function or comorbidities, has not been shown to influence response rates. Therefore, it is likely that therapy will benefit only the healthy segment of the aged population with additional life expectancy of greater than 10 to 15 years.

Chronic Hepatitis B Infection

Interferon-alpha therapy is the treatment of choice for chronic hepatitis B infection. It is administered as an injection of 5 to 20 million units thrice weekly for 12 weeks. Response to interferon is highest (40–50%) in patients with infection acquired during adulthood with inflammatory liver disease consistent with chronic active infection who are not immunocompromised. Additional approved regimens include lamivudine 150 mg daily and adefovir 10 mg daily, each given for a minimum of one year. Combination therapy is of limited value in chronic HBV and indicated only in patients with evidence of resistance.

Chronic Hepatitis C Infection

Combination therapy with interferon and ribavirin has been proved to be more effective than interferon therapy alone. Studies using combination therapy for chronic HCV infection have demonstrated sustained response rates up to 40% to 50%, compared with 15% to 25% seen with interferon alone. Patients with genotypes 2 or 3 typically have favorable response rates to chemotherapy. However, patients with genotype 1, the most common genotype found in the United States, have significantly lower response rates. Combination therapy should not be used in patients with anemia, renal insufficiency, coronary artery disease, cerebral vascular disease, or gouty arthropathy. Due to these limitations, it is clear that many elderly patients may not be candidates for combination therapy. A recent study of 33 elderly (mean age 70.2) patients received pegylated interferon-alpha-2b plus ribavirin for 24 to 52 weeks. Compared with younger patients, elderly patients had significantly lower virological response at the end of treatment and higher likelihood of side effects (40).

The recommended dose of interferon-alpha is 3 million units three times a week and ribavirin 1000 to 12,000 mg/day for 24 or 48 weeks, based on the viral genotype and the serum HCV RNA level measured at week 24.

INFECTION CONTROL AND PREVENTION

Infection control in any specific setting must reflect the nature of the health-care activities and the biology of potential pathogens. It is obvious that there will be differences in emphasis on certain measures necessary for control of infection in LTCFs compared with those for acute care or for the operating theater. Nevertheless, there are requisite conditions for all sites for successful transmission: in each instance it is necessary to have an infectious agent, a transmission vector, and a susceptible host.

Infection control has become more complex in recent decades and is subject to regulation by various federal and state government agencies. Each LTCF is required to have coordinated infection control policies and procedures that address sick employees, hand washing, and surveillance, as well as other infection control issues. Isolation practice guidelines are fundamental components of infection control, and the CDC has formulated one that calls for a two-tiered system. The first, *standard precautions*, are recommended for all patients and was formerly called "universal precautions." These guidelines emphasize hand washing, use of gloves when handling body fluids, masks, eye protection, and gowns when splashing of body fluids is likely. Avoidance of needlestick and other "sharps" injuries are also emphasized. *Transmission-based precautions*, the second type of isolation practice, are recommended for patients with suspected contagious pathogens, with emphasis on droplet or contact transmission (41).

Numerous investigators have identified the most common pathogens that afflict residents in LTCFs, as well as the epidemiology of these agents. Urinary tract infections, respiratory infections, tuberculosis, and skin infections have comprised the greatest number of clinical problems in recent decades, but diarrheal illness and antibiotic-resistant bacteria have also posed challenges to physicians (42). In comparison, viral hepatitis is much less common. However, because of the serious nature of the disease, and because individuals may harbor inapparent infections, it deserves close attention.

The biology of the three major types of viral hepatitis has been described in previous sections. For the purposes of discussion, infection control measures for viral hepatitis can be divided into those that address agents involving transmission predominantly by the oral (e.g., hepatitis A virus) or the parenteral route (e.g., hepatitis B or hepatitis C virus).

Hepatitis A Virus

Frequency of HAV infection in LTCFs: In recent decades, the occurrence of acute HAV in LTCFs has been rare. Clearly, the potential remains for transmission from infected food handlers to patients, patients to health-care workers (HCW) (e.g., fecal incontinence), and even from patient to patient by the classic fecal–finger–oral route. However, current food preparation systems and a significant prevalence of host immunity in patients and HCW seem to have been sufficient to minimize this threat. In patients over 70 years of age in the United States, more than 75% have been found to have antibody to HAV, confirming previous infection or vaccination (42). However, before dismissing HAV as a potential problem we must acknowledge the uncertain impact of ongoing economic pressures on regulatory compliance of long-term health-care facilities, with the resulting potential for a loosening of current infection control standards.

Screening for HAV: Acute hepatitis due to HAV in older adults is unusual, and no testing for it is indicated in asymptomatic patients admitted to an LTCF. Furthermore, in contrast to HBV and HCV, HAV does not produce a chronic, infectious form of disease that could serve as a rationale for testing.

Vaccination: Clinical guidelines have been developed to identify patients who should receive vaccination against HAV as primary prevention (Table 4). It has been recommended that patients with chronic liver disease should be vaccinated in order to prevent possible infection with HAV that could produce diagnostic confusion and could result in a poor outcome because of diminished hepatic reserve. It may be difficult to make a definitive diagnosis of chronic liver disease in the setting of an LTCF, given the many causes of minor liver function test abnormalities. In some clinical situations additional testing may be unwarranted, and physicians may wish to proceed with vaccination without additional interventions and X-rays.

Consideration should also be given to vaccination of food handlers who work in LTCFs. However, in one investigation, rates of hepatitis A among food handlers were found to be similar to rates among the general population, and, in general, the frequency of outbreaks in hospitals, institutions, and

Table 4 Hepatitis A Vaccine: Indications and Schedule

Persons who should receive hepatitis A vaccine
    Persons traveling to or working in countries outside of the United States (except
        for Northern and Western Europe, New Zealand, Australia, Canada, and Japan)
    Children (>2 yr) in communities that have high rates of hepatitis A and periodic
        hepatitis A outbreaks
    Men who have sex with men
    Illegal drug users (injecting and noninjecting)
    Persons who have occupational risk for infection
    Persons who have chronic liver disease
    Persons who have clotting factor disorders
    Food handlers, where health authorities or private employers determine
        vaccination to be cost-effective
Vaccination schedule
    Two doses are required
    The minimal interval between doses is 6 mos

Vaccinee's age (yr)	Dose (EL.U.)	Volume (mL)	No. doses	Schedule (mos)
Recommended dosages of HAVRIX (Merck)				
2–18	720	0.5	2	0, 6–12
>18	1440	1.0	2	0, 6–12
Recommended dosages of VAQTA (Merck)				
2–17	25	0.5	2	0, 6–18
>17	50	1.0	2	0, 6

Abbreviation: EL.U., enzyme-linked immunosorbent assay units.
Source: From Ref. 42.

schools is not high enough to warrant routine hepatitis A vaccination of persons specifically because they are in these settings (42,43).

    Postexposure protection against HAV infection: In the rare instance in which an active case of hepatitis A is identified in an LTCF, use of immune globulin and vaccination with hepatitis A vaccine is recommended for susceptible persons in close contact with infected patients. Persons identified as candidates for postexposure management should receive a single intramuscular dose of immune globulin (0.02 mL/kg) as soon as possible, and not later than two weeks following exposure. Hepatitis A vaccination should also be given, with the first vaccination to be given as early as possible after exposure, and a second and final vaccination six to 12 months later.

Hepatitis B Virus

Transmission of blood-borne pathogens presents a more complicated picture than orally transmitted infections. Generally, administration of blood products are not an important infection control issue in LTCFs, because they are given infrequently in this setting and because current blood banking practices have been very effective in eliminating this source of HBV and HCV. Infection control measures must address issues that affect HCW, such as injuries from sharps, as well as patient-to-patient transmission caused by contaminated instruments. Several examples of the latter have been reported over the past several years in diabetics who have contracted viral hepatitis from contaminated lancets used for fingerstick glucose monitoring (44).

Although a highly effective vaccine against HBV has been available for more than 20 years, this infection remains a threat to both HCW and patients. Federal regulations require all hospitals and LTCFs to offer vaccination to employees at no cost; yet a determined few decline and remain at risk of infection, Although the majority of residents in LTCFs are also susceptible. Infection control measures must be in place to minimize risk for HBV transmission in these two populations.

 Frequency of HBV infection in the LTCF setting: The frequency of HBV infection in LTCFs varies greatly, according to the cultural and socio-economic background of the population in the facility. The likelihood that persons will be chronic carriers of HBV will vary from less than 1% for healthy, American-born individuals to 5% to 15% for recent immigrants, dialysis patients, and users of illicit parenteral drugs.

 Screening for HBV: Screening for HBV infection in persons admitted to LTCFs is not indicated on a routine basis but should be part of an evaluation of patients with acute and chronic liver disease or abnormal liver function tests. The critical issue to resolve, both for the individual resident and for LTCFs, is whether the resident is an infectious carrier of HBV. Of the many serologic tests available in the laboratory, only the detection of HBsAg and anti-HBc provides useful information about the infectious status of the individual.

 Screening HCW in LTCFs for HBV infection or immunity is not routinely necessary because vaccination during professional training or at the time of employment is almost universal.

 Vaccination: HCW should be encouraged to undergo vaccination for HBV as early as possible in their professional training. Published guidelines recommend that all HCW who perform tasks involving contact with blood, blood-contaminated body fluids, other body fluids, or sharps should be vaccinated (Table 5). Prevaccination serologic screening for previous infection is not indicated for persons being vaccinated because of occupational risk (13). For patients, those with chronic liver disease or unexplained abnormal liver function tests should be vaccinated in order to prevent a possible infection with HBV that could produce diagnostic confusion and could have a poor outcome because of diminished hepatic reserve.

 Postexposure protection against HBV infection: Prophylaxis should be considered for HCW for any percutaneous, ocular, or mucous membrane exposure to blood, and is determined by the HBsAg status of the source

Table 5 Hepatitis B Vaccination—Indications and Schedule

Persons who should receive hepatitis B vaccine
   All babies at birth
   Persons at occupational risk for exposure to blood
   All adolescents
   High-risk adults, including the following conditions or behaviors:
      Household contacts and sex partners of HBsAg-positive persons
      Users of injectable drugs
      Heterosexuals with more than one sex partner in 6 months
      Men who have sex with men
      People with recently diagnosed sexually transmitted disease
      Patients receiving or likely to receive hemodialysis
      Recipients of certain blood products
      Health-care workers and public safety workers who are exposed to blood
      Inmates of long-term correctional facilities
      Clients and staff of institutions for the developmentally disabled
Vaccination schedule
   Three doses are needed on a 0, 1, 6 mo schedule
   Alternative timing options for vaccination include:
      0, 2, 4 mo
      0, 1, 4 mo
   There must be 4 wk between doses 1 and 2, and 8 wk between doses 2 and 3.
      Overall there must be at least 4 mo between doses 1 and 3
   Recommendations for vaccination:

	Recombivax HB		Engerix HB	
Group	Dose (μg)	(mL)	Dose (μg)	(mL)
Infants of HBsAg-negative mothers and children aged <11 yr	2.5	(0.5)	10.0	(0.5)
Infants of HbsAg-positive mothers; prevention of perinatal infection	5.0	(0.5)	10.0	(0.5)
Children and adolescents aged 11–19 yr	5.0	(0.5)	20.0	(1.0)
Adults aged >19 yr	10.0	(1.0)	20.0	(1.0)
Dialysis patients and other immunocompromised persons	40.0	(1.0)	40.0	(2.0)

Abbreviations: HBsAg, hepatitis B surface antigen; HB, hepatitis B.
Source: From Refs. 45, 46.

patient and vaccination status of the exposed person. Treatment of unvaccinated HCW following an exposure will include hepatitis B immune globulin
and the initiation of a hepatitis B vaccine series if the source patient is
unknown or has evidence of infection with HBV. The effectiveness of
postexposure prophylaxis is related to the interval after exposure to time
of prophylaxis. The maximal established delay in prophylaxis is seven days

for needlestick exposures and 14 days for sexual exposures. [The reader is referred to specific guidelines for more details (12,47).]

Hepatitis C Virus

Most of the principles and practices described above for HBV may be applied to infection control strategies for HCV. Unhappily, and in contrast to HBV, the prevalence of HCV is greater than HBV, immunization is not available, and postexposure treatment is unsatisfactory. HCV infection is the most common chronic blood-borne infection in the United States, and, in general, transmission patterns and population risk-groups are similar to those for HBV. The frequency of HCV found among residents in LTCFs has ranged from 1% to 3% (47).

Screening for HCV: Policies concerning screening for HCV infection in persons admitted to LTCF are similar to those given in the previous section for HBV. Thus, screening is not indicated on a routine basis but should be part of an evaluation of patients with acute and chronic liver disease or abnormal liver function tests. Persons considered at high risk for HCV should also be tested; this includes individuals who have injected illegal drugs, persons who received clotting factor concentrates, persons on chronic hemodialysis, and recipients of organ transplants and transfusions prior to 1992. It is not necessary to screen HCW for HCV because of the rarity of transmission of HCV infection from HCW to patients.

Vaccination: No vaccination is available for HCV.

Postexposure protection against HCV infection: HCW should be tested routinely for HCV infection after needlesticks, sharps injury, or mucosal exposure to HCV-positive blood. However, prophylaxis following HCV exposure with immunoglobulin or antiviral treatment has not been shown to be effective and is not recommended. For the 2% to 10% of HCW who will have anti-HCV seroconversion after exposure to an HCV-positive source, combination treatment with interferon and another antiviral drug should be considered (48,49).

CONCLUSION

A knowledge of the epidemiology and biology of the various types of viral hepatitis is essential for primary prevention and optimal management of patients exposed to infection in LTCFs facilities. It is encouraging to consider that effective vaccines are now available for two of the three major types of viral hepatitis, and numerous, specific serologic tests facilitate diagnosis of these infections. It is hoped that the information and clinical approach to patient care contained in this chapter will be helpful to healthcare professionals in LTCFs who face a myriad of complex management issues concerning viral hepatitis.

SUGGESTED READING

Baldo V, Floreani A, Menegon T, Angiolelli G, Trivello R. Prevalence of antibodies against hepatitis C virus in the elderly: a seroepidemiological study in a nursing home and in an open population. The Collaborative Group. Gerotonology 2000; 46:194–198.

Chien N, Dundoo G, Horani M, Osmack P, Morley J, Di Bisceglie A. Seroprevalence of viral hepatitis in an older nursing home population. J Am Geriatr Soc 1999; 47:1110–1113.

Floreani A, Minola E, Carderi E, Ferrara F, Rizzotto ER, Baldo V. Are elderly patient poor candidates for pegylated interferon plus ribavirin in the treatment of chronic hepatitis C? J Am Geriatr Soc 2006; 54:549–550.

REFERENCES

1. Centers for Disease Control. Hepatitis Surveillance Report No. 57. Atlanta: Centers for Disease Control, 2000.
2. Alter M, Mast E. The epidemiology of viral hepatitis in the United States. Gastroenterol Clin North Am 1994; 23:437–455.
3. Shapiro C, Coleman P, McQuillan G, Alter M, Margolis H. Epidemiology of hepatitis A: seroepidemiology and risk groups in the USA. Vaccine 1992; 10(suppl 1):S59–S62.
4. Szmuness W, Dienstag J, Purcell R, et al. The prevalence of antibody to hepatitis A antigen in various parts of the world: a pilot study. Am J Epidemiol 1977; 106:392–398.
5. Papaevangelou G. Epidemiology of hepatitis A in Mediterranean countries. Vaccine 1992; 10(suppl 1):S63–S66.
6. Floreani A, Chiaramonte M. Hepatitis in nursing homes. Incidence and management strategies. Drugs Aging 1994; 5:96–101.
7. Lednar W, Lemon S, Kirkpatrick J, Redfield R, Fields M, Kelley P. Frequency of illness associated with epidemic hepatitis A virus infections in adults. Am J Epidemiol 1985; 122:226–233.
8. Forbes A, Williams R. Increasing age: an important adverse prognostic factor in hepatitis A virus infection. J R Coll Physicians Lond 1988; 22:237–239.
9. Lindsay KL, Hoofnagle JH. Serological tests for viral hepatitis. In: Kaplowitz N, ed. Liver and Biliary Diseaser. Baltimore: Williams & Wilkins, 1992:195–206.
10. Braconier J, Nordenfelt E. Serum hepatitis at a home for the aged. Scand J Infect Dis 1972; 4:72–82.
11. Wright R. Hepatitis B and the HbBAg carrier: an outbreak related to sexual contact. JAMA 1975; 232:717–721.
12. Chiaramonte M, Floreani A, Naccarato R. Hepatitis B virus infection in homes for the aged. J Med Virol 1982; 9:247–255.
13. Centers for Disease Control and Prevention. Nosocomial hepatitis B virus infection associated with reusable fingerstick blood sampling devices—Ohio and New York City, 1996. MMWR 1997; 46(RR-10):217–221.
14. Alter MJ, Margolis HS, Krawcynski K. The natural history of acquired hepatitis C in the United States. N Engl J Med 1992; 327:1899–1905.

15. Goodson J, Taylor P, Campion E, Richter J, Wands J. The clinical course of acute hepatitis in the elderly patient. Arch Intern Med 1982; 142:1485–1488.
16. Sonnenblick M, Oren R, Tur-Kaspa R. Non A, non B hepatitis in the aged. Postgrad Med J 1990; 66:462–464.
17. Laverdant C, Algayres J, Daly J, et al. Viral hepatitis in patients over 60 years of age: clinical, etiologic and developmental aspects. Gastroenterol Clin Biol 1989; 13:499–504.
18. Alter M. Epidemiology of hepatitis C in the West. Semin Liver Dis 1995; 15: 5–14.
19. Floreani A, Bertin T, Soffiati G, Naccarato R, Chiaramonte M. Anti-hepatitis C virus in the elderly: a seroepidemiological study in a home for the aged. Gerontology 1992; 38:214–216.
20. Simor A, Gordon M, Bishai F. Prevalence of hepatitis B surface antigen, hepatitis C antibody, and HIV-1 antibody among residents of a long-term care facility. J Am Geriatr Soc 1992; 40:218–220.
21. Rabicetta M, Attili A, Mele A, et al. Prevalence of hepatitis C virus antibodies and hepatitis C virus RNA in an urban population. J Med Virol 1992; 37:87–92.
22. Chien N, Dundoo G, Horani M, Osmack P, Morley J, Di Bisceglie A. Seroprevalence of viral hepatitis in an older nursing home population. J Am Geriatr Soc 1999; 47:1110–1113.
23. Marcus E, Dahoudi N, Tur-kaspa R. Hepatitis C virus infection among elderly patients in a geriatric hospital. Arch Gerontol Geriatr 1994; 19:213–221.
24. Baldo V, Floreani A, Menegon T, Angiolelli G, Trivello R. Prevalence of antibodies against hepatitis C virus in the elderly: a seroepidemiological study in a nursing home and in an open population. The Collaborative Group. Gerontology 2000; 46:194–198.
25. Sampietro M, Caputo L, Corbetta N, et al. Hepatitis G virus infection in the elderly. Ital J Gastroenterol Hepatol 1998; 30:524–527.
26. Dienstag JL, Issenlbacher KJ. Acute viral hepatitis. In: Kasper DL, Braunwald E, Hauser SL, Longo DL, Jameson JL, Fauci AS, eds. Harrison's Principles of Internal Medicine. 16th ed. New York: McGrow-Hill, 2005:1831–1833.
27. Lee W. Acute liver failure. N Engl J Med 1993; 329:1862–1872.
28. Bernuau J, Goudeau A, Poynard T, et al. Multivariate analysis of prognostic factors in fulminant hepatitis B. Hepatology 1986; 6:648–651.
29. Takahashi Y, Kumada H, Shimizu M, et al. A multicenter study on the prognosis of fulminant viral hepatitis: early prediction for liver transplantation. Hepatology 1994; 19:1065–1071.
30. MacMahon M, James O. Liver disease in the elderly. J Clin Gastroenterol 1994; 18:330–334.
31. Horiike N, Masumoto T, Nakanishi K, et al. Interferon therapy for patients more than 60 years of age with chronic hepatitis C. J Gastroenterol Hepatol 1995; 10:246–249.
32. Yamada G, Takatani M, Kishi F, et al. Efficacy of interferon alfa therapy in chronic hepatitis C patients depends primarily on hepatitis C RNA level. Hepatology 1995; 22:1351–1354.
33. Tong M, El-Farra N, Reikes A, Co RL. Clinical outcomes after transfusion-associated hepatitis C. N Engl J Med 1995; 332:1463–1466.

34. Sallie T, Di Bisceglie A. Viral hepatitis and hepatocellular carcinoma. Gastroen-
    terol Clin North Am 1994; 19:1065–1071.
35. McMahon B, Alberts S, Wainwright RB, Bulkow L, Lanier A. Hepatitis B-
    related sequelae: prospective study in 1400 hepatitis B surface antigen-positive
    Alaska native carriers. Arch Intern Med 1990; 150:1051–1054.
36. Mazzalla G, Accogli E, Sottili S. Alfa interferon treatment may prevent hepato-
    cellular carcinoma in HCV-related liver cirrhosis. J Hepatol 1996; 24:141–147.
37. Beasley R. Hepatitis B virus: the major etiology of hepatocellular carcinoma.
    Cancer 1988; 61:1942–1956.
38. Collier J, Curless R, Bassendine M, James O. Clinical features and prognosis of
    hepatocellular carcinoma in Britain with respect to advancing age. Age Ageing
    1994; 23:22–27.
39. National Institutes of Health. Management of hepatitis C. NIH consensus state-
    ment No. 105. 1997 March 24–26; 15(3):1–41.
40. Floreani A, Minola E, Carderi E, Ferrara F, Rizzotto ER, Baldo V. Are elderly
    patient poor candidates for pegylated interferon plus ribavirin in the treatment
    of chronic hepatitis C? J Am Geriatr Soc 2006; 54:549–550.
41. Smith PW, Rusnak PG. Infection prevention and control in the long-term
    facility. Am J Infect Control 1997; 25:488–512.
42. Centers for Disease Control and Prevention. Prevention of hepatitis A through
    active or passive immunization: recommendations of the Advisory Committee
    on Immunization Practices (ACIP). 1999; 48(RR-12):1–37.
43. Bader T. Hepatitis A vaccine. Am J Gastroenterol 1996; 91:217–222.
44. Centers for Disease Control and Prevention. Immunization of health-care work-
    ers: recommendations of the Advisory Committee on Immunization Practices
    (ACIP) and the Hospital Infection Control Practices Advisory Committee
    (HICPAC). MMWR 1997; 46(RR-18):1–42.
45. Centers for Disease Control and Prevention. Update on adult immunization:
    recommendations of the Immunization Practices Advisory Committee (ACIP).
    MMWR 1991.
46. Centers for Disease Control and Prevention. A comprehensive immunization
    strategy to eliminate transmission of hepatitis B virus infection in the United
    States MMWR December 2005.
47. Lok AS, McMahon BJ. Chronic Hepatitis B. Alexandria, VA: American Asso-
    ciation for the Study of Liver Diseases, 2004.
48. Centers for Disease Control and Prevention. Recommendations for prevention
    and control of Hepatitis C virus (HCV) infection and HCV-related chronic
    disease. MMWR 1998; 47(RR-19):1–39.
49. National Institutes of Health. Management of Hepatitis C; 2002. Rockville, MD:
    NIH, August 2002.

20

Conjunctivitis, Otitis, and Sinusitis

Deborah Moran

*Department of Internal Medicine, Charles R. Drew University of Medicine and
Science, and Martin Luther King, Jr.–Charles R. Drew Medical Center,
Los Angeles, California, U.S.A.*

Made Sutjita

*Division of Infectious Disease, Department of Internal Medicine,
Charles R. Drew University of Medicine and Science, and
Martin Luther King, Jr.–Charles R. Drew Medical Center,
Los Angeles, California, U.S.A.*

Kathleen Daretany

*Center for Psycho-Oncology Research, Dartmouth-Hitchcock Medical Center,
Dartmouth College, Lebanon, New Hampshire, U.S.A.*

KEY POINTS

1. A thorough medical history, physical examination, and medication history are necessary when evaluating a patient in a long-term care facility with a "red eye."
2. Chronic suppurative otitis media is only second in frequency to impacted cerumen among elderly patients with ear disease.
3. Malignant otitis externa in elderly patients with diabetes mellitus is a life-threatening infection.
4. Care providers must carefully consider the use of antibiotics for the treatment of sinusitis in the elderly population.
5. The utilization of the interdisciplinary team in the diagnosis and treatment of infectious disease in the elderly should not be overlooked.

CONJUNCTIVITIS

Epidemiology and Clinical Relevance

Conjunctivitis is a common infection in long-term care facilities (LTCFs). It is the most common inflammation of the eye and ocular adnexa (1). The frequency, however, varies between institutions (2). A prevalence of 0.3% to 3.4% has been reported in different studies (3), and there tends to be an increased frequency in more highly functionally impaired residents (3). Long-term care facilities provide an environment that is ideal to acquire and spread infection (4). Residents in these settings oftentimes share sources of air, food, water, and health care with visitors, staff, and residents who bring pathogens from both the hospital and community.

The various forms of infectious conjunctivitis are caused by viruses, *Chlamydia*, bacteria, parasites, and fungi (5). It can be difficult to determine a cause of conjunctivitis (i.e., differentiate between infectious, allergens, chemicals); however, conjunctivitis is usually benign and self-limited. Table 1 lists the various infectious causes of conjunctivitis.

The normal flora of the conjunctiva include *Staphylococcus epidermidis*, diphtheroids, and anaerobic flora. Coliforms are found in elderly debilitated patients. The conjunctiva does not usually have fungal organisms (5).

Similar to mucous membranes elsewhere in the body, the conjunctiva is a mucous membrane whose surface is composed of nonkeratinizing squamous epithelium, intermixed with goblet (mucous) cells, Langerhans cells (dendritic-appearing cells expressing class II antigen), and occasional dendritic melanocytes (7). Degenerative changes, which occur during the aging process, may affect conjunctival function and alter epithelial and stromal morphology. Consequent disorders include absorption of toxic irritants, amyloidosis, pinguecula, pterygium, and xerosis (5).

Clinical Manifestations

Given the frequent nonclassic presentation of acute illness in the frail elderly, the clinician should pay attention to any inciting events, time course, and any recent medication use. The physical examination focuses on the appearance of the periorbital skin, as well as other mucous membranes (nasal/oral), appearance of the conjunctiva, discharge, and any facial, lid, or corneal involvement (6). Table 2 lists the possible clinical presentation of a patient with conjunctivitis.

Diagnostic Approach

A thorough medical history, physical examination, and medication history are necessary when evaluating a patient in an LTCF with a "red eye." Though beyond the scope of this text, the clinician should consider and exclude possible sight-threatening conditions, such as a corneal ulcer, uveitis,

Table 1   Causes of Infectious Conjunctivitis

Viral conjunctivitis
  Adenovirus
  Herpes simplex virus
  Rubella
  Rubeola
  Influenza
  Epstein–Barr virus
  Papillomavirus
  Molluscum contagiosum
Bacterial conjunctivitis
  Staphylococcus spp.
  Corynebacterium diphtheriae
  Streptococcus pneumoniae
  Haemophilus influenzae
  Moraxella
  Neisseria spp.
  Enteric gram-negative rods
  Chlamydia trachomatis
Parasitic conjunctivitis
  Leishmania
  Encephalitozoon
  Phthirus pubis
  Demodex
Fungal conjunctivitis
  Candida spp.
  Blastomyces spp.
  Sporothrix schenckii

Source: From Ref. 6.

Table 2   Clinical Presentation of Infectious Conjunctivitis

Itching—common
Discharge—common
Conjunctival hyperemia (redness/injection)—common
Skin changes—some cases
Visual acuity—usually normal or mildly decreased
Preauricular adenopathy—often present
Eye pain—not common
Photophobia—not common
Visual loss—not common

Source: From Ref. 6.

and angle-closure glaucoma. Most residents with conjunctivitis will present with a painless discharge, normal vision, and normally reactive pupil. A mucopurulent or purulent discharge strongly suggests a bacterial infection (and the possibility of *Neisseria gonorrhoeae* infection should be considered when the discharge is copiously purulent) (8). A serous discharge is most commonly associated with a viral infection (8).

Therapeutic Interventions

In the absence of a culture or smear, the patient's age, environment, and ocular findings must be considered for the etiologic agent. In most cases, broad-spectrum topical antibiotics are the treatment of choice (9). Although most cases of bacterial conjunctivitis are self-limiting, treatment with antibiotics can lessen the patient's symptoms and the duration and chances of recurrence of the disease (9).

Cold compresses, lubricants, and ocular decongestants comprise the supportive therapy recommended for adenoviral infections (9). Topical antibiotics are not routinely used to treat viral conjunctivitis unless there is evidence of secondary bacterial infection (9). The treatment of herpes simplex conjunctivitis may include the use of antiviral agents, although there is no evidence that this results in a lower incidence of recurrent disease. Topical corticosteroids are specifically contraindicated for treating herpes simplex conjunctivitis (9). Effective management of conjunctivitis requires appropriate patient and staff education (see section "Prevention").

Prevention

Conjunctivitis is a common infection among nursing home residents. The hands of residents and nursing staff, and washing and bathing equipment may expose residents to an increased risk of infection (10). There has been little evaluation of methods to limit infection despite the high prevalence and incidence of infections in nursing homes (2). The practitioner should stress the importance of frequent hand washing by patients, family members, and staff; of using separate linens, towels, and washcloths; and of avoiding direct contact with infected material or individuals (9). Clear guidelines on the prevention of cross-infection are needed in LTCFs.

OTITIS MEDIA

Epidemiology and Clinical Relevance

Though oftentimes classified as a disease of children, otitis media also occurs in the frail elderly. Accordingly, chronic suppurative otitis media is only second in frequency to impacted cerumen among elderly patients with ear disease (11). It is important to differentiate between otitis media with effusion (OME) and acute bacterial otitis media. OME is defined as fluid in the middle ear without local or systemic illness (12). Because OME may often occur after a viral upper respiratory tract infection, fluid may become "trapped" in the middle ear. In contrast, symptoms and signs of acute bacterial otitis media occur when fluid in the middle ear becomes infected (12,13). Acute bacterial otitis media is characterized by purulent fluid behind a bulging tympanic membrane (12). The required criteria for acute otitis media include inflammation of and fluid in the middle ear (14,15). Acute otitis media usually occurs after a viral upper respiratory infection. The congestion causes occlusion of the eustachian tubes and creates a negative pressure with resultant serous effusion. This effusion may act as a medium for microbial growth, leading to bacterial overgrowth and bacterial otitis media. The most common microorganisms causing otitis media include *Streptococcus pneumoniae*, nontypable *Haemophilus influenzae*, and *Moraxella catarrhalis* (12,16). Untreated infection may cause tympanic membrane perforation, extension into adjacent tissues causing mastoiditis, or spread to the central nervous system causing meningitis.

Clinical Manifestations

Patients with acute otitis media usually complain of earache, ear drainage, hearing loss, and dizziness. Though the elderly patient may not always present with "classic" findings, the presence of dizziness and facial nerve paralysis suggests erosion of the labyrinthine bone. Labyrinthitis or vestibular neuritis is usually caused by a viral infection. It occasionally may be secondary to extension of bacterial otitis media. Signs of vestibular neuritis include spontaneous nystagmus and unsteadiness (17). Patients with labyrinthitis require referral to an audiologist or otoneurologist for an audiogram or electronystagmography.

Diagnostic Approach

Removal of cerumen and other debris from the auditory canal allows optimal visualization of the entire tympanic membrane. In bacterial otitis media, otoscopy usually reveals a bulging tympanic membrane and purulent fluid behind this membrane. Culture and sensitivity testing of the middle ear discharge assists in the microbiological diagnosis and in guiding antibiotic therapy of otitis media in the elderly patient. Occasionally, high-resolution computed tomography (CT) of the temporal bone assists in demonstrating the status of the middle ear and the surrounding anatomy. CT also assists with excluding an underlying cholesteatoma. Cholesteatoma is an epithelial growth that occurs in the middle ear behind the tympanic membrane. Over time, the cholesteatoma can increase in size and destroy the surrounding delicate hearing bones of the middle ear ossicles and may further contribute to sensory impairment of the long-term care resident. Table 3 lists common organisms and therapeutic treatment for otitis.

Table 3 Most Common Organisms and Therapy for Otitis

Site	Organism	Recommended antibiotic therapy
Otitis media	*Streptococcus pneumoniae*	High-dose amoxicillin or amoxicillin–clavulanate
	Haemophilus influenzae	Alternate: cephalosporins (e.g., cefuroxime or cefdinir)
	Moraxella catarrhalis	Penicillin or beta-lactam allergy: fluoroquinolone, treatment duration = 10–14 day
Otitis externa	Usually: *Pseudomonas aeruginosa*	Usually use two antibiotics of different classes: ceftazidime ciprofloxacin cefepime carbapenems or piperacillin with tobramycin

Source: From Refs. 12, 16, 18, and 19.

Therapeutic Interventions

High-dose amoxicillin or amoxicillin–clavulanate are the preferred agent(s) in the treatment of patients who are not allergic to penicillin. The alternative antibiotics are the cephalosporins (e.g., cefuroxime or cefdinir). For penicillin or beta-lactam allergic patients, fluoroquinolones (such as levafloxacin or moxifloxacin) are reasonable choices. Duration of antibiotic therapy in the elderly with otitis media is usually between 10 and 14 days.

OTITIS EXTERNA

Epidemiology and Clinical Relevance

Elderly patients with diabetes mellitus are prone to a progressive outer ear infection: malignant otitis externa or necrotizing otitis externa. This infection is usually caused by *Pseudomonas aeruginosa* and is isolated from aural drainage in more than 90% of cases (20). Other organisms (such as *Klebsiella oxytoca* and *S. epidermidis*) have been reported to cause malignant otitis externa (18,19). One study (21) demonstrated in patients with a mean age of 62 years that the main risk factor for acquiring malignant otitis externa is diabetes mellitus. A state of immunodeficiency and microangiopathy in uncontrolled diabetes mellitus may allow for the invasiveness of the infecting organism. Changes in the aging skin, including dryness, increased epithelial sloughing, and increased production of thicker and drier cerumen, may increase local debris, allow obstruction, and lead to development of ear canal infection.

The patient's ear may be exposed to *Pseudomonas* during bathing or during ear irrigation for cerumen impaction. Once the organism penetrates the skin of the auditory canal, it may spread along the cartilage, vascular and fascial planes, causing facial nerve (and other adjacent cranial nerves) paralysis, sinus thrombosis, temporal bone osteomyelitis, and even death (22). The mortality rate is high if not managed promptly.

Clinical Manifestations

Malignant otitis externa should be suspected in patients with diabetes mellitus who do not respond promptly to treatment for routine external otitis. It may also be suspected in patients with otalgia disproportionate to their clinical findings. The involved ear may be pruritic, erythematous, edematous, increasingly painful, and associated with a purulent drainage. Subsequently, a conductive hearing loss can be observed.

Diagnostic Approach

Culture and sensitivity testing of the ear discharge, preferably prior to the start of antibiotic therapy, is important for microbiologic diagnostic confirmation. In most cases, *P. aeruginosa* is detected. Imaging studies, such as CT scan (23) of the temporal bone, can be performed quickly on admission. Opacification of the mastoid air cell spaces or demineralization of bone on CT scan suggests a more invasive infection. Technetium-99m bone scan detects temporal bone osteomyelitis early in the course of the disease process. It is considered to be the gold standard for diagnosing malignant otitis externa (24). If granulation tissue is present, it should be biopsied to exclude other inflammatory or neoplastic processes.

Therapeutic Interventions

Treatment of malignant otitis externa generally includes antibiotic therapy and surgical debridement of the ear canal. Any necrotic cartilage and adjacent bone should be debrided. The antibiotic of choice should be active against *P. aeruginosa* and other responsible organisms. Due to the seriousness of this infection and potential of antibiotic resistance among many *Pseudomonas* strains, it is a common practice to begin treatment of *P. aeruginosa* infection with two antibiotics. Treatment, however, with a single agent, such as ceftazidime (25) or ciprofloxacin (26), has been successful. Cefepime, the so-called fourth-generation cephalosporin, can also be prescribed. Carbapenems or piperacillin, in combination with tobramycin, has been shown to be effective. However, due to its nephrotoxicity and ototoxicity, particularly in elderly patients, close monitoring of tobramycin levels and side effects are required. As in osteomyelitis, the length of antibiotic treatment is generally six weeks or longer (depending on the clinical response). Erythrocyte sedimentation rate and gallium-67 single photon emission CT scanning have been useful in accessing treatment response and for selecting therapy endpoints (27). Therapy with other ear preparations (e.g., polymixin B + neomycin + hydrocortisone suspension) alone is not recommended for life-threatening malignant otitis externa.

Prevention

Optimal blood sugar control in elderly patients with diabetes mellitus and proper hand washing techniques may play a role in the prevention of malignant otitis externa.

SINUSITIS

Epidemiology and Clinical Relevance

It is estimated that sinusitis affects 32 million adults in the United States each year (28). Among these individuals, the elderly and others with immunosuppression are at high risk for invasive sinus infection. "Infections are responsible for 30% of deaths in the elderly and are the most frequent reason for hospitalization" (29). Among those infected, there happens to be about 0.5% to 2% of colds and influenza-like infections that have complications of acute bacterial sinusitis (30). Therefore, due to its prevalence, the discussion of sinusitis in the geriatric population is significant.

A viral infection is the most prevalent condition linked with acute bacterial sinusitis. However, infections that impair sinus drainage and changes, such as mechanical obstruction of the nose, can increase a person's risk of bacterial sinusitis (30).

It is important for the treating clinician to differentiate between bacterial and viral etiologies in order to correctly diagnosis and treat a sinus infection. Although true bacterial sinusitis may present in only a small number of patients, along with viral sinusitis it remains a severe health matter (28). When formulating differential diagnoses, we are challenged to decipher if the presenting infection has a bacterial or viral etiology in order to provide appropriate usage of antibacterial therapies. The concern of the growing problem of antimicrobial resistance among common bacterial infections may be accredited to the inappropriate use of antibiotics for viral infections (28).

Clinical Manifestations

Sinusitis refers to an inflammatory process concerning the four structures surrounding the nasal cavities; the maxillary sinus is the most commonly involved. In a normally functioning sinus cavity, the respiratory epithelium (which produces mucus that is transported out by ciliary action) lines the cavity. The sinuses remain sterile in normal circumstances regardless of the close proximity to the bacterium-filled nasal passages, and mucus does not usually accumulate. Typical symptoms and signs of infection present when the secretions are retained due to impaired or absent ciliary clearance, or obstructed sinus ostia (31).

It is challenging to distinguish acute sinusitis from chronic sinusitis due to the fact that both produce similar symptoms and signs. Table 4 lists the common clinical manifestations of sinusitis.

Diagnostic Approach

It is believed that sinus involvement is present in most cases of the common cold. The difficulty is recognizing the small percentage of cases that are compounded with secondary bacterial infection (30). Clinically, decision making is often guided by illness duration (31). Be aware that acute bacterial sinusitis is rare in patients whose symptoms have lasted less than seven days. It is now the recommendation to diagnose a bacterial infection in individuals with appropriate symptoms, such as facial or tooth pain combined with purulent nasal discharge, which have continued for greater than seven days (31). "There is general agreement that the diagnosis of acute bacterial sinusitis is based on clinical criteria and that imaging studies are not routinely necessary for diagnosis" (28). Sinus radiography or CT is not recommended for standard cases. If one is evaluating a recurrent or chronic sinusitis, CT is the gold standard for diagnosis.

Therapeutic Intervention

One study identified the elderly at risk for respiratory tract infections. The authors of this study examined the safety and efficacy of gatifloxacin in adults with a diagnosis of community-acquired pneumonia, acute bacterial exacerbation of chronic bronchitis, or acute uncomplicated maxillary sinusitis. Participants were given gatifloxacin 400 mg once daily for 7 to 14 days. Cure rates for community-acquired pneumonia, acute bacterial exacerbation of

Table 4   List of Common Clinical Manifestations of Sinusitis

Common clinical manifestations of sinusitis
  The area over the affected sinus may be tender or swollen
  Maxillary pain, toothache, headache
  Pain behind and between the eyes
  Malaise—general
  Yellow or green purulent rhinorrhea
  Swollen mucous membranes may cause the affected sinus to
    appear opaque on X-ray
  Halitosis (usually associated with bacterial infection)

Source: From Refs. 31 and 36.

chronic bronchitis, and sinusitis ranged from 91.1% to 96.2% for those aged 65 to 79 and 89.5% to 94.8% for those at least 80 years old (29).

There are few studies published evaluating the use of short-term oral therapy for acute sinusitis (32). However, the management of sinusitis presents a challenge to clinicians, because of the difficulty in establishing when to prescribe antibiotic therapy (28). "Although there are no consistent recommendations regarding treatment of choice for acute bacterial sinusitis, there is general agreement that the antimicrobial agent should be active against *S. pneumoniae* and *H. influenzae*" (28).

Although it is necessary for physicians to diagnose and prescribe antibiotics when appropriate, it is also imperative that they utilize the entire interdisciplinary team, including other physicians, nurses, and pharmacists in the process. Consultation with a pharmacist should take place when considering the use of antibiotics in the frail elderly in a long-term care setting. Bearing in mind the vulnerability of the frail elderly and the possibility of adverse reactions to the antimicrobial agent, the physician should consult with a pharmacist and follow up with education for the other staff, particularly nurses, who will be administering the medication (32). Table 5 outlines the basic approach to treatment of sinusitis in the adult population.

Control in Long-Term Care/Infection Control

It is known that infections are common in LTCFs. This presents a great challenge for clinicians who take responsibility for protecting patients and at times inadvertently expose them to more pathogens. In the near future, there will be an increase in the number of individuals living in extended care facilities secondary to the aging of the population. It is our duty to be mindful of infection

Table 5 Treatment Approach to Sinusitis

Acute sinusitis	Focus on comfort therapy to treat symptoms Nasal saline lavage Decongestants/antihistamines NSAIDs and acetaminophen
Sinusitis (<7 day duration)	Focus on comfort therapy to treat symptoms Nasal saline lavage Decongestants/antihistamines NSAIDs and acetaminophen
Bacterial sinusitis (>7 day duration)	Antibiotic therapy Amoxicillin for mild to moderate cases; consultation with ENT

Abbreviations: NSAIDs, nonsteroidal anti-inflammatory drugs; ENT, ear, nose, and throat.
Source: From Refs. 31 and 33.

control and measures to control infections in these settings. "In the last two decades, an increasing number of LTCFs have developed infection control programs with surveillance and control activities" (34).

Because of the population and environmental setting, LTCFs provide an exceptional opportunity for the transmission of infections. All LTCFs should have infection control programs. However, it is imperative that the program be designed around the needs of the residents in the specific institution, taking into consideration available resources as well (35) (see Chapter 9).

Prevention

Recent publications of clinical trials in long-term care settings with respect to infection prevention have been uniformly negative. These trials have been helpful, however, in focusing on the extent to which infections are preventable. One must not forget that prevention strategies should also focus on the increasing complexity of medicine in LTCFs (34).

The most effective manner in which to prevent infections among the elderly in LTCFs is to maintain universal precautions and provide residents and staff with appropriate education. All facilities should have written procedures and guidelines regarding isolation precautions, hand washing, and the handling of sharps.

SUGGESTED READING

Guay D. Short-course antimicrobial therapy for bacterial respiratory tract infections: staving off resistance and enhancing adherence in the elderly. Elder Care 2004; 4:1–4.

Rubin Grandis J, Branstetter BF IV, Yu VL. The changing face of malignant (necrotising) external otitis: clinical, radiological, and anatomic correlations. Lancet Infect Dis 2004; 4:34–39.

Strausbaugh LJ, Sukumar SR, Joseph CL. Infectious disease outbreaks in nursing homes: an unappreciated hazard for frail elderly persons. Clin Infect Dis 2003; 36:870–876.

REFERENCES

1. O'Brien TP. Conjunctivitis. In: Mandell GL, Bennett JE, Dolin R, eds. Principles and Practice of Infectious Diseases. Vol. 1. 5th ed. New York, NY: Churchill Livingstone, 2000:1249–1257.
2. Nicolle LE, Strausbaugh LJ, Garibaldi RA. Infections and antibiotic resistance in nursing homes. Clin Microbiol Rev 1996; 9:1–17.
3. Bousthca E, Nicolle LE. Conjunctivitis in a long-term care facility. Infect Control Hosp Epidemiol 1995; 16:210–216.
4. Strausbaugh LJ, Sukumar SR, Joseph CL. Infectious disease outbreaks in nursing homes: an unappreciated hazard for frail elderly persons. Clin Infect Dis 2003; 36:870–876.

5. Rodrigues MM, Hidayat AA. Conjunctival and corneal pathology. In: Albert DA, Jakobiec FA, eds. Principles Practice of Ophthalmology. 2nd ed. Philadelphia, PA: W.B. Saunders Company, 2000:3609–3634.

6. Barnes SD, Pavan-Langston D, Azar DT. Microbial conjunctivitis. In: Mandell GL, Bennett JE, Dolin R, eds. Principles and Practice of Infectious Diseases. 6th ed. Philadelphia, PA: Elsevier Inc., 2005:1387–1394.

7. Jakobiec FA, Iwamoto T. The ocular adnexa: lids, conjunctiva, and orbit. In: Fine BS, Yanoff M, eds. Ocular Histology: a Text and Atlas. 2nd ed. Hagerstown: Harper & Row, 1979:308–310.

8. Jackson WB. Differentiating conjunctivitis of diverse origins. Surv Ophthalmol 1993; 38(suppl):91–104.

9. American Optometric Association. Care of the Patient with Conjunctivitis. Vol. 11. 2nd ed. St. Louis, MO: American Optometric Association, 2002:1–55.

10. Hu M. Preventing conjunctivitis in nursing homes. Prof Nurse 1997; 12:875–877.

11. Ologe FE, Segun-Busari S, Abdulraheem IS, Afolabi AO. Ear diseases in elderly hospital patients in Nigeria. J Gerontol A Biol Sci Med Sci 2005; 60A:404–406.

12. Hendley JO. Otitis media. N Engl J Med 2002; 347:1169–1174.

13. Cook K, Walsh M. Otitis media. (Accessed August 2005, at http://www.emedicine.com/emerg/topic351.htm.)

14. Dowell SF, Marcy SM, Phillips WR, Gerber MA, Schwartz B. Otitis media—principles of judicious use of antimicrobial agents. Pediatrics 1998; 101(suppl): 165–171.

15. Takata GS, Chan LS, Shekelle P, Morton SC, Mason W, Marcy SM. Evidence assessment of management of acute otitis media. The role of antibiotics in treatment of uncomplicated acute otitis media. Pediatrics 2001; 108:239–247.

16. Block SL. Causative pathogens, antibiotic resistance and therapeutic considerations in acute otitis media. Pediatr Infect Dis J 1997; 16:449–456.

17. Silvoniemi P. Vestibular neuronitis: an otoneurological evaluation. Acta Otolaryngol 1988; 453:1–72.

18. Garcia Rodriguez JA, Montes Martinez I, Gomez Gonzalez JL, Ramos Macias A, Lopez Alburquerque T. A case of malignant external otitis involving *Klebsiella oxytoca*. Eur J Clin Microbiol Infect Dis 1992; 11:75–77.

19. Barrow HN, Levenson MJ. Necrotizing 'malignant' external otitis caused by *Staphylococcus epidermidis*. Arch Otolaryngol Head Neck Surg 1992; 118:94–96.

20. Rubin Grandis J, Branstetter BF IV, Yu VL. The changing face of malignant (necrotising) external otitis: clinical, radiological, and anatomic correlations. Lancet Infect Dis 2004; 4:34–39.

21. Lasisi OA, Nwaorgu OG. Behavioural pattern of malignant otitis externa: 10-year review in Ibadan. Afr J Med Sci 2001; 30:221–223.

22. Rubin J, Yu VL. Malignant external otitis: insights into pathogenesis, clinical manifestations, diagnosis, and therapy. Am J Med 1988; 85:391–398.

23. Guy RL, Wylie E, Hickey A, Tonge KA. Computed tomography in malignant external otitis. Clin Radiol 1991; 43:166–170.

24. Parisier SC, Lucente FE, Som PM, Hirschman SZ, Arnold LM, Roffman JD. Nuclear scanning in necrotizing progressive "malignant" external otitis. Laryngoscope 1982; 92:1016–1019.

25. Johnson MP, Ramphal R. Malignant external otitis: report on therapy with ceftazidime and review of therapy and prognosis. Rev Infect Dis 1990; 12:173–180.
26. Gehanno P. Ciprofloxacin in the treatment of malignant external otitis. Chemotherapy 1994; 40(suppl 1):35–40.
27. Stokkel MP, Boot CN, van Eck-Smit BL. SPECT gallium scintigraphy in malignant external otitis: initial staging and follow-up. Laryngoscope 1996; 106: 338–340.
28. Sande M, Gwaltney J. Acute community-acquired bacterial sinusitis: continuing challenges and current management. Clin Infect Dis 2004; 39:S151–S158.
29. Nicholoson S, High K, Gothelf S, et al. Gatifloxacin in community-based treatment of acute respiratory tract infections in the elderly. Diagn Microbiol Infect Dis 2005; 44:109–116.
30. Gwaltney J. Acute sinusitis and rhinosinusitis. Up To Date online 13.2. (Accessed July 2005, at www.utdol.com.)
31. Kasper DL, Braunwald E, Fauci AS, et al. Infections of the upper respiratory tract. Harrison's online. (Accessed July 2005, at www.accessmedicine.com.)
32. Guay D. Short-course antimicrobial therapy for bacterial respiratory tract infections: staving off resistance and enhancing adherence in the elderly. Elder Care 2004; 4:1–4.
33. Gonzales R, Kulner J. Current practice guidelines in primary care 2005. (Accessed July 2005, at www.accessmedicine.com.)
34. Nicolle L. Preventing infections in non-hospital settings: long-term care. Emerg Infect Dis 2001; 7:205–207.
35. Richards M, Cordell R. Principles of infection control in long term care facilities. Up To Date online 13.2. (Accessed July 2005, at www.uptodate.com.)
36. Beers M, and Berkow R, (eds). Merck manual of diagnosis and therapy. Section 7: Ear, Nose, and Throat Disorders. 2005.

21

Human Immunodeficiency Virus Infection in the Nursing Home

Allen S. Funnyé

Department of Internal Medicine, Charles R. Drew University of Medicine and Science, and Martin Luther King, Jr.–Charles R. Drew Medical Center, Los Angeles, California, U.S.A.

KEY POINTS

1. The aging of the population and increasing prevalence of human immunodeficiency virus/acquired immune deficiency syndrome (HIV/AIDS) in older patients will lead to an increase in the number of residents in nursing homes with HIV/AIDS.
2. HIV/AIDS may be a chronic disease and have prominent effects on functional capacity and psychosocial issues in elder nursing home residents.
3. In elderly nursing home residents, clinical manifestations of AIDS may be atypical or more severe and progressive.
4. Comorbid diseases, such as diabetes mellitus, coronary heart disease, and hyperlipidemia, complicate AIDS in older patients and may affect the choices of antiretrovirals and other therapy.
5. Trends in substance abuse, racial disparities in AIDS cases, gender, and regional issues will affect the landscape of future nursing home care for AIDS residents.

INTRODUCTION

Acquired immune deficiency syndrome (AIDS) was first reported in 1981, and in 1983 the virus causing AIDS was identified. AIDS—a syndrome of immunodeficiency affecting primarily the CD4+ lymphocytes—has a wide spectrum of disease manifestations. It has gone from a disease in which the life span averaged 10 years to a more chronic disease with increasing prevalence (1). Human immunodeficiency virus (HIV) has been known to affect primarily younger individuals and most research has addressed the needs of this group; however, HIV is becoming increasingly known as a cause of morbidity and death in the older population. The aging of the population makes AIDS more likely to be encountered in individuals aged 65 years and older. With the increasing prevalence of HIV/AIDS and the aging of the population, the numbers of HIV infections are likely to increase in long-term care facilities (LTCFs) (1,2). HIV infection in the nursing home population involves significant psychosocial issues, and special considerations for rehabilitation, may present with atypical clinical manifestations, and may be associated with comorbidities that may affect therapy.

GENERAL EPIDEMIOLOGY

An estimated 1,039,000 to 1,185,000 persons at the end of 2003 in the United States were living with HIV/AIDS. Upwards of 40,000 persons may become infected with HIV yearly according to Centers for Disease Control and Prevention estimates (3). The decreases previously seen in the number of AIDS cases began to level off during the years 1999–2003. During that period there was a 15% decrease in AIDS cases reported in the age group 25 to 34, but other age groups shown in Table 1 increased. The 35 to 44 age group accounted for 41% of AIDS cases in 2003. At the end of 2003, 405,926 persons were living with AIDS in the United States and, of this, 41% were in the age group 35 to 44, 23% in the age group 45 to 54, 7% in the age group 55 to 64, and 2% aged 65 and older (4). The general epidemiology of HIV/AIDS has implications for the long-term care of individuals. Trends in the epidemic that may necessitate or affect nursing home care include substance abuse, racial disparities, the regions of residence, and gender issues.

Drug Abuse

Drug abuse continues to be a major cause of HIV infection. In the year 2003, 11% of male and 12% of female HIV infections were related to substance abuse. The cumulative totals through 2003 were 14%. In addition, 4% of infections resulted from sex with an intravenous drug abuser (4). Behaviors can have a direct effect on contracting the virus through needle exposures or indirectly by increasing risky behaviors leading to the acquisition of the virus. In the early and middle phases of the HIV epidemic, many AIDS patients with substance abuse were admitted to a skilled nursing facility. Movements were under way to provide special HIV sections in nursing

Table 1 Estimated Numbers and Percentages of Acquired Immune Deficiency Syndrome Cases by Year of Diagnosis in United States, 1999–2003

Age at diagnosis	Year of diagnosis										Cumulative through 2003[a]	
	1999		2000		2001		2002		2003			
	Number	w/%	Number	w/%	Number	w/%	Number	w/%	Number	w/%	Number	w/%
<13	187	0.45	117	0.28	119	0.29	105	0.25	59	0.14	9419	1.01
13–14	57	0.14	56	0.14	76	0.14	68	0.16	59	0.14	891	0.10
15–24	1541	3.73	1642	3.98	1625	4.02	1810	4.38	1991	4.61	37,599	4.04
25–34	11,349	27.44	10,385	25.17	9947	25.43	9504	23.02	9605	22.25	311,137	33.46
35–44	17,165	41.51	17,295	41.91	16,890	42.36	17,008	41.19	17,633	40.84	365,432	39.29
45–54	8099	19.58	8566	20.76	8929	20.98	9310	22.55	10,051	23.28	148,347	15.95
55–64	2218	5.36	2422	5.87	2468	5.93	2724	6.60	2888	6.69	43,451	4.67
>65	739	1.79	783	1.90	779	1.92	759	1.84	886	2.05	13,711	1.47
Total	41,355		41,266		40,833		41,288		43,172		929,987	

[a]Includes persons with a diagnosis of AIDS from the beginning of the epidemic through 2003.
Source: From Ref. 4.

homes in anticipation of the rising incidence and prevalence of AIDS (5). The introduction of protease inhibitors (PIs) in the 1990s had a dramatic effect on both survival and AIDS disabilities, such as myopathies, dementias, and wasting syndromes. Nevertheless, some substance abusers, because of a late diagnosis or a lack of adherence to medications, still develop these clinical manifestations and may need the services of a LTCF.

Racial Disparities

The burden of HIV has disproportionately impacted blacks and hispanics. For the period 1999–2003, AIDS cases by year of diagnosis for blacks went from 48% of the reported AIDS cases in 1999 to 50% in 2003. Blacks represented 39% of the cumulative total of AIDS cases through 2003. AIDS in Hispanics remained stable during that period, with 20% of the yearly AIDS totals and 18% of the cumulative totals through 2003. The incidence in whites during the same period decreased from 31% to 28% (4). Table 2 shows the yearly totals of AIDS cases for the period and the cumulative totals through 2003. Whereas blacks make up approximately 12% of the population and Hispanics 13%, they are disproportionately affected with HIV/AIDS. As the population ages, the number of blacks and Hispanics in long-term care (LTC) will increase. In comparison to traditional nursing home residents, older African Americans may have more complex comorbidities and more acute symptoms.

Gender Issues

The majority of current and cumulative AIDS cases are in men. Seventy-five percent of all AIDS cases were males in 2003; however, during the period of 1999–2003 there was a 15% increase in the number of female AIDS cases reported (4).

Regional Issues

The southern region of the United States has the highest proportion of HIV/AIDS cases. In 2003 compared with 2002, there was a 9% increase in AIDS cases in the Northwest, 6% increase in the South, 4% in the Midwest. There was a decrease of new AIDS cases by 3% in the West. The regional increases of AIDS cases are shown in Table 3. Increased rates are expected to occur in rural areas, especially in the rural South (4,5).

EPIDEMIOLOGY IN OLDER ADULTS

As illustrated in Table 1, from 1999 through the year 2003 the number of AIDS cases went from 739 to 886 in persons aged 65 and older. This represents a 16% increase. The total for the age group 55 to 64 went from 2218 to

Table 2 Estimated Numbers of Acquired Immune Deficiency Syndrome Cases by Year of Diagnosis and Race, 1999–2003

Race/ethnicity	Year of diagnosis											Cumulative through 2003[a]	
	1999		2000		2001		2002		2003				
	Number	w/%	Number	w/%	Number	w/%	Number	w/%	Number	w/%		Number	w/%
White, not Hispanic	12,626	31	12,047	29	11,620	29	11,960	29	12,222	28		376,834	40.60
Black, not Hispanic	19,960	48	20,312	49	20,291	50	20,476	50	21,304	50		368,169	39.67
Hispanic	8141	20	8233	20	8204	20	8021	20	8757	20		172,993	18.64
Asian/Pacific Islander	369	1	373	1	409	1	452	1	497	1		7166	0.77
American-Indian/Alaska native	162	0	186	0	179	0	196	0	196	0		3026	0.33
Totals	41,258		41,151		40,703		41,105		42,976			928,188	

[a]Includes persons with a diagnosis of AIDS from the beginning of the epidemic through 2003.
Source: From Ref. 4.

Table 3 Estimated Number of Acquired Immune Deficiency Syndrome Cases by Region of Residence in United States, 1999–2003

Region of residence	Year of diagnosis										Cumulative through 2003[a]	
	1999		2000		2001		2002		2003			
	Number	w/%	Number	w/%	Number	w/%	Number	w/%	Number	w/%	Number	w/%
Northeast	11,885	29	12,516	30	11,350	28	10,551	26	11,461	27	285,040	31
Midwest	4069	10	4139	10	4094	10	4337	11	4498	10	91,926	10
South	17,224	42	16,757	41	17,693	43	18,482	45	19,609	45	337,409	36
West	6892	17	6661	16	6468	16	6843	17	6667	15	186,100	20
Other[b]	1286	3	1194	3	1228	3	1075	3	935	2	29,511	3
Total	41,356		41,267		40,833		41,289		43,171		929,985	

[a]Includes persons with a diagnosis of AIDS from the beginning of the epidemic through 2003.
[b]U.S. dependencies, possessions, and associated nations.
Source: From Ref. 4.

2888, an increase of 23%. The cumulative totals for ages 55 to 64 were 43,451 and for those aged 65 and older through 2003 were 13,711. During the mid-1990s, the rate of increase in AIDS cases in the over-50 age group was among the highest in the United States. Through December of 2000, the percentage of AIDS cases reported in the United States in those over-50 years of age at the time of diagnosis was approximately 11%. Racial disparities continue in the older age groups. Older African American males and females are disproportionately affected by AIDS, representing 50% of female cases over 50 and 35% of male cases over 50, while representing only 12% of the population (6). Tables 4 and 5 illustrate the cumulative numbers of AIDS cases by older age and race through 2001.

Drug abuse and its association with HIV infection in older individuals have not been frequently appreciated. The percentage of those over 50 with HIV infection related to drug abuse was 8% in 1988, 11% in 1991, and 17% in 2000 (6). The prevalence of older people living with HIV infection is difficult to ascertain. Older people at risk do not get tested as often as younger people, and until recently HIV infection has not been a reportable disease in many states. This may underestimate the true prevalence of disease. It is possible that as many as 60,000 people over the age of 60 are now living with HIV infection. Because by the year 2030 the number of individuals aged 65 and older will double to more than 70 million (20% of the population), in the future this may result in an even higher prevalence of HIV infection in this older age group (7). The numbers of individuals in nursing homes who are elderly and have HIV/AIDS are difficult to ascertain. The 1999 National Nursing Home Survey found that less than 1% of surveyed nursing homes in the United States provided specialty HIV/AIDS services. The higher

Table 4 Acquired Immune Deficiency Syndrome Cases > Age 50 by Male Sex, Age at Diagnosis, and Race/Ethnicity, Reported Through December 2001, United States

Male age at diagnosis (yr)	White, not Hispanic		Black, not Hispanic		Hispanic		Grand total	
	No.	Male grand total (%)	No.	Male grand total (%)	No.	Male grand total (%)	No.	%
50–54	17,498	23.16	12,959	17.15	5861	7.76	36,318	48.07
55–59	9337	12.36	6987	9.25	3242	4.29	19,566	25.90
60–64	5139	6.80	3819	5.05	1769	2.34	10,727	14.20
65 or older	4249	5.62	3242	4.29	1455	1.93	8946	11.84
Male total	36,223	47.94	27,007	35.74	12,327	16.31	75,557	100.00

Source: From Ref. 6.

Table 5 Acquired Immune Deficiency Syndrome Cases > Age 50 by Female Sex, Age at Diagnosis, and Race/Ethnicity, Reported Through December 2001, United States

Female age at diagnosis (yr)	White, not Hispanic		Black, not Hispanic		Hispanic		Grand total	
	No.	Female grand total (%)	No.	Female grand total (%)	No.	Female grand total (%)	No.	%
50–54	1309	9.27	3447	24.42	1245	8.82	6062	42.94
55–59	816	5.78	1865	13.21	750	5.31	3479	24.64
60–64	519	3.68	1103	7.81	411	2.91	2069	14.66
65 or older	1044	7.40	1073	7.60	355	2.51	2507	17.76
Female total	3688	26.12	7488	53.04	2761	19.56	14,117	100.00

Source: From Ref. 6.

prevalence of HIV in older Americans may create a situation where LTCFs may care for or be required to treat more HIV/AIDS residents. This is of increasing concern to those who manage nursing homes. Increased rates will occur in rural areas whose ability to provide care may be limited (5).

LONG-TERM CARE FACILITIES

Long-term care includes a broad range of services to individuals with decreased functional capacity and chronic disabilities. Demand for nursing home care is driven by the number of frail elderly with functional and psychosocial disabilities, social support systems, and the availability of community-based resources (8). The long-term care system is being transformed by alternatives to nursing homes, such as assisted living and continuing-care retirement communities, community-based centers, and the home. Less than 5% of elderly individuals, approximately 1.4 million, live in nursing homes. The transformation is being driven in part by consumer demand, which is expected to grow as the population ages. LTCFs meet primarily the needs of the elderly, but other groups, such as those with disabilities and AIDS, also benefit from these services (9).

AIDS Residents in LTCFs

Limited data are available on elderly residents of nursing homes with HIV infection. Using the Minimum Data Set, one study analyzed data for residents admitted with HIV with and without dementia to nursing homes during the period from June 22, 1998, through January 17, 2000 (10). There were 1074 residents admitted with dementia (other than Alzheimer's) with

HIV and 4040 with HIV without dementia. The total number of HIV admissions was 5114 during the period. Of the HIV residents with dementia, 72% were men, and the mean age was 48.5 years. The majority were in the age group 31 to 40 (27%), and 17.5% were older than 60. Blacks made up the majority with 53.2%, whites 31.9%, and Hispanics 14.2%. Of the HIV residents without dementia, 68.7% were men, and the mean age was 43.4 years. The majority were in the age group 41 to 50 (38%), and 7.5% were older than 60. Blacks comprised the majority with 60.9%, whites 21.3%, and Hispanics 16.7%. Twenty-five percent of all residents with HIV/AIDS residing in nursing homes during the study period were over the age of 50.

The minimum data set from 175,000 assessments has been used to calculate the activities of daily living (ADL) scores for general nursing home residents. The average for the ADL long scale was 15.24, and 8.73 for the ADL short scale. The higher the value the more dependent the resident. In contrast to general nursing home residents, residents with HIV were less physically dependent at the time of their admission. Recently admitted residents with HIV who had dementia averaged 11.0 on the ADL long scale and 6.6 on the ADL short scale. Other residents with HIV and without dementia recently admitted to nursing homes were even less physically dependent according to ADL scales, averaging 7.6 on the ADL long scale and 4.5 on the ADL short scale. These results show that residents with HIV tended to be much less physically dependent at admission than other nursing home residents. This may reflect the younger average age for HIV patients; nevertheless, HIV residents with dementia were substantially more physically dependent than other residents with HIV, as measured by these same ADL scales.

HIV-associated dementia affects between 15% and 20% of people with HIV disease and is characterized by disabling cognitive, behavioral, and motor impairments. Only one of five HIV residents with dementia was independent in cognitive skills for daily decision making, compared with three of five other residents with HIV who were independent in these skills (10). The prospect of an increasing prevalence of HIV-associated dementia due to longer life expectancies for people with HIV increases the role of the nursing home in the treatment of late-stage HIV disease. Nursing homes can provide a cost-effective alternative to the acute care hospital when people with HIV can no longer receive appropriate care using only home- and community-based services. A secondary analysis of data obtained from three nursing home studies identified key issues addressing older African Americans with HIV/AIDS residing in nursing homes. These issues included: (i) physical health and well-being, which was linked to their energy level, functional capacity and ADLs; older persons had more comorbidities and opportunistic infections, physical symptomatology, and pain; (ii) mental health and well-being: emotional stressors included admission to the nursing home, separation from family and friends, and fears related to death; emotional issues were critical but not recognized by many staff members; (iii) spirituality and religious beliefs, which was integral to a sense of well-being and encouraged by staff; bedbound residents were less likely to participate in organized religious activities; (iv) family: residents benefited from active family support and visitations; residents without family involvement adjusted poorly to the nursing home environment, and (v) institutional resources: staffing levels and empathetic caring affected residents' well-being and impacted the nursing home capacity to meet residents' needs; limitations of insurance coverage affected the types of medications covered and residents' sense of well-being (2).

PATHOGENESIS OF HIV IN THE ELDERLY

Studies in the early and mid part of an epidemic showed that older people with HIV did not do as well as younger people. CD4+ cell counts were lower at initial diagnosis and the stage of the disease was more advanced; there were more comorbidities and the clinical course was more aggressive (11). Older age was related to a more rapid progression of HIV disease and higher rates of opportunistic diseases and death. The causes of the more rapid progression include a higher viral set point at initial infection, selective infection of memory T cells that increase proportionally in the elderly, more rapid destruction of T cells, impaired replacement of HIV-infected CD4 T cells, progressive increase in T cells with shortened telomeres that may be destroyed faster, and less effective anti-HIV cytotoxic T-lymphocyte activity than younger persons (12). With highly active antiretroviral therapy (HAART) the CD4 cells should increase. In the elderly, this recovery is blunted and is negatively correlated with age. Nevertheless, the effect of HAART substantially improves the survival rate for older individuals and supports the importance of treatment in this group. Older HIV-infected patients have responded well to HAART, with a significantly greater percentage achieving a plasma HIV RNA below detectable limits than younger patients. This greater viral suppression may be secondary to the greater rate of adherence in older people (11).

Most studies on progression of HIV disease in older individuals were done before the advent of HAART. A post-HAART study showed that older patients had increases in CD4+ T-lymphocyte counts comparable to younger patients. These results provide evidence that there should be no difference in the management of older and younger HIV-infected patients (14). One study compared outcomes in higher age groups of 66 to 84 year-olds versus 55 to 65 year-olds. Mean drop in viremia was nearly 1 log10 among the younger group and 0.5 log10 among older patients. Immune recovery was significantly blunted in patients aged 65 years or older. The older age group also had a less rapid and effective virologic response and complete viral suppression over time (14).

CLINICAL ISSUES IN NURSING HOME AIDS RESIDENTS

Comorbidities, decreased functional capacity, and frailty significantly affects the management of residents in nursing homes. Elderly residents with AIDS diagnosis progress to death more rapidly, and advanced age is associated with decreased survival. Prophylactic therapies and antiretroviral agents have reduced short-term mortality. More persons are living with chronic diseases and may have associated dementing encephalopathies and severe peripheral neuropathies. Two studies help elucidate some of the diseases and complications associated with AIDS in nursing home residents.

A case-series review in a 242-bed teaching nursing home described the initial 26 months care for patients admitted with AIDS (15). There were 42 admissions by 32 patients and 13 discharges. Twenty-nine patients died (69% mortality rate). Relevant AIDS clinical diagnosis included (i) generalized wasting/weakness (76%), (ii) HIV-related dementia (64%), (iii) active seizure disorder (36%), and (iv) Kaposi's sarcoma (19%). Problematic management issues included (i) recurrent falling (67%), (ii) episodic severe diarrhea (55%), (iii) narcotic analgesic usage (48%), and (iv) progressive weight loss (43%). The frequency of AIDS-related clinical diagnoses, such as HIV dementia, generalized wasting and weight loss, Kaposi's sarcoma, and the 69% mortality rate were similar to prior reports of nursing home AIDS care. Terminal care was often provided. The mean age of this study population was low (33.5) compared with the mean age of 78.3 years for the average nursing home patient. Nevertheless, the data illustrate some of the problems encountered in elderly patients of particular import to the nursing home AIDS resident including falls, weight loss, weakness, and dementia. Another study used the Minimum Data Set to describe HIV patients with and without dementia as previously noted (10). A significant portion of these patients was greater than age 51. Clinical conditions more common in HIV patients with dementia, as opposed to those without dementia included incontinence, pain, depression, anemia, tuberculosis, paraplegia/quadriplegia, and renal failure.

AIDS and Geriatric Syndromes

Advanced AIDS patients may share several clinical features seen in the elderly with geriatric syndromes, including dementia, delirium, frailty, failure to thrive, dizziness, falls, and syncope. HIV dementia and frailty from wasting aspects of AIDS and sarcopenia may be prominent. Delirium may result from infections or central nervous system causes and dizziness, falls and syncope may also result from central nervous system effects of AIDS. These manifestations make the recognition and management of frail elderly with HIV infection, as well as differential diagnosis of geriatric syndromes, especially challenging.

Dementia and AIDS

Between 15% and 20% of people with advanced HIV disease eventually develop HIV-associated dementia. Older age at the time of AIDS diagnosis is a significant risk factor. HIV-associated dementia typically develops late in the course of HIV disease. It is characterized by disabling cognitive, behavioral, and motor impairments. Among the cognitive symptoms of HIV-associated dementia are decreased short-term memory and concentration, loss of spontaneity, increased distractibility, and mental slowing. Changes in behavior include apathy, withdrawal, irritability, and depression. Clumsiness, tremor, and leg weakness are motor impairments that occur and increase the tendencies for falls (7).

HIV dementia may mimic Alzheimer's disease or vascular dementia. Some important differences are that HIV dementia is associated with ataxia, motor slowing, tremors, reflex abnormalities, weakness, and peripheral neuropathy, whereas Alzheimer's disease is not generally associated with these characteristics. Aphasia, a language disorder that may occur with Alzheimer's disease, is not generally present in HIV dementia. HIV dementia often responds to antiretroviral therapy, whereas Alzheimer's does not. The impact of HIV-associated cognitive decline on psychosocial interactions, adherence to medications, and ability to benefit from educational intervention can be profound (7).

Opportunistic Infections

Infections in the nursing home, such as pneumonia and urinary tract infections, are a frequent source of morbidity. These infections plus the range of opportunistic infections (OIs) that advanced AIDS patients acquire make infection surveillance particularly important. The range of OIs in nursing home residents with AIDS is similar in the young and old. The elderly may progress more rapidly, and they may be frequently misdiagnosed. Symptoms, such as fatigue, anorexia, weight loss, and memory impairment, may be attributed to old age. These same symptoms frequently occur in OIs, such as tuberculosis, cryptococcal meningitis, and *Pneumocystis carinii* pneumonia. As in younger individuals, the most frequent OIs include *P. carinii* pneumonia and *Candida* esophagitis. Treatment and prophylaxis should take into account altered pharmacokinetics, drug interactions, and comorbidities.

In spite of the benefits of antiretrovirals, some patients continue to develop AIDS-related complications such as *Mycobacterium avium* complex and tuberculosis, neurologic impairment from HIV neuropathy, and vacuolar myelopathy of the spinal cord. These disorders may produce chronic disability and require special forms of rehabilitation (1).

Comorbid Diseases

Many chronic diseases, such as diabetes mellitus, hypertension, coronary artery disease, and congestive heart failure, occur in older HIV-infected patients. Patients older than 55 have four times more comorbid conditions than those under 45. Lipid abnormalities become more prevalent and of significant importance. When these diseases occur on the backdrop of HIV infection, the clinical presentation and treatment may be significantly impacted. Diabetes mellitus, for example, is frequently associated with dyslipidemia. Patients who do not take their medications or who develop infections may develop diabetic ketoacidosis, and patients given nucleoside reverse transcriptase inhibitors (NRTIs) may develop lactic acidosis.

TREATMENT OF HIV INFECTION IN THE NURSING HOME

The approach to treatment of HIV infection in elderly nursing home residents is similar to that of younger patients with this infection but also should include assessing functional capacity, the potential for polypharmacy and adherence, altered pharmokinetics, and the effect of comorbidities. The viral load, CD4 cell count, electrolytes, complete blood count, liver enzymes, and urinalysis should be routinely monitored (3–6 months). A tuberculin skin test, serology for syphilis, *Toxoplasma gondii* IgG, hepatitis A, B, and C serologies, and chest radiographs should be performed if not initially obtained. Fasting glucose and lipid analysis should be done before initiation of therapy and monitored regularly.

The elderly frequently take multiple medications for comorbid conditions. Age-related pharmacological changes may result in increased therapeutic effect of drugs and potential toxicity including HIV medications.

HIV Drug Classes

Nucleoside Analog Reverse Transcriptase Inhibitors

NRTIs were the first drugs approved for the treatment of HIV infection. They inhibit the synthesis of DNA by reverse transcriptase (RT), which results in the decrease or prevention of HIV replication. NRTIs may cause mitochondrial toxicity with a potentially fatal syndrome of lactic acidosis and hepatic steatosis (16).

Non-nucleoside Analog Reverse Transcriptase Inhibitors

Non-nucleoside analog reverse transcriptase inhibitors (NNRTIs) also inhibit the synthesis of viral DNA but do so by a different mechanism from NRTIs that act as false nucleoside analogs. They bind to RT and inhibit the RT directly. They may induce or inhibit cytochrome P450. Resistance develops rapidly and cross-resistance is common in this class (16).

Nucleotide Reverse Transcriptase Inhibitor

These are phosphorylated nucleosides and do not require intracellular phosphorylation. They inhibit RT and viral replication and function the same as NRTIs (16).

Protease Inhibitors

PIs prevent the processing of viral proteins into functional forms by binding the viral protease enzyme. This prevents cleavage of precursor proteins necessary for HIV maturation, infection of new cells, and viral replication. PIs are metabolized by cytochrome P450 and may cause hepatotoxicity, lipodystrophy, gastrointestinal distress, increased bleeding, and insulin resistance with hyperglycemia and hyperlipidemia (16).

Fusion Inhibitors

HIV fuses into the target cell by utilizing the HIV envelop protein gp41. This protein undergoes a conformational change (folds), which allows HIV to fuse into the target cell membrane. Fusion inhibitors bind to this protein and interfere with the conformational change, thereby preventing the entry of HIV into target cells. Enfuvirtide (Fuzeon) must be given by subcutaneous injections twice a day, and there is a high incidence of local reactions (16).

Principles of HIV Treatment in the Elderly

In general, the elderly should be treated like the young with knowledge of important comorbidities. Antiretroviral therapy should be started in all those with symptomatic HIV infection and those with CD4+ T cells < 200 and individualized in those with CD4+ T cells between 200 and 350. Plasma viremia, a strong prognostic indicator for HIV infection, should be used to help determine initiation of therapy for CD4 counts between 200 and 350 (17).

Patient understanding, willingness to adhere to treatment, their current and future pill burden, severity of HIV infection, potential adverse drug reactions and interactions, and comorbidities are significant factors in deciding whether to initiate treatment. Dementia with decreased life expectancy in elderly HIV nursing home residents presents ethical dilemmas for the initiation and/or continuation of therapy. If there is a component of HIV dementia, then the benefits versus risks of antiretrovirals become more apparent. Most nursing home residents have been admitted with HIV and thus many are not medication naïve; nevertheless, the provider should set parameters before initiating treatment and analyze the risk–benefit ratio of treatment and present this to the resident and/or caregiver. The resident's current drugs should be reviewed, and the potential for drug–drug interactions assessed.

All PIs and NNRTIs are metabolized in the liver by the cytochrome P450 (CYP) system. Therefore, the range of possible interactions can be considerable. NRTIs do not undergo hepatic transformation through the CYP metabolic pathway and may have less interactions. Table 6 lists some common drug interactions of significance for elderly and nursing home residents. Contraindicated antiretrovirals or combinations are noted in Table 7.

Table 6 Important Antiretroviral and Drug Interactions in the Elderly

Drug	Interactions	Mechanism/effects	Comments
St. John's wort	All PIs and NNRTIs	Induces cytochrome p450 and decreases concentrations of PIs and NNRTIs	Should not be used
Bepridil (type 4 calcium channel blocker)	PIs: ritonavir, amprenavir fosamprenavir, atazanavir	Peak concentration and T1/2 markedly increased in those over 74 yr	Arrhythmias, heart block, and prolonged QT interval on EKG. Do not use with PIs
Simvastatin, lovastatin	PIs, NNRTIs, and delavirdine	Increased statin levels	Increased risk of myopathy and rhabdomyolysis
Sildenafil, vardenafil, tadalafil	PIs	Increased levels of erectile dysfunction drugs	Increased risk of myocardial ischemia
Rifamycins (rifampin and rifabutin)	PIs, NNRTIs	CYP3A4 inducers reduce plasma levels of PIs and NNRTIs. Increased levels of rifabutin	Rifabutin less potent inducer; alternative to rifampin for tuberculosis treatment for patients on PIs, NNRTIs. Downward dose adjustment for rifabutin

Abbreviations: PIs, protease inhibitors; NNRTIs, non-nucleoside reverse transcriptase inhibitor; EKG, electrocardiogram.
Source: From Ref. 18.

In general, combinations should always be used and include (i) an NNRTI with two NRTIS (NNRTI-based regimens that are PI sparing), (ii) a PI with low-dose ritonavir and two NRTIS (PI-based regimens that are NNRTI sparing), and (iii) three NRTIs (triple NRTI regimens that are both PI and NNRTI sparing) (17).

Important Side Effects of HAART in Older Adults

Lactic Acidosis/Hepatic Steatosis and Hyperglycemia

Chronic hyperlactatemia can occur with NRTIs. Cases of severe lactic acidosis with hepatomegaly and steatosis are rare but associated with a high

Table 7 Contraindicated Antiretrovirals or Combinations

Drug therapy/ combination	Effects	Comments
Monotherapy	Inadequate	Leads to rapid resistance
Dual nucleoside therapy	Leads to rapid resistance	Antiviral activity less than 3 drug combinations
Didanosine plus stavudine	High incidence of toxicities: peripheral neuropathy, pancreatitis, lactic acidosis	Diabetics and patients at risk for falls would be at considerable risk
Stavudine plus zidovudine	Stavudine antagonizes zidovudine	May cause lactic acidosis and severe hepatomegaly with steatosis
Zalcitabine plus stavudine	Overlapping toxicities	Increased rates and severity of peripheral neuropathy
Zalcitabine plus didanosine	Overlapping toxicities	Increased rates and severity of peripheral neuropathy
Atazanavir plus indinavir	Can cause grade 3–4 hyperbilirubinemia	Additive when used together. Indinavir causes kidney stones
Abacavir + tenofovir + lamivudine (or emtricitabine)	High rate of early virologic nonresponse	Do not use as initial treatment
Tenofovir + didanosine + lamivudine (or emtricitabine)	High rate of early virologic nonresponse	Do not use as initial treatment

Source: From Ref. 18.

mortality rate. This may be related to mitochondrial toxicity. Nevirapine, an NNRTI, has the greatest potential for causing clinical hepatitis.

Hyperglycemia has been reported in 3% to 17% of patients receiving HAART. A retrospective study involving 1011 HIV-positive patients found that older age and regimens including stavudine or indinavir were associated with a higher risk of developing diabetes mellitus (18). Insulin resistance associated with PI use results in hyperglycemia, diabetes mellitus, worsening of preexisting diabetes mellitus, and diabetic ketoacidosis.

Hyperlipidemia and Fat Maldistribution

HIV infection and antiretroviral therapy have been associated with altered fat distribution. There may be fat wasting (lipoatrophy) or fat accumulation (hyperadiposity). These changes have been called lipodystrophy. It may be associated with dyslipidemias, glucose intolerance, or lactic acidosis. There are no clear effective therapies for lipodystrophy.

Dyslipidemia can be the direct result of HIV infection or a consequence of antiretroviral therapy. Cardiovascular risk factors associated with HIV infection and HAART include plasma lipid abnormalities (decreased high-density lipoprotein cholesterol, increased low-density lipoprotein cholesterol, increased triglycerides), increased visceral fat, insulin resistance, chronic inflammation, and endothelial dysfunction/atherosclerosis. Before HAART, cachexia, low total cholesterol, and high triglyceride levels were reported in HIV patients. Several features of the metabolic syndrome overlap with common features of HIV treatment-associated lipodystrophy, such as hyper-insulinemia, glucose intolerance, an atherogenic lipoprotein phenotype, a prothrombotic state, and central obesity (19).

Hypertriglyceridemia is common and severe in patients taking ritonavir. Lipid abnormalities tend to be most marked with ritonavir and lopinavir-ritonavir. NNRTs cause alterations in lipid profiles but less than with PIs. The PI atazanavir has little effect on lipids. Patients with risk factors for hyperlipidemia should be monitored closely. Statins may be necessary, but one should use agents less affected by cytochrome P450 such as pravastatin. Switching from a PI to nevirapine or abacavir results in improved total cholesterol and triglycerides. PIs have been associated with myocardial infarctions; consequently, clinicians must weigh the risks and benefits of switching therapy versus the risks of hyperlipidemia including myocardial infarction, and the need to initiate statin therapy. PI-associated insulin resistance and altered expression of apolipoprotein C-III gene may mediate PI-associated dyslipidemia (20). In HIV-infected patients with elevated cholesterol or triglyceride levels, nonpharmacologic interventions should be tried first unless the patient has existing coronary heart disease or total cholesterol levels > 400 mg/dL.

Avascular Necrosis and Osteoporosis

Avascular necrosis, also known as osteonecrosis, has been associated with HIV infection, and the incidence has been rising among HIV-infected patients. This may be in part due to better recognition, prolonged survival, and/or direct or indirect effects of antiretroviral agents. Musculoskeletal pain and osteoarthritis involving the hips and other joints is common in elderly patients, and thus the risk and diagnosis for osteonecrosis in cases of residents with HIV infection should be entertained (20). Several studies have linked osteonecrosis to PI therapy; however, two case control studies and one case series have not shown HAART to be a consistent risk factor for the development of osteonecrosis (21). HIV infection in and of itself may cause bone loss. The mechanism is largely unknown but may be related to cytokines, such as tumor necrosis factor and interleukin-6, which may be increased and may lead to osteoclast activation. Biochemical markers of bone metabolism in HIV-infected patients, such as increased C-telopeptide, may be high and associated with advanced disease and high viral loads. Osteoclastin levels, which indicate bone turnover, may be increased after initiation of HAART (20). Osteoporosis has been associated with PI use and this has been documented by dual-energy X-ray absorptiometry scans. PIs may inhibit conversion of 25-hydroxy vitamin D to 1,25-dihydroxy vitamin D, which may contribute to the development of osteoporosis (22). Risk factors for the development of osteoporosis include advanced age, low body weight, a long duration of HIV infection, and PIs. Fragility fractures have been known to occur in patients with HIV/AIDS and antiretroviral treatment (23). This may be of particular importance in older and frail nursing home residents and residents at risk for falls. Residents should have an adequate intake of calcium and vitamin D. For residents with prolonged HIV infection, hypogonadal patients, and those on antiretroviral therapy, a dual-energy X-ray absorptiometry scan should be performed and alendronate should be prescribed if consistent with osteopenia and there are no contraindications (22,23).

Dermatologic Problems

Many frail nursing home residents are already at risk of or have developed pressure ulcers. Complications of skin rashes from medications may add to the risk of pressure ulcers. Rashes range from mild to severe, including Stevens–Johnson syndrome and toxic epidermal necrosis. NNRTIs are more prone to cause skin rashes and should prompt permanent discontinuation. Nevirapine in particular causes more frequent and severe skin rashes; however, rashes are NNRTI class-specific and may occur with other NNRTIs. Abacavir, an NRTI, is associated with a systemic hypersensitivity reaction. Therapy should be discontinued and not restarted. Aprenavir is the PI that causes skin rashes most frequently. It is a sulfonamide and has the potential for cross-reactivity with sulfur drugs and should be used with caution in cases of sulfur allergies.

PSYCHOSOCIAL CONCERNS AND PREVENTION

Older people with HIV infection have significant emotional distress and may have thoughts of suicide, suggesting a need for targeted interventions to improve mental health. In terminally ill residents, issues related to death and dying and adequate pain control need to be addressed. The nursing home-based hospice may provide for better physical, emotional, and mental health care to these residents (2).

Though the risk of HIV transmission and acquisition in the nursing home may be low, there is still a risk. Interventions are needed for both primary and secondary prevention of HIV infection. Mucosal disruptions from thinned anal and vaginal mucosa increase the risk of HIV transmission. The magnitude of undiagnosed and unrecognized HIV infection in the elderly in nursing homes is not known. Providers may be reluctant to consider AIDS as a possibility in older individuals until late in the course of the disease. Long-term care providers will be more likely to encounter elderly people living with AIDS in need of their services. Prevention programs may be more difficult in the face of cognitive, visual, and auditory declines that occur with age. An individualized approach may be necessary to address such challenging issues in the elderly. Prevention efforts that are done individually have been found to be more effective. This allows for questions and concerns to be more readily answered, and provides an opportunity to monitor the residents' alertness (24).

SUGGESTED READING

Benjamin AE. Long-term care and AIDS: perspectives from experience with the elderly. Milbank Q 1988; 66:415–443.

Cohen MA. Psychiatric care in an AIDS nursing home. Psychosomatics 1998; 39:154–161.

Funnyé AS, Akhtar AJ, Biamby G. Acquired immunodeficiency syndrome in older African Americans. J Natl Med Assoc 2002; 94:209–214.

Waysdorf SL. The aging of the AIDS epidemic: emerging legal and public health issues for elderly persons living with HIV/AIDS. Elder Law 2002; 10:47–89.

REFERENCES

1. Schmitt JK, Stuckey CP. AIDS—no longer a death sentence, still a challenge [editorial]. South Med J 2004; 97:329–330.
2. Fox-Hill EJ, Gibson DV, Engle VF. Nursing home experiences of older African Americans with HIV/AIDS: issues for future research. In: Emlet CA, ed. HIV/AIDS and Older Adults, Challenges for Individuals, Families, and Communities. New York: Springer Publishing Company, 2004:111–129.
3. Centers for Disease Control and Prevention. HIV/AIDS fact sheet: a glance at the HIV/AIDS epidemic. www.cdc.gov/Hiv/resources/factsheets/At-A-Glance. htm April 2006:1–2.
4. Centers for Disease Control and Prevention. *HIV/AIDS Surveillance Report* 2003. (Vol. 15). Atlanta: US Department of Health and Human Services, Centers for Disease Control and Prevention; 2004:1–46.
5. Pearson WS, Hueston WJ. Treatment of HIV/AIDS in the nursing home: variations in rural and urban long-term care settings. South Med J 2004; 97:338–341.
6. Centers for Disease Control and Prevention. AIDS among persons aged ≥50 years—United States, 1991–1996. Morb Mortal Wkly Rep 1998; 47:21–27.
7. Shah SS, McGowan JP, Smith C, Blum S, Klein RS. Comorbid conditions, treatment, and health maintenance in older persons with human immunodeficiency virus infection in New York City. Clin Infect Dis 2002; 35:1238–1243.
8. Lesesne AJ, Ouslander JG. Demographics and economics of long-term care. In: Ouslander JG, Yoshikawa TT, eds. Infection Management for Geriatrics in Long-Term Care Facilities. New York: Marcel Dekker, Inc., 2002:1–13.

9. Gallagher RM. How long-term care is changing. Am J Nurs 2000; 100:65–67.

10. Buchanan RJ, Wang S, Huang C. Analyses of nursing home residents with HIV and dementia using the Minimum Data Set. JAIDS 2001; 26:246–255.

11. Wellons MF, Sanders L, Edwards LJ, Bartlett JA, Heald AE, Schmader KE. HIV infection: treatment outcomes in older and younger adults. J Am Geriatr Soc 2002; 50:603–607.

12. Bender BS. HIV and aging as a model for immunosenescence. J Gerontol A Biol Sci Med Sci 1997; 52A:M261–M263.

13. Grimes RM, Otiniano E, Rodriguez-Barradas MC, Lai D. Clinical experience with human immunodeficiency virus infected older patients in the era of effective antiretroviral therapy. Clin Infect Dis 2002; 34:1530–1533.

14. Manfredi R, Calza L, Davide C, Chiodo F. Antiretroviral treatment and advanced age: epidemiologic, laboratory, and clinical features in the elderly. JAIDS 2003; 33:112–120.

15. Heath JM. Care of persons with AIDS in the nursing home. Fam Med 1998; 30:436–440.

16. Anonymous. Drugs for HIV infection. Med Lett Drugs Ther. 2001; 43(1119): 103–108.

17. Panel on Clinical Practices for Treatment of HIV Infection. Guidelines for the use of antiretroviral agents in HIV-1 infected adults and adolescents. US Department of Health and Human Services; April 7, 2005:1–108.

18. Brambilla AM, Novati R, Calon G, et al. Stavudine- or indinavir-containing regimens are associated with an increased risk of diabetes mellitus in HIV-infected individuals. AIDS 2003; 17:1993–1995.

19. Currier JS. Cardiovascular risk associated with HIV therapy. JAIDS 2002; 31:S16–S23.

20. Thomas J, Doherty SM. HIV infection—a risk factor for osteoporosis. JAIDS 2003; 33:281–291.

21. Allison GT, Bostrom MP, Glesby MJ. Osteonecrosis in HIV disease: epidemiology, etiologies, and clinical management. AIDS 2003; 17:1–9.

22. Montessori V, Press N, Harris M, Akagi L, Montaner JSG. Adverse effects of antiretroviral therapy for HIV infection. Can Med Assoc J 2004; 170:229–238.

23. McComsey GA, Huang JS, Woolley IJ, et al. Fragility fractures in HIV-infected patients: need for better understanding of diagnosis and management. JIAPAC 2004; 3:86–91.

24. Williams E, Donnelly J. Older Americans and AIDS: some guidelines for prevention. Social Work 2002; 47:105–111.

22

Vaccinations

Rex Biedenbender and Stefan Gravenstein

Division of Geriatrics, The Glennan Center for Geriatrics and Gerontology, Department of Medicine, Eastern Virginia Medical School, Norfolk, Virginia, U.S.A.

Arvydas Ambrozaitis

Clinic of Infectious Diseases and Microbiology, Vilnius University, Vilnius, Lithuania

KEY POINTS

1. Immunosenescence in aging increases infectious morbidity and mortality.
2. Nursing home residents often present with attenuated symptoms and signs of infection.
3. Vaccination of older adults remains cost effective for prevention of infectious disease.
4. Vaccination rates >80% reduce spread (herd immunity), morbidity, and mortality.
5. Influenza, pneumococcal, and tetanus/diphtheria vaccinations are recommended for nursing home residents. Hepatitis and, for those without prior infection ("chicken pox"), herpes zoster virus vaccination are also recommended for caregivers.

INFECTION, AGING, AND IMMUNE RESPONSE

The greatest effect of immunosenescence and its interaction with chronic illness is increased infectious morbidity and mortality (see also Chapter 5) (1–5). The impact of many infections increases with age, including influenza, pneumonia, *Clostridium difficile*, nosocomial infections, and such recrudescent latent infections as herpes zoster. Use and abuse of antibiotics select resistant microorganisms that may spread from the primary source patient. This is especially true for methicillin-resistant *Staphylococcus aureus* and *Streptococcus pneumoniae* and also extended-spectrum beta-lactamase organisms and vancomycin-resistant enterococci. *S. pneumoniae* is increasingly resistant to antibiotics, is a leading cause of morbidity and mortality, and stands out among resistant organisms in that the most important pathogenic strains are vaccine preventable. Immunosenescence increases frequency and duration of infections and leads to atypical clinical presentations that can obscure the diagnosis.

Because of immunosenescence and coexisting chronic diseases, the elderly fail to respond efficiently to therapy for infections (e.g., *C. difficile* or influenza), may be infected by unusual pathogens (e.g., *Listeria monocytogenes*), or have reactivation of quiescent diseases (e.g., shingles). Immunosenescence is a major factor of impaired response to infection and attenuated clinical signs. Despite attenuation, the immune reaction is believed to be paradoxically responsible for much of the morbidity and mortality following some infections, such as influenza, mostly as consequences of inflammation. Typical signs of infection can be absent and requires a high index of suspicion for an adequately inclusive differential diagnosis. The elderly may not develop high fever, leucocytosis, or prominent infiltrates on chest X-ray as younger patients with pneumonia (6–8). Lower baseline temperatures from decreased thermoregulation and reset hypothalamic thermostat in frail elders may require monitoring change rather than absolute temperature in old age (see also Chapter 8) (9). The availability of effective vaccines in elders is essential, as vaccination is one of the few cost-effective defenses against antibiotic-resistant organisms in long-term care facilities (LTCFs) where transmissibility contributes to disease impact. LTCF employee vaccination is also important, as staff may be vectors of disease transmission to residents.

VACCINE UTILIZATION IN LONG-TERM CARE FACILITIES

Despite evidence of morbidity and mortality from vaccine-preventable diseases in LTCFs, vaccination rates remain suboptimal. A survey of Canadian LTCFs compared vaccination rates for influenza and pneumococcus in 1991 versus 1999 (10). Average rate of influenza vaccination in 1999 was 83% for residents and 35% among staff. Average resident pneumococcal vaccination rate was 71%. These rates were significantly higher than those in 1991 (10). In a survey of Minnesota LTCFs in 1993, it showed 12-month resident immunization rates for influenza, pneumococcal, and tetanus/diphtheria vaccine of 84%, 11.9%, and 2.9%, respectively. One third of LTCFs did not offer influenza vaccine to residents admitted during the influenza season. Policies for influenza vaccine existed in 69%, but only one third for pneumococcal vaccine, and under 20% for tetanus/diphtheria administration.

EFFORTS TO INCREASE VACCINE UTILIZATION

Steps to improve vaccine use in LTCFs include implementing standing orders for routine vaccination in a sustainable immunization program (11,12). Consensus among staff, infection control nurse, medical director, and administration about importance of vaccination in this setting improves use. A vaccination program team with defined roles and responsibilities and setting-specific measurable goals helps create that consensus (13,14).

Other methods improving vaccine utilization include having a written, well-defined plan (13,14). Plans should include assessing immunization status of new residents, offering residents vaccination via standing order protocols, and performing annual vaccination campaigns, perhaps in conjunction with influenza vaccination. Immunization programs should include annual in-service of staff, physicians, and medical directors providing overview of vaccination policy, vaccine effectiveness, recommendations, record-keeping requirements, infection control, and indications and contraindications to vaccination.

Improving vaccination utilization may depend on past success of the programs. Periodic review of resident and staff vaccination status and comparison with baseline status, assessing efficiency of administration, and evaluating residents and staff not vaccinated and the reason why can identify areas of improvement.

INFLUENZA

Older adults, aged ≥ 65 years, currently account for >90% of the deaths attributed to pneumonia, and influenza and is the seventh leading cause of death (15). In an evaluation of influenza-related deaths from 19 epidemics occurring from 1972–1973 through 1994–1995, the influenza-related death rate ranged from 30 to 150 per 100,000 persons aged $\geq$65 years. Influenza-related illness (ILI) costs more health-care dollars and causes more life losses than any other viral illness in the United States. National hospital discharge data indicate an average of 114,000 excess hospitalizations annually related to influenza. Since 1968, the greatest number of hospitalizations have occurred during epidemics caused by type A (H3N2) viruses, where an estimated 142,000 influenza-related hospitalizations occurred per year and more than 40% of those were in individuals $\geq$65 years old (see also Chapter 13).

Influenza outbreaks relate to two phenomena: antigenic drift and antigenic shift. Because the influenza virus genome is segmented, different segment combinations yield phenotypically different viruses. Recombination of the genetic segments from two dissimilar influenza A viruses make antigenic shift possible. Antigenic drift due to single nucleic acid substitutions of the genome also occurs even in the course of individual infections. These phenomena enable the influenza virus to escape immune recognition and allow annual epidemics (with antigenic drift) or pandemics (with antigenic shift) to occur.

Elderly persons are at increased risk for influenza complications related to secondary bacterial infection, and their likelihood of hospitalization and mortality rate is higher than among younger people. In LTCFs, up to 70% of the residents may contract ILIs during an outbreak; during non-epidemic years the attack rate is 5% to 20%. The case-fatality ratio during outbreaks may be as high as 30%. Because the U.S. population is aging, the impact of influenza will continue to intensify unless better control is attained.

Vaccine Effectiveness

The cornerstone to influenza prevention remains vaccination, a far more cost-effective alternative to chemoprophylaxis. A well-matched vaccine is effective in reducing incidence and severity of influenza illness, but even poorly matched vaccines provide benefit. Vaccinations reduce influenza-related hospitalizations, radiologically diagnosed cases of pneumonia, and deaths (16).

Despite high resident vaccination rates in LTCFs, outbreaks occur annually. The influenza vaccine can fail to provide protection due to immunosenescence, underlying chronic diseases, weak vaccine immunogenicity, lack of herd immunity, antigenic drift, or antigenic shift. Because of advanced age and comorbidity, one half of LTCF residents develop "protective" vaccine-induced antibody titers, compared with 70% to 90% of young healthy adults, and fewer develop substantial cellular immunity. Supplemental vaccination and vaccines with higher concentrations of antigen have not consistently shown increased antibody response (immunogenicity) in elderly persons but have shown more side effects (reactogenicity). Nevertheless, elderly persons may benefit from vaccination despite low antibody titers; the influenza illness may be less severe and the risk of complications, hospitalization, and death may be reduced.

Results from retrospective studies show vaccine efficacy varying from 30% to 80%. One prospective study suggested that the Centers for Disease Control and Prevention (CDC) case definition for influenza might only be 61% sensitive and 63% specific for detecting laboratory-confirmed H3N2 influenza. Retrospective studies reporting vaccine efficacy relying on clinical symptoms for case detection may underestimate the ability of the vaccine to prevent infection. When infection does occur in vaccinated individuals, morbidity and death is reduced in community and LTCF settings (16).

Indications

Annual influenza vaccination is recommended for high-risk individuals, their caregivers, and those in close contact. High-risk individuals include LTCF residents, persons ≥50 years old, those with chronic pulmonary or cardiovascular disorders, and those requiring frequent follow-up or hospitalization during the preceding year due of chronic metabolic disorders, renal dysfunction, hemoglobinopathies, or immunosuppression.

Annual U.S. LTCF influenza vaccination rates range from 0% to 100%, with an estimated average of 80% nationwide. The rate of vaccinated LTCF staff is often less than 30% (16). Increasing staff and resident vaccination depends on the implementation of the program by the medical director, director of nursing, and infection control practitioner, as well as implementation of LTCF education programs and vaccination policies.

A positive outcome of high rates of influenza immunization in LTCFs is herd immunity, which reduces probability of virus transmission within a population. Vaccination rates of 80% for residents and staff are calculated to generate herd immunity and should be a minimum goal. Residents of LTCFs should be the highest priority for vaccination during periods of vaccine shortage.

Administration and Revaccination

An intramuscular (IM) injection of 0.5 mL of the trivalent influenza vaccine via a 1-in needle is recommended in the United States for those age ≥ 50. Half-inch needles may fail to reach muscle due to reduced lean muscle mass and increased fat. Subcutaneous and intradermal routes have been used, but efficacy has not been adequately compared. Live attenuated influenza vaccine (LAIV) is now available (i.e., Flumist™, MedImmune, Inc.) but is approved only for ages 5 to 49 years and is specifically contraindicated in many chronic conditions (see Table 1 for current commercially available

Table 1 Approved Influenza Vaccines for Different Age Groups in the United States

Vaccine	6 mos–3 yrs	4 yrs	5–49 yrs	≥ 50 yrs
Fluzone® (Sanofi Pasteur, Inc.)	X[a]	X	X	X
Fluvirin™ (Chiron)		X	X	X
FluMist™ (MedImmune, Inc.)			X	

[a]Children aged 6 to 35 months should receive 0.25 mL/dose. Children aged > 35 months should receive 0.50 mL/dose.

influenza vaccines). Annual vaccination is needed, as protective response to current influenza vaccines is short-lived and the virus's rapid antigenic change reduces the previous year's vaccine effectiveness. Optimum timing of the influenza vaccine is important and not easily determined. Vaccination performed too early may result in protective antibody titers falling prior to virus circulation. Late vaccination permits viral exposure before protective antibody develops. Because it may take four to six weeks to develop optimum antibody titers in the elderly, vaccinating four to six weeks prior to the expected influenza season is advisable. In most states, vaccination in November is reasonable, whereas vaccination before October is usually premature. Influenza typically circulates from December to March, justifying vaccination of new staff and residents in January or later. When an influenza outbreak is identified, unvaccinated staff and residents should be offered the vaccine. Those accepting vaccination during influenza A outbreaks should be offered adjunctive therapy with an antiviral agent (amantadine, rimantadine, zanamivir, or oseltamivir) for two weeks following vaccination allowing time to develop vaccine-induced immunity. Neuraminidase inhibitors (zanamivir and oseltamivir) effectively reduce also influenza B illness. Unvaccinated persons should be offered chemoprophylaxis with amantadine (if at low risk for side effects), rimantadine, or neuraminidase inhibitors during the influenza A outbreak. However, recent data are showing an increased incidence of current strains of influenza A resistant to amantadine and rimantadine. Neuraminidase inhibitor therapy for outbreak control appears to be more effective in vaccinated populations (17,18). Most outbreaks are associated with influenza A, but if influenza B is identified, only neuraminidase inhibitors are effective. Dosing information is presented in Table 2.

Clinical trials of new vaccines have had variable success. Approaches to enhance immunogenicity have included use of biologic response modifiers, adjuvants, protein conjugates, and cold-adapted vaccine constructs. Although some of these have shown evidence of improved immunogenicity and clinical efficacy, none has yet demonstrated a sufficient advantage for manufacturers to bring them to market in the United States.

Safety

Fear of adverse effects of influenza vaccine, particularly influenza illness, has reduced vaccination rates. The current, commercially available split virion IM vaccine is made of noninfectious particles and is incapable of causing influenza infection. Respiratory illness occurring after vaccination is coincidental. About 30% of recipients have injection site tenderness for one to two days following administration. Fever, malaise, or myalgia occur in <10% of individuals and most often in persons naïve to the influenza vaccine. Rates of systemic reactions in the elderly are similar to saline placebo recipients.

Table 2 Daily Dosage of Influenza Antiviral Medications for Prophylaxis in LTCF Residents During an Outbreak

Antiviral agent	Daily dose		Duration (day)
	< 65 yrs	≥ 65 yrs	
Treatment[a]			
Amantadine[b] (influenza A only)	100 mg twice daily	100 mg/day	3–5
Rimantadine[c] (influenza A only)	100 mg twice daily	100 mg/day	3–5
Zanamivir[d]	10 mg twice daily	10 mg twice daily	5
Oseltamivir[e]	75 mg twice daily	75 mg twice daily	5
Prophylaxis[f]			
Amantadine[b] (influenza A only)	100 mg twice daily	100 mg/day	≥14
Rimantadine[c] (influenza A only)	100 mg twice daily	100 mg/day	≥14
Zanamivir[d]	N/A	N/A	N/A
Oseltamivir[e]	75 mg/day	75 mg/day	≥14

[a]Treatment must begin within two days of symptom onset to be effective.
[b]Consult the drug package insert for dosage recommendations for administering amantadine to persons with creatinine clearance ≤50 mL/min/1.73 m^2.
[c]A reduction in dosage to 100 mg/day of rimantadine is recommended for persons who have severe hepatic dysfunction or those with creatinine clearance ≤10 mL/min. Other persons with less severe hepatic or renal dysfunction taking 100 mg/day of rimantadine should be observed closely, and the dosage should be reduced or the drug discontinued, if necessary.
[d]Zanamivir is not approved for prophylaxis.
[e]A reduction in dose is recommended for persons with creatinine clearance <30 mL/min.
[f]Continued prophylaxis is recommended to begin within two days of exposure and/or facility outbreak declaration. Prophylaxis should continue a minimum of two weeks or until clinical disease activity has ended at the facility. All residents should be offered chemoprophylaxis regardless of vaccination status.
Abbreviation: N/A, not applicable.

Rare hypersensitivity reactions to vaccine components, residual egg proteins, or preservatives are possible. Influenza vaccine is contraindicated in those with anaphylactic hypersensitivity to eggs. Only the 1976 influenza vaccine was significantly associated with Guillain–Barré syndrome. This relationship appears real, but its impact was small (<1/1,000,000 vaccinated) and has not recurred.

Influenza viral shedding from staff vaccinated with LAIV to residents is now an issue. Currently, the CDC recommends that staff and visitors receiving LAIV refrain from contact for at least seven days from severely immunocompromised patients, such as those receiving hematopoietic stem cell transplant during periods requiring a special protective environment. The attenuated virus theoretically could still be virulent in this situation.

Previous recommendations to avoid all potentially immunosuppressed contacts for 21 days following LAIV administration have been demonstrated to be unnecessary (19).

PNEUMOCOCCAL DISEASE

Immunosenescence, comorbid disease, and drug therapy should be considered when assessing risk for pneumococcal disease. One study found the incidence of pneumococcal disease to be 70 cases per 100,000 in individuals over the age of 70, compared with five cases per 100,000 in younger adults. *S. pneumoniae*, a gram-positive bacterium, also referred to as pneumococcus and diplococcus, colonizes the nasopharynx. Prior to widespread availability of antibiotics, *S. pneumoniae* was frequently isolated from the nasopharynx (up to 70%). The rate of colonization is much lower today (i.e., <40%). Microbiologically, pneumococci are gram-positive, nonsporulating, encapsulated, lancet-shaped diplococci, although they may also grow in chains. The capsule is the antigenic determinant in the current pneumococcal vaccine.

Historically, pneumococci have been exquisitely sensitive to penicillin antibiotics. However, the prevalence of penicillin- and other antibiotic-resistant pneumococci is on the rise worldwide (20,21). This has implications for antimicrobial treatment of these infections and reinforces prevention as a primary management strategy for pneumococcal disease.

The presence of *S. pneumoniae* in the nasopharynx is usually harmless. In immunocompetent individuals infection is usually avoided. However, when the bacterium invades the lung, pneumonitis follows, which progresses to pneumonia. Risk factors include conditions that predispose to aspiration, including dementia, delirium, stupor, stroke with abnormal swallowing, chronic obstructive pulmonary disease, alcoholism, and seizure disorders. Also, certain therapeutics, such as nasogastric tubes, sedatives, antipsychotics, and anxiolytics, should be considered in assessing aspiration risk. These conditions are common in LTCFs, placing this population at considerable risk for pneumococcal infections (see also Chapter 14). Prevention of pneumococcal disease holds promise for affecting the incidence of disease in the elderly and immunocompromised populations.

Pneumonia is the most common expression of *S. pneumoniae* infection. Other infections include otitis media, sinusitis, meningitis, septic arthritis, pericarditis, endocarditis, peritonitis, cellulitis, glomerulonephritis, and sepsis (especially postsplenectomy). Underutilization of pneumococcal vaccine has resulted in outbreaks in LTCFs, showing the need for increasing vaccination rates.

Pneumococcal Vaccine

Studies have documented efficacy of the current 23-valent vaccine in preventing invasive pneumococcal pneumonia and bacteremia in elderly persons and have shown these vaccines to be cost-effective (22,23). Still, the public health benefits have been received with little enthusiasm. The Advisory Committee on Immunization Practices of the Centers for Disease Control and Prevention recommends pneumococcal vaccine for the individuals at risk of pneumococcal disease (Table 3) (24,25). Revaccination is recommended for persons ≥65 years old if vaccinated ≥5 years previously and were <65 years of age at time of vaccination.

Currently available vaccines, Pneumovax® 23 and Pnu-Imune® 23, contain 25 μg of capsular polysaccharide antigen for each of the 23 most prevalent and pathogenic *S. pneumoniae* serotypes in a 0.5 mL dose. The 23-valent vaccine was developed to provide a broader spectrum of coverage against the *S. pneumoniae* serotypes implicated in pneumococcal disease over the older 14-valent vaccine. The makeup of the current vaccine was recently compared against the respiratory isolates obtained in a national surveillance study conducted in 1987–1988. The most common pneumococcal serotype encountered was type 3 (13.1%), followed by 19F, 23F, 6B, 14, 4, and 6A. These serotypes, comprising 74.9% of the respiratory isolates in the study, were all included in the current 23-valent vaccine. When cross-reactivity (i.e., when antibody specific for one serotype or pneumococcal strain will cross-react with or also bind another serotype or pneumococcal strain) was considered, 89% of respiratory disease isolates were included. This was confirmed in a study with 93% of serotypes implicated in infections in their population being represented in the 23-valent vaccine. Current studies are suggesting a possible shift in serotypes isolated from elderly patients (26,27). Theoretically, the 23-valent pneumococcal vaccine should provide ability to develop immunity against *S. pneumoniae* strains most commonly implicated in disease. Clinical experience has generated controversy regarding vaccine efficacy and cost-effectiveness.

Efficacy

Efficacy has been measured in clinical and serologic terms (see Section, "Antibody Response") with numerous clinical trials showing efficacy ranging from negligible to three fourths of patients (28). The Veterans Affairs Cooperative Study was one of the few randomized controlled trials of pneumococcal vaccine efficacy; however, it has been criticized for lack of power to draw generalized conclusions. In a study population of 2295, one case of pneumococcal infection in 1175 vaccine recipients was observed, whereas 42 infections of proven and probable cause were identified in the control group. In two other trials conducted in individuals >50 years of age, efficacy was 69% and 70%, respectively. A recent randomized trial in Finland comparing pneumococcal and influenza vaccination to influenza vaccine alone demonstrated a protective efficacy for pneumonia of 71% in individuals over 70 years of age with an additional risk (other than age alone) for contracting pneumonia (i.e., those also with heart disease, lung disease, bronchial asthma,

(*Text continues on page 382.*)

Table 3 Recommendations for Adult Immunization in Long-Term Care Facilities

Vaccine name and route	For whom it is recommended	Schedule	Contraindications and precautions (mild illness is not a contraindication)
Influenza Give IM	Adults who are 50 yrs of age or older. Adults <50 yrs of age with medical problems, such as heart disease, lung disease, diabetes, renal dysfunction, hemoglobinopathies, immuno-suppression, and/or those living in chronic care facilities People working or living with at-risk people All health-care workers and those who provide key community services	Given every year October through November is the optimal time to receive an annual flu shot to maximize protection, but the vaccine may be given at any time during the influenza season (typically December–March) or at other times when the risk of influenza exists May be given anytime during the influenza season	Moderate or severe acute illness May be given with all other vaccines but at a separate site Previous anaphylactic reaction to this vaccine, to any of its components, or to eggs Live attenuated influenza vaccine (Flumist™) not approved for patients >49 yrs old
Pneumococcal polysaccharide Given IM or SQ	Adults who are 65 yrs of age or older Adults <65 yrs of age who have chronic illness or other risk factors, including chronic cardiac or pulmonary diseases, chronic liver disease, alcoholism, diabetes mellitus, CSF leaks, as well as persons living in special environments or social settings (including Alaska natives and certain American Indian populations). Those at highest risk of	Routinely given as a one-time dose; administer if previous vaccination history is unknown One-time revaccination is recommended 5 yrs later for people at highest risk of fatal pneumococcal infection or rapid antibody loss (e.g., renal disease) and for people ≥65 yrs if the 1st dose was given prior to age 65 and	May be given with all other vaccines but at a separate site Previous anaphylactic reaction to this vaccine or to any of its components Moderate or severe acute illness

fatal pneumococcal infection are persons with anatomic or functional asplenia, sickle cell disease, immunocompromised persons, including those with HIV infection, leukemia, lymphoma, Hodgkin's disease, multiple myeloma, generalized malignancy, chronic renal failure, or nephrotic syndrome, those receiving immunosuppressive chemotherapy (including corticosteroids), and those who received an organ or bone marrow transplant

> 5 yrs have elapsed since previous dose

Td (tetanus, diphtheria)
Give IM   All adolescents and adults

After the primary series has been completed, a booster dose is recommended every 10 yrs.
Determine if patients have received a primary series of 3 doses
A booster dose as early as 5 yrs later may be needed for the purpose of wound management
Booster dose every 10 yrs after completion of the primary series of 3 doses

Previous anaphylactic or neurologic reaction to this vaccine or to any of its components
Moderate or severe acute illness
May be given with all other vaccines but at a separate site

(Continued)

Table 3 Recommendations for Adult Immunization in Long-Term Care Facilities (*Continued*)

Vaccine name and route	For whom it is recommended	Schedule	Contraindications and precautions (mild illness is not a contraindication)
		For those who have fallen behind: the primary series is 3 doses Give dose #2 4 wks after #1; #3 is given 6–12 mos after #2	
Varicella Give SQ	All susceptible adults and adolescents should be vaccinated. Make special efforts to vaccinate susceptible persons who have close contact with persons at high risk for serious complications (e.g., health-care workers and family contacts of immunocompromised persons) and susceptible persons who are at high risk of exposure (e.g., teachers of young children, day care employees, residents and staff in institutional settings, such as colleges and correctional institutions, military personnel, adolescents and adults living with children, nonpregnant women of childbearing age, and international	Two doses are needed Dose #2 is given 4–8 wks after dose #1	If varicella vaccine and MMR are both needed and are not administered on the same day, space them at least 4 wks apart If the second dose is delayed, do not repeat dose #1. Just give dose #2 Previous anaphylactic reaction to this vaccine or to any of its components Pregnancy, or possibility of pregnancy within 1 mo If blood products or immune globulin have been administered during the past 5 mos, consult the ACIP recommendations regarding

travelers who do not have evidence of immunity).

Note: People with reliable histories of chickenpox (such as self or parental report of disease) can be assumed to be immune. For adults who have no reliable history, serologic testing may be cost effective because most adults with a negative or uncertain history of varicella are immune

Immunocompromised persons due to malignancies and primary or acquired cellular immunodeficiency, including HIV/AIDS.

Note: For those on high-dose immunosuppressive therapy, consult ACIP recommendations regarding delay time Unlabeled use: prevention of herpes zoster and postherpetic neuralgia in the elderly

time to wait before vaccinating Moderate or severe acute illness.

Note: Manufacturer recommends that salicylates be avoided for 6 wks after receiving varicella vaccine because of a theoretical risk of Reyes syndrome

Abbreviations: IM, intramuscular; CSF, cerebrospinal fluid; ACIP, Advisory Committee on Immunization Practices; MMR, measles, mumps, and rubella; SQ, subcutaneous.
Source: From Ref. 24.

alcoholism, or who were institutionalized or permanently bedridden). Individuals with acquired immune deficiency syndrome, young adults, children, and the elderly may all respond differently to the vaccine and require individual study to demonstrate efficacy.

Antibody Response

Vaccine efficacy can also be assessed by antibody response to vaccination. In theory, if an individual develops antibody response to vaccine antigen, the individual is protected from infection. Most healthy adults generate satisfactory antibody response to serotypes in pneumococcal vaccine. In immunocompromised adults or persons who are ≥ 65 years of age, antibody responses have been variable (29–31). Healthy elderly patients have been observed to have lower antibody responses compared with young healthy adults. This would not have been predicted, as pneumococcal vaccine consists of polysaccharide antigens that should generate a T-cell–independent B-cell response, which is less affected by advancing age. However, T-cell–dependent B-cell responses do decline with age, such as for peptides and glycoproteins (e.g., influenza vaccine), suggesting that there may be a T-cell–dependent component to pneumococcal vaccine response.

Currently available pneumococcal vaccines are composed of purified capsular polysaccharide antigens. Polysaccharide vaccines are less immunogenic than other vaccines composed primarily of protein antigens (i.e., live or killed bacteria, viruses, or toxoids). Several advances in the knowledge of protein conjugate technology, immunobiologics, and also antigenic determinants that relate to protection by pneumococcal vaccines are in various stages of development, and promise to improve pneumococcal vaccine efficacy. A pneumococcal conjugate vaccine, Prevnar® by Wyeth-Lederle Laboratories, has been approved for use in children but not in adults.

Cost-Effectiveness

Clinical decision makers are increasingly conditioned to cost of therapeutics before acceptance into general practice. Pneumococcal vaccine has been scrutinized, and negative perceptions may help explain low utilization. Until recently, population-specific efficacy data have been equivocal, with high-risk populations having variable antibody response, compromising measures of efficacy. Health-care providers therefore may not consider pneumococcal vaccination a therapeutic priority, based on available data. Several studies showing cost savings potential of the vaccine have since been published and support its use (32).

The cost savings of the vaccine was evaluated in a retrospective study of Blue Cross/Blue Shield recipients in Minnesota using medical and pharmaceutical claims information. In persons at risk of developing pneumonia, or greater than 50 years of age, the cost savings associated with use of the vaccine was $141 per person or a total observed cost savings of $141,098 for each 1000 persons vaccinated.

Safety

Currently available pneumococcal vaccines are safe. Reactions to initial administration has shown erythema and pain at injection site in 50%; fever, myalgia, and severe local reactions <1%; and anaphylaxis that was reported to occur in approximately five cases per million. Neurologic complications, reported with vaccines derived from whole, killed, or live-attenuated organisms, have not been associated with pneumococcal vaccine. Product information of current pneumococcal vaccines reports temporal association with neurological disorders, such as paresthesias, and acute radiculopathy, including Guillain–Barré. There are no case reports in the medical literature to support this observation, specifically with regard to Guillain–Barré, a presumed but unproven adverse effect of some other vaccines.

Revaccination with pneumococcal vaccine has been reported to result in more severe local reactions when administration time between the primary and secondary doses was ≤13 months but low in those unable to recall when prior vaccination occurred. The incidence of adverse effects is similar for revaccination and primary immunization when revaccination occurs >4 years after the initial dose. Revaccination should be considered for those at highest risk of pneumococcal disease and complications (Table 3).

Drug Interactions

Administration of pneumococcal and influenza vaccines in separate IM sites has not caused increased adverse effects or reduced immunogenicity and is accepted by the CDC, when necessary to administer two or more vaccines concurrently. Corticosteroids and other immunosuppressant drugs (e.g., alkylating agents, antimetabolites, antithymocyte antibodies, cyclosporine, and radioisotopes) may interfere with antibody response to vaccine. Vaccination should be delayed for 3 to 12 months after discontinuing immunosuppressant therapy.

Tetanus and Diphtheria

Tetanus

Tetanus is one of the oldest diseases known. National surveillance began in the United States in 1947, when the incidence of tetanus was 0.39 per 100,000 person-years. The incidence has declined to 0.01 per 100,000 person-years (based on 2003 data; 20 reported cases, including two deaths) (33–35). The risk of tetanus is doubled in individuals ≥60 years old, compared with those aged 20 to 59 years and is >12-fold that of those aged five to 19.

Tetanus is caused by *Clostridium tetani,* a spore-forming, gram-positive, anaerobic bacillus. As part of the intestinal microbial flora in humans and animals, it is widely distributed in fecally contaminated soil. *C. tetani* toxin results in prolonged muscular spasm of flexor and extensor muscle groups. Advanced tetanus shows generalized flexion contractures and prolonged masseter muscle spasm ("lockjaw"). Respiratory failure from involvement of the respiratory muscles can lead to death.

The risk of tetanus and associated mortality increases with age. The case-fatality ratio for elderly was 40%, compared with 8% in patients aged 20 to 59 years (CDC data from 1998 to 2000) (35). Elders are more prone to tetanus mostly because protective antitoxin levels decline with age and frailty. Healthy, independent living elders have vaccine immune responses similar to younger populations. Pressure ulcers, vascular ulcers, and surgical wounds are more common in elders placing hospitalized and institutionalized persons at risk. Fecal incontinence, common in many frail elderly, increases risk of pressure ulcers and potential contamination with *C. tetani.*

A U.S. population-based serologic survey of immunity to tetanus showed prevalent immunity of 28% in persons ≥70 years old, compared with 80% in younger individuals. In LTCF studies of those with average age of 80 years, protective antitetanus antibodies occur in 29% to 51% of the residents. Protective antibody titers decline with age, especially in women, whereas men with previous military service show better tetanus immunity.

Besides immunization, better care of wounds reduces incidence of tetanus. Those lacking primary vaccination series, particularly elderly women, are occasionally identified. These persons should receive tetanus immune globulin for contaminated wounds. Booster alone is appropriate if the patient received a primary series but not tetanus toxoid within five years. An attempt should be made to determine the primary immunization status of LTCF residents. Patients with uncertain immunization history are considered tetanus toxoid naive. Military veterans since 1941 are considered to have received at least one dose. Most have completed a primary series, but this cannot be assumed. The number of people at risk will increase unless elders are more conscientiously given tetanus toxoid.

Diphtheria

Diphtheria was described in 1821 by Pierre Brettonneau. It is an illness caused by *Corynebacterium diphtheriae* and is now very rare in the United States, with few cases reported per year, mostly in nonimmunized elders. Only one fatal, confirmed case was reported in 2003: an elderly man never vaccinated to diphtheria, who had traveled to Haiti (34). Pathogenesis of diphtheria begins with *C. diphtheriae* mucosal colonization of the nose or mouth. Toxin elaboration causes tissue necrosis and local inflammation followed by absorption of toxin, which has tropism for cardiac, neural, and renal cells. Clinical manifestations appear after toxin tissue fixation with myocarditis in 10 to 14 days and peripheral neuritis three to seven weeks after disease onset. Tonsillar and pharyngeal diphtheria is characterized by anorexia, malaise, low-grade fever, and sore throat. Severe cases are associated with toxemia, myocarditis, arrhythmias, congestive heart failure, stupor, coma, and death within 6 to 10 days. Cutaneous diphtheria is indolent and often occurs at burn sites or other wounds and is more common in warmer climates and in poverty, overcrowding, and poor hygiene.

Widespread use of diphtheria toxoid in the United States limits annual incidence to practically nil, with one case reported to the CDC in 2003 (34). More than 90% of diphtheria cases occur in unvaccinated adults. Susceptibility reflects reduced lifetime exposure (to *C. diphtheriae*) and failure to administer the primary vaccine series and decadal boosters throughout life.

Vaccine Effectiveness

Tetanus-diphtheria toxoids (Td) are among the most immunogenic of vaccines indicated for older adults, and they are almost 100% effective in immunocompetent persons with up-to-date vaccination status. Naturally acquired immunity to tetanus toxin does not occur, and natural immunity to diphtheria occurs in only 50% of infected individuals. Primary immunization with tetanus toxoid provides 10 or more years of protection. Appropriately timed boosters are needed to maintain antitoxin titers.

Recent outbreaks of diphtheria abroad highlight risk of diphtheria. After a 23-year period without reported cases, the disease reemerged in Sweden. Although 95% to 99% of children were vaccinated and 81% of the population <20 years old had protective immunity, only 19% of women and 44% of men >60 years old had protective immunity. Individuals who died or had neurological complications had low antibody levels, whereas 33 of 36 symptom-free carriers of the same strain had protective antibody titers. In Kyrgyzstan in 1995, the case-fatality ratio of 676 of hospitalized diphtheria cases was 3%. In the United States, the number of older adults with protective antibody to both tetanus and diphtheria is low, making an experience similar to Sweden's likely if we are unable to better vaccinate our population.

Indications

Elders should be immunized against both tetanus and diphtheria with the initial primary series and revaccination every 10 years. Anyone not having received the complete primary series should complete it with combined Td vaccine, although earlier doses do not need repeating if the schedule is delayed. A booster dose even 30 years after primary vaccination results in protection for tetanus and diphtheria. Getting the series up to date is especially relevant if travel to developing countries is anticipated.

Td prophylaxis is recommended for clean, minor wounds if the primary series is incomplete or the last booster vaccination was >10 years ago. Serious wounds require active and passive immunization with tetanus immune globulin.

Cost effectiveness of tetanus immunization, specifically booster doses, has been questioned. Because tetanus is rare, the cost of each case prevented and associated year of life gained is high. Some experts have recommended targeting high-risk adults, such as those with vascular ulcers or at time of injury, for revaccination.

Administration and Revaccination

Tetanus toxoid is produced singly or in combination with diphtheria toxoid (Td) with or without whole-cell or acellular pertussis vaccine. In LTCF elders, Td is recommended. The primary series in adults is two 0.5 mL doses of Td given IM one to two months apart, followed by a third 0.5 mL dose 6 to 12 months later. The Td vaccine contains 10% of the diphtheria toxoid in the pediatric DTP, making it much less reactogenic.

Adverse Reactions

Current vaccines are well tolerated. High reactogenicity of childhood DTP vaccines are attributed to the pertussis component, and that has been minimized with transition to acellular formulation of pertussis antigen. Contraindication to tetanus and diphtheria toxoid is a history of neurological or severe hypersensitivity reaction after a previous dose, or sensitivity to the preservative.

Previously immunized adults have local reactions in 40% to 50% of vaccinations. Less than 10% of those vaccinated have redness or swelling >5 cm. Side effects include local reactions, fever, chills, hypersensitivity, arthralgia, rash, and encephalopathy. Reactions are related to high anti-toxin titers or by hypersensitivity to the mercury preservative.

Td vaccination occurred without major sequelae following a vaccination program for 161 institutionalized veterans. Nine percent of the participants had local reactions generally considered insignificant. A fall in one individual was attributed to a sore deltoid muscle. A sore arm may be only a minor inconvenience in a healthy adult; however, an individual who depends on arm support for environmental stability and transfers may be placed at risk for falls and fractures.

VARICELLA VACCINE

Varicella immunization is recommended for all LTCF residents and staff without a history of primary varicella infection ("chicken pox"). It has been suggested that as varicella incidence declines due to increased pediatric use of varicella vaccine the rate of herpes zoster virus (HZV) infection will increase (see also Chapter 17) (36). However, the incidence of herpes zoster has remained stable so far (37). HZV is a prevalent condition in LTCF residents, with high rate of complication, most notably postherpetic neuralgia with high patient suffering and cost. Varicella vaccine boosts cell-mediated immunity to HZV in elders and can reduce the incidence of herpes zoster and its complications (38); however, it is not yet approved by the Food and Drug Administration for zoster prevention in LTC residents.

VACCINATION OF HEALTH-CARE WORKERS IN LTCFs

Immunization of health-care staff is recommended to prevent spread of infection to frail elders in LTCFs. The recommended vaccination rate for staff with direct patient contact is 80%. Immunization rates in LTCF staff remain low despite these recommendations.One study evaluated the effects of vaccinating health-care staff in geriatric LTC hospitals on incidence of influenza, lower respiratory tract infections, and death. When staff were vaccinated, ILI occurred in 7.7% of unvaccinated patients, compared with 0.9% of vaccinated patients. Fewer patients died in hospitals where health-care staff were vaccinated than where not vaccinated (10% vs. 17%, respectively).

Clinical data on efficacy of health-care staff vaccination with respect to resident benefit are primarily on influenza vaccination. It is still reasonable to encourage pneumococcal vaccination to reduce carriage of pathogenic- and antibiotic-resistant strains and hepatitis vaccination to protect staff, in addition to annual influenza vaccination. To maximize compliance, vaccination should be free to employees, and vaccine status reviewed upon employment and annually at the time influenza vaccination. A formal policy of vaccination status review and annual education regarding importance of vaccination to staff and residents will help compliance. Policy review and enforcement should be assigned to the infection control practitioner, backed with authority from administration, and consistent with local, state, and federal statutes.

SUMMARY

Infectious diseases are an important cause of morbidity and mortality in LTCFs. Risk is partially due to enclosed setting, close living conditions affecting disease transmissibility, and immunosenescence. Vaccination is important in infection control for LTCFs. Pneumococcal, tetanus/diphtheria, and influenza vaccines should be part of admission standing orders. Standing orders and policy should address past vaccination status, initial and repeat vaccination timing, and contraindications. For health-care staff, these three vaccines, plus hepatitis vaccine, should be included in infection control policy, be readily available, and be provided in employee benefits to improve use. New vaccines being developed may have better safety and immunogenicity. Shingles from HZV now appears to be a vaccine-preventable disease (38). The role of vaccines is expanding from prevention to include treatment for various diseases including osteoporosis and Alzheimer's disease. LTCF practitioners should follow development of vaccine benefits, policy and strategies to maximize uptake in residents and staff.

SUGGESTED READING

Centers for Disease Control and Prevention (CDC). Recommended adult immunization schedule—United States, October 2005–September 2006. MMWR Morb Mortal Wkly Rep 2005; 54:Q1–Q4.
Oxman MN, Levin MJ, Johnson GR, et al. A vaccine to prevent herpes zoster and postherpetic neuralgia in older adults. N Engl J Med 2005; 352:2271–2284.

REFERENCES

1. Tarazona R, Solana R, Ouyang Q, Pawelec G. Basic biology and clinical impact of immunosenescence. Exp Gerontol 2002; 37:183–189.
2. Gavazzi G, Krause KH. Ageing and infection. Lancet Infect Dis 2002; 2:659–666.
3. Ginaldi L, Loreto MF, Corsi MP, Modesti M, De Martinis M. Immunosenescence and infectious diseases. Microbes Infect 2001; 3:851–857.
4. Castle SC. Clinical relevance of age-related immune dysfunction. Clin Infect Dis 2000; 31:578–585.
5. Castle SC. Impact of age-related immune dysfunction on risk of infections. Z Gerontol Geriatr 2000; 33:341–349.
6. Norman DC, Yoshikawa TT. Fever in the elderly. Infect Dis Clin North Am 1996; 10:93–99.
7. Roghmann MC, Warner J, Mackowiak PA. The relationship between age and fever magnitude. Am J Med Sci 2001; 322:68–70.
8. Monto AS, Gravenstein S, Elliott M, Colopy M, Schweinle J. Clinical signs and symptoms predicting influenza infection. Arch Intern Med 2000; 160:3243–3247.
9. Castle SC, Norman DC, Yeh M, Miller D, Yoshikawa TT. Fever response in elderly nursing home residents: are the older truly colder? J Am Geriatr Soc 1991; 39:853–857.
10. Stevenson CG, McArthur MA, Naus M, Abraham E, McGeer AJ. Prevention of influenza and pneumococcal pneumonia in Canadian long-term care facilities: How are we doing? CMAJ 2001; 164:1413–1419.
11. Thiry N, Beutels P, Van Damme P, Van Doorslaer E. Economic evaluations of varicella vaccination programmes: a review of the literature. Pharmacoeconomics 2003; 21:13–38.
12. Shefer A, McKibben L, Bardenheier B, Bratzler D, Roberts H. Characteristics of long-term care facilities associated with standing order programs to deliver influenza and pneumococcal vaccinations to residents in 13 states. J Am Med Dir Assoc 2005; 6:97–104.
13. Bardenheier B, Shefer A, McKibben L, Roberts H, Bratzler D. Characteristics of long-term-care facility residents associated with receipt of influenza and pneumococcal vaccinations. Infect Control Hosp Epidemiol 2004; 25:946–954.
14. Bardenheier BH, Shefer A, McKibben L, Roberts H, Rhew D, Bratzler D. Factors predictive of increased influenza and pneumococcal vaccination

coverage in long-term care facilities: the CMS-CDC Standing Orders Program project. J Am Med Dir Assoc 2005; 6:291–299.

15. Anderson RN, Smith BL. Deaths: leading causes for 2002. Natl Vital Stat Rep 2005; 53:1–89.
16. Barker WH, Mullooly JP. Influenza vaccination of elderly persons. Reduction in pneumonia and influenza hospitalizations and deaths. JAMA 1980; 244: 2547–2549.
17. Gravenstein S, Drinka P, Osterweil D, et al. Inhaled zanamivir versus rimantadine for the control of influenza in a highly vaccinated long-term care population. J Am Med Dir Assoc 2005; 6:359–366.
18. Ambrozaitis A, Gravenstein S, van Essen GA, et al. Inhaled zanamivir versus placebo for the prevention of influenza outbreaks in an unvaccinated long-term care population. J Am Med Dir Assoc 2005; 6:367–374.
19. Glezen WP. Cold-adapted, live attenuated influenza vaccine. Expert Rev Vaccines 2004; 3:131–139.
20. Pottumarthy S, Fritsche TR, Sader HS, Stilwell MG, Jones RN. Susceptibility patterns of *Streptococcus pneumoniae* isolates in North America (2002–2003): contemporary in vitro activities of amoxicillin/clavulanate and 15 other antimicrobial agents. Int J Antimicrob Agents 2005; 25:282–289.
21. Porat N, Arguedas A, Spratt BG, et al. Emergence of penicillin-nonsusceptible *Streptococcus pneumoniae* clones expressing serotypes not present in the antipneumococcal conjugate vaccine. J Infect Dis 2004; 190:2154–2161.
22. Ament A, Fedson DS, Christie P. Pneumococcal vaccination and pneumonia: even a low level of clinical effectiveness is highly cost-effective. Clin Infect Dis 2001; 33:2078–2079.
23. De Graeve D, Beutels P. Economic aspects of pneumococcal pneumonia: a review of the literature. Pharmacoeconomics 2004; 22:719–740.
24. Recommended Adult Immunization Schedule—United States, October 2004–September 2005. MMWR 2004; 53(45):Q1–Q4.
25. Whitney CG. Preventing pneumococcal disease. ACIP recommends pneumococcal polysaccharide vaccine for all adults age > or = 65. Geriatrics 2003; 58: 20–22, 25.
26. Feikin DR, Klugman KP, Facklam RR, Zell ER, Schuchat A, Whitney CG. Active Bacterial Core surveillance/Emerging Infections Program network. Increased prevalence of pediatric pneumococcal serotypes in elderly adults. Clin Infect Dis 2005; 41:481–487.
27. Kellner JD, Mandell L. Pneumococcal serotypes in the elderly. Clin Infect Dis 2005; 41:488–489.
28. Conaty S, Watson L, Dinnes J, Waugh N. The effectiveness of pneumococcal polysaccharide vaccines in adults: a systematic review of observational studies and comparison with results from randomised controlled trials. Vaccine 2004; 22:3214–3224.
29. Mufson MA. Antibody response of pneumococcal vaccine: need for booster dosing? Int J Antimicrob Agents 2000; 14:107–112.
30. Lackner TE, Hamilton RG, Hill JJ, Davey C, Guay DR. Pneumococcal polysaccharide revaccination: immunoglobulin g seroconversion, persistence, and safety in frail, chronically ill older subjects. J Am Geriatr Soc 2003; 51:240–245.
31. Brandao AP, de Oliveira TC, de Cunto Brandileone MC, Goncalves JE, Yara TI, Simonsen V. Persistence of antibody response to pneumococcal capsular

polysaccharides in vaccinated long term-care residents in Brazil. Vaccine 2004; 23:762–768.

32. Melegaro A, Edmunds WJ. The 23-valent pneumococcal polysaccharide vaccine. Part II. A cost-effectiveness analysis for invasive disease in the elderly in England and Wales. Eur J Epidemiol 2004; 19:365–375.

33. Bardenheier B, Prevots DR, Khetsuriani N, Wharton M. Tetanus surveillance—United States, 1995–1997. MMWR CDC Surveill Summ 1998; 47:1–13.

34. Hopkins RS, Jajosky RA, Hall PA, et al. Summary of notifiable diseases—United States, 2003. MMWR Morb Mortal Wkly Rep 2005; 52:1–85.

35. Pascual FB, McGinley EL, Zanardi LR, Cortese MM, Murphy TV. Tetanus surveillance—United States, 1998–2000. MMWR Surveill Summ 2003; 52:1–8.

36. Wagenpfeil S, Neiss A, Wutzler P. Effects of varicella vaccination on herpes zoster incidence. Clin Microbiol Infect 2004; 10:954–960.

37. Jumaan AO, Yu O, Jackson LA, Bohlke K, Galil K, Seward JF. Incidence of herpes zoster, before and after varicella-vaccination-associated decreases in the incidence of varicella, 1992–2002. J Infect Dis 2005; 191:2002–2007.

38. Oxman MN, Levin MJ, Johnson GR, et al. A vaccine to prevent herpes zoster and postherpetic neuralgia in older adults. N Engl J Med 2005; 352:2271–2284.

23

Methicillin-Resistant *Staphylococcus aureus*

Thomas T. Yoshikawa

Office of Research, Charles R. Drew University of Medicine and Science, Los Angeles, California, U.S.A.

Larry J. Strausbaugh

Portland Veterans Affairs Medical Center and Oregon Health Sciences University School of Medicine, Portland, Oregon, U.S.A.

KEY POINTS

1. MRSA prevalence in LTCFs ranges from 5% to 34%; however, the vast majority of residents carrying MRSA are colonized and not infected.
2. Person-to-person contact accounts for most cases of MRSA transmission, with transiently colonized health-care workers passing on the organism to residents.
3. Skin, soft tissue, and respiratory tract are the most common sites of MRSA colonization and infection.
4. MRSA infections are best treated with vancomycin, with quinipristin–dalfopristin and linezolid being effective alternative agents.
5. During outbreaks of MRSA in an LTCF, segregation of colonized and infected residents should be instituted. The role and success of decolonization therapy with antimicrobial agents are unclear and unproven.

INTRODUCTION

Methicillin-resistant *Staphylococcus aureus* (MRSA) is defined by minimum inhibitory concentrations of methicillin of $16\,\mu g/mL$ or more or oxacillin $4\,\mu g/mL$ or more (1). Strains of MRSA possess the *mecA* gene (1,2). This chromosomal gene encodes an altered enzyme, termed penicillin-binding protein 2a (or PBP2′), which has a low affinity for all beta-lactam antibiotics. As a rule, strains of MRSA also possess resistance determinants for many other antimicrobial agents.

Strains of MRSA emerged soon after methicillin became commercially available in the early 1960s (2,3). They became increasingly prevalent in the United States in the late 1970s (2,4). By the year 2000, MRSA strains accounted for 53% of all *S. aureus* clinical isolates obtained from patients with nosocomial infections that were acquired in U.S. intensive care units (5). As MRSA became more prevalent in acute care settings, the continual interchange of patients between hospitals and long-term care facilities (LTCFs) ensured their spread into the latter. The first report of MRSA in a U.S. nursing home appeared in 1970 (6); however, strains of MRSA remained uncommon in this setting until 1985.

EPIDEMIOLOGY AND CLINICAL RELEVANCE

Frequency of MRSA Colonization

Prevalence surveys that targeted both infected and colonized residents offer the most comprehensive assessment of MRSA infiltration into LTCFs, because the ratio of colonized residents to infected residents generally exceeds 20 to 1 (4). Counting only infected residents underestimates the magnitude of a facility's MRSA burden. Colonization denotes asymptomatic persons who harbor MRSA at some body site, for example, the anterior nares (7). Detection requires bacterial cultures of the colonized site. In contrast, infected individuals have symptoms and signs of disease with positive cultures from the affected site.

Rates of MRSA colonization in LTCFs have ranged from 5% to 34% in prevalence studies (8–18) reported from facilities in nine states (Table 1). These studies have detected nasal carriage most frequently, but rectal, perineal, wound, urine, and sputum cultures occasionally yielded MRSA. Although Veterans Affairs (VA) facilities often have higher colonization rates than community nursing homes, considerable overlap is noted.

Three prevalence studies reported MRSA colonization rates in LTCF health-care workers ranging from 2.3% to 7% (Table 1). As in other health-care settings, colonized workers serve as both reservoir and vector for MRSA (1–4,7).

Natural History of MRSA in LTCF

New residents who are already colonized or infected with MRSA bring this organism into LTCFs at the time of their admission and serve as the initial

Table 1 Prevalence of Methicillin-Resistant *Staphylococcus aureus* in Long-Term Care Facilities

Ref	LTCF location	Study period	No. beds (LTCF type)	% Residents colonized with MRSA	Comment
8	St. Louis, Missouri	3/85	82 (Comm NH)	12	Nasal cultures of 74 residents; 7% of nursing home staff colonized
9	Los Angeles, California	5/87 and 8/87	170 (Comm NH)	7.3 and 6.0	Nasal and wound cultures from all residents on 2 separate occasions; 3.4% and 2.3% staff colonized
10	Pittsburgh, Pennsylvania	1/86–12/88	432 (VA NHCU)	13.1	981 total nasal cultures (obtained at monthly and bimonthly intervals); 32 residents persistently colonized
11	Vancouver, Washington	3/89	120 (VA NHCU)	34	Nasal and wound cultures from all residents; 7% of staff colonized
12	Chicago, Illinois	8/88–11/89	150 (Comm NH)	4.9–15.6	Eight facility-wide nasal culture surveys over 15 mo; overall 8.7% of 994 nasal cultures positive for MRSA
13	Ann Arbor, Michigan	6/89–5/90	120 (VA NHCU)	23 + 1.0 (mean monthly rate)	Monthly cultures of nose, perineum, rectum, and wounds; 25% of residents colonized on admission; only 10% of newly admitted patients acquired MRSA
14	Baltimore, Maryland	1/89–1/90	233 (Comm NH)	22	Culture of nares, pressure ulcers, ostomy sites, urine and sputum; 25% of new admissions in 4 mo after prevalence survey found to be MRSA colonized

(Continued)

Table 1 Prevalence of Methicillin-Resistant *Staphylococcus aureus* in Long-Term Care Facilities (*Continued*)

Ref	LTCF location	Study period	No. beds (LTCF type)	% Residents colonized with MRSA	Comment
15	Ann Arbor, Michigan	6/89–5/91	120 (VA NHCU)	22.7 + 1.0 (year 1) 11.5 + 1.8 (year 2)(mean monthly rate)	Monthly cultures of nose, perineum, rectum, and wounds; mupirocin intervention introduced in year 2
16	Durham, North Carolina	12/91–1/92	120–125 beds (1 VA and 3 Comm NHs)	27.3 (VA NHCU) 8.1 (3 Comm NHs)	Nasal cultures performed on all consenting residents; differences between VA NHCU and 3 community nursing homes persisted over time
17	Orange County, California	1990–1992 (20 months)	149 (Comm NH)	7.5 (cumulative during study period)	Cultures of nares and rectum obtained quarterly over 20 mo; 4.1% of nares and 2.5% of rectal cultures
18	Orange County, California	1993–1994 (12 months)	149 (Comm NH)	9.7 (overall mean)	Cultures of nares and rectum obtained on admission and quarterly; overall 35% of residents colonized at least once with *Staphylococcus aureus*–72% with MSSA and 25% with MRSA; 13% of carriers detected only with rectal cultures

Abbreviations: VA, veterans affairs; NHCU, nursing home care unit; Comm, community; NH, nursing home; MSSA, methicillin-susceptible *Staphylococcus aureus*; MRSA, methicillin-resistant *Staphylococcus aureus*, LTCF, long-term care facility reservoir (7,11). Asymptomatic residents transferred directly from acute care facilities where MRSA strains are prevalent probably account for most of this spread. Screening cultures in various types of facilities have indicated that 2% to 25% of new residents harbor this organism in their nose or at some other body site (12–14,17).

Once it has entered an LTCF, MRSA tends to spread and persist. Spread may be dramatic. For example, 15 months after the introduction of MRSA into a VA nursing home care unit in Vancouver, Washington, a prevalence study indicated that 34% of residents and 7% of staff were colonized with the out-break strain (11). A nasal prevalence study conducted almost three years later indicated that 10% of the facility's residents remained colonized (19). Serial prevalence studies in other LTCFs also testify to MRSA's persistence in this environment. Individual residents may remain colonized for months to years.

As in other health-care settings, colonized or infected residents and colonized staff constitute the reservoir for MRSA. Person-to-person spread accounts for most transmission, and direct contact of residents with the hands of transiently colonized health-care workers probably represents the principal mode of acquisition (20). Although uncommon, hand carriage of MRSA by health-care workers has been documented in LTCFs (21). Resident-to-resident transmission may also occur. In a one-year prevalence study, nine residents—approximately 25% of residents acquiring MRSA in the facility that year—became colonized with the same phage type as their roommate (13). In that situation, direct contact with the roommate or indirect contact with contaminated objects in the environment or colonized health-care workers represents the likely means of spread. It is not known how frequently resident contacts with MRSA lead to prolonged colonization, but carriage rates in LTCFs suggest that it occurs commonly.

Infection Caused by MRSA

Skin and soft tissue infections, urinary tract infections, and respiratory tract infections account for the majority of infections. Because these three types of infections predominate in LTCFs (22), MRSA's involvement is not unexpected. Like methicillin-susceptible *S. aureus* (MSSA) in LTCFs, MRSA causes skin and soft tissue infections with greater frequency than any other types of infections.

Generally, MRSA infections arise in residents who have been colonized for various lengths of time. The risk of colonized residents developing infection varies considerably and depends to some extent on cormorbid conditions, such as pressure ulcers and influenza. In one VA report, 25% of 32 persistently colonized residents developed staphylococcal infections (10). In contrast, only 4% of residents persistently colonized with MSSA, and 4.5% of residents not colonized with *S. aureus* became infected. Thus, in this study, persistent colonization with MRSA carried a significantly greater risk of subsequent infection.

Other VA studies have reported much lower percentages of infection in MRSA-colonized individuals. For example, in a one-year study, only 3% of 341 patients at risk developed MRSA infection, even though MRSA carriage rates exceeded 20% (13).

In another study, the risk of infection in MRSA-colonized residents in one VA facility and three community nursing homes was 6.4 times [95% confidence interval (CI), 2.3–18.0] greater in residents colonized at baseline (16). No statistically significant increased risk in the VA facility was detected. However, the risk of infection in MRSA-colonized residents in the three community nursing homes was 15 times (95% CI, 13.3–73.3) that seen in noncolonized residents. The rates of MRSA infection in the VA facility and three community nursing homes did not differ significantly in the one-year of study, even though colonization rates were higher in the former.

In sum, MRSA infections usually arise in colonized residents, but only a small percentage of colonized residents become infected. Infections caused by MRSA in LTCFs are similar to those caused by MSSA in this environment. Unlike other common bacterial pathogens in LTCFs, they cause skin and soft tissue infections with greater frequency than urinary or respiratory tract infections.

Risk Factors for Colonization and Infection by MRSA in LTCFs

Risk factors for MRSA colonization and infection in LTCFs mirror those associated with other antimicrobial-resistant bacteria (7). In general terms, these include poor functional status, conditions that cause skin breakdown, presence of invasive devices, prior antimicrobial therapy, and a history of antecedent colonization. Studies have identified the following specific risk factors for MRSA colonization in LTCFs: male gender, urinary incontinence, fecal incontinence, presence of wounds, pressure ulcers, nasogastric intubation, antibiotic therapy, and hospitalization within previous six months.

Only two VA studies have examined risk factors for MRSA infection in LTCFs. Using stepwise logistic regression analysis, one study found persistent MRSA colonization and dialysis to be significantly associated with infection with odds ratio (ORs) of 5.9 (95% CI, 2.2–15) and 4.7 (95% CI, 1.8–12), respectively. Another study used similar methods and identified diabetes mellitus (OR = 5.1; 95% CI, 2.1–18.6) and peripheral vascular disease (OR = 4.3; 95% CI, 1.3–14.3) as risk factors for MRSA infection (15).

CLINICAL MANIFESTATION

Syndromes and Pathogenesis

MRSA and MSSA appear to have equivalent virulence for humans (1,2,4). Accordingly, the kinds of infections caused by MRSA and their clinical features are virtually identical to those caused by MSSA (Table 2).

Table 2 Clinical Infections Associated with Methicillin-Resistant *Staphylococcus aureus* and Methicillin-Susceptible *S. aureus* in Elderly Persons

Clinical site	Types of infection
Lung	Pneumonia, empyema, abscess
Urinary tract	Intrarenal abscess, perinephric abscess, pyelonephritis, catheter-related UTI
Skin/soft tissue	Cellulitis, abscess (furuncles, carbuncles), postsurgical wound
Bone and joint	Septic arthritis, acute, and chronic osteomyelitis
CNS	Meningitis, brain abscess, epidermal abscess, subdural empyema
Heart	Endocarditis, pericarditis
Prosthetic devices	Heart valves, joints, CNS shunts, hemodialysis shunts, IV catheter

Abbreviations: IV, intravenous, CNS, central nervous system; UTI, urinary tract infection.

S. aureus on cutaneous surfaces combined with breeches in the integrity of skin and mucous membranes likely gives rise to skin and soft tissue infections, which may include cellulitis, surgical site and other wound infections, bursitis, perianal and skin abscesses, infected pressure ulcers, infected leg ulcers, and paronychia. Nasal colonization in association with aspiration probably contributes to the development of pneumonia. *S. aureus* on perineal skin or genital membranes and the presence of indwelling urinary catheters likely predispose LTCF residents to staphylococcal urinary tract infections.

Both MRSA and MSSA can invade the bloodstream and give rise to distant site infections, such as arthritis, endocarditis, osteomyelitis, visceral abscesses, and others. Bacteremias and distant site infections account for a small percentage of staphylococcal infections in LTCF residents. In some cases, bone and joint involvement may result from local invasion, for example contiguous spread from infected pressure ulcers.

Clinical Features

The manifestations of various infectious syndromes caused by MRSA in LTCF resident are similar to those caused by other pyogenic bacteria. However, elderly nursing home residents often have atypical presentations for MRSA infections, as they do for those caused by other etiological agents. Local and systemic inflammatory responses may be diminished, resulting in decreased temperature elevations and blunting of local manifestations (22,23). Neurological deficits and cognitive impairment, which are common in elderly nursing home residents, may also obscure symptoms and signs of MRSA and other types of infection. Accordingly, LTCF practitioners maintain a high index of suspicion for infection and subtle signs, such as minor changes in mental or functional status, as possible indicators of MRSA and other types of infections.

DIAGNOSTIC APPROACH

Recognition and Delineation of Clinical Syndrome

MRSA-infected LTCF residents come to clinical attention in the usual ways. Reports from nursing staff about temperature elevation or other alteration in vital signs often prompt evaluation, as do those that describe specific symptoms or signs of infection. Diminished cognitive function and inability to perform usual activities of daily living also bring patients to clinical attention (23). Often the residents' history and a limited physical examination disclose the presence of MRSA infection. For example, residents with a new cough, tachypnea, and rales over one lung field probably have pneumonia. Pneumonia caused by MRSA enters the differential diagnosis from the outset in known carriers and in facilities with high rates of colonization or infection. Similarly, the resident with a colonized pressure ulcer who develops fever and redness, swelling, and tenderness extending out from the margins of the ulcer likely has an MRSA secondary infection of that site.

The use of laboratory tests, radiography, and other ancillary procedures in the diagnosis of MRSA infections conforms to current guidelines (23). Leukocytosis, infiltrates on chest radiographs, pyuria, and bacteriuria (especially in uncatheterized residents), and meaningful Gram stain results from respiratory secretions or cutaneous exudates, all help to define syndromic diagnoses.

Etiological Diagnosis

On gram-stained smears, both MSSA and MRSA appear as gram-positive cocci, often in clumps, or grapelike clusters. Gram-stain findings do not distinguish between the two. Strains of both bacteria grow easily on most nonselective media, such as blood agar, yielding white to yellowish colonies within a day or less (1). Rapid test for coagulase production readily distinguish *S. aureus* from other species of *Staphylococcus*. Distinguishing MRSA from MSSA usually requires antimicrobial susceptibility tests, which typically necessitate a second day for completion. Therefore, isolation of MRSA strains generally requires 36 to 48 hours. Some clinical laboratories offer faster service by identifying MRSA strains with gene probes that detect *mec*A.

The etiologic diagnosis awaits finalization of culture results and their interpretation in the context of the resident's illness and course. Isolation of MRSA from the blood cultures of symptomatic residents virtually always indicates MRSA infection, whereas isolation from respiratory secretions, cutaneous exudates, and urine require interpretation to distinguish colonization from infection. In residents with strong clinical evidence for a specific infectious syndrome, isolation of MRSA in pure culture often solidifies the etiologic diagnosis, especially when Gram stain results indicate that the bacterium is present in large numbers. Isolation of MRSA with other potential pathogens in the same culture and isolation of MRSA from a site not clearly involved by an infectious process, for example, from urine in a catheterized resident with no genitourinary symptoms, provoke the greatest diagnostic uncertainty. Nevertheless, from a therapeutic standpoint, few practitioners can dismiss such isolates obtained from symptomatic residents, because MRSA may be an etiological participant.

THERAPEUTIC INTERVENTIONS

Antimicrobial Therapy

Antimicrobial therapy with systemic antibiotics should be reserved for MRSA infections and not be prescribed for colonization. Isolation of MRSA from mucocutaneous surfaces (e.g., rectum, skin) in the absence of symptoms or signs of infection is generally due to colonization and does not require antimicrobial therapy unless it is associated with an outbreak of MRSA. Under these circumstances, topical mupirocin ointment applied to skin, wounds, or mucosa for short periods may temporarily eradicate the organism and halt the outbreak (24).

Table 3 summarizes the antibiotics that are recommended for treating systemic infections caused by MRSA (24). Vancomycin is the antibiotic of choice, but it can only be administered by the intravenous route. Similarly, quinipristin–dalfopristin is available for only intravenous administration (25). Linezolid has the advantage of having both an oral and an intravenous formulation, which could facilitate therapy in the LTCF setting (25). Daptomycin, given intravenously, may be considered for skin and soft-tissue

Table 3 Antibiotics Recommended for Methicillin-Resistant *Staphylococcus aureus* Infections

Antibiotic	Dosage	Route	Toxicity/comments
Vancomycin	500–1000 mg	IV	Potential otoxocicity; "red man" syndrome; adjust dose for renal function
Quinupristin– dalfopristin	75 mg/kg q 8 hr	IV	Pheblitis; arthralgias; potential drug interactions (e.g., quinidine; nifedipine)
Linezolid	400–600 mg q 12 hr	IV, PO	Leukopenia, thrombocytopenia; neuropathy; potential drug interactions (e.g., pseudoephedrine, SSRI)
Daptomycin	4 mg/kg	IV	Potential rhabdomyolysis; adjust for renal function

Abbreviations: IV, intravenous; PO, oral (per OS), SSRI, selective serotonin receptor inhibitor.

infections caused by MRSA. Most infections require 10 to 14 days of therapy, with more severe infections, such as osteomyelitis and endocarditis, necessitating treatment for as long as four to six weeks.

Role of Drainage, Debridement, and Other Surgical Procedures

Cure of MRSA and MSSA infections associated with abscesses, devitalized tissue, and closed spaces, such as joints or pleural cavity, usually requires drainage or debridement (1). Abscesses, depending on their location and size, require either drainage from percutaneously placed catheters or needles or drainage from an open surgical procedure. Repeated needle aspirations generally suffice for infected joints, except for the hip, which requires open surgical drainage. Pleural empyemas require chest tube thoracostomies and, rarely, decortication procedures. Surgical debridement is necessary to cure chronic osteomyelitis or osteomyelitis associated with peripheral vascular disease. Also, MRSA-infected arthroplasties and other infections involving prosthetic material generally necessitate removal of foreign material and surgical debridement. Management of endocarditis may require valve replacement surgery. It is apparent that management of these infections will generally require transfer to an acute care facility.

INFECTION CONTROL MEASURES

General Considerations

In LTCFs, opinions about appropriate measures for controlling MRSA run the gamut from those favoring do-nothing, laissez-faire approaches on one extreme to those favoring do-everything, hospital-like approaches on the other. Unfortunately, there are virtually no controlled trials of different strategies to focus on the discussion or to inform the development of policy (see Chapters 9, 10). Nevertheless, the last decade has witnessed the emergence of consensus on key principles for management of MRSA in LTCFs (Table 4). Some areas of controversy persist, but there is general agreement on the following points (7,20,26–31):

1. Virtually all LTCFs can provide good care for MRSA-colonized and -infected residents without jeopardizing the well-being of other residents. In a review of the literature, the author noted, "In five nursing homes where MRSA was endemic, 95 infections with five deaths occurred during 12 years of surveillance with 12,000 admissions" (20). Efforts to restrict admission of colonized or infected residents usually fail because detection of carriage can be difficult. In one LTCF study, nasal cultures failed to identify 13% of MRSA carriers (18). Restricting or delaying transfers also

Table 4 Infection Control Measures for Management of Methicillin-Resistant *Staphylococcus aureus* Colonization and Infections in Long-Term Care Facilities

Endemic situation—few infections	Outbreak or high endemic infection rate
Surveillance	Consultation
From microbiology reports on established residents	With experienced epidemiologist from local/regional hospital or state/local health department
From hospital records of new residents or returning transfers	Consultant to advise on use of measures below
Establish baseline rates of colonization and infection	Enhanced surveillance
Education and communication	Consider screening cultures of residents or staff
Create awareness and alleviate fear of MRSA	Consider typing MRSA isolates
Emphasize importance of standard precautions	Patient placement
Use of antimicrobial agents	Consider using private rooms for MRSA cases
Avoid unnecessary usage	Consider cohorting MRSA-positive residents and staff
Monitor for appropriateness	Otherwise place MRSA cases in rooms with residents who lack risk factors for colonization
Precautions	Other measures
Standard precautions for most residents	Consider greater use of contact precautions
Contact precautions for residents whose drainage or respiratory secretions cannot be contained	Consider (rarely) decolonization therapy

Abbreviation: MRSA, methicillin-resistant *Staphylococcus aureus*.

imposes an unnecessary burden on other sectors of the health-care system. There is no evidence to suggest that screening potential admissions for MRSA and decolonizing those who are positive reduce LTCF colonization or infection rates, and this approach is not recommended (7).

2. LTCFs are not hospitals. Few facilities have more than a few private rooms for isolation. Few have laboratory resources necessary for screening. Rehabilitation and socialization needs of residents and communal activities, such as eating in dining rooms, limit use of isolation and stringent barrier precautions that are often used in hospitals. Moreover, some control measures may affect residents' quality of life adversely (32). Rapid discharge of colonized residents is seldom possible. Accordingly, control strategies in LTCFs necessarily differ from those used in hospitals (7,20).

3. Prudent use of antimicrobial agents by providers plays a key role in facility management of MRSA and other antimicrobial-resistant pathogens (33,34).
4. Once in LTCFs, MRSA will likely persist. Aggressive approaches after MRSA's first appearance occasionally drive it out; however, this result is the exception to the rule.
5. LTCFs need to perform enough surveillance to determine their status with regard to MRSA and other antimicrobial-resistant pathogens.
6. Judicious uses of the limited infection control resources in LTCFs necessitate distinguishing between endemic and epidemic MRSA situations, as well as between MRSA colonization and infection.
7. LTCF settings with predominantly endemic cases of MRSA colonization primarily require appropriate use of standard precautions.
8. LTCF settings with MRSA outbreaks, especially those with substantial morbidity due to MRSA infections, require more stringent infection control measures in addition to standard precautions.

Surveillance

Some workers in this field have advocated routine cultures of all new admissions to identify MRSA carriers (28,31), whereas others question the utility of this practice in non-outbreak settings. Few LTCFs have the resources to perform this task. Because identification of all MRSA carriers requires multiple cultures from different sites, including the rectum, a universal screening policy is generally regarded as onerous. Finally, screening only makes sense if it dictates changes in management for MRSA-positive residents, and in most non-outbreak settings it does not alter room assignment, precautions, or medications. In their position paper, the Society for Healthcare Epidemiology (SHEA) Long-Term Care Committee specifically recommends against this practice in non-outbreak settings (7).

Precautions

Standard precautions, which combine elements of universal precautions and body substance isolation, entered the world of medicine with publication of the 1996 guideline for isolation precautions in hospitals by the Hospital Infection Control Practices Advisory Committee (35). Standard precautions embody the concept that all patients and all patient specimens should be handled as if they were infectious, capable of transmitting disease. They would seem ideal for prevention of MRSA transmission, which almost exclusively involves person-to-person spread by direct contact and often involves contact between health-care workers and asymptomatic carriers. They emphasize hand washing after direct contact with patients and potentially infectious material, especially between contacts with different patients. Standard precautions also dictate use of gloves, masks, eye protection, and gowns when necessary to prevent contact between infectious material and the health-care worker. When used appropriately and consistently, these measures should interrupt transmission from one resident to another by the transiently contaminated hands of the health-care workers. The additional value of using antimicrobial soaps remains unclear. Hand-cleansing agents offer an alternative to soap and water (36).

The position paper from the SHEA Long-Term Care Committee (7) recommends that "routine precautions in LTCFs include adequate sinks, education, and incentives to ensure good hand-washing practices throughout the facility at all times... and adequate supplies and education to ensure that appropriate barrier precautions are used in the management of all wounds and invasive devices." Attention to these considerations facilitates the use of standard precautions in LTCFs.

In non-outbreak settings, most residents colonized or infected with MRSA do not require use of additional precautions in their care. Moreover, as long as they do not have large wounds or other lesions that cannot be contained by dressings or tracheostomies with excessive secretions, most authorities would not limit their movement within the LTCF or their participation in LTCF activities. Nevertheless, residents known to be colonized or infected with MRSA should not be placed in rooms with debilitated, nonambulatory residents, that is, those at greatest risk for subsequent colonization and infection. Residents with large wounds or draining lesions that cannot be contained and those with tracheostomies and difficulty handling secretions generally require a higher level of scrutiny and, often, additional precautions. If such residents can be linked epidemiologically to MRSA infection in other residents, then placing them in a private room or cohorting them with similar residents is prudent, as is restriction of their movement and participation in group events. In addition, contact precautions, which require gowns and gloves for all persons entering the room, as well as hand washing after glove removal, should be strongly considered (35).

Outbreak Management Issues

Definition

Fundamentally, an outbreak represents an increase in caseload that exceeds the baseline rate (see also Chapter 10). The more accurate baselines reflect several years of experience and delineate an expected range of random variation. The SHEA position paper advocates defining outbreaks in terms of infections, not in terms of colonization (7). As examples, it suggests that more than three infections in a week or twice the number of infections in a month than had been observed in each of the three preceding months qualify as an outbreak. Lastly, this paper suggests that situations with high endemic rates of infection, which it defines as more than one infection per 1000 resident car days, be treated like outbreaks.

Consultation

Once an MRSA outbreak or high endemic rate of infection is recognized, the SHEA position paper recommends consultation with an experienced epidemiologist. Hospital epidemiologists at local or regional hospitals, senior infection control practitioners, state or local health officials, and others may qualify for this role, especially if they are knowledgeable about infection control issues in LTCFs. Consulting epidemiologists can offer independent confirmation of the problem, provide an analysis of possible causes, and offer potential solutions. Ideally, they customize their approaches to the specific circumstances and needs of a given facility. As a rule, their judgments will dictate consideration of enhanced surveillance, additional isolation precautions, and decolonization efforts.

Enhanced Surveillance

Outbreaks and high endemic rates of infection usually precipitate some discussion about culturing newly admitted residents, established residents, or staff to identify symptomatic carriers who might be playing a pivotal role in transmission. Costs and uncertainty about management of identified carriers generally discourage such screening, except in the presence of severe and protracted outbreaks.

Typing of MRSA strains can solidify epidemiological links between cases and generate hypotheses about transmission. Investigations of hospital outbreaks frequently involve molecular typing methods (2); investigations of a few LTCF outbreaks also have used them (11,13,17). Cost, availability, and time issues preclude their use in most LTCF settings. Of note, antibiograms perform poorly in comparison to molecular typing methods (2,37).

Isolation and Cohorting

In the setting of outbreaks and high endemic rates of infection, segregation of MRSA-colonized and -infected residents may diminish transmission (7,29,30). Depending on the facility layout, segregation could involve use of single rooms for MRSA-colonized or -infected individuals, especially for those linked epidemiology to other cases and those likely shedding large numbers of bacteria (from large, uncovered wounds, for example). Although disruptive, cohorting MRSA-colonized and -infected residents and, possibly, colonized staff may protect susceptible residents from additional exposure. When private rooms and cohorting fails to provide adequate segregation, placing MRSA cases in rooms occupied by healthier individuals without risk factors for colonization or infection may limit transmission.

Control of outbreaks and reduction of high endemic rates may also require limiting admissions, restricting movement of MRSA-positive residents, and selective use of contact precautions (35). Because these actions disrupt the functioning of most LTCFs and cause considerable hardship for residents, their use requires sufficient provocation and justification. Individual facilities should modify or adjust the use of such measures to their specific circumstances.

Decolonization

Because a large percentage of MRSA infections arise in colonized individuals, various investigators have attempted to eradicate the carrier state with antimicrobial therapy. If successful, this therapy would reduce an individual's risk of infection and diminish a facility's reservoir of MRSA. Unfortunately, when used to quell outbreaks or reduce high endemic rates of colonization in LTCFs or hospitals, the combined use of several different control measures has obscured evaluation of decolonization therapy, per se (7,8,15). Consequently, the concept of decolonization lacks supporting evidence of efficacy.

There are several other problematic considerations. First, decolonization is not always successful; it frequently fails in debilitated patients with significant underlying disease, especially in those with open wounds or invasive devices. Paradoxically, decolonization often fails in those who have the greatest risk of infection. Second, use of various agents in decolonization regimens invariably induces resistance to the agents used. For example, in one study using rifampin-containing regimens, rifampin-resistant isolates were recovered from 80% of the 20 residents who remained persistently colonized or became recolonized with MRSA during the 30-day follow-up period (38). Likewise, during a seven-month mupirocin intervention trial in one facility, mupirocin-resistant MRSA was isolated from 10.8% of residents (39).

Finally, decolonization entails considerable expense, and it exposes residents to various toxicities of the agents used. For these reasons, routine use of decolonization therapy is not recommended in health-care settings. Long-term care facilities should consider this strategy only in the setting of an outbreak associated with substantial morbidity, and even then, with careful monitoring by an experienced epidemiologist.

In the rare circumstance when an LTCF uses a decolonization strategy, mupirocin would probably be the agent of choice. Topical application of 2% mupirocin ointment to nares for five days and to colonized cutaneous sites for two weeks will eradicate colonization in 90% of residents (1,15). However, colonization commonly recurs in 20% to 30% of residents during the weeks and months that follow treatment. Orally administered antimicrobial regimens for decolonization usually contain rifampin with or without one or two other agents (1,2,38). After a week of such therapy, follow-up cultures are negative in 60% to 90% of recipients. More than one-half will become recolonized in the weeks and months that follow. Therefore, decolonization therapy is effective in the short run, a period of one to two weeks. For a sizeable percentage of residents, however, the effect is not sustained, and resistance to the agent used appears in isolates obtained subsequently.

PREVENTION

No single measure can prevent MRSA colonization or infection. However, attention to several basic principles will likely minimize acquisition by uncolonized residents. Prudent use of antimicrobial therapy, avoidance of invasive devices, such as nasogastric tubes, and efforts to prevent pressure ulcers will probably lower an individual's risk for colonization. Consistent use of standard precautions and contact precautions, when indicated, will interrupt the cycle of transmission. All of these efforts require a knowledgeable and compliant staff, underscoring the need for education, communication, and feedback in the infection control program. Surveillance activity helps to maintain awareness and serves to identify trends that may require additional attention.

Although controversial, on occasion an elective surgical procedure on an LTCF resident may prompt consideration of preoperative decolonization and prophylactic antimicrobial therapy with vancomycin (40,41). For example, known MRSA carriers scheduled for total hip arthroplasty may have reduced risks of postoperative surgical site infections if they receive decolonization therapy preoperatively. This same possibility applies to MSSA-colonized residents, and the results of a trial that used preoperative therapy with mupirocin to eradicate staphylococcal carriage are eagerly awaited. No formal recommendation currently supports its use (41). Using vancomycin instead of a first-generation cephalosporin antibiotic for perioperative prophylaxis may also reduce postoperative MRSA infection rates, but this approach is generally reserved for hospitals with high rates of MRSA surgical site infections (40,41). Its routine use is not recommended (41). Both the preoperative decolonization and vancomycin prophylaxis strategies await additional evidence of benefit before they can receive a firm endorsement for use as a preventive measure in LTCF residents undergoing elective surgical procedures.

SUGGESTED READING

Bradley SF. Methicillin-resistant *Staphylococcus aureus*: long-term care concerns. Am J Med 1999; 106(5A):2S–10S.

Moreillon P, Que Y-A, Glauser HP. *Staphylococcus aureus* (including staphylococcal toxic shock). In: Mandell GL, Bennett JE, Dolin R, eds. Mandell, Douglas, and Bennett's Principles and Practice of Infectious Diseases. 6th ed. Philadelphia: W.B. Saunders, Company, 2005:2321–2357.

Strausbaugh LJ, Jacobson C, Sewell DL, Potter S, Ward TT. Methicillin-resistant *Staphylococcus aureus* in extended care facilities: experience in a Veterans Affairs nursing home and a review of the literature. Infect Control Hosp Epidemiol 1991; 12:36–45.

REFERENCES

1. Moreillon P, Que Y-A, Glauser HP. *Staphylococcus aureus* (including staphylococcal toxic shock). In: Mandell GL, Bennett JE, Dolin R, eds. Mandell, Douglas, and Bennett's Principles and Practice of Infectious Diseases. 6th ed. Philadelphia: W.B. Saunders, Company, 2005:2321–2357.
2. Hartstein AI, Strausbaugh LJ. Methillicin-resistant *Staphylococcus aureus*. In: Mayhall CG, ed. Hospital Epidemiology and Infection Control. 3rd ed. Philadelphia: Lippincott Williams & Wilkins, 2004:471–494.
3. Kuehnert MJ, Hill HA, Kupronis BA, Tokars JL, Solomon SL, Jernigan DB. Methicillin-resistant *Staphylococcus aureus* hospitalizations, United States. Emerging Infect Dis 2005; 11:868–872.
4. Bradley SF. Methicillin-resistant *Staphylococcus aureus* infection. Clin Geriatr Med 1992; 8:853–868.
5. Centers for Disease Control and Prevention NNIS System. National Nosocomial Infections Surveillance (NNIS) system report, date summary from January 1992–April 2000, issued June 2000. Am J Infect Control 200; 28:429–448.
6. O'Toole RD, Drew WL, Dahlgren BJ, Beaty HN. An outbreak of methicillin-resistant *Staphylococcus aureus* infection: observations in hospital and nursing home. JAMA 1970; 213:257–263.
7. Strausbaugh LJ, Crossley KB, Nurse BA, Thrupp LD, SHEA Long-Term Care Committee. Antimicrobial resistance in long-term care facilities. Infect Control Hosp Epidemiol 1996; 17:129–140.
8. Storch GA, Radcliff JL, Meyer PL, Hinrichs JH. Methicillin-resistant *Staphylococcus aureus* in a nursing home. Infect Control 1987; 8:24–29.
9. Thomas JC, Bridge J, Waterman S, Vogt J, Kilman L, Hancock G. Transmission and control of methicillin-resistant *Staphylococcus aureus* in a skilled nursing facility. Infect Control Hosp Epidemiol 1989; 10:106–110.
10. Muder RR, Brennen C, Wagener NM, et al. Methicillin-resistant staphylococcal colonization and infection in a long-term care facility. Ann Intern Med 1991; 114:107–112.
11. Strausbaugh LJ, Jacobson C, Sewell DL, Potter S, Ward TT. Methicillin-resistant *Staphylococcus aureus* in extended care facilities: experience in a Veterans Affairs nursing home and a review of the literature. Infect Control Hosp Epidemiol 1991; 12:36–45.
12. Hsu CCS. Serial survey of methicillin-resistant *Staphylococcus aureus* nasal carriage among residents in a nursing home. Infect Control Hosp Epidemiol 1991; 12: 416–421.
13. Bradley SF, Terpenning MS, Ramsey MA, et al. Methicillin-resistant *Staphylococcus aureus*: colonization and infection in a long-term care facility. Ann Intern Med 1991; 115:417–422.
14. Murphy S, Denman S, Bennett RG, Greenough WB III, Lindsay J, Zelesnick LB. Methicillin-resistant *Staphylococcus aureus* colonization in a long-term care facility. J Am Geriatric Soc 1992; 40:213–217.
15. Terpenning MS, Bradley SF, Wan JY, Chenoweth CE, Jorgensen KA, Kauffman CA. Colonization and infection with antibiotic-resistant bacteria in a long-term care facility. J Am Geriatr Soc 1994; 42:1062–1069.

16. Mulhausen PL, Harrell LJ, Weinberger M, Lochersberger GG, Feussner JR. Contrasting methicillin-resistant *Staphylococcus aureus* colonization in veterans affairs and community nursing homes. Am J Med 1996; 100:24–31.

17. Lee Y-L, Gupta G, Cesario T, et al. Colonization by *Staphylococcus aureus* resistant to methicillin and ciprofloxacin during 20 months' surveillance in a private skilled nursing facility. Infect Control Hosp Epidemiol 1996; 17:649–653.

18. Lee Y-L, Cesario T, Gupta G, et al. Surveillance of colonization and infection with *Staphylococcus aureus* susceptible or resistant to methicillin in a community skilled-nursing facility. AJIC Am J Infect Control 1997; 25:312–321.

19. Strausbaugh LJ, Jacobson C, Yost T. Methicillin-resistant *Staphylococcus aureus* in a nursing home and affiliated hospital: a four-year perspective. Infect Control Hosp Epidemiol 1993; 14:331–336.

20. Bradley SF. Issues in the management of resistant bacteria in long-term-care facilities. Infect Control Hosp Epidemiol 1999; 20:362–366.

21. Lee YI, Cesario T, Lee R, et al. Colonization by *Staphylococcus* species resistant to methicillin or quinolone on hand of medical personnel in skilled nursing facility. AJIC Am J Infect Control 1994; 22:3346–3351.

22. Strausbaugh LJ, Joseph C. Epidemiology and prevention of infections in residents of long-term care facilities. In: Mayhall CG, ed. Hospital Epidemiology and Infection Control. 3rd ed. Philadelphia: Lippincott-Williams and Wilkins, 2004:1855–1880.

23. Bentley DW, Bradley S, High K, Schoenbaum S, Taler G, Yoshikawa TT. Practice guideline for evaluation of fever and infection in long-term care facilities. Clin Infect Dis 2000; 31:640–653.

24. Yoshikawa TT. Antibiotic-resistant bacterial infections. In: Yoshikawa TT, Rajagopalan S, eds. Antibiotic Therapy for Geriatric Patients. New York: Taylor & Francis, 2006:617–624.

25. Marer S, Rajagopalan S. Oxazolidinones and streptogramins. In: Yoshikawa TT, Rajagopalan S, eds. Antibiotic Therapy for Geriatric Patients. New York: Taylor & Francis, 2006:289–300.

26. Cahill CK, Rosenberg J. Guideline for prevention and control of antibiotic-resistant microorganisms in California long-term care facilities. J Gerontol Nurs 1995; May:40–47.

27. Yoshikawa TT. VRE, MRSA, PRP, and DRGNB in LTCF: lessons to be learned from this alphabet. J Am Geriatr Soc 1998; 46:241–243.

28. Bonomo RA, Rice LB. Emerging issues in antibiotic-resistant infections in long-term care facilities. J Gerontol A Biol Sci Med Sci 1999; 54A:B260–B267.

29. Sioux Falls Task Force on Antimicrobial Resistance. Guideline for the prevention and control of methicillin-resistant *Staphylococcus aureus* in long-term care facilities. South Dakota Med J 1999; (52):235–240.

30. Bradley SF. Methicillin-resistant *Staphylococcus aureus*: long-term care concerns. Am J Med 1999; 106(5A):2S–10S.

31. Bonomo RA. Multiple antibiotic-resistant bacteria in long-term care facilities. An emerging problem in the practice of infectious diseases. Clin Infect Dis 2000; 31:1414–1422.

32. Loeb M, Moss L, Stiller A, et al. Colonization with multiresistant bacteria and quality of life in residents of long-term care facilities. Infect Control Hosp Epidemiol 2001; 22:67–68.

33. Nicolle LE, Bentley DW, Garibaldi R, Neuhas EG, Smith PW. SHEA Long-Term-Care Committee. Antimicrobial use in long-term-care facilities. Infect Control Hosp Epidemiol 2000; 21:537–545.
34. Loeb M. Antibiotic use in long-term-care facilities: many unanswered questions. Infect Control Hosp Epidemiol 2000; 21:680–683.
35. Garner JS. Hospital Infection Control Practices Advisory Committee. Guideline for isolation precautions in hospitals. Infect Control Hosp Epidemiol 1996; 17:53–80.
36. Guilhermetti M, Hernandes SED, Fukushige Y, Garcia LB, Cardoso CL. Effectiveness of hand-cleansing agents for removing methicillin-resistant *Staphylococcus aureus* from contaminated hands. Infect Control Hosp Epidemiol 2001; 22:105–108.
37. Lee Y-L, Thrupp L. Genotyping by restriction endonuclease analysis compared to phenotyping by antibiogram for typing methicillin-resistant *Staphylococcus aureus* strains colonizing patients in a nursing home. Infect Control Hosp Epidemiol 2000; 21:218–221.
38. Strausbaugh LJ, Jacobson C, Sewell DL, Potter S, Ward TT. Antimicrobial therapy for methicillin-resistant *Staphylococcus aureus* colonization in residents and staff of a veterans affairs nursing home care unit. Infect Control Hosp Epidemiol 1992; 13:151–159.
39. Kauffman CA, Terpenning MS, He X, et al. Attempts to eradicate methicillin-resistant *Staphylococcus aureus* from a long-term-care facility with the use of mupirocin ointment. Am J Med 1993; 94:371–378.
40. Talbot TR, Kaiser AB. Postoperative infections and antimicrobial prophylaxis. In: Mandell GL, Bennett JE, Dolin R, eds. Mandell, Douglas, and Bennett's Principles and Practice of Infectious Diseases. 6th ed. Philadelphia: W. B. Saunders Company, 2005:3533–3547.
41. Mangram AJ, Horan TC, Pearson ML, Silver LC, Jarvis WR. Hospital Infection Control Practices Advisory Committee. Guideline for prevention of surgical site infection, 1999. Infect Control Hosp Epidemiol 1999; 20:247–278.

24

Vancomycin (Glycopeptide)-Resistant Enterococci in the Long-Term Care Setting

Suzanne F. Bradley

Divisions of Infectious Diseases and Geriatric Medicine, Veterans Affairs Ann Arbor Healthcare System, The University of Michigan Medical School, Ann Arbor, Michigan, U.S.A.

KEY POINTS

1. If VRE are present in referring hospitals, they will be found in local LTCFs.
2. LTCF residents who carry VRE also are commonly colonized with methicillin-resistant *Staphylococcus aureus*, *Clostridium difficile*, and resistant gram-negative bacilli.
3. If VRE infections occur in LTCF residents, they are typically less severe than hospital-acquired infection and involve infection of the urinary tract or skin and soft tissue.
4. Fewer effective antibiotics are available to treat VRE infection.
5. Infection control procedures are effective in controlling VRE in LTCF.

EPIDEMIOLOGY AND CLINICAL RELEVANCE

The Enterococcus: An Overview

The *Enterococcus* is a normal component of the endogenous gastrointestinal and perineal flora. Overall, the ability of enterococci to cause disease

411

(virulence) is quite limited relative to other common pathogens, such as *Staphylococcus aureus*, group A beta-hemolytic streptococci, or aerobic gram-negative bacilli. As a result, enterococcal infections occur primarily when normal host defenses are impaired.

When the host is compromised, the *Enterococcus* becomes a significant opportunistic pathogen causing many of the major clinical infectious syndromes affecting humans. *E. faecalis*, and less often *E. faecium*, is frequent cause of urinary tract infection (UTI), intra-abdominal and pelvic infection, soft tissue infection, bacteremia, and endocarditis. Enterococci commonly coexist with other pathogens in the setting of gastrointestinal and soft tissue infection. Other enterococcal species, such as *E. gallinarum* and *E. casseliflavus*, rarely cause infection (Table 1). The emergence of resistance to glycopeptide antibiotics (vancomycin and teicoplanin) in enterococci is important primarily because effective treatment for serious infection is very difficult (2,3).

Significance of Glycopeptide Resistance in Enterococci

Not unexpectedly, enterococci resistant to glycopeptide antibiotics predominate among the most seriously ill patients in the acute care setting, primarily in intensive care units (ICUs), in association with lengthy hospital stays, prolonged use of broad-spectrum antibiotics, and frequent use of invasive devices. In those settings, vancomycin-resistant enterococci (VRE) are frequent causes of blood stream infection (BSI), with urinary tract and wound infections occurring less often (1). VRE BSI has been associated with very high mortality in this very seriously ill patient population, but vancomycin resistance has not been clearly shown to be an independent risk factor for death. Increased mortality may be due to the lack of effective antibiotic

Table 1 Prevalence of Enterococcal Species Among Clinical Isolates

		Vancomycin-resistant strains in 1997–1999 (%)				
All clinical isolates	(%)	United States	Canada	Latin America	Europe	Asia-Pacific
Enterococcus faecalis	57–77	14–17	0–2	0–2	1–3	1–2
Enterococcus faecium	5–20					
Enterococcus casseliflavus	2–6					
Enterococcus gallinarum						
Enterococcus durans						
Enterococcus avium						
Enterococcus raffinosus						
Other enterococcal species						

Source: From Ref. 1.

treatment and the severity of illness in populations at risk of VRE rather than due to an increase in the virulence (4).

E. faecalis remains the most common species recovered among all hospital enterococcal isolates worldwide (1). The incidence of *E. faecium*, the predominant species manifesting vancomycin resistance, continues to increase (Table 1). In the United States, VRE are still found less commonly in non-ICU and outpatient settings (3,5). Healthy health-care workers are rarely colonized with vancomycin-resistant *E. faecium* or *E. faecalis*. In parts of Europe, VRE commonly colonize healthy humans and pets in the community, but most are rarely pathogenic enterococcal species (2,3).

It is thought that VRE have emerged due to the selective pressure of antibiotic use. Enterococci resistant to antibiotics, such as glycopeptides, exist in nature, albeit in small numbers. These clones are selected in the gastrointestinal tract when a patient is exposed to antibiotics and normal flora is suppressed, allowing resistant enterococci to emerge. In Europe, community-based strains emerged initially in livestock because of the use of glycopeptide antibiotics, such as avoparicin, in animal feeds. Ingestion of meat contaminated with these enterococci may have contributed to widespread colonization in humans. In the United States, specific antibiotics, such as the glycopeptides themselves, third-generation cephalosporins, and antibiotics with anaerobic activity have been particularly associated with the emergence of VRE. Enterococci also thrive quite readily on inanimate surfaces. In hospital, patients may acquire antibiotic-resistant enterococci from other VRE-colonized patients or from contaminated hands of health-care workers or environmental sources (2,3).

The Epidemiology of VRE in Long-Term Care Facilities

Colonization with antibiotic-resistant enterococci in long-term care facility (LTCF) residents is not a new or uncommon problem. More than a decade ago, high-level gentamicin-resistant enterococci (HGRE) colonization was common in residents of LTCF; rates of 35% to 47% were observed in a single nursing home. More residents were already colonized with HGRE at the time of admission to hospital and had strains closely related to those found in the attached acute care facility, suggesting that acquisition might have occurred in hospital. Infections with HGRE were not severe and often involved the urinary tract or skin and soft tissue; most occurred in residents with known colonization (6).

Similar findings have been noted for VRE in LTCF. However, the precise prevalence and epidemiology of VRE infection among residents of LTCF are still being established. Most of the information on VRE rates in the long-term care setting is based on studies of asymptomatic rectal carriage rather than infection. In studies of nursing home residents admitted to hospital, rates of colonization have ranged from 10% to 47% (7). Rates of rectal or fecal VRE colonization based on point prevalence surveys have been assessed in Michigan (9–22%), the Siouxland region of Iowa, Nebraska, South Dakota (1.7%), Western New York (1%), Chicago (4%), and Melbourne, Australia (3%) (7–12). One study found that 4% of LTCF residents remained colonized for more than one year with the same strain; one resident was persistently positive for up to five years (13).

Residents of LTCF with VRE colonization tend to be functionally impaired; comorbid illnesses, wounds, urinary devices, and feeding tubes are significant risk factors. Many of these patients are also colonized with organisms, such as methicillin-resistant *S. aureus* (MRSA), multidrug-resistant gram-negative bacilli, or *Clostridium difficile*, that have those risk factors in common (7,9,14,15). Most have received recent treatment with vancomycin, antianaerobic agents, or a third-generation cephalosporin (7,10,13,15,16).

Many of the residents colonized with VRE have been recently hospitalized and may have introduced VRE into the LTCF (8,10,16–20). One study found that 67% of residents were already positive upon admission to the LTCF (16). Residents of LTCF with VRE were fourfold more likely to have been recently discharged from hospitals where the organism was endemic than uncolonized residents (17). Strains obtained from those LTCF residents were closely related genetically to VRE strains that predominated in the transferring hospitals (17).

High VRE rates in an LTCF may not represent the same organism or be proof that spread is occurring. The prevalence of VRE may remain high in LTCF, because carriage can persist for months and can be prolonged by the use of antimicrobial therapy (8,13,16). Multiple, rather than single, strains often circulate in an LTCF at the same time (8,10,21). Individual residents may carry multiple strains of VRE that emerge when antibiotic therapy is initiated (21). Although roommates have not been shown to share the same strain of VRE in one study, spread could theoretically occur from the environment or the hands of personnel who were frequently colonized with multiple strains of VRE (8,19).

Data on VRE infection, rather than colonization in LTCF residents, are still scant and commonly represent microbiological surveys of cultures obtained for clinical purposes; whether these clinical isolates represented true infection or asymptomatic carriage often cannot be determined. In 1992, clinical isolates from 100 nursing homes revealed that 3% of 243 *E. faecalis* and 12% of 32 *E. faecium* were resistant to vancomycin (22). In Western New York, only one of 139 enterococci obtained over a two-year period was vancomycin-resistant (12). Over two years, 18/153 (12%) LTCF residents were admitted to two Chicago hospitals with VRE infection (23).

VRE colonization is associated with some risk of infection; 6/27 (22%) colonized LTCF residents developed symptomatic UTI (22%) (15). However, in contrast to hospitals, severe infection with VRE seems uncommon relative to rates of colonization. In two nursing homes where VRE colonization

Table 2 Clinical Syndromes Associated with Enterococci

Asymptomatic colonization
Urinary tract infection
Skin/soft tissue infection
Intra-abdominal infection
Bloodstream infection
Endocarditis
Meningitis/pneumonia (true infections extremely rare)

was common, seven UTIs, one bacteremia, and no deaths were seen (8,16). So, VRE infections do occur in LTCF but with less severity and frequency than described in the acute care setting.

CLINICAL MANIFESTATIONS

The clinical manifestations of vancomycin-susceptible enterococci and VRE are identical (Table 2). UTI are the most common infections in long-term care residents. Whereas gram-negative bacilli clearly predominate as the major causes of UTI in residents of LTCF, infections with enterococci are more common in older adults requiring hospitalization than in healthy community dwellers. Enterococcal UTIs are similarly more common among nursing home residents, and urethral catheterization may be an important risk factor for colonization (24).

Skin and soft tissue infections associated with enterococci are rarely mentioned in the long-term care setting. Despite the fact that enterococci are commonly isolated from diabetic polymicrobial foot infections, and diabetes mellitus and its complications are common in older adults, enterococcal infections have been rarely reported in series of soft tissue infection among residents of LTCF (25). Enterococci have also been recovered from the polymicrobial flora of pressure ulcers (26). Whether enterococci are significant pathogens in polymicrobial soft tissue infections and require specific antimicrobial therapy is controversial.

Aging is associated with increased prevalence of hepatobiliary disease, diverticulosis, and other gastrointestinal pathology with a risk of infectious complications. Polymicrobial infection, including enterococci from biliary sources, and following intra-abdominal surgery is not uncommon. Although enterococcal infections specifically associated with intra-abdominal/gastrointestinal sources have not been noted in surveys of infection in LTCF, clinicians should be vigilant that older adults may develop intra-abdominal sources of enterococcal infection during their stay (27).

In hospitals, VRE BSI was most common in patients over 50 years of age (5). Fortunately, bacteremia is uncommonly reported in the nursing home-acquired infections. Enterococci have been noted in 1% to 7% of blood-stream infections (28). Isolation of enterococci occurred most commonly in the setting of polymicrobial bacteremia with another organism and with the use of a urinary device (28). Native valve enterococcal endocarditis is classically associated with instrumentation of a colonized urinary tract or gastrointestinal tract in an older man. Whether enterococcal endocarditis actually occurs more often in older adults remains a subject of debate (29).

DIAGNOSTIC APPROACH

Enterococci can be easily isolated from cultures of urine, stool, wounds, blood, abscess material, and rectal swabs using standard culture media. It is important for the laboratory to speciate all enterococci and screen for the presence of vancomycin resistance. Detection of vancomycin resistance in colonizing or infecting strains of enterococci requires the use of appropriate microbiologic methods. Standard broth microdilution methods, disk diffusion, or E-test methods can be used. However, some automated methods are unreliable in detecting VRE (3,30). Different VRE species also vary in their antimicrobial susceptibility patterns (Tables 1,3,4).

Patterns of resistance to vancomycin and teicoplanin and the level of resistance to those antibiotics have been used as phenotypic markers for the five mechanisms of resistance currently described in enterococci (Table 3). These six VRE phenotypes are termed VanA, VanB, VanC, VanD, VanE, and VanG. These phenotypes provide additional information regarding the likelihood that vancomycin resistance might spread or respond to certain antibiotics (2,3).

Vancomycin resistance in enterococci is defined by a minimum inhibitory concentration of $\geq 2\,\mu g/mL$. Resistance to vancomycin at low levels

Table 3 Phenotypes of Vancomycin-Resistant Enterococci Based on Antimicrobial Susceptibilities to Vancomycin and Teicoplanin

Phenotype	Resistance element	Common species	Vancomycin resistance	Teicoplanin susceptible
VanA	Acquired/ transferable	*E. faecium, E. faecalis*	High level	No
VanB	Acquired/ transferable	*E. faecium, E. faecalis*	High level	Yes
VanC	Intrinsic/ not transferable	*E. gallinarum, E. casseliflavus*	Low level	Yes
VanD	Acquired/ not transferable	*E. faecium*	High level	No
VanE	Acquired/ not transferable	*E. faecalis*	Low level	Yes

Table 4 Treatment of Vancomycin-Resistant Enterococcal Infection[a]

Antibiotic	Route	Indication
Ampicillin	IV, PO	Efficacious in susceptible *E. faecalis* strains
		Bactericidal for *E. faecalis* in combination with gentamicin or streptomycin unless high-level aminoglycoside resistance is present
		E. faecium strains generally resistant to normal regimens of ampicillin
		High-dose IV ampicillin/beta-lactamase inhibitor regimens experimental
Quinupristin/ dalfopristin	IV	*E. faecium,* only use in serious infections
		E. faecalis not susceptible
		Bacteriostatic agent for enterococci
		Toxicities common: myalgias, phlebitis
		Resistance described but rare
Linezolid	PO, IV	*E. faecium* or *E. faecalis*, only use in serious infections
		Oral formulation 100% bioavailable
		Bacteriostatic
		Thrombocytopenia, anemia, peripheral neuropathy reported
		Resistance described
Nitrofurantoin	PO	Efficacious for urinary tract infection only
Doxycycline	PO, IV	May be effective in treatment of urinary tract infections. Efficacy in serious infections unpredictable
Quinolones	PO, IV	May be effective in treatment of urinary tract infections
		Efficacy in serious infections unpredictable
Chloramphenicol	IV	Many *E. faecium* susceptible
		Efficacy in serious infection not established
		Significant hematologic toxicities
Teicoplanin	IV	Serious infections VanB strains only
		Not available in the United States

[a]Enterococcal strains must demonstrate sensitivity to an agent using approved antimicrobial susceptibility methods.
Abbreviations: IV, intravenous; PO, oral.

(2–32 µg/mL) and susceptibility to teicoplanin are typical of *E. casseliflavus*, *E. gallinarum*, and *E. flavescens*. These species are referred to phenotypically as VanC strains and rarely cause clinically significant disease. VanC-mediated resistance is an intrinsic and chromosomally mediated characteristic of these organisms, which is not transferable to other bacteria (2,3).

Vancomycin resistance also can be acquired from other organisms by some enterococci. VanA and VanB strains are found most commonly and are important epidemiologically, because they can spread or transfer vancomycin resistance elements to other bacteria. Acquisition of resistance elements can lead to high-level resistance to vancomycin ($\geq 64\,\mu g/mL$) and teicoplanin ($\geq 16\,\mu g/mL$) in strains that have required the VanA gene. Acquired resistance to vancomycin with susceptibility to teicoplanin is referred to as a VanB strain. VanA and VanB strains are most often found among strains of *E. faecium* and *E. faecalis*. VanA strains are found widely throughout the United States, whereas VanB strains are present on a regional basis (2,3).

The diagnosis of infection with VRE is based on the isolation of the organism in association with symptoms and signs consistent with an appropriate clinical syndrome (Table 2) (31). The clinical presentation of these syndromes is addressed elsewhere. Isolation of VRE in the absence of clinically apparent symptoms or signs represents asymptomatic colonization of urine, skin, or stool, or contamination of wounds or blood cultures. In the appropriate clinical setting, vancomycin-resistant *E. faecium* and *E. faecalis* are more likely to represent true pathogens. Isolation of *E. casseliflavus, E. gallinarum, E. flavescens,* and other species likely represents colonization unless obtained from a sterile site, on multiple occasions, and in high inoculum (3,4).

THERAPEUTIC INTERVENTIONS

Compared with other gram-positive cocci, the *Enterococcus* is relatively resistant to the bactericidal effects of cell-wall active antibiotics. Even among vancomycin-susceptible enterococci, intrinsic resistance to many antibiotic classes is common. Penicillins and vancomycin remain the most reliable treatments for infections due to susceptible enterococci, but their activities are bacteriostatic rather than bactericidal. Currently, only the addition of an aminoglycoside to vancomycin or penicillins provides reliable and effective bactericidal activity for the treatment of serious enterococcal infections (32).

Unfortunately, resistance to vancomycin in enterococci is usually associated with resistance to multiple antibiotics, including penicillins and aminoglycosides. Most vancomycin-resistant *E. faecium* and many *E. faecalis* are resistant to normally achievable levels of penicillin and ampicillin and high levels of gentamicin or streptomycin (Table 4) (32). In the event of resistance to penicillin in VRE, antimicrobial susceptibilities to other antibiotic classes should be assessed. If susceptible, nitrofurantoin may be effective in treating UTI with VRE. However, despite in vitro susceptibility to tetracyclines, chloramphenicol, and quinolones, clinical success in the treatment of serious VRE infections has been infrequent (32).

Newer agents may be effective in treating less serious infections, but most remain bacteriostatic. A streptogramin, quinupristin/dalfopristin

(Synercid®), is active against *E. faecium*, but not *E. faecalis*, whereas the oxazolidinone, linezolid (Zyvox®), is active against both species. Teicoplanin is active only against VanB and VanC strains but is not approved for use in the United States. Newer antibiotic classes, such as the cyclic lipopeptides (daptomycin or Cubicin) and glycylcyclines (Tigecycline or Tygacil), have not been approved for treatment of VRE. The lipoglycopeptides (ramoplanin) are still investigational. Many of the agents have significant toxicities and may not be bactericidal for the *Enterococcus*. Surgical incision and drainage with removal of foreign devices whenever possible remains a mainstay of treatment for infection due to VRE (32).

INFECTION CONTROL MEASURES

In the acute care setting, infection due to VRE leads to increased morbidity and mortality from infection and increased costs of treatment. The extensive use of infection control resources in the hospital setting can, therefore, be easily justified (33). It is still not clear that VRE are a cause of serious infection or that transmission of VRE is common in the LTCF setting. In addition, a significant proportion of residents of LTCF may be colonized with more than one drug-resistant bacterium for prolonged periods of time. If hospital-based infection control procedures were used, long-term confinement in a private room would have a significant impact on the psychological, social, and physical needs of LTCF residents.

The controversies surrounding the control of VRE and other antibiotic-resistant bacteria in LTCF have been addressed by the Society for Healthcare Epidemiology of America (SHEA) Committee on Long-Term Care and the Centers for Disease Control and Prevention (Table 5) (31,34). Hospital Infection Control Practices Advisory Committee recommendations for contact precautions for drug-resistant bacteria have been recently revised to address the needs of all health-care facilities and are under review (35). SHEA and Centers for Disease Control and Prevention precautions acknowledge the limited infection control resources in nursing homes and are achievable in facilities that provide long-term care. Use of screening measures and aggressive isolation procedures in a referring acute care hospital along with use of procedures similar to those advocated by SHEA not only led to a reduction of infection in hospital but also reduction in colonization rates in those LTCF (10).

Screening for VRE

The essential element of an infection control program to minimize the spread of VRE includes the routine use of barrier precautions in all residents of LTCF. Routine screening of patients for VRE has been recommended as means to prevent transmission and infection, particularly in hospitals (10,33). The benefits of such a routine screening policy to the LTCF is unclear (34,35).

Table 5 Strategies and Procedures for the Control of Vancomycin-Resistant Enterococci in Long-Term Care Facilities

Employee education
Surveillance of cultures obtained for clinical reasons/symptomatic infection
   Establishes the rate of VRE infections in an individual LTCF
   Establishes what is the normal infection rate for a LTCF
   Defines when an infection rate is abnormal and potential epidemic transmission
   Defines when to start procedures to control an outbreak
Maintain listing of VRE carriers that are already known
   Useful information if an outbreak of infection suspected in LTCF or hospitals
   Transferring facilities should routinely provide this information to receiving
     facilities if known
Use of routine surveillance cultures specifically to detect asymptomatic VRE
  colonization
   May be falsely reassuring if negative
   Increased cultures, need for isolation not cost effective unless documented that
     infections are prevented
Isolation procedures
   Private room/cohorting with other colonized residents recommended, but
     efficacy in LTCF not established
   VRE-colonized residents with good hygiene, no diarrhea, or draining wounds
     may room/share bathrooms with uncolonized residents who are not severely
     compromised, do not have urinary catheters, drainage devices, or wounds, and
     are not on broad-spectrum antibiotics
   VRE-colonized resident with good hygiene, no diarrhea, and draining wounds
     contained by a dressing need not be confined to their rooms
   Isolation can be discontinued after 2 successive negative cultures of stool or
     wounds
Hand washing
   Mandatory before and after caring for all resident
   Antimicrobial soaps and hand disinfectants suggested, but efficacy not
     established in LTCF
Gloves/gowns
   Use if contact with body fluids for all residents
   Use in the room prior to contact with a VRE-colonized or infected resident or the
     inanimate environment
   Gowns recommended if contamination of health-care worker clothes likely
Environmental disinfection
   Daily cleaning of room surfaces and equipment recommended, but efficacy and
     optimum germicide not established in LTCF
   Dedicated equipment for VRE-colonized or infected residents if available
Antibiotic use
   Monitor antibiotic use
   Reduce unnecessary use of antibiotics
   Follow guidelines for appropriate use of vancomycin use

(Continued)

Table 5 Strategies and Procedures for the Control of Vancomycin-Resistant Enterococci in Long-Term Care Facilities (*Continued*)

Serious gram-positive infections resistant to beta-lactam antibiotics
Serious allergies to beta-lactam antibiotics
C. difficile infections unresponsive to metronidazole
Prophylaxis for residents at high risk of endocarditis
Prophylaxis for surgical procedures with prosthetic devices and risk of methicillin-resistant staphylococcal infection
Limit vancomycin prophylaxis to only two doses
Decolonization regimens for VRE
Frequent relapses
No evidence of efficacy, particularly in residents of LTCF
Emergence of resistance likely

Abbreviations: VRE, vancomycin-resistant enterococci; LTCF, long-term care facilities.
Source: From Ref. 34.

Routine screening by standard stool culture cannot completely exclude that VRE are present in stool at low levels; levels may increase to detectable levels only if the patient is on therapy with certain antibiotics (13). The SHEA guidelines outlined below recommend discontinuation of VRE precautions in LTCF if two rectal or wound cultures are negative on successive days. However, if VRE are present in referring hospitals or in the LTCF itself, it may be prudent to be vigilant and to assume that all residents are potential VRE carriers. Moreover, given the limits of detection of VRE, it makes little sense to accept residents with negative stool cultures for VRE into a nursing home while refusing others with positive cultures if VRE are clearly known to be present in referring institutions. Routine use of screening procedures to detect carriers for the purposes of elimination of VRE from an LTCF in an endemic geographic locale is unlikely to be cost effective and is not recommended. Routine surveillance cultures to detect VRE colonization in residents in LTCF is only recommended if rates of VRE infection are increasing despite routine infection control precautions and transmission is suspected (34).

In light of scant data regarding transmission of VRE in LTCF, the SHEA guidelines recommend that VRE-colonized or -infected patients should optimally be placed in a private room or share a room with a roommate colonized with the same organism (34). Given that residents may be colonized with various combinations of VRE, MRSA, resistant gram-negative bacilli, and *C. difficile*, these isolation recommendations can pose a significant logistic problem for infection control practitioners in LTCF. The SHEA Committee on Long-Term Care alternatively recommends that VRE-colonized residents can be placed with or can share bathrooms with noncolonized individuals if the colonized resident is continent of stool and does not have diarrhea or open wounds. In addition, the noncolonized roommate should not be severely compromised, receiving broad-spectrum antibiotics, or should not have a urinary catheter, drainage device, or open wounds (34). Careful hand washing by colonized and noncolonized residents is emphasized. Restriction to rooms is not recommended in residents who are continent, use good hygiene, and have draining wounds contained by bandages. Private rooms or cohorting techniques have been used in LTCF, but most of these facilities allowed VRE-colonized residents to participate freely in social activities (19,20,36). Direct contact between colonized and noncolonized residents was restricted in only one facility (36). Lack of further transmission of VRE could not be directly attributed to the use of these cohorting techniques.

Precautions to disrupt the transmission of antibiotic-resistant pathogens recognize body fluids and the environment as major reservoirs of VRE and the hands of personnel as potential vectors. Therefore, routine hand washing by personnel before and after providing care to a patient is essential. Some studies have shown that standard soaps may not remove VRE from hands as effectively as hand disinfectants with antimicrobial activity. Antimicrobial soaps and alcohol disinfectants have been used in LTCF with VRE, but whether these interventions are effective in preventing transmission has not been established (37).

It is accepted that clean, nonsterile gloves be worn as part of standard infection control precautions when contact with body fluids from any patient is likely (33). In LTCF, it has been recommended that gloves also be worn within the room of a VRE-colonized or infected resident prior to initiating any direct contact with the patient or the patient's inanimate environment (34). The efficacy of donning gowns prior to entry into the rooms of VRE-colonized or infected patients in acute care hospitals remains controversial (33,35). In LTCF, it has been recommended that gowns be worn only if the clothes of health-care workers are likely to become soiled with body fluids (34). In uncontrolled studies, no transmission of VRE was documented in six LTCFs where the use of gowns and gloves was required (16,19,20,36). In one facility, gloves were also required for any casual contact with colonized residents outside of their room (36). However, universal gloving for care of uncolonized as well as colonized resident in LTCF may be just as effective as identifying and restricting colonized patients to their rooms and requiring the use of gowns and gloves in preventing transmission of VRE, MRSA, and multidrug-resistant gram-negative bacilli (38).

Because VRE is most likely transmitted by environmental sources, the SHEA guidelines recommend the use of dedicated equipment for colonized or infected patients (34). Although the optimum methods and frequency of disinfection have yet to be defined in hospitals or LTCF, daily cleaning of environmental surfaces within the resident's room with an appropriate germicide were recommended (33,36). In uncontrolled studies of four LTCFs, environmental cleaning of the resident's room ranged from thrice weekly to twice daily with a quaternary ammonium compound or germicide (19,36).

Small equipment/wheelchairs were left in the rooms (19,20) and/or wheelchairs were decontaminated with 1:10 dilution of bleach twice daily (20,36).

More randomized, controlled trials are necessary to define the minimum, least costly, and most effective means of infection control in LTCF. Despite the diversity of infection control measures employed above, the superiority of one approach in preventing colonization has not been established (16,19,20,36). No infections and deaths could be attributed directly to VRE in these studies (16,19,20,36).

PREVENTION

In the hospital setting, oral antimicrobial agents, such as bacitracin, doxycycline, and novobiocin, alone or in combination, have been tried to eradicate VRE from urine, stool, or wounds with frequent recurrences and emergence of further resistance (32). As a result, experts have generally not recommended attempts at VRE decolonization except in patient populations at extreme risk of infection (32). In the long-term care setting, decolonization of VRE-colonized residents with oral bacitracin regimens has been tried with variable success (20,36). However, it should be recognized that many colonized residents clear their colonization with resistant enterococci spontaneously after decolonization failed or without antibiotics (8,19,36).

It is likely that increased antibiotic use will perpetuate the problem of VRE. Prevention of the emergence of VRE in susceptible populations requires reducing the unnecessary use of antibiotics in animal feed, the hospital, and the long-term care setting. Hospital Infection Control Practices Advisory Committee recommends that vancomycin use be limited to treatment of serious gram-positive infections resistant to beta-lactam antibiotics, treatment of patients with serious beta-lactam allergy, and treatment of *C. difficile* unresponsive to metronidazole. Brief courses of vancomycin prophylaxis should be limited to high-risk endocarditis prevention or surgical procedures involving prosthetic devices with high rates of infection due to methicillin-resistant staphylococci (32). Restriction of the use of third-generation cephalosporins and antibiotics with antianaerobic activity has been associated with declines in rates of VRE infection (32). Further studies need to be done to see if antibiotic restriction leads to declines in the burden of VRE colonization in LTCF. Antibiotics are frequently continued in the long-term care setting, even if cultures are negative, the infection is resistant to the antibiotic chosen, or the organism is likely to represent contamination (39). Therefore, significant improvements in antibiotic use in the long-term care setting can be achieved in the meantime. Modification of risk factors that predispose residents of LTCF to colonization and infection with antibiotic resistant bacteria, such as use of feeding tubes, urinary catheters, intravenous devices, presence of wounds, and *C. difficile* infection, can be made with appropriate geriatric assessments and interventions.

SUGGESTED READING

Bradley SF. Issues in the management of resistant bacteria in long-term-care facilities. Infect Control Hosp Epidemiol 1999; 20:362–366.
Crossley K. The Long-Term-Care Committee of the Society for Healthcare Epidemiology of America. Vancomycin-resistant enterococci in long-term care facilities. Infect Control Hosp Epidemiol 1998; 19:521–525.
Patel R. Clinical impact of vancomycin-resistant enterococci. J Antimicrob Chemother 2003; 51(suppl 3):iii13–iii21.

REFERENCES

1. Low DE, Keller N, Barth A, Jones RN. Clinical prevalence, antimicrobial susceptibility, and geographic resistance patterns of enterococci: results from the SENTRY antimicrobial surveillance program, 1997–1999. Clin Infect Dis 2001; 32(suppl 2):S133–S145.
2. Bonten MJM, Willems R, Weinsein RA. Vancomycin-resistant enterococci: why are they here, and where do they come from? Lancet Infect Dis 2001; 1: 314–326.
3. Cetinkaya F, Falk P, Mayhall CG. Vancomycin-resistant enterococci. Clin Microbiol Rev 2000; 13:686–707.
4. Patel R. Clinical impact of vancomycin-resistant enterococci. J Antimicrob Chemother 2003; 51(suppl 3):iii13–iii21.
5. Diekema DJ, Pfaller MA, Jones RN. SENTRY Participants Group. Age-related trends in pathogen frequency and antimicrobial susceptibility of bloodstream isolates in North America SENTRY Antimicrobial Surveillance Program, 1997–2000. Int J Antimicrob Agents 2002; 20:412–418.
6. Bradley SF. Issues in the management of resistant bacteria in long-term-care facilities. Infect Control Hosp Epidemiol 1999; 20:362–366.
7. Elizaga ML, Weinstein RA, Hayden MK. Patients in long term care facilities: a reservoir for vancomycin-resistant enterococci. Clin Infect Dis 2002; 34:441–446.
8. Bonilla HF, Zervos MA, Lyons MJ, et al. Colonization with vancomycin-resistant *Enterococcus faecium*: comparison of a long-term care unit with an acute-care hospital. Infect Control Hosp Epidemiol 1997; 18:333–339.
9. Trick WE, Weinstein RA, DeMarais PL, et al. Colonization of skilled-care facility residents with antimicrobial-resistant pathogens. J Am Geriatr Soc 2001; 49:270–276.
10. Ostrowsky BE, Trick WE, Sohn AH, et al. Control of vancomycin-resistant *Enterococcus* in health care facilities in a region. N Engl J Med 2001; 344:1427–1433.
11. Padiglione AA, Grabsch E, Wolfe R, Gibson K, Grayson ML. The prevalence of fecal colonization with VRE among residents of long-term-care facilities in Melbourne, Australia. Infect Control Hosp Epidemiol 2001; 22:576–578.
12. Mylotte JM, Goodnough S, Tayara A. Antibiotic-resistant organisms among long-term care facility residents on admission to an inpatient geriatrics unit: retrospective and prospective surveillance. Am J Infect Control 2001; 29:139–144.
13. Baden LR, Thiemke W, Skolnik A, et al. Prolonged colonization with vancomycin-resistant *Enterococcus faecium* in long-term care patients and the significance of "clearance." Clin Infect Dis 2001; 33:1654–1660.

14. Donskey CJ, Ray AJ, Hoyen C, et al. Colonization and infection with multiple nosocomial pathogens among patients colonized with vancomycin-resistant *Enterococcus*. Infect Control Hosp Epidemiol 2003; 24:242–245.
15. Pacio GA, Visintainer P, Maguire G, Wormser GP, Raffalli J, Montecalvo MA. Natural history of colonization with vancomycin-resistant enterococci, methicillin-resistant *Staphylococcus aureus*, and resistant gram-negative bacilli among long-term-care facility residents. Infect Control Hosp Epidemiol 2003; 24:246–250.
16. Brennen C, Wagener MM, Muder RR. Vancomycin-resistant *Enterococcus faecium* in a long-term care facility. J Am Geriatr Soc 1998; 46:157–160.
17. Trick WE, Kuehnert MJ, Quirk SB, et al. Regional dissemination of vancomycin-resistant enterococci resulting from interfacility transfer of colonized patients. J Infect Dis 1999; 180:391–396.
18. Quale J, Patel K, Zaman M, et al. Fecal carriage of vancomycin-resistant enterococci in long-term care facility and hospitalized patients. Clin Infect Dis 1995; 21:733.
19. Greenaway CA, Miller MA. Lack of transmission of vancomycin-resistant enterococci in three long-term-care facilities. Infect Control Hosp Epidemiol 1999; 20:341–343.
20. Silverblatt FJ, Tibert C, Mikolich D, et al. Preventing the spread of vancomycin-resistant enterococci in a long-term care facility. J Am Geriatr Soc 2000; 48:1211–1215.
21. Schoonmaker DJ, Bopp LH, Baltch AL, Smith RP, Rafferty ME, George M. Genetic analysis of multiple vancomycin-resistant *Enterococcus* isolates obtained serially from two long-term care patients. J Clin Microbiol 1998; 36:2105–2108.
22. Flournoy DJ. Antimicrobial susceptibilities of bacteria from nursing home residents in Oklahoma. Gerontology 1994; 40:53–56.
23. Toubes E, Singh K, Yin D, et al. Risk factors for antibiotic-resistant infection and treatment outcomes among hospitalized patients transferred from long-term care facilities: does antimicrobial choice make a difference? Clin Infect Dis 2003; 36:724–730.
24. Nicolle LE. The chronic indwelling catheter and urinary infection in long-term-care facility residents. Infect Control Hosp Epidemiol 2001; 22:316–321.
25. Temple ME, Nahata MC. Pharmacotherapy of lower limb diabetic ulcers. J Am Geriatr Soc 2000; 48:822–828.
26. Livesley NJ, Chow AW. Infected pressure ulcers in elderly individuals. Clin Infect Dis 2002; 35:1390–1396.
27. Podnos YD, Jimenez JC, Wilson SE. Intra-abdominal sepsis in elderly persons. Clin Infect Dis 2002; 35:62–68.
28. Mylotte JM, Tayara A, Goodnough S. Epidemiology of bloodstream infection in nursing home residents: evaluation of a large cohort from multiple homes. Clin Infect Dis 2002; 35:1484–1490.
29. Dhawan VK. Infective endocarditis in elderly patients. Clin Infect Dis 2002; 34:806–812.
30. Wendt C, Krause C, Floss H. Validity of screening procedures for glycopeptide-resistant enterococci. Eur J Clin Microbiol Infect Dis 1999; 18:422–427.
31. Centers for Disease Control and Prevention. Multidrug-resistant organisms in non-hospital healthcare settings December 2000 (http://www.cdc.gov/ncidod/dhqp/ar_multidrug.FAQ.html.).

32. Kauffman CA. Therapeutic and preventative options for the management of vancomycin-resistant enterococcal infections. J Antimicrob Chemother 2003; 51: iii23–iii30.
33. Muto CA, Jernigan JA, Ostrowsky BE, et al. SHEA guideline for preventing nosocomial transmission of multi-drug resistant strains of *Staphylococcus aureus* and *Enterococcus*. Infect Control Hosp Epidemiol 2003; 24:362–386.
34. Crossley K. The Long-Term-Care Committee of the Society for Healthcare Epidemiology of America. Vancomycin-resistant enterococci in long-term care facilities. Infect Control Hosp Epidemiol 1998; 19:521–525.
35. Garner JS. The Hospital infection Control Practices Advisory Committee, Centers for Disease Control and Prevention. Guidelines for isolation precautions in hospitals. Infect Control Hosp Epidemiol 1996; 17:53–80.
36. Armstrong-Evans M, Litt M, McArthur MA, et al. Control of transmission of vancomycin-resistant *Enterococcus faecium* in a long-term-care facility. Infect Control Hosp Epidemiol 1999; 20:312–317.
37. Mody L, McNeil SA, Sun R, Bradley SE, Kauffman CA. Introduction of waterless alcohol-based hand rub in a long-term care facility. Infect Control Hosp Epidemiol 2003; 24:165–171.
38. Trick WE, Weinstein RA, DeMarais PL, et al. Comparison of routine glove use and contact-isolation precautions to prevent transmission of multidrug-resistant bacteria in a long-term care facility. J Am Geriatr Soc 2004; 52:2003–2009.
39. Loeb M, Bentley DW, Bradley S, et al. Development of minimum criteria for the initiation of antibiotics in residents of long-term-care facilities: results of a consensus conference. Infect Control Hosp Epidemiol 2001; 22:120–124.

25

Gram-Negative Bacteria

Vinod K. Dhawan

*Division of Infectious Diseases, Department of Internal Medicine, Charles R. Drew
University of Medicine and Science, Martin Luther King, Jr.–Charles R. Drew Medical
Center, and UCLA School of Medicine, Los Angeles, California, U.S.A.*

KEY POINTS

1. Gram-negative bacteria are common causes of infection among
   the residents of long-term care facilities. Emergence of antimicrobial resistance in the gram-negative bacteria has been a growing
   problem in nursing homes. Bacterial resistance to antimicrobial
   agents negatively impacts the outcome of infections.
2. Mechanisms of resistance to antibiotics in gram-negative bacilli
   include the production of β-lactamase by the organism, decreased
   membrane permeability, and the efflux mechanisms that pump the
   antimicrobial agent out of the cell.
3. Risk factors for acquisition of gram-negative bacilli in the elderly
   include poor functional status; increased patient morbidity; prior
   antibiotic use; presence of wounds, foreign bodies, and percutaneous devices; mechanical ventilation; emergency abdominal
   surgery; and longer hospital stay.
4. Appropriate therapy of infections due to antibiotic resistance
   gram-negative bacilli is critical to patient survival. Antimicrobial
   therapy should take into account the prevalent resistance patterns
   of organisms and the antimicrobial susceptibility data. Carbapenems are highly effective in the treatment of bacteria containing
   extended-spectrum β-lactamases. Trimethoprim–sulfamethoxazole

is the treatment of choice for infections due to *Stenotrophomonas maltophilia*.

5. Measures for control of antibiotic resistance in the long-term care facilities include appropriate planning for identifying, isolating, and treating patients. Better staffing, hand washing, and optimal use of antimicrobials are important components of such a strategy.

EPIDEMIOLOGY AND CLINICAL RELEVANCE

Gram-negative bacteria are common causes of infection among the residents of long-term care facilities (LTCFs). Emergence of antimicrobial resistance in the gram-negative bacteria has been a growing problem in nursing homes, hospitals, and even the community. Antibiotic-resistant organisms may be introduced into nursing homes with the admission of new residents who are already colonized or infected. Alternatively, bacterial resistance may emerge in the endogenous flora of residents upon exposure to antimicrobial agents, either through selection of resistant strains or through spontaneous mutation or gene transfer. There is ample evidence that bacterial resistance negatively impacts the outcome of infections. Data from the Centers for Disease Control and Prevention have linked bacterial resistance with higher rates of mortality and morbidity.

Mechanisms of Resistance

The development of antimicrobial resistance in microorganisms is a perfect example of contemporary biological evolution. Over the years, the introduction of new antibiotics has been matched by the development of new mechanisms of resistance by the bacteria. Gram-negative bacteria use a variety of strategies to avoid the inhibitory effect of antibiotics and have evolved highly efficient means for dissemination of resistance traits (Table 1).

Table 1 Mechanisms of Antibiotic Resistance Among Gram-Negative Bacteria

Mechanism	Antibiotics affected
Enzymatic inhibition	β-Lactams, aminoglycosides, chloramphenicol
Decreased membrane permeability	β-Lactams, aminoglycosides, chloramphenicol, trimethoprim, sulfonamides
Active efflux of antibiotic	Quinolones, tetracyclines
Altered ribosomal target	Aminoglycosides, chloramphenicol, tetracyclines
Altered target enzymes	β-Lactams, quinolones, trimethoprim, sulfonamides
Overproduction of target enzymes	Trimethoprim, sulfonamides
Bypass of inhibited steps by organisms	Trimethoprim, sulfonamides

Among the mechanisms that create resistance to antibiotics in gram-negative bacilli, the production of β-lactamase is the single most important factor. β-Lactamases are enzymes that hydrolyze the amide bond in the β-lactam ring of the antibiotic, leading to its inactivation. The ability of a β-lactamase to cause resistance varies with its activity, quantity, and its cellular location within the gram-negative bacteria. A variety of β-lactamases encoded chromosomally or by plasmids (TEM, SHV, or Oxa β-lactamases) has been described in gram-negative bacteria. The β-lactamases have been classified based on their sequences into evolutionary distinct classes A, B, C, and D. In addition, Bush, Jacoby, and Medeiros have proposed a functional classification of β-lactamases (Group 1 2, 3, and 4) based on their substrate and inhibitor profiles (Table 2) (1).

Extended-Spectrum β-Lactamases

The originally discovered β-lactamases (TEM-1, TEM-2, and SHV-1) had a rather restricted spectrum of activity against antibiotics. Resistance of some gram-negative bacilli to broad-spectrum cephalosporins has been noted to be mediated by the extended-spectrum β-lactamases (ESBLs) designated as Group 2be. Extended-spectrum β-lactamases are a group of enzymes that confer resistance to oxyimino cephalosporins (e.g., cefotaxime, ceftazidime, and ceftriaxone) and monobactams. The ESBLs are not capable of hydrolyzing cephamycins and carbapenems. Most ESBLs found in gram-negative bacilli are plasmid-borne variants of the original TEM-1 and SHV-1 enzymes in which one or more amino acid substitutions have expanded the substrate specificity. The ESBLs are most commonly expressed in *Klebsiella*

Table 2 The Bush-Jacoby-Medeiros Classification of β-Lactamases

Group	Preferred substrate	Inhibition by clavulanate	Molecular class
1	Cephalosporins	No	C
2a	Penicillins	Yes	A
2b	Penicillins, cephalosporins	Yes	A
2be	Penicillins, narrow- and extended-spectrum cephalosporins, monobactams	Yes	A
2br	Penicillins	Diminished	A
2c	Penicillins, carbenicillin	Yes	A
2d	Penicillins, cloxacillin	Yes	D
2e	Cephalosporins	Yes	A
2f	Penicillins, cephalosporins, carbapenems	Yes	A
3	Most β-lactams, including carbapenems	No	B
4	Penicillins	No	Not determined

Source: From Ref. 1.

pneumoniae, *Klebsiella oxytoca*, and *Escherichia coli*, although they have been detected in other organisms including *Salmonella* spp., *Pseudomonas aeruginosa*, *Proteus mirabilis*, and other Enterobacteriacea. More than 100 of these variants have been described. An updated list of ESBLs is maintained (2).

Different substitutions in ESBLs produce variable effects on the susceptibility of cefotaxime, ceftazidime, and aztreonam to the β-lactamases. Most ESBLs have increased activity against ceftazidime and aztreonam and diminished activity against cefotaxime. However, a serine substitution for glycine at amino acid 238 in SHV and TEM β-lactamases causes decreased hydrolytic activity against ceftazidime but increased activity against cefotaxime. TEM-1 ESBLs have decreased catalytic activity compared with TEM-2 β-lactamases. TEM-1 β-lactamases frequently mutate to TEM-2 lactamases, resulting in improved activity. An emerging mechanism of resistance to β-lactamase inhibitors, mediated by the derivatives of TEM and SHV enzymes with a limited number of nucleotide substitutions, has occurred in Europe. These types of β-lactamases have been designated Bush–Jacoby–Medeiros Group 2br or inhibitor-resistant TEM. Plasmid-encoded β-lactamases can be transmitted among different gram-negative bacteria, resulting in the horizontal spread of antimicrobial resistance. Such plasmids often carry resistance to other antibiotics, including tetracyclines, aminoglycosides, chloramphenicol, trimethoprim, and sulfonamides.

Inducible Chromosomal β-Lactamases AmpC

Another important mechanism of resistance in gram-negative organisms is the production of inducible chromosomal β-lactamases, most notably AmpC (Bush–Jacoby–Medeiros group 1). The presence of a β-lactam can cause depression of regulatory genes in these organisms, resulting in β-lactamase hyperproduction and inducible resistance to third-generation cephalosporins. Such enzymes are present in 24% to 48% of *Enterobacter* strains (3). They have also been noted in some strains of *Serratia marcescens*, *Pseudomonas*, *Citrobacter*, and indole-positive *Proteus*. This results in cross-resistance to other β-lactams except carbapenems, such as imipenem or the fourth-generation cephalosporin cefepime. Concomitant aminoglycoside therapy does not prevent the emergence of this resistance. The appearance of plasmid-mediated β-lactamases similar to AmpC in some strains of *K. pneumoniae* has resulted in their resistance to cephamycins, oxyimino-β lactams, and β-lactam inhibitors. Their potential plasmid-mediated transfer has raised concerns about horizontal spread of this resistance trait.

Metallo-Beta-Lactamases

Inducible chromosomal enzymes, called metallo-β-lactamases, confer resistance to β-lactam antibiotics in organisms, such as *Stenotrophomonas maltophilia*. Two major functional groups of metallo-β-lactamases have been identified (4). One group is a set of enzymes with broad substrate specificities capable of hydrolyzing most β-lactams except monobactams. A second group is composed of the "true" carbapenemases—enzymes that exhibit poor hydrolysis of penicillins and cephalosporins. This latter group has been found primarily in *Aeromonas* species. Although metallolactamases have been recovered from *Bacteroides fragilis*, *S. marcescens*, *Aeromonas* species, and *P. aeruginosa* in Japan, resistance to imipenem has not become widespread. Carbapenem resistance in *K. pneumoniae* also can be modulated by plasmid-mediated metallo-β-lactamase production, raising concerns about widespread dissemination of this resistance mechanism. Plasmid-mediated resistance to carbapenems is likely to increase and limit the use of these agents as a therapeutic option.

Porin Channels

Resistance of some gram-negative bacilli to the β-lactam antibiotics may also occur through the loss of porin channels in the outer cellular membrane, which decreases antibiotic entry into in periplasmic space. This often leads to increased resistance to cephalosporins, cephamycins, and β-lactam inhibitors. In *P. aeruginosa*, carbapenem resistance can occur by mutational loss of a porin channel. Similarly, decreased membrane permeability secondary to porin mutations often leads to quinolone resistance in gram-negative bacilli.

Efflux Pump Mechanisms

A set of multidrug efflux systems in some gram-negative bacteria enables them to survive in a hostile environment. The efflux mechanisms pump the antimicrobial agent out of the cell, preventing its access to the target site. Each efflux pump of gram-negative bacteria consists of three components: the inner membrane transporter, the outer membrane channel, and the periplasmic lipoprotein. The molecular mechanism of the drug extrusion across a two-membrane envelope of gram-negative bacteria may involve the formation of the membrane adhesion sites between the inner and the outer membranes. Quinolone resistance is often modulated by antibiotic efflux systems in addition to alteration in the DNA gyrase, topoisomerase II, and, to a lesser extent, toporisomerase IV.

Aminoglycoside Resistance

Aminoglycoside resistance is modulated by bacterial enzymes, which inactivate the aminoglycoside by variously acetylating, adenylating, or phosphorylating the antibiotic molecule.

Prevalence of Antibiotic-Resistant Gram-Negative Bacteria

Antimicrobial resistance among gram-negative bacteria is a problem worldwide. The Study for Monitoring Antimicrobial Resistance Trends surveillance program reported the antimicrobial susceptibility of 5658 aerobic and facultative gram-negative bacteria from intra-abdominal infections collected from 74 medical centers from 23 countries in 2003 (5). Enterobacteriaceae composed 84% of the total isolates. *E. coli* was the most common isolate (46%), and the susceptibility rate to the quinolone (70–90% susceptible), cephalosporin (80–97% susceptible), aminoglycoside (77–100% susceptible), and carbapenem (99–100% susceptible) agents tested varied among geographic regions, with isolates from the Asia/Pacific region generally being the most resistant. Extended-spectrum β-lactamases were detected phenotypically in 9% of *E. coli*, 14% of *Klebsiella* spp., and 14% of *Enterobacter* spp. worldwide. The carbapenems—ertapenem, meropenem, and imipenem—were highly active in vitro against Enterobacteriaceae isolated from intra-abdominal sites, including organisms that produce ESBLs.

Gram-negative bacilli are commonly associated with hospital-acquired infections in intensive care units (ICUs). One study recently analyzed >410,000 nosocomial bacterial isolates in ICUs reported to the National Nosocomial Infections Surveillance system from 1986 to 2003 (6). The study reported that in 2003, gram-negative bacilli were associated with 23.8% of bloodstream infections, 65.2% of pneumonia episodes, 33.8% of surgical site infections, and 71.1% of urinary tract infections in the ICU patients. The proportion of *Acinetobacter* species associated with ICU pneumonia increased from 4% in 1986 to 7.0% in 2003. Significant increases in resistance rates were uniformly seen for selected antimicrobial–pathogen combinations.

Most of the information regarding the prevalence of antibiotic-resistant organisms in nursing homes and other LTCFs is derived from surveillance studies of infections or outbreak investigations. The available data suggest that antibiotic-resistant organisms, including gram-negative bacilli, are frequent in the nursing home population. Antibiotic resistance among gram-negative bacteria has steadily increased over the years. Rates of prevalence of ampicillin or amoxicillin resistance in strains of *E. coli* are approximately 40% in the United States, 40% to 50% in the United Kingdom and in France, 58% in Spain, and 63% in Israel (7). Amicillin-resistant isolates of *E. coli* and cephalothin-resistant isolates of *Klebsiella* spp. are common in nursing homes. Aminoglycoside resistance has been noted in a significant proportion of uropathogens isolated from nursing home patients. One study reported colonization of urine or perineum with trimethoprim-resistant gram-negative bacilli in 52% of patients at a Department of Veterans Affairs nursing home (8). Resistance of gram-negative bacilli to fluoroquinolones has also been described. Prospective surveillance in seven skilled nursing facilities in Southern California found about a third of the urinary *Pseudomonas* isolates, and 12% of isolates of the family Enterobacteriaceae were resistant to norfloxacin (9).

ESBL-producing organisms, which are being identified worldwide, are probably more prevalent than are currently recognized because they are often undetected by routine susceptibility testing methods. These organisms are commonly encountered in nosocomial infections and have been implicated in several nursing home outbreaks. The prevalence of ESBL-producing *K. pneumoniae* is on the incline with rates approaching as high as 40% in some hospitals in northeastern United States (10). Teaching hospitals have been shown to have a higher prevalence of resistant organisms.

Organisms producing AmpC frequently are associated with infections in the ICU, representing 8% of ICU-related pneumonia isolates, 11% of urinary tract infection (UTI) isolates, and 4% central line-associated bacteremia isolates. As a group, AmpC-producing organisms may represent more than 30% of isolates in ICU patients with pneumonia in some institutions (11).

Risk Factors

Several studies have evaluated the risk factors for colonization and infection with antibiotic-resistant pathogens in nursing home patients. These risk factors include poor functional status, prior antibiotic use, presence of wounds (such as pressure ulcers), and presence of foreign bodies, such as urinary catheters (12). Exposure to any cephalosporin and log percentage of residents using gastrostomy tubes within the nursing home have been associated with having a clinical isolate resistant to third-generation cephalosporins (13). Other risk factors include mechanical ventilation, emergency abdominal surgery, the presence of percutaneous devices, longer hospital stay, and increased patient morbidity (14–16). Activity of daily living score and previous use of antibiotics were considered to predict the presence of antimicrobial-resistant pathogens in severe nursing home-acquired pneumonia in a recent study (17).

Risk factors for acquisition of ESBLs are generally similar to those reported for other hospital-acquired organisms (Table 3). Emergence of ESBL has also been associated with use of third-generation cephalosporins, particularly ceftazidime, as well as aztreonam, and trimethoprim–sulfamethoxazole.

Table 3 Factors Associated with Increased Antimicrobial Resistance in Gram-Negative Bacteria

Antibiotic use
Prolonged hospitalization
Stay in intensive care unit
Severely ill patient status
Immunocompromised status
Use of intravenous catheters
Ineffective infection control
Interhospital transfer of patients colonized with antibiotic-
    resistant organisms

CLINICAL SYNDROMES

Gram-negative bacilli are common causes of a variety of infections in the hospitals and long-term care facilities. Therefore, the development of resistance in these organisms is quite worrisome. ESBL-producing organisms have been implicated in a broad range of clinical syndromes. *E. coli* is the most common gram-negative pathogen associated with nosocomial infections, isolated from 12% of such infections. It is the leading cause of UTIs in nursing home populations and among patients with nosocomial UTIs. *K. pneumoniae* is also common, representing 5% of nosocomial infection site isolates, and 8% of hospital-acquired UTI and pneumonia isolates (18). *P. aeruginosa* has been associated with 9% of all hospital-acquired infection site isolates and is the most common cause of nosocomial gram-negative pneumonia, representing 17% of isolates. *Enterobacter* spp. represents 6% of all hospital-acquired isolates and 11% cases of pneumonia isolates (18). *S. maltophilia* (formerly *Xanthomonas maltophilia*) is a gram-negative bacilli that has been associated with bacteremia, respiratory tract infections, skin and soft-tissue infections, and endocarditis (19). *Acinetobacter*, a gram-negative coccobacillus, has emerged as an important nosocominal pathogen. The most common site of isolation is the respiratory tract. Hospital outbreaks are often related to contaminated respiratory equipment. *Acinetobacter* also has been associated with other types of nosocomial infection, including blood stream, soft tissue, UTIs, abdominal infections, meningitis, and endocarditis. Patients with impaired host defenses or central venous lines, and patients in the intensive care unit are particularly susceptible. *Burkholderia cepacia* (formerly, *Pseudomonas cepacia*) is an uncommon cause of infections. This organism has been reported in isolated patients with pneumonia, bacteremia, and invasive otitis. It is an important opportunistic agent of pneumonia in patients with cystic fibrosis (20). It can cause life-threatening infections in patients with chronic granulomatous disease.

DIAGNOSTIC APPROACH

The laboratory diagnosis of ESBL-producing gram-negative bacilli requires special methods. Simple screening for ceftazidime or aztreonam resistance is not adequate and misses approximately 15% to 20% of ESBL-producing organisms (21). Although some ESBL-containing bacteria might display in vitro susceptibility to these antibiotics, their minimum inhibitory concentrations often are at the borderline of susceptibility and the inoculum effect may lead to treatment failure in the presence of high in vivo bacterial concentrations. Resistance to cefpodoxime has been studied as a screening method. Using sensitivity breakpoints of $\geq 2\,\mu g/mL$ by minimum inhibitory concentration or $<22\,mm$ by disk diffusion (for a $30\,\mu g$ cefpodoxime disk) has a sensitivity of $\geq 98\%$ for ESBL detection (22,23).

ESBLs are susceptible in vitro to β-lactamase inhibitors, such as clavulanic acid. The most effective way to detect ESBLs is to test for synergy between ceftazidime or cefotaxime and clavulanic acid, as is recommended by the National Committee for Clinical Laboratory Standards for confirmation of ESBLs. Disks containing cefotaxime and ceftazidime alone and disks containing the combination of clavulanic acid with these antibiotics are placed on Mueller-Hinton agar. A 5 mm or greater increase in size of the zone diameter for either cefotaxime or ceftazidime tested in combination with clavulanic acid versus the zone for either antibiotic tested alone indicates the presence of an ESBL (24,25). An effective screening strategy might be a cefpodoxime screen followed by the confirmatory double disk diffusion test for isolates screening positive.

The Vitek ESBL test is reliable single-test alternative. It is an automated broth microdilution test using cefotaxime and ceftazidime alone and in combination with clavulanic acid. The test has been shown to be both sensitive ($\geq$99.5%) and specific (100%) for the detection of ESBLs (26,27). The E-test method, which involves testing third-generation cephalosporins with and without a β-lactamase inhibitor, is another method. However, the test is relatively expensive and the reliability of the commercially available version of this test is questionable.

THERAPEUTIC INTERVENTIONS

The rapidly evolving antimicrobial resistance in gram-negative bacilli poses a significant therapeutic challenge, and multiresistance is of particular concern. The elderly patients infected with multiresistant organisms are at higher risk of death. It has been noted that patients with ESBL-producing *K. pneumoniae* or *E. coli* bacteremia were significantly more likely to survive if they received appropriate therapy within three days of the onset of infection (27). Aproriate therapy of infections due to antibiotic-resistant gram-negative bacilli is, therefore, critical to patient survival. Currently available treatment options for the common antibiotic-resistant gram-negative bacteria are summarized in Table 4. The ESBL-producing *K. pneumoniae* and *E. coli* strains are often resistant to quinolones and aminoglycosides, leaving few therapeutic alternatives. In one study, ceftazidime-resistant isolates were resistant to gentamicin and ciprofloxacin in 67% and 45% of cases, respectively, compared with rates of 3.6% and 2.0% for ceftazidime-susceptible organisms (28). For susceptible isolates, however, aminoglycosides and quinolones remain effective treatment options. Carbapenems are highly effective in the treatment of bacteria containing ESBLs, with susceptibility rates ranging from 93% to 100% (29–31).

Gram-negative bacilli producing AmpC may initially test as "susceptible" to third-generation cephalosporins, but resistance can emerge during treatment with these antibiotics. It is important for the clinician to realize

Table 4 Treatment Options for Antibiotic-Resistant Gram-Negative Bacilli

Organism	Potential treatment options
ESBL-producing *Klebsiella*, *E. coli*	Imipenem or meropenem, cefepime, quinolones (for susceptible strains)
Enterobacter spp.	Imipenem or meropenem, cefepime, quinolones
Pseudomonas aeruginosa	Imipenem or meropenem, cefepime, quinolones
Stenotrophomonas maltophilia	Trimethoprim/sulfamethoxazole, ticarcillin-clavulanic acid, quinolones
Acinetobacter spp.	Imipenem-cilastatin, colistin
Burkholderia cepacia	Trimethoprim/sulfamethoxazole

Abbreviation: ESBL, extended-spectrum beta-lactamases.

that even when these organisms display in vitro susceptibility to the third-generation cephalosporins, treatment failures often occur in vivo. In one study, 20% of blood stream isolates of *E. cloacae* developed resistance to third-generation cephalosporins upon exposure to these agents (32). In contrast to other cephalosporins, cefepime, a new aminothiazolylacetamido, has a wider spectrum and a greater potency against the ESBL-producing organisms. Cefepime penetrates the gram-negative cell more rapidly, targets multiple essential penicillin-binding proteins, and escapes the effects of many β-lactamases due to the enzymes' low affinity for the drug. Cefepime is a much weaker inducer of AmpC production. The latter characteristic is most apparent in studies of Bush group 1 β-lactamases. De-repression of this class of β-lactamases has lesser effect on the in vitro activity of cefepime as compared with other cephalosporins. In one study, 80% of *Pseudomonas* isolates and >99% of other AmpC-producing Enterobacteriaceae tested sensitive to cefepime (30). The carbapenems represent another treatment option. Eighty-four percent of *Pseudomonas* isolates and >99% of *Enterobacter* and *Citrobacter* isolates remain sensitive (30). Cephamycins are a treatment option, but plasmid-mediated AmpC β-lactamase production and porin channel mutations may limit their clinical utility. Quinolones and aminoglycosides are often effective, although resistance is emerging. Ceftibuten, an oral oxyimino-β-lactam that binds less tightly to ESBLs compared to other cephalosporins, has demonstrated reasonable in vitro activity, but clinical experience with this antibiotic is limited. β-Lactam/β-lactamase inhibitor antibiotics have good in vitro activity against some ESBL-expressing organisms and have been shown to protect against ESBL acquisition (33). However, bacterial mutation may lead to decreased susceptibility to these agents. AmpC is not susceptible to β-lactamase inhibitors. Because of the high prevalence of antibiotic resistance and because of the potential for emergence of resistance during therapy, *Pseudomonas* infections are usually treated with two active agents.

The management of infections due to *S. maltophilia* is problematic because many strains manifest resistance to multiple antibiotics. Trimethoprim–sulfamethoxazole (TMP–SMX) is the treatment of choice for infections due to *S. maltophilia*. Ticarcillin–clavulanate is the only β-lactam/β-lactamase inhibitor combination antibiotic that is reliably effective in the treatment of *S. maltophilia*. It has been suggested as the treatment of choice for patients who are unable to tolerate TMP–SMX. However, resistance to both of these agents is increasing. Aminoglycosides generally are not active against *S. maltophilia*, possibly due to aminoglycoside-mediating enzymes, and alterations in cell surface. Resistance rates to imipenem approach 100% (34). Cefepime has greater in vitro activity against *S. maltophilia* than does ceftazidime, with susceptibility rates of blood stream isolates reported to be 88.7% and 35.3%, respectively, in one United States study (34). Some of the newer quinolones, notably clinafloxacin, sparfloxacin, and trovafloxacin, have better in vitro activity than ciprofloxacin. In one study, 94% of isolates were susceptible to clinafloxacin (35). Minocycline has good in vitro activity (36), but its use in clinical settings is limited. Antibiotic combinations, including TMP–SMX plus ticarcillin/clavulanate or a third-generation cephalosporin and TMP–SMX plus minocycline and ticarcillin/clavulanate, might be effective in the treatment of serious *S. maltophilia* infections.

Acinetobacter infections are most reliably treated with carbapenems although resistance to these agents is emerging (30). Quinolones may be effective treatment options for some strains. One study noted that only 17% of clinical *A. baumannii* isolates were susceptible to this antibiotic class (36). Aminoglycoside resistance is common in *A. baumannii*, occurring in approximately 85% of isolates (36). β-Lactam/β-lactamase antibiotics have good in vitro activity against *A. lwoffi* (<10% are resistant) but are less effective against *A. baumannii*, with 30% strains being resistant. Sulbactam has intrinsic bactericidal activity against many multidrug-resistant *Actinetobacter* strains via its penicillin-binding protein 2 properties that are separate from its inhibition of β-lactamases. Ceftazidime and cefepime are active against *A. lwoffi* but have lesser activity against *A. baumannii*, resistance rates approaching 12% and 30%, respectively, in the two isolates (30,37).

Intrinsic resistance of *B. cepacia* to several antibiotics complicates treatment of infections due to this organism. Trimethoprim–sulfamethoxazole has historically been the drug of choice. Ceftazidime, meropenem, and ciprofloxacin are also active for most of the strains. Doripenem has somewhat better activity against *B. cepacia* and multidrug-resistant strains of mucoid *P. aeruginosa* than established antimicrobial agents and, thus, may provide an alternative to therapy (38).

Colistin therapy should be considered in severe infections with multiresistant gram-negative bacilli. It has an acceptable safety profile. Clinical response to colistin was observed for 73% of such cases in a recent report (39). Tigecycline is a newly approved glycylcycline. Its spectrum of activity includes enteric gram-negative bacilli and anacrobes, thus making it a viable option for the monotherapy of intra-abdominal infections (40).

Infection Control Measures

Nursing home patients may be an important reservoir of multiple antibiotic-resistant organisms including ESBL-producing gram-negative bacteria. Control of antibiotic-resistant pathogens is important for both the patients and the society in general. There has been little evaluation of methods to limit the spread of infections in nursing home population. Most of the recommendations are extrapolated from programs considered effective in the acute care facilities. The role of ESBL-producing organisms in hospital and nursing home outbreaks, as well as the ability of their plasmid DNA to be transferred to other bacterial species, makes effective control a growing challenge. Nursing home outbreaks can occur through either clonal spread of a specific plasmid-carrying strain or through transfer of a particular plasmid to a variety of bacterial strains or even different bacterial genera. Use of broad-spectrum antibiotics and poor infection control practices facilitate the spread of this plasmid-mediated resistance.

Efficient monitoring of antimicrobial resistance can produce timely and important data and information that will benefit patients. One of the reasons cited for the spread of the organism in the largest outbreak of ESBL-producing *K. pneumoniae*, which occurred at a Brooklyn, New York, hospital, was a failure of initial detection of the organism. Implementation of effective screening methods for the detection of ESBLs is a key factor in the control of hospital outbreaks and is necessary for accurate surveillance. Resistant organisms can be passed from patient to patient by the hands of health-care providers. A recent outbreak of *Enterobacter aerogenes* in a geriatric acute unit was attributed to the failure to institute contact isolation (41). Patients infected or colonized with antibiotic-resistant bacteria, including ESBL-producing gram-negative bacteria, should be isolated and barrier precautions should be instituted to prevent the spread of these organisms in the LTCFs. Limitation in patient movement and interaction within the facility, and specific therapy of patients infected with antibiotic-resistant bacteria are important control measures. Appropriate planning for identifying, transferring, discharging, and readmitting patients with antibiotic-resistant gram-negative bacilli to long-term care facilities constitute important control measures (see also Chapter 10).

Restriction of cephalosporin use has been associated with control of hospital outbreaks. Class restriction of all cephalosporins at a New York hospital was associated with significant reduction in the prevalence of ceftazidime-resistant *K. pneumoniae* (42). Unfortunately, there was a significant increase in imipenem-resistant *P. aeruginosa* during the study period, presumably related to increased use of imipenem. Discontinuation of ceftazidime use at a hospital in Massachusetts resulted in a significant decrease in the prevalence of ESBL-producing *K. pneumoniae*. Education of health-care providers, application of clinical practice guidelines, and audit and feedback activities have all been shown to have a salutary effect in altering antibiotic prescribing. Nursing homes should monitor and control antibiotic use and regularly survey antibiotic resistance patterns among pathogens. Pharmacists can play a major role through clinician education and focused clinical services. With the cooperation of health-care teams, the effectiveness of available antibiotics may be sustained, and the threat of resistance minimized.

PREVENTION

To control the emergence of resistant pathogens, Centers for Disease Control and Prevention guidelines and infection control guidelines must be adhered to. Prevention of emergence of resistance and the spread of antibiotic-resistant gram-negative bacilli require prudent use of antimicrobials and strict adherence to infection control measures. Better staffing, more hand-washing sinks, and use of antimicrobial soap reduce resistance to antimicrobial agents in LTCFs (43). There is intense antimicrobial use in the LTCFs, and studies have repeatedly documented that much of this use is inappropriate (44). Attempts to improve antimicrobial use in the LTCFs are complicated by characteristics of the patient population, limited availability of diagnostic tests, and the virtual absence of relevant clinical trials. Optimal use of antimicrobials is essential in the face of escalating antibiotic resistance and requires cooperation from all sectors of the health care system (see also Chapter 11).

Clinicians must alter their antibiotic prescribing habits for the treatment of infectious diseases, and patients must change their perception of the need for antibiotics. Important strategies for the prevention of antimicrobial resistance with regard to antibiotic use include monitoring of antibiotic use, improving antimicrobial prescribing by educational and administrative means, optimizing perioperative prophylaxis, optimizing the choice and duration of empiric therapies, and developing guidelines for the optimal use of antibiotics for common indications.

Cycling of currently available antibiotics to reduce resistance is an attractive concept, because it periodically removes from the institutional environment certain classes or specific agents that could induce or select for resistance. Rotation of antibiotics was noted to help to avoid ventilator-associated pneumonia and improve the susceptibilities of the potentially antibiotic-resistant gram-negative bacilli responsible for late-onset ventilator-associated pneumonia (45). For cycling strategies to be successful, their implementation must have a demonstrable impact on the prevalence of resistance determinants already dispersed throughout the patient environment.

Rotational usage practices are likely to be most appropriate for drugs active against gram-negative bacilli because of the wide choices available for rotation. Although antibiotic use provides an obvious stimulus for the emergence of resistance, it is by no means the only important factor. Antibiotic recycling must be evaluated in the context of other concomitant attempts to improve antimicrobial usage and must take into account other factors influencing resistance (46). Large-scale, cooperative studies on a national basis may provide data on this important issue.

There has been an increasing appreciation of the role played by the use of antibiotics in agriculture, aquaculture, and veterinary settings in the emergence of antimicrobial resistance. For example, fluoroquinolone use in aquaculture has been associated with the emergence of a variety of gram-negative bacilli, including *E. coli*, *Aeromonas salmonicida*, and other organisms. Subtherapeutic concentrations of tetracyclines have been shown to increase the frequency of the transfer of resistance plasmids in the guts of animals. Global control of antimicrobial resistance must address the non-human use of antimicrobials.

SUGGESTED READING

Gaynes R, Edwards JR. Overview of nosocomial infections caused by gram-negative bacilli. Clin Infect Dis 2005; 41:848–854.

Loeb MB, Craven S, McGeer AJ, et al. Risk factors for resistance to antimicrobial agents among nursing home residents. Am J Epidemiol 2003; 157:40–47.

Paterson DL, Rossi F, Baquero F, et al. In vitro susceptibilities of aerobic and facultative gram-negative bacilli isolated from patients with intra-abdominal infections worldwide: the 2003 Study for Monitoring Antimicrobial Resistance Trends (SMART). J Antimicrob Chemother 2005; 55:965–973.

Sandoval C, Walter SD, McGeer A, et al. Nursing home residents and Enterobacteriaceae resistant to third-generation cephalosporins. Emerg Infect Dis 2004; 10:1050–1055.

REFERENCES

1. Bush K, Jacoby GA, Medeiros AA. A functional classification scheme for beta-lactamases and its correlation with molecular structure. Antimicrob Agents Chemother 1995; 39:1211–1233.
2. http://www.lahey.org/studies/webt.htm.
3. Drusano GL. Infection in the intensive care unit: beta-lactamase-mediated resistance among Enterobacteriaceae and optimal antimicrobial dosing. Clin Infect Dis 1998; 27(suppl 1):S111–S116.
4. Bush K. Metallo-beta-lactamases: a class apart. Clin Infect Dis 1998; 27(suppl 1): S48–S53.
5. Paterson DL, Rossi F, Baquero F, et al. In vitro susceptibilities of aerobic and facultative gram-negative bacilli isolated from patients with intra-abdominal

infections worldwide: the 2003 Study for Monitoring Antimicrobial Resistance Trends (SMART). J Antimicrob Chemother 2005; 55:965–973.

6. Gaynes R, Edwards JR. Overview of nosocomial infections caused by gram-negative bacilli. Clin Infect Dis 2005; 41:848–854.

7. Wiederman B, Grimm H. Susceptibility to antibiotics: species incidence and trends. In: Lorian V, ed. Antibiotics in Laboratory Medicine. New York: Williams & Wilkins, 1996.

8. Wingard E, Shlaes JH, Mortimer EA, Shlaes DM. Colonization and cross-colonization of nursing home patients with trimethoprim-resistant gram-negative bacilli. Clin Infect Dis 1993; 16:75–81.

9. Lee YL, Thrupp LD, Friis RH, Fine M, Maleki P, Cesario TC. Nosocomial infection and antibiotic utilization in geriatric patients: a pilot prospective surveillance program in skilled nursing facilities. Gerontology 1992; 38:223–232.

10. Burwen DR, Banerjee SN, Gaynes RP. Ceftazidime resistance among selected nosocomial gram-negative bacilli in the United States. National Nosocomial Infections Surveillance System. J Infect Dis 1994; 170:1622–1625.

11. Fridkin SK, Welbel SF, Weinstein RA. Magnitude and prevention of nosocomial infections in the intensive care unit. Infect Dis Clin North Am 1997; 11:479–496.

12. Nicolle LE, Strausbaugh LJ, Garibaldi RA. Infections and antibiotic resistance in nursing homes. Clin Microbiol Rev 1996; 9:1–17.

13. Sandoval C, Walter SD, McGeer A, et al. Nursing home residents and Enterobacteriaceae resistant to third-generation cephalosporins. Emerg Infect Dis 2004; 10:1050–1055.

14. De Champs C, Rouby D, Guelon D, et al. A case-control study of an outbreak of infections caused by *Klebsiella pneumoniae* strains producing CTX-1 (TEM-3) beta-lactamase. J Hosp Infect 1991; 18:5–13.

15. Pena C, Pujol M, Ricart A, et al. Risk factors for faecal carriage of *Klebsiella pneumoniae* producing extended spectrum beta-lactamase (ESBL-KP) in the intensive care unit. J Hosp Infect 1997; 35:9–16.

16. Wiener J, Quinn JP, Bradford PA, et al. Multiple antibiotic-resistant *Klebsiella* and *Escherichia coli* in nursing homes. JAMA 1999; 281:517–523.

17. El Solh AA, Pietrantoni C, Bhat A, Bhora M, Berbary E. Indicators of potentially drug-resistant bacteria in severe nursing home-acquired pneumonia. Clin Infect Dis 2004; 39:474–480.

18. National Nosocomial Infections Surveillance (NNIS) report, data summary from October 1986–April 1996, issued May 1996. A report from the National Nosocomial Infections Surveillance (NNIS) System. Am J Infect Control 1996; 24:380–388.

19. Denton M, Kerr KG. Microbiological and clinical aspects of infection associated with *Stenotrophomonas maltophilia*. Clin Microbiol Rev 1998; 11:57–80.

20. Spencer RC. The emergence of epidemic, multiple-antibiotic-resistant *Stenotrophomonas (Xanthomonas) maltophilia* and *Burkholderia (Pseudomonas) cepacia*. J Hosp Infect 1995; 30(suppl):453–464.

21. Jacoby GA, Han P. Detection of extended-spectrum beta-lactamases in clinical isolates of *Klebsiella pneumoniae* and *Escherichia coli*. J Clin Microbiol 1996; 34:908–911.

22. Cullmann W. Antibiotic susceptibility and outer membrane proteins of clinical *Xanthomonas maltophilia* isolates. Chemotherapy 1991; 37:246–250.
23. Emery CL, Weymouth LA. Detection and clinical significance of extended-spectrum beta-lactamases in a tertiary-care medical center. J Clin Microbiol 1997; 35:2061–2067.
24. Jacoby GA. Extended-spectrum beta-lactamases and other enzymes providing resistance to oxyimino-beta-lactams. Infect Dis Clin North Am 1997; 11:875–887.
25. NCCLS. Performance Standards for Antimicrobial Susceptibility Testing: Ninth Informational Supplement Document M100-S9. Wayne, PA: National Committee for Clinical Laboratory Standards, 1999.
26. Sanders CC, Barry AL, Washington JA, et al. Detection of extended-spectrum-beta-lactamase-producing members of the family Enterobacteriaceae with Vitek ESBL test. J Clin Microbiol 1996; 34:2997–3001.
27. Spargo J. Enhanced detection of extended-spectrum beta-lactamases by the Vitek ESBL test. In: 38th Interscience Conference on Antimicrobial Agents and Chemotherapy. San Diego, CA: American Society of Microbiology, 1998:41.
28. Schiappa DA, Hayden MK, Matushek MG, et al. Ceftazidime-resistant *Klebsiella pneumoniae* and *Escherichia coli* bloodstream infection: a case-control and molecular epidemiologic investigation. J Infect Dis 1996; 174:529–536.
29. Itokazu GS, Quinn JP, Bell-Dixon C, Kahan FM, Weinstein RA. Antimicrobial resistance rates among aerobic gram-negative bacilli recovered from patients in intensive care units: evaluation of a national postmarketing surveillance program. Clin Infect Dis 1996; 23:779–784.
30. Jones RN, Pfaller MA, Doern GV, Erwin ME, Hollis RJ. Antimicrobial activity and spectrum investigation of eight broad-spectrum beta-lactam drugs: a 1997 surveillance trial in 102 medical centers in the United States. Cefepime Study Group. Diagn Microbiol Infect Dis 1998; 30:215–228.
31. Pfaller MA, Jones RN, Doern GV. Multicenter evaluation of the antimicrobial activity for six broad-spectrum beta-lactams in Venezuela using the Etest method. The Venezuelan Antimicrobial Resistance Study Group. Diagn Microbiol Infect Dis 1998; 30:45–52.
32. Chow JW, Fine MJ, Shlaes DM, et al. *Enterobacter bacteremia*: clinical features and emergence of antibiotic resistance during therapy. Ann Intern Med 1991; 115:585–590.
33. Piroth L, Aube H, Doise JM, Vincent-Martin M. Spread of extended-spectrum beta-lactamase-producing *Klebsiella pneumoniae*: are beta-lactamase inhibitors of therapeutic value? Clin Infect Dis 1998; 27:76–80.
34. Jones RN, Pfaller MA, Marshall SA, Hollis RJ, Wilke WW. Antimicrobial activity of 12 broad-spectrum agents tested against 270 nosocomial blood stream infection isolates caused by non-enteric gram-negative bacilli: occurrence of resistance, molecular epidemiology, and screening for metallo-enzymes. Diagn Microbiol Infect Dis 1997; 29:187–192.
35. Pankuch GA, Jacobs MR, Appelbaum PC. Susceptibilities of 123 *Xanthomonas maltophilia* strains to clinafloxacin, PD 131628, PD 138312, PD 140248, ciprofloxacin, and ofloxacin. Antimicrob Agents Chemother 1994; 38:369–370.
36. Vartivarian S, Anaissie E, Bodey G, Sprigg H, Rolston K. A changing pattern of susceptibility of *Xanthomonas maltophilia* to antimicrobial agents: implications for therapy. Antimicrob Agents Chemother 1994; 38:624–627.

37. Seifert H, Strate A, Pulverer G. Nosocomial bacteremia due to *Acinetobacter baumannii*. Clinical features, epidemiology, and predictors of mortality. Medicine (Baltimore) 1995; 74:340–349.
38. Chen Y, Garber E, Zhao Q, et al. In vitro activity of doripenem (S-4661) against multidrug-resistant gram-negative bacilli isolated from patients with cystic fibrosis. Antimicrob Agents Chemother 2005; 49:2510–2511.
39. Markou N, Apostolakos H, Koumoudiou C, et al. Intravenous colistin in the treatment of sepsis from multiresistant Gram-negative bacilli in critically ill patients. Crit Care 2003; 7:R78–R83.
40. Zinner SH. Overview of antibiotic use and resistance: setting the stage for tigecycline. Clin Infect Dis 2005; 41(suppl 5):S289–S292.
41. Piagnerelli M, Kennes B, Brogniez Y, Deplano A, Govaerts D. Outbreak of nosocomial multidrug-resistant *Enterobacter aerogenes* in a geriatric unit: failure of isolation contact, analysis of risk factors, and use of pulsed-field gel electrophoresis [in process citation]. Infect Control Hosp Epidemiol 2000; 21:651–653.
42. Rahal JJ, Urban C, Horn D, et al. Class restriction of cephalosporin use to control total cephalosporin resistance in nosocomial *Klebsiella*. JAMA 1998; 280:1233–1237.
43. Loeb MB, Craven S, McGeer AJ, et al. Risk factors for resistance to antimicrobial agents among nursing home residents. Am J Epidemiol 2003; 157:40–47.
44. Nicolle LE, Bentley DW, Garibaldi R, Neuhaus EG, Smith PW. Antimicrobial use in long-term-care facilities. SHEA Long-Term-Care Committee [in process citation]. Infect Control Hosp Epidemiol 2000; 21:537–545.
45. Gruson D, Hilbert G, Vargas F, et al. Strategy of antibiotic rotation: long-term effect on incidence and susceptibilities of gram-negative bacilli responsible for ventilator-associated pneumonia. Crit Care Med 2003; 31:1908–1914.
46. McGowan JE Jr. Strategies for study of the role of cycling on antimicrobial use and resistance. Infect Control Hosp Epidemiol 2000; 21:S36–S43.

26

Fungal Infections

Carol A. Kauffman

Division of Infectious Diseases, Department of Internal Medicine, Veterans Affairs Ann Arbor Healthcare System, University of Michigan Medical School, Ann Arbor, Michigan, U.S.A.

Sara A. Hedderwick

Department of Infectious Diseases, Royal Victoria Hospital, Belfast, Northern Ireland, U.K.

KEY POINTS

1. Candiduria is common, generally reflects colonization and not infection, and rarely requires antifungal treatment.
2. Mucocutaneous *Candida* infections usually can be treated effectively with antifungal creams, troches, solutions, or powders.
3. Onychomycosis cannot be treated with local therapy; systemic antifungal agents are required.
4. Good infection control practices can prevent transmission of dermatophyte infections among residents of LTCFs.
5. Oral azole antifungal agents have significant drug–drug interactions that must be taken into account before starting treatment with one of these agents.

INTRODUCTION

The prominent fungal infections that are encountered in residents of long-term care facilities (LTCFs) are mostly local infections of skin and mucous membranes. Invasive fungal infections are uncommon. Older adults in LTCFs are chronically ill and have many underlying illnesses, but most are not overtly immunosuppressed and thus not at risk for invasive fungal infections.

Most infections in the long-term care setting are due to dermatophytes, which infect only the superficial skin and hair structures, and *Candida* species, which normally colonize the gastrointestinal and genitourinary tracts of humans. Filamentous fungi, such as *Aspergillus* and the Zygomycetes, and *Cryptococcus neoformans*, an opportunistic yeast, are almost always acquired from the environment and cause disease mostly, but not entirely, in those who are immunosuppressed.

Although systemic fungal infections are uncommon in the long-term care setting, increasingly, patients are transferred to such facilities for continuation of intravenous (IV) antimicrobial agents, including antifungal agents, initiated in the hospital. Thus, knowledge of modes of administration, side effects, and drug–drug interactions of systemic antifungal agents will be important for the care of these patients. Because these infections are uncommon in the long-term care setting, the diagnosis and initiation of therapy for a systemic fungal infection should be undertaken only after consultation with an infectious diseases physician.

EPIDEMIOLOGY AND CLINICAL RELEVANCE

Dermatophyte Infections

Dermatophytes normally infect the keratinized layers of the skin and the hair shafts. They are responsible for tinea corporis (ringworm), tinea pedis ("athlete's foot"), tinea cruris ("jock itch"), tinea capitis, and onychomycosis. The prevalence of onychomycosis increases with age. However, scalp infection is predominantly a childhood disease and is rarely seen in the elderly. Although uncommon, outbreaks of tinea corporis have been described in long-term care facilities (1,2).

The genera of dermatophytes that cause disease in humans are *Trichophyton, Microsporum*, and *Epidermophyton*. Many dermatophytes cause disease only in humans and are transmitted directly by person-to-person contact or by fomites, such as hairbrushes. A few species cause infection in cats and dogs and can be transmitted from pets (Table 1).

Yeast Infections

Tinea Versicolor

Malassezia furfur, previously known as *Pityrosporum orbiculare*, is the cause of tinea versicolor, a superficial fungal infection of the head, neck, and chest. This organism is frequently part of the normal flora found on the skin of humans.

Table 1 Epidemiology of Fungal Infections in Long-Term Care Facilities

Fungal organism	Pertinent epidemiologic characteristics
Dermatophytes	Usually single cases, men more than women, chronic, relapsing infections; rarely outbreaks occur with spread among patients and health-care workers; potential for outbreaks from pets brought into the facility
Candida	Infection almost always from patient's own endogenous flora; *Candida glabrata* more common in urinary tract and in older persons; infection more likely in those with indwelling intravenous and urinary catheters
Cryptococcus	Acquired from outside environment; may present years later as chronic meningitis or dementia in long-term care resident
Aspergillus	Acquired from outside environment; rare in long-term care facility
Zygomycoses	Acquired from outside environment; rare in long-term care facility

Candida

The most common systemic fungal infections in older patients are those due to *Candida* species. *Candida* species colonize the human gastrointestinal and genitourinary tracts. *C. albicans* is the most common colonizing species and is the cause of most infections. *C. glabrata* (formerly *Torulopsis glabrata*) is an important cause of urinary tract infections and candidemia in older adults. In some hospitals, the proportion of fungemias due to *C. glabrata* is strikingly higher in patients over age 60 (3). *C. glabrata* is also disproportionately increased in the oropharynx of octogenarians compared with those who are 60 to 80 years old and is a cause of denture stomatitis (Table 1) (4).

Risk factors and patterns of yeast colonization among residents of LTCFs have been assessed in few studies. Hedderwick et al. noted that 84% of residents of a veterans LTCF were colonized with yeasts on at least one occasion, 42% had intermittent colonization, and 16% were persistently colonized (5). Risk factors independently associated with colonization included neurogenic bladder, lower extremity amputation, and low serum albumin.

Cryptococcosis

Infection with *C. neoformans* is uncommon in the long-term care setting. The infection is almost always acquired from the outside environment. This heavily encapsulated yeast is inhaled, causing pulmonary infection, which is usually asymptomatic. Because of the organism's neurotropism, the most common clinical manifestations of cryptococcosis are those that occur after spread to the central nervous system. Development of cryptococcal meningitis in a patient in an LTCF is most likely due to reactivation of infection acquired years earlier.

Cryptococcosis is noted most often in older adults who have been treated with corticosteroids, have received an organ transplant, or who have diabetes mellitus, renal failure, liver dysfunction, or chronic obstructive pulmonary disease. However, approximately 20% to 30% of patients, most of whom are older, have no underlying risk factors (6).

Invasive Filamentous Fungal Infections

Aspergillus and the Zygomycetes, *Mucor* and *Rhizopus,* are ubiquitous molds found in the environment. Only rarely do these fungi infect patients in the long-term care setting (Table 1). Almost always, invasive infections with these fungi occur in immunosuppressed patients, especially those who are taking corticosteroids and are neutropenic. However, there are more indolent forms of infection with *Aspergillus* that do occur in older adults who are not immunosuppressed (7). The Zygomycetes have a propensity to cause infection in patients with diabetes mellitus complicated by ketoacidosis and in those with iron overload states that require treatment with the iron chelator, deferoxamine.

CLINICAL MANIFESTATIONS

Dermatophyte Infections

Tinea Corporis (Ringworm)

The dermatophytes characteristically produce annular lesions that have prominent edges, and contain pustules, central clearing, and scaling. Pigmented skin can become hyperpigmented. The lesions are single or multiple and tend to occur on the trunk or legs. Pruritus may be present but is often mild. The rash should be differentiated from contact dermatitis, eczema, and psoriasis.

Tinea Cruris

This manifestation is seen almost exclusively in men. The rash, which is erythematous, scaling, and pustular, usually starts in the groin and then extends to involve the anterior thighs. The rash must be differentiated from that of intertrigenous candidiasis, erythrasma due to *Corynebacterium*, and psoriasis, which can occasionally present as a rash in the groin. The absence of satellite lesions beyond the edge of the rash points toward a dermatophyte infection, rather than candidiasis; erythrasma and psoriasis generally are not pustular.

Tinea Capitis

Dermatophyte infections of the scalp vary depending on the infecting species. The main clinical manifestation is scaling of the skin of the scalp;

erythema, pustules, and alopecia can occur. Tinea capitis is rarely seen in elderly patients.

Tinea Pedis

This dermatophyte infection is more common in men than in women. It is very common in institutions that use common bathing facilities. The infection usually starts in the web spaces of the lateral toes with characteristic peeling, fissures, maceration, and pruritus. The soles and lateral borders of the feet are also involved, showing erythema and scaling. Patients who have recurrent lower extremity cellulitis should be examined carefully for signs of tinea pedis, as this is a frequent point of ingress of streptococci and staphylococci.

Onychomycosis

Fungal infection of the nails is predominantly caused by dermatophytes (8). Almost always, patients with onychomycosis due to dermatophytes also have chronic tinea pedis. Commonly, the nail bed is invaded from the distal and lateral borders and becomes thickened and discolored. The distal part of the nail can completely crumble. In contrast to *Candida* nail infections, fingernails are much less commonly affected than toenails.

Yeast Infections

Tinea Versicolor

This benign skin infection usually presents as flat round patches of hypo- or hyperpigmented skin on the neck, chest, or upper arms. Mild pruritus may be present, and fine scales are noted. The lesions should be differentiated from those associated with vitiligo, in which scaling does not occur.

Candida Infections

Oropharyngeal candidiasis: Oropharyngeal candidiasis (thrush) is associated with a number of different local and mechanical factors (Table 2) (9). These include the use of broad-spectrum antibiotics, inhaled corticosteroids, and radiation therapy to the head and neck areas. Additionally, xerostomia, related to a variety of systemic diseases and medications, is associated with increased colonization and infection with *Candida*. Age alone is not sufficient for the development of oropharyngeal candidiasis. If thrush is present in an older adult who has no obvious risk factors, the possibility of underlying immunosuppression due to cancer or acquired immunodeficiency syndrome should be explored.

White plaques appear on the buccal, palatal, and oropharyngeal mucosa; these usually are not painful and can be scraped off with a tongue depressor revealing erythematous mucosa. With or without oropharyngeal lesions, patients may have painful cracks at the corners of the mouth (perleche or angular cheilitis).

Table 2 Major Clinical Manifestations of Infection with *Candida*

Manifestation	Major characteristics
Oropharyngeal (thrush)	White plaques on buccal mucosa, palate, tongue; under upper dentures appears as diffuse erythema
Cutaneous (intertrigo)	Erythematous, pustular, pruritic rash in warm moist areas; satellite lesions beyond primary border common
Onychomycosis	Thickened, opaque nails with onycholysis
Vulvovaginitis	Erythema, white exudate, and discharge; vulvar pruritus
Urinary tract infection	Lower tract infection–dysuria, increased frequency
	Upper tract infection–fever, flank pain, nausea, vomiting
	Fungus ball may form and obstruct collecting system
Candidemia	Fever, chills, hypotension, tachycardia, "toxic" appearance
	Pustular skin lesions, retinal lesions, vitritis
Invasive candidiasis	Depends on organ involved—includes osteoarticular infections, endocarditis, meningitis, hepatosplenic candidiasis

Denture stomatitis (chronic atrophic candidosis) is a variant of oral candidiasis that has been noted in as many as 65% of patients who wear dentures and occurs particularly in those with full upper dentures (10). Lower dentures are rarely linked to the development of candidiasis. Patients who have poor oral hygiene and who do not remove their dentures at night are more likely to develop this form of oropharyngeal candidiasis. Plaques are rarely observed under the dentures; more often, diffuse erythema is seen on the hard palate when upper dentures are removed. Patients may be asymptomatic but often complain of pain and irritation associated with their dentures.

Candida infections of the skin and nails: Candida infection of the skin (intertrigo) occurs mostly under pendulous breasts or pannus and in the perineum. The erythematous, pruritic, frequently pustular lesions have a distinct border; smaller satellite lesions provide a clue to the diagnosis of candidiasis. However, scratching may distort the typical lesions and make the diagnosis more difficult. The main differential diagnosis is tinea cruris or tinea corporis.

Although most cases of onychomycosis are due to dermatophytes, *Candida* also can infect the nails, especially those of the hand. The nails become thickened, opaque, and wrinkled, the condition may be painful, and onycholysis is frequent. The thickened nails are difficult to trim, predisposing patients to subsequent bacterial infections, such as paronychia and cellulitis. *Candida* itself also causes paronychia; this occurs most often in those whose occupation involves frequent immersion of their hands in water and is an unlikely infection among patients in a long-term care setting.

Vulvovaginitis: Candida vulvovaginitis is not increased in older women. After the menopause, *Candida* vulvovaginitis actually becomes less common. This decrease is likely related, at least in part, to the estrogen dependence of vaginal epithelial colonization by *Candida*. Among older women with *Candida* vulvovaginitis, risk factors include diabetes mellitus, corticosteroid therapy, and broad-spectrum antibiotic therapy (10).

Candida vulvovaginitis is manifested as vulvar pruritus, vaginal discomfort, and discharge; classically the discharge is described as curdlike, but it can also be thin and watery. External burning is experienced with urination. The labia are often erythematous and swollen; the vaginal walls show erythema, and white plaques and discharge usually are evident.

Candida urinary tract infections: Candiduria is a frequent finding in residents of LTCFs. Factors predisposing to candiduria include diabetes mellitus, the use of broad-spectrum antibiotics, the presence of an indwelling urinary catheter, and genitourinary tract abnormalities (11,12).

Most patients with candiduria are asymptomatic and probably do not have infection but merely colonization. Patients with lower urinary tract infection can have symptoms similar to those seen with bacterial cystitis: suprapubic discomfort, dysuria, and frequency. Those who have upper urinary tract infection may present with fever, flank pain, nausea, and vomiting, which is indistinguishable from acute bacterial pyelonephritis. Uncommonly, a fungus ball composed of fungal hyphae may form and obstruct the collecting system at any level.

Systemic Candida infections: Risk factors for infection in older adults include broad-spectrum antibiotics, indwelling urinary and central vascular catheters, parenteral nutrition, renal failure, and surgical procedures involving the gastrointestinal tract. In the long-term care setting, this is an unusual infection except in those who are receiving hemodialysis or have a central IV catheter in place for another reason. The attributable mortality from candidemia approaches 40% and appears to be higher in the elderly population (13). The patient with candidemia often appears "toxic," and the clinical presentation cannot be distinguished reliably from that caused by bacteremia.

Cryptococcosis

Cryptococcosis typically presents as subacute meningitis, but in older patients mental status changes without fever, headache, or focal neurological findings may be the only manifestation. Isolated pulmonary cryptococcosis occurs more often in older adults than in their younger counterparts (14). A recent retrospective review of 316 patients noted that mortality rates for patients with either meningitis or pulmonary crytococcosis were higher for those over age 60 (6).

Invasive Filamentous Fungal Infections

Older adults who develop sino-orbital aspergillosis usually are not overtly immunosuppressed, although some have had prior corticosteroid therapy. Orbital pain and loss of vision are the most common presenting symptoms; proptosis, ophthalmoplegia, and decreased visual acuity are noted on examination. The infection often arises in adjacent sinuses and then extends behind the orbit entrapping the optic nerve; further extension into cerebral vessels and brain may occur.

Chronic necrotizing pulmonary aspergillosis occurs mostly in middle-aged and elderly men who have underlying chronic obstructive pulmonary disease. Patients generally are not immunosuppressed. Symptoms are those of a progressive pneumonia that is unresponsive to antibacterial agents and that progresses to include cavitation and pleural involvement. Patients have a cough productive of purulent sputum with occasional hemoptysis, pleuritic chest pain, and increasing dyspnea. Fever, night sweats, anorexia, weight loss, and fatigue are common. The differential diagnosis includes other fungal pneumonias, such as histoplasmosis and blastomycosis, atypical mycobacterial infections, nocardiosis, and less commonly chronic bacterial pneumonias.

Among older adults, those likely to develop zygomycosis are diabetics who have poor glycemic control and are prone to ketoacidosis and those who have myelodysplastic syndromes, are transfusion-dependent, and require treatment with an iron chelator. Patients present with rapidly progressive painful necrotic lesions of the palate, nares, sinuses, or orbit or have pulmonary involvement. If this diagnosis is suspected, the patient must be transferred immediately to an acute care hospital for diagnosis and treatment.

DIAGNOSTIC APPROACH

Localized Mucocutaneous Infections

Skin Infections

The diagnosis of most dermatophyte and cutaneous yeast infections is made by clinical appearance. However, if no improvement is noted within one to two weeks of initiating local therapy or if the lesions are extensive enough to warrant systemic therapy, microscopic examination of scrapings from the lesion should be performed. This will ensure that noninfectious causes of rash are not treated inappropriately and that the appropriate antifungal agent is used for treatment. Scrapings should be taken from the edge of the lesion with a scalpel blade, collected on a piece of dark paper, and transferred to a slide, on which is added a drop of potassium hydroxide. Microscopic examination reveals hyphae in cases of dermatophyte infection and yeast when *Candida* or *Malessezia* are the cause of the infection. When there is suspicion of an outbreak of dermatophyte infection, skin scrapings should be sent for culture (in a paper packet, not in a culture transport tube as used for bacterial infections), and consultation should be sought with a dermatologist.

Nail Infections

For patients with onychomycosis, full thickness nail clippings taken as close to the nail bed as possible may show fungal elements when viewed under direct microscopy after potassium hydroxide digestion. However, for up to 50% of clinically diagnosed cases of onychomycosis, fungi will not be seen. Culture of the nail is especially useful for cases of onychomycosis because treatment courses are long and not without side effects and drug–drug interactions.

Mucous Membrane Infections

Oropharyngeal and vaginal candidiasis are diagnosed primarily by clinical appearance. Scrapings of the exudates that are then stained with Gram stain or visualized as a wet preparation reveal budding yeasts and often pseudo-hyphae. Culture is usually not necessary unless there is a poor response to therapy or multiple recurrent episodes. In that situation, fungal culture will show whether an unusual drug-resistant species is the cause of the infection and will guide further therapy.

Candida Urinary Tract Infections

A major dilemma arises in determining whether yeasts in a urine sample represent contamination, colonization, or infection (Table 3) (11). Contamination may be detected by repeating the collection and culture of the urine. In older women, catheterization may be needed to obtain an uncontaminated urine specimen.

The difference between colonization and infection is less clearly defined. This problem has arisen, in part, because candiduria is usually an asymptomatic condition. Currently, no test on urine can differentiate *Candida* colonization from infection. The presence of a urinary catheter in most patients with candiduria limits the usefulness of pyuria. Yeast quantitation has not proved helpful in separating infection from colonization. The presence of pseudohyphae, although once thought to indicate urinary tract infection, also has not been proved useful.

For patients suspected of having upper tract infection, imaging studies are necessary. Ultrasonography, computerized tomography, or retrograde pyelography can be used to ascertain the presence of hydronephrosis; fungus balls are seen as masses obstructing the collecting system or filling the bladder.

Systemic Infections

Candidiasis

The diagnosis of candidiasis should be entertained in any patient in the long-term care setting who appears septic and who has the risk factor of having a central IV catheter in place. Blood should be cultured using the same techniques as used for bacteria. A single positive culture yielding yeast is adequate for a diagnosis of candidemia. Patients who are suspected of possibly having systemic *Candida* infection should be transferred to an acute care facility where further diagnostic procedures can be performed.

Table 3 Approach to the Patient with Candiduria in the Long-Term Care Setting

Repeat culture to be sure not a contaminant:
  If cannot obtain clean-catch urine, do straight catheterization to obtain urine
If repeat culture is (+) and patient is asymptomatic:
  Assess predisposing factors (diabetes mellitus, antibiotics, indwelling catheters,
    GU tract abnormalities) and correct if possible
  If patient remains asymptomatic, observe, do not treat
If repeat culture is (+) and patient has mild symptoms suggesting lower urinary tract
  infection:
  Culture urine for bacteria and treat if found; check whether symptoms resolve
  Assess predisposing factors as listed above and correct if possible
  If bacterial infection not present and predisposing factors removed, observe
    clinical response and repeat urine culture to see whether funguria has cleared
  If patient remains symptomatic and funguria persists, treat with fluconazole
    14 days
If repeat culture is (+) and patient appears ill:
  Image the GU tract to be sure no obstruction present (ultrasound,
    computed tomography scan)
  If obstruction present, urology consult for options to relieve obstruction
  Obtain blood cultures to be sure not fungemic
  Correct predisposing factors when possible
  Treat with fluconazole 14 days
Follow urine cultures at end of therapy, if clinical condition worsens at any time
  during treatment, and several weeks after therapy has ended to be certain
  funguria has cleared

Abbreviation: GU, genitourinary.

Cryptococcosis

Patients suspected of having cryptococcal meningitis should have a lumbar puncture, including measurement of cerebrospinal fluid (CSF) opening pressure, performed. The typical CSF findings are those of a lymphocytic meningitis with elevated protein and decreased glucose. Increased intracranial pressure is common. A latex agglutination test for cryptococcal polysaccharide capsular antigen is available in most hospitals. This assay, which should be performed on both CSF and blood, is very sensitive and specific for cryptococcal infection. Cultures of blood and CSF readily yield *C. neoformans*, using standard techniques.

Filamentous Fungi

Many filamentous fungi are ubiquitous in the environment. Although easily grown from sputum, proof of infection, except in markedly immunosuppressed patients, almost always requires biopsy evidence of tissue invasion. When suspicion of invasive aspergillosis or zygomycosis arises, the patient should be immediately transferred to an acute care facility so that appropriate histopathological and microbiological tests can be performed.

THERAPEUTIC INTERVENTIONS

Localized Mucocutaneous Infections

Skin Infections

Both dermatophyte and yeast infections of the skin usually respond to topical therapy with creams or lotions. Lotions or sprays are easier to apply to large or hairy areas. Particularly for tinea cruris and intertrigenous candidiasis, the affected area should be kept as dry as possible; otherwise, recurrence is likely following discontinuation of the antifungal agent. Tinea versicolor often responds to the application of selenium sulfide shampoo. For patients who have extensive skin lesions, oral azole agents or terbinafine can be used to clear the lesions more quickly (15). Terbinafine or itraconazole are generally used for dermatophyte infections, and itraconazole or fluconazole for *Candida* infections. Terbinafine has fewer drug–drug interactions than itraconazole, and for that reason should be used first for those older adults who require systemic therapy for dermatophyte infections.

Nail Infections

Onychomycosis does not respond to topical therapy (Table 4). Either itraconazole or terbinafine, both of which accumulate in the nail plate, can be used to treat onychomycosis (15,16). Toenail infection is harder to cure than fingernail infection. Itraconazole or terbinafine, given either as pulsed therapy for one week out of each month for four to six months or daily for three months, is more efficacious than griseofulvin or ketoconazole.

Oropharyngeal Candidiasis

Oropharyngeal candidiasis is usually easily treated with clotrimazole troches or nystatin suspension (17). However, unless the underlying cause is removed,

Table 4   Recommended Management of Onychomycosis

Keep nails short and straight to avoid ingrown toenails
File nails that have become hypertrophic
Wash feet daily and dry well, especially between the toes, after bathing
Keep feet dry with use of antifungal powder and cotton socks
Avoid sharing instruments for nail clipping and filing among patients
Make a diagnosis of fungal infection by looking at nail clippings for fungal elements
    and if the diagnosis is questionable, by culture of nail clippings, prior to treatment
Treat with oral itraconazole or terbinafine for 3–6 months

the infection often returns after treatment is discontinued. Oral fluconazole or itraconazole suspension should be reserved for patients with more severe disease, such as might occur following chemotherapy or radiation therapy. Treatment of denture stomatitis requires removal of the dentures at night and vigorous brushing and disinfection of the appliance, along with topical antifungal solutions or lozenges. For recalcitrant cases, systemic therapy with oral fluconazole, in addition to local measures related to the appliance, are usually effective. Treatment options have been extensively reviewed previously (9).

Vulvovaginitis

The successful treatment of *Candida* vaginitis is usually accomplished by the application of topical creams or suppositories (10). Older women who are frail or suffering from dementia may find topical agents difficult to apply. Single-dose fluconazole is an attractive, easily tolerated alternative for these patients and is preferred by many women. Removing any precipitating factors is important to prevent recurrence. However, some women will continue to have recurrent infection; treatment with suppressive doses of fluconazole is helpful in this circumstance.

Candiduria

Given the benign nature of candiduria and our inability to differentiate colonization from infection, antifungal therapy should not be given unless the patient appears to have symptomatic urinary tract infection and/or obstruction of the collecting system due to *Candida* (Table 3) (11,12). Candiduria will often disappear with removal of the predisposing factors. Thus, the first step is to remove the indwelling urinary catheter and stop antibiotics when feasible or clinically appropriate. When treatment is deemed necessary, fluconazole, 400 mg for the first dose, then 200 mg daily for two weeks, has been shown to be effective (18). Bladder irrigation with amphotericin B is not recommended (17,19).

Systemic Infections

Candidiasis

Patients who develop invasive candidiasis while in the long-term care setting should be transferred to an acute care hospital. However, patients with complications of candidemia, such as osteomyelitis or endophthalmitis, often are transferred from an acute care hospital to an LTCF to finish a long course of antifungal therapy. In this situation, it is recommended that consultation with an infectious diseases physician be obtained. Invasive candidiasis can be treated with amphotericin B, fluconazole, caspofungin, or voriconazole (17).

Cryptococcosis

Initial treatment of cryptococcal meningitis with amphotericin B and flucytosine should be given in hospital. The patient may return to the LTCF to finish therapy with oral fluconazole. Pulmonary cryptococcosis without evidence of disseminated infection can be treated with oral fluconazole in most cases.

Invasive Filamentous Fungi

Chronic necrotizing pulmonary and sino-orbital aspergillosis are usually treated initially with voriconazole or amphotericin B. Patients are almost always in hospital during the initiation of antifungal therapy, but may continue with long-term oral voriconazole treatment in the LTCF.

Patients with zygomycoses are treated with amphotericin B given in high dosages because *Rhizopus* and *Mucor* species are only modestly susceptible to this drug and resistant to other antifungal agents. Surgical debridement of all necrotic tissue is essential.

Specific Antifungal Agents

Azoles

Azole agents have become the preferred treatment for localized yeast infections when topical agents have not been proved effective and also play an important role in the treatment of systemic infections (17,20,21). There are four azole agents currently available: ketoconazole, itraconazole, fluconazole, and voriconazole. Ketoconazole has been largely supplanted by itraconazole and will not be discussed further. Fluconazole is an important agent in the treatment of candidiasis and cryptococcosis. Voriconazole is used mostly in immunosuppressed patients with filamentous fungal infections; it will be used rarely in the long-term care setting.

Fluconazole has superior pharmacological attributes in that the oral formulation is almost 100% bioavailable; the drug distributes into most compartments, including the eye and the CSF, and it is excreted as active drug in the urine. The oral formulation of voriconazole is 95% bioavailable if given on an empty stomach and distributes to all compartments with the exception of the urine. Itraconazole differs in that absorption is problematic; it is lipophilic and accumulates in the skin and nails. Like voriconazole, itraconazole is metabolized by the liver and not excreted as active drug into the urine.

Itraconazole capsules require gastric acid and food for absorption. Therefore, histamine receptor antagonists (H_2 blockers), antacids, and proton pump inhibitors should not be administered to patients requiring therapy with itraconazole (Table 5). In older adults, who are more likely to have achlorhydria than younger adults, absorption of this agent may be erratic. The oral suspension of itraconazole, given on an empty stomach,

Table 5 Drugs that Decrease Serum Azole Levels

Azole	Drugs that decrease azole levels
Ketoconazole	Rifampin, isoniazid, phenytoin and all drugs that decrease gastric acid[a]
Itraconazole capsules	Rifampin, rifabutin, phenytoin, carbamazepine and all drugs that decrease gastric acid[a]
Itraconazole suspension	Rifampin, rifabutin, phenytoin, carbamazepine
Fluconazole	Rifampin
Voriconazole	Rifampin, rifabutin, phenytoin, carbamazepine

[a]Includes antacids, histamine-2 blockers, proton pump inhibitors.

has approximately 30% better absorption than the capsule formulation. Whether this is also true for older adults has not been established. This formulation should always be used in those patients who must also take agents that inhibit gastric acid secretion.

Azoles have relatively few side effects. Rash can occur with all azoles but appears to be most common with voriconazole. Fluconazole causes reversible alopecia. Hepatitis is possible with all of the azoles. Liver function tests should be measured at baseline and after several weeks of therapy. Mild elevations of serum alanine transamenase or serum aspartate transaminase (two- to three-fold increase over normal) do not require stopping the drug, but do require careful follow-up. If the levels increase further, the drug should be discontinued. Itraconazole causes hypertension, edema, and hypokalemia; although uncommon, this complication occurs most often in older adults and requires stopping the drug. Itraconazole also has been noted to cause myocardial dysfunction and should be used carefully, if at all, in a patient with a history of congestive heart failure. Voriconazole is unique in its ability to cause photopsia in which patients complain of bright lights, wavy lines, or blurring of vision about 30 to 60 minutes after taking the drug. These visual effects do not cause retinal damage and immediately cease when voriconazole is stopped.

The azoles have the potential to produce serious and even life-threatening drug–drug interactions through their actions on the cytochrome P450 system (Table 6) (20–22). Itraconazole and voriconazole are the most problematic. Patients receiving cholesterol-lowering agents, such as simvastatin and lovastatin, can develop life-threatening rhabdomyolysis when given itraconazole and probably should not be given any azole. If the antifungal agent is needed, the "statin" should be stopped temporarily. Increased serum levels of warfarin, phenytoin, and oral hypoglycemic agents occur when azoles are given along with these commonly used drugs in older adults. Itraconazole increases serum levels of digoxin in some, but not all, patients. Coadministration of an azole with cisapride is contraindicated

Table 6 Effects of Azole Antifungal Drugs on Serum Levels of Other Drugs

Drug affected	Ketoconazole	Itraconazole	Fluconazole	Voriconazole
Cyclosporine	Increased[a]	Increased[a]	Increased[a]	Increased[a]
Tacrolimus	Increased[a]	Increased[a]	Increased[a]	Increased[a]
Warfarin	Increased[a]	Increased[a]	Increased[a]	Increased[a]
Phenytoin	Increased[a]	None	Increased[a]	Increased[a]
Carbamazepine	None	None	Increased[a]	None
Cisapride	Increased[b]	Increased[b]	Increased[b]	Increased[b]
Digoxin	None	Increased[a]	None	None
Oral hypoglycemics	Increased[a]	None	Increased[a]	Increased[a]
Isoniazid	Decreased	None	None	None
Rifampin	Decreased	None	None	None
Rifabutin	None	None	Increased[a]	Increased[b]
Triazolam, alprazolam, midazolam	Increased[a]	Increased[a]	None	Increased[a]
Lovastatin, simvastatin, etc.	None	Increased[b]	None	Increased[b]

[a]Significant interaction, monitor serum levels of drug and/or clinical status.
[b]Life-threatening interaction; avoid the combination.

because the azole potentiates the QT prolongation on electrocardiogram induced by this and similar drugs. Thus, in older adults who take many medications and may have multiple health-care providers, careful attention to existing drug regimens before adding an azole is important in order to avoid serious and life-threatening drug–drug interactions.

Terbinafine

Oral terbinafine is readily absorbed and concentrates in the stratum corneum, hair follicles, and nails. The drug is usually well tolerated, although changes in taste perception can occur and can be distressing (23). Stevens–Johnson syndrome and neutropenia are serious but rare side effects. Hepatitis is common enough such that patients with known liver disease should not receive this agent, and those who are given this agent should have liver enzymes monitored at weeks 2 and 4 and then monthly. Terbinafine is metabolized by cytochrome P450 enzymes in the liver, but it does not affect the metabolism of other drugs, such as warfarin, as is noted with the azoles. However, rifampin will increase the metabolism of terbinafine, thus decreasing serum terbinafine levels.

Amphotericin B

This agent will rarely be used in the long-term care setting. However, patients may be transferred to a long-term care unit in order to administer this agent after the initial phase of the infection has been treated in hospital.

Nephrotoxicity, manifested by a rising serum creatinine, hypokalemia, and/or hypomagnesemia, is seen in almost all older adults who receive amphotericin B. Patients with underlying renal disease show a more rapid rise in serum creatinine. Concomitant use of other nephrotoxic drugs should be avoided. During amphotericin B treatment, salt restriction should be stopped, and diuretics should be used very judiciously, because enhanced nephrotoxicity, presumably related to sodium depletion and hypovolemia, is likely to occur. Sodium loading can decrease nephrotoxicity, but this can be problematic in older adults who have preexisting heart failure.

Potassium and magnesium losses can be large and can contribute to other organ dysfunction; for this reason, electrolytes should be monitored carefully and replaced as soon as the serum levels show even a slight decrease. In many patients, IV repletion is ultimately required in order to keep pace with the renal loss.

Infusion-related reactions are commonly experienced by patients treated with amphotericin B. Chills or rigors, fever, nausea, headache, and myalgias occur in the majority of patients treated. Many of these side effects can be diminished or eliminated by administering acetaminophen and diphenhydramine prior to the infusion.

Three lipid formulations of amphotericin B are currently available: liposomal amphotericin B (AmBisome), amphotericin B lipid complex (Abelcet), and amphotericin B colloidal dispersion (Amphotec or Amphocil). Each differs from the others and from standard amphotericin B in respect to composition, pharmacological parameters, recommended dosages, toxicities, and cost, but all are less nephrotoxic. Because most older patients who require more than a few days of therapy with amphotericin B will develop some degree of renal failure, one of these less nephrotoxic lipid formulations should be used.

Echinocandins

Echinocandins are a new class of antifungal agent that acts on the fungal cell wall, a structure not shared with mammalian cells (24). There are currently three echinocandins available: caspofungin, anidulafungin, and micafungin. These agents will rarely be administered in the long-term care setting but might possibly be used in someone for whom therapy is continuing after hospital discharge. The echinocandins are available only as IV formulations.

The echinocandins are exceedingly safe drugs. Flushing with rapid administration and rash have been reported but are uncommon. Hepatotoxicity may occur, but this has not been well established.

INFECTION CONTROL MEASURES

Dermatophyte Infections

Isolation of patients with tinea infections is not recommended. Transmission of dermatophytes from person to person is uncommon, although rare outbreaks of tinea corporis have occurred in LTCFs (1,2). Tinea capitis can be spread by fomites, such as hats or hairbrushes; thus, sharing of these items should be avoided. Dogs and cats, increasingly common in LTCFs, have been documented as a source for dermatophyte infections. All animals that are brought into LTCFs for pet therapy should be certified as being free of skin lesions.

Tinea pedis can be spread in common bathing facilities. Private tubs and showers help obviate spread within a facility. Simple measures, such as drying the feet well after washing, will decrease the potential for infection. Disinfecting the tub or shower after each patient use with an appropriate agent, such as a quaternary product, will help decrease spread.

Yeast Infections

There is no evidence of intrafacility spread of the yeasts causing tinea versicolor, candidiasis, or cryptococcosis, and thus there is no need for isolation precautions to be used. Scrupulous care of IV catheters, especially indwelling dialysis catheters and those used for parenteral nutrition, is important to help prevent candidemia.

Invasive Filamentous Fungal Infections

These infections are not transmitted from person to person or by health-care workers. There is no need for isolation precautions for patients with aspergillosis or zygomycosis in LTCFs.

PREVENTION

Dermatophyte Infections

Prevention of dermatophyte infections involves mostly good local hygiene. Skin should be kept dry and maceration avoided. The feet should be washed and dried between the toes every day; heavy socks and shoes that increase sweating should be avoided, and socks should be changed daily. Routine visits by a podiatrist will lead to improved care of toenails, early diagnosis of tinea pedis and onychomycosis, and appropriate therapy. Prophylactic use of antifungal agents has no role to play in preventing dermatophyte infections.

Yeast Infections

Cutaneous yeast infections, such as intertrigo, onychomycosis, and paronychia, can be prevented by the measures described for dermatophytes. Prevention of oropharyngeal candidiasis is related directly to decreasing those factors that contribute to growth of *Candida* in the mouth. Avoiding drugs that cause xerostomia, decreasing the use of inappropriate broad-spectrum antibiotics, and emphasizing good dental hygiene will help to decrease the risk of thrush. The care of dentures is exceedingly important in the prevention of denture stomatitis (9). Dentures should always be removed at night and should be cleaned daily by brushing with a denture brush and soaking in a disinfectant solution, such as chlorhexidine, or a commercially available denture cleanser.

Prevention of *Candida* vulvovaginitis and urinary tract infections should focus on removal of those factors that are associated with infection. In the case of vulvovaginitis, hyperglycemia, corticosteroid use, and broad-spectrum antibiotic therapy may contribute to development of vaginitis and should be modified when feasible. *Candida* urinary tract infections rarely occur in the absence of indwelling urethral catheters and broad-spectrum antibiotic use. One option that can be used is the use of intermittent rather than chronic catheterization; however, it has not been proved that this will decrease *Candida* urinary tract infections.

Because most cases of candidemia and invasive candidiasis in the long-term care setting will likely occur in patients undergoing chronic hemodialysis or those with central IV catheters in place for nutritional supplementation or other reasons, prevention rests with scrupulous care of the catheter.

Prophylactic use of azole agents to prevent *Candida* infections should be reserved for those patients who have frequent recurrent episodes of thrush or vulvovaginitis and for whom risk factors cannot be modified (25).

Invasive Filamentous Fungal Infections

These infections are acquired from the environment. Preventive measures are recommended only for institutions that care for patients who have hematological malignancies and who have received transplants. There are no special preventive measures that should be used in the long-term care setting.

SUGGESTED READING

Kauffman CA. Fungal infections in older adults. Clin Infect Dis 2001; 33:550–555.
Kauffman CA, Hedderwick S. Opportunistic fungal infections: filamentous fungi and cryptococcosis. Geriatrics 1997; 52:40–49.
Kauffman CA, Hedderwick SA. Treatment of systemic fungal infections in older patients: achieving optimal outcomes. Drugs Aging 2001; 18:213–223.

REFERENCES

1. Lewis SM, Lewis BG. Nosocomial transmission of *Trichophyton tonsurans* tinea corporis in a rehabilitation hospital. Infect Control Hosp Epidemiol 1997; 18:322–325.

2. Kane J, Leavitt E, Summerbell RC, Krajden S, Kasatiya SS. An outbreak of *Trichophyton tonsurans* dermatophytosis in a chronic care institution for the elderly. Eur J Epidemiol 1988; 4:144–149.
3. Malani PN, Bradley SF, Little RS, Kauffman CA. Trends in species causing fungemia in a tertiary care medical center over 12 years. Mycoses 2001; 44: 446–449.
4. Wilkieson C, Samaranayake LP, MacFarlane TW, Lamey PJ, MacKenzie D. Oral candidosis in the elderly in long term hospital care. J Oral Pathol Med 1991; 20:13–16.
5. Hedderwick SA, Wan JY, Bradley SF, Sangeorzan JA, Terpenning MS, Kauffman CA. Risk factors for colonization with yeast species in a veterans affairs long-term care facility. J Am Geriatr Soc 1998; 46:849–853.
6. Pappas PG, Perfect JR, Cloud GA, et al. Cryptococcosis in HIV-negative patients in the era of effective azole therapy. Clin Infect Dis 2001; 33:690–699.
7. Kauffman CA. Fungal infections in older adults. Clin Infect Dis 2001; 33:550–555.
8. Baran R, Hay RJ, Tosti A, Haneke E. A new classification of onychomycosis. Br J Dermatol 1998; 139:567–571.
9. Shay K, Truhlar MR, Renner RP. Oropharyngeal candidosis in the older patient. J Am Geriatr Soc 1997; 45:863–870.
10. Sobel JD. Treatment of vaginal *Candida* infections. Expert Opin Pharmacother 2002; 3:1059–1065.
11. Kauffman CA, Vazquez JA, Sobel JD, et al. Prospective multicenter surveillance study of funguria in hospitalized patients. The National Institute for Allergy and Infectious Diseases (NIAID) Mycoses Study Group. Clin Infect Dis 2000; 30:14–18.
12. Lundstrom T, Sobel J. Nosocomial candiduria: a review. Clin Infect Dis 2001; 32:1602–1607.
13. Pappas PG, Rex JH, Lee J, et al. A prospective observational study of candidemia: epidemiology, therapy, and influences on mortality in hospitalized adult and pediatric patients. Clin Infect Dis 2003; 37:634–643.
14. Aberg JA, Mundy LM, Powderly WG. Pulmonary cryptococcosis in patients without HIV infection. Chest 1999; 115:737–740.
15. Del Rosso JQ. Current management of onychomycosis and dermatomycoses. Curr Infect Dis Rep 2000; 2:438–445.
16. Crawford F, Young P, Godfrey C, et al. Oral treatments for toenail onychomycosis. Arch Dermatol 2002; 138:811–816.
17. Pappas PG, Rex JH, Sobel JD, et al. Guidelines for the treatment of candidiasis. Clin Infect Dis 2004; 38:161–189.
18. Sobel JD, Kauffman CA, McKinsey D, et al. Candiduria: a randomized, double-blind study of treatment with fluconazole and placebo. Clin Infect Dis 2000; 30:19–24.
19. Jacobs LG. Fungal urinary tract infections in the elderly: treatment guidelines. Drugs Aging 1996; 8:89–96.
20. Kauffman CA, Carver PL. Use of azoles for systemic antifungal therapy. Adv Pharmacol 1997; 39:143–189.
21. Kauffman CA. Antifungal drugs. In: Yoshikawa TT, Rajagopalan S, eds. Antibiotic Therapy for Geriatric Patients. Chapter 25. New York: Marcel Dekker, Inc., 2005:337–351.

22. Johnson LB, Kauffman CA. Voriconazole: a new triazole antifungal agent. Clin Infect Dis 2003; 36:630–637.
23. Balfour JA, Faulds D. Terbinafine. A review of its pharmacodynamic and pharmacokinetic properties and therapeutic potential in superficial mycoses. Drugs 1992; 43:259–284.
24. Deresinski SC, Stevens DA. Caspofungin. Clin Infect Dis 2003; 36:1445–1457.
25. Sobel JD, Wiesenfeld HC, Martens M, et al. Maintenance fluconazole therapy for recurrent vulvovaginal candidiasis. N Engl J Med 2004; 351:876–883.

27

Severe Acute Respiratory Syndrome

Mark B. Loeb

*Departments of Pathology and Molecular Medicine, and Clinical
Epidemiology and Biostatistics, McMaster University,
Hamilton, Ontario, Canada*

KEY POINTS

1. Clinical presentation of SARS is nonspecific.
2. Diagnosis of such emerging infections as SARS is an important clinical challenge.
3. Older adults are at high risk of complications of SARS.
4. At present, there is no effective therapy for SARS.
5. Although efforts are under way, there are presently no effective vaccines for SARS.

INTRODUCTION

The Institute of Medicine in 1992 defined emerging infections as "new, reemerging or drug-resistant infections whose incidence in humans has increased within the past two decades or whose incidence threatens to increase in the near future" (1). Recently, it has become evident that severe acute respiratory syndrome (SARS) is an emerging infection that can pose an important threat to the health of older adults. This chapter will focus on SARS and will summarize available evidence of the impact of these infections on older adults.

SARS: EPIDEMIOLOGY AND CLINICAL RELEVANCE

SARS has been documented in more than 8400 persons globally, with cases in Asia, Europe, and North America. A novel coronavirus has been identified as the etiologic agent. The first cases of SARS arose from Guandong province, in the south of China, in November 2002. The outbreak was officially recognized by the World Health Organization on February 13, 2003, based on initial reports from the Chinese government. Unfortunately, many more deaths ensued over the next five months.

Both the global and local spread of SARS is related to the so-called "super-spreading" events. A critical event for the global spread of SARS occurred at the Hotel Metropol in Hong Kong in late February 2003. A physician who had treated hospitalized patients in the city of Guangzhou and who was symptomatic with SARS while staying in Hong Kong became the source of infection for 12 people, the majority of whom were staying on the same floor as the physician. These individuals, also tourists, eventually sought medical care in hospitals in Hong Kong, Vietnam, Singapore, Ireland, United States, and Canada. There was secondary spread in all these countries with the exception of United States and Ireland.

Spread of SARS occurred primarily within the health-care setting. The secondary spread that occurred, predominantly in acute care hospitals, was largely due to a failure to recognize a new respiratory syndrome, along with the associated delay in assuming appropriate infection control precautions soon enough. Fortunately, spread of SARS to elderly residents of long-term care facilities was limited. However, transfer of patients to a nursing home did lead to secondary spread in Hong Kong (2). Nursing homes may be especially at risk to cross-infection because of potential crowded living environment, inadequate ventilation, less than optimal hygiene, and limited number of staff.

The incubation period of SARS, estimated to range from 2 to 10 days with a mean incubation period of 6 days is long enough for some people to be presymptomatic on admission and to develop symptoms later. Importantly, there is no evidence that individuals who are asymptomatic can transmit the virus. The incidence of asymptomatic infection appears to be very low. In fact, in the Toronto outbreak fewer than 2% of health-care workers with multiple exposures to SARS patients developed serological evidence of infection.

The reproductive number of the SARS coronavirus, which is the expected number of infectious secondary cases generated by an average infectious case in a completely susceptible population, has been estimated to range from 2.2 to 3.7 (3). This figure is not particularly high compared with the reproductive numbers of other respiratory viruses spread by respiratory droplet aerosol, such as influenza or measles. The clinical experience with SARS reflects this, i.e., once appropriate infection control precautions are instituted, the virus can promptly be contained and transmission can be stopped. The fact that SARS, unlike influenza for example, is not efficiently transmitted in the community supports this as well. The notable exceptions to the lack of community transmission was the spread at the Hotel Metropol, where it was hypothesized that virus detected by polymerase chain reaction (PCR) in vomit near the index case's room or elevator might have been the source of environmental transmission. Community spread also occurred at Amoy Garden in Hong Kong, an apartment complex, where the leading hypothesis was that sewage contaminated with small virus-containing droplets entered bathrooms of the apartment complex, through dried-up U traps (4). A comprehensive review of all the cases of SARS in Hong Kong showed that the transmissibility of viral infection was low, with the exception of settings where intimate contact or clinically significant contamination occurred (5).

The epidemiologic evidence suggests that within hospitals, the transmission mode was by droplet, although limited aerosol transmission might also have played a role. Super-spreading events, defined as spread from one source patient to many others, played an important role. In one report of SARS transmission in a Beijing hospital, patients linked to super-spreading tended to be older, more ill, had more contacts, and were more efficient at spreading the virus compared with other source patients not linked to super-spreading (6).

To date, there have been a number of studies that have addressed risk factors for acquiring SARS. There is no evidence to suggest that the elderly are prone to infection with SARS; however, there is ample evidence that outcomes are worse. A consistent finding is that exposure to aerosol generating procedures is high risk. For example, a retrospective cohort study in a Toronto hospital revealed that assisting with intubation, as well as suctioning, prior to intubation was associated with a fourfold risk of acquiring SARS among critical care nurses (7). Manipulation of an oxygen mask resulted in a ninefold increased risk to nursing staff. Studies to further define risk factors among household contacts and hospitalized patients are ongoing.

MICROBIOLOGY

SARS is caused by a novel strain of coronavirus (SARS-CoV) believed to have originated from an animal in southern China, such as a masked palm civet. Coronavirus are single-stranded RNA viruses, known to cause illness in both animals and humans. The virus belongs to a new group within the coronavirus family. An important feature of the SARS-CoV is that, unlike other respiratory viruses, the viral load increases until about the 10th day of illness and then diminishes (4). This has implications both for infection control precautions and clinically. The chance of secondary transmission occurring if a case is put into isolation before the viral load has peaked can be lessened. Clinically, one often sees a worsening of symptoms after the first week of illness. Molecular epidemiologic studies reveal that the SARS-CoV from outbreaks in Hong Kong, Vietnam, Singapore, Toronto, and Taiwan are clonally related, whereas those from Guangdong province are more

Table 1 Clinical Case Definition of Severe Acute Respiratory Syndrome

Radiological evidence of infiltrates consistent with pneumonia
Temperature >38°C or history of such temperature at any time in
  the previous 2 days
At least two of the following:
  History of chills in the previous 2 days
  Cough (new or increased) or breathing difficulty
  General malaise or myalgia
  Known history of exposure

Source: From Ref. 8.

diverse genetically (4). This may imply that some molecular lineages are more likely to be transmitted than others.

CLINICAL DISEASE

At presentation, SARS is characterized by fever, myalgia, cough, chills, or rigors (Table 1). Unfortunately, this syndrome is nonspecific, and the clinical features cannot be used to distinguish it from other viral or bacterial respiratory syndromes. The most common symptom is fever, occurring in virtually all cases. Shortness of breath occurs later in the illness. Some patients have diarrhea, others nausea and vomiting. In the elderly, SARS may present as an afebrile illness, where malaise and decreased appetite are the main features. Alternatively, it can present with a low-grade fever with few respiratory symptoms (9). When compared with younger patients with SARS, older patients are less likely to present with fever, chills, and diarrhea (Table 2) (8). This pattern is similar to community-acquired pneumonia, where symptoms and signs of pneumonia are less distinct in older adults.

There are a number of factors associated with a poor prognosis in SARS. An important factor is older age. Studies have shown that older patients are

Table 2 Comparative Clinical Features of Severe Acute Respiratory Syndrome Between Older and Young Adults

Clinical feature	Age ≤ 60 (%)	Age > 60 (%)
Fever	88	56
Chills	52	24
Malaise	17	16
Myalgia	31	12
Cough	37	32
Dyspnea	17	36

Source: From Ref. 8.

at substantially higher risk of death. In a study from China, the mortality rate among patients aged 50 years and over was 13 times that for patients aged below 50 years (10). In another study, every 10-year increase in age was associated with twofold increase in death (11). In a study from Hong Kong, multivariate analysis revealed that age more than 60 years [relative risk, 5.10; confidence interval (CI), 2.30–11.31; $P < 0.001$] and serum lactate dehydrogenase level greater than 3.8 μkat/L at presentation (relative risk, 2.20; CI, 1.03–4.71; $P = 0.04$) were independent predictors of mortality (12). Comorbidity, especially diabetes mellitus but heart disease as well, have also been repeatedly demonstrated to be risk factors for adverse outcomes in SARS (4). The aforementioned risk factors were noted in a Toronto study of 196 patients with SARS (13). Thirty-eight (19%) SARS patients became critically ill. The interquartile range of age of the 38 patients was 57.4 (39.0 to 69.6) years. The median duration between initial symptoms and admission to the intensive care unit was eight (5–10) days. Twenty-nine (76%) patients required mechanical ventilation. Mortality at 28 days was 13 (34%) of 38 patients, and for those requiring mechanical ventilation mortality was 13 (45%) of 29. Six patients (16%) remained mechanically ventilated at 28 days. Two of these patients had died by eight weeks' follow-up. Patients who died were more often older, had preexisting diabetes mellitus, and on admission to hospital were more likely to have bilateral radiographic infiltrates (13). High viral load at presentation can also be associated with poor outcomes. In a prospective study from Hong Kong, the following factors were independently associated with worse survival: older age (61 to 80 years) [adjusted hazard ratio (HR) 5.24; 95% CI, 2.03 to 13.53], presence of an active comorbid condition (adjusted HR 3.36; 95% CI, 1.44 to 7.82), and higher initial viral load of SARS coronavirus, according to quantitative PCR of nasopharyngeal specimens (adjusted HR 1.21 per log10 increase in number of RNA copies per millilitre; 95% CI, 1.06 to 1.39) (14).

Along with increased lactate dehydrogenase, elevated serum creatine kinase and alanine aminotransferase are often seen in SARS. However, these laboratory indices cannot discriminate SARS from other respiratory infections. The chest radiograph is abnormal in the majority of patients with SARS, the most common abnormalities being ground-glass opacifications. Again however, these findings are not specific for SARS.

DIAGNOSIS

One of the most important challenges of SARS has been making the diagnosis. The lack of an accurate real-time diagnostic test allowed SARS to be spread in hospitals around the world. SARS can be diagnosed very accurately retrospectively using serology. That is, antibodies to the virus will appear in more than 95% of infected patients at least 21 days (but preferably 28 days) or longer after onset of symptoms. Although this is of important epidemiologic value, it is not helpful to the front-line clinician who must decide if a patient has SARS. A number of groups are working on developing nucleic acid amplification tests, such as reverse transcription-PCR; however, none of these tests has proven to have a sufficiently high positive or negative predictive value to date. For example, in one recent report the highest detection rate was 75% between days five and seven of illness (15). Although SARS-CoV is readily cultured, the infection control risks to laboratory workers do not make routine culturing of the virus an attractive option. Other types of assays being studied, including immunoblot assays and radioimmunoassays, are still in a development phase. The utility of individual clinical symptoms in diagnosing SARS is limited. However, clinical prediction rules, where constellation of symptoms and signs are used, can be of benefit to clinicians in the setting of a SARS outbreak. For example, in a study from Hong Kong the sensitivity of a clinical prediction rule was 90%; however, specificity was lower at 62% (16).

TREATMENT

Once a case of SARS is diagnosed or presumptively diagnosed, the infected resident must be isolated either in the nursing home or in an acute care facility. Health-care workers in the nursing home who have contact with residents must use personal protective equipment (N95 mask, gown, gloves, and goggles). There must be restriction of visitors, and restriction of health-care workers in movement to other health-care facilities. Daily temperatures need to be recorded for all residents, and any resident with a fever or respiratory symptoms must be cohorted with other presumed cases of SARS or transferred to a hospital.

There are a number of agents that have been proposed as therapy for SARS. However, there have not been any randomized controlled trials of therapy to document efficacy. Ribavirin, a synthetic nucleoside antiviral agent with inhibitory activity against both DNA and RNA viruses, was commonly used during the SARS outbreak. Usually in an aerosolized form, it has been used for the treatment of respiratory syncytial virus pneumonitis in both adults and children. The combination of oral ribavirin and interferon has also been shown to be efficacious in the treatment of chronic hepatitis C. High-dose intravenous ribavirin has been used in the treatment of Lassa fever and hemorrhagic fever with renal syndrome. The theoretical rationale for using this agent was that it was known to have in vitro activity against other respiratory viruses, including respiratory syncytial virus and influenza, and its use began before the agent of SARS was fully defined. There are no systematic evaluations of efficacy of ribavirin for SARS. However, there are reports of toxicity. In Toronto, 61% of patients with SARS who were treated with ribavirin developed hemolytic anemia. Hypocalcemia and hypomagnesmia were reported in 58% and 46% of patients, respectively (17).

There have been reports of benefit with treatment from high-dose corticosteroids; however, there have been no randomized controlled trials to substantiate efficacy (18). One concern about these regimens is long-lasting adverse reactions, such as avascular necrosis and neuromuscular sequelae. One study has confirmed that cumulative dose of prednisone is an important risk factor for developing osteonecrosis of the hip and knee in patients with SARS who were treated with corticosteroids (19).

There are theoretical and limited clinical data to suggest a role for interferon-alpha in the treatment of SARS. Evidence exists that prophylactic treatment of SARS coronavirus-infected macaques with the pegylated interferon-alpha significantly reduces viral replication and excretion, viral antigen expression by Type 1 pneumocytes, and pulmonary damage compared with untreated macaques (20). In a study of 22 patients with probable SARS, interferon treatment was associated with a shorter time to resolution of radiologic infiltrates, better oxygen saturation, less of an increase in creatine kinase, and more rapid resolution of lactate dehydrogenase (21).

PREVENTION

There are many groups that are presently working on a vaccine against the SARS-CoV. One of the obstacles has been the inability to find an animal model where the disease manifestations are reliably reproduced when the animal is challenged with the virus. Once an animal model can be found, then testing vaccinated animals challenged with the SARS-CoV can begin. Research groups are currently working on vaccines using inactivated virus, recombinant virus, and plasmid DNA.

In the absence of a vaccine, surveillance measures are an important strategy for preventing the spread of SARS. Use of personal protective equipment is also important. Evidence exists suggesting that use of a mask can reduce the relative risk of SARS by 80% in critical care units (7).

SUGGESTED READING

Lederberg J, Shope RE, Oaks SC Jr., eds. Emerging Infections: Microbial Threats to Health in the United States. Washington, D.C.: National Academy Press, 1992.
Peiris JS, Yuen KY, Osterhaus AD, Stohr K. The severe acute respiratory syndrome. N Engl J Med 2003; 349:2431–2441.

REFERENCES

1. Lederberg J, Shope RE, Oaks SC Jr., eds. Emerging Infections: Microbial Threats to Health in the United States. Committee on Emerging Microbial Threats to Health, Institute of Medicine. Washington, D.C.: National Academy Press, 1992.
2. Ho Wency W, Hui Elsie, Kwok Timothy C, Woo J, Leung NW. An outbreak of severe acute respiratory syndrome in a nursing home. J Am Geriatr Soc 2003; 51:1504–1505.

3. Lipsitch M, Cohen T, Cooper B, et al. Transmission dynamics and control of severe acute respiratory syndrome. Science 2003; 300:1966–1970.

4. Peiris JS, Yuen KY, Osterhaus AD, Stohr K. The severe acute respiratory syndrome. N Engl J Med 2003; 349:2431–2441.

5. Leung GM, Hedley AJ, Ho LM, et al. The epidemiology of severe acute respiratory syndrome in the 2003 Hong Kong epidemic: an analysis of all 1755 patients. Ann Intern Med 2004; 141:662–673.

6. Shen Z, Ning F, Zhou W, et al. Superspreading SARS events, Beijing, 2003. Emerg Infect Dis 2004; 10:256–260.

7. Loeb M, Henry B, Ofner M, et al. SARS among critical care nurses, Toronto. Emerg Infect Dis [serial online] Feb 2004.

8. Chan TY, Miu KY, Tsui CK, Yee KS, Chan MH. A comparative study of clinical features and outcomes in young and older adults with severe acute respiratory syndrome. J Am Geriatr Soc 2004; 52:1321–1325.

9. Cheng HM, Kwok T. Mild SARS in elderly patients. Can Med Assoc J 2004; 16(170):927.

10. Zou Z, Yang Y, Chen J, et al. Prognostic factors for severe acute respiratory syndrome: a clinical analysis of 165 cases. Clin Infect Dis 2004; 38:483–489.

11. Lee N, Hui D, Wu A, et al. A major outbreak of severe acute respiratory syndrome in Hong Kong. N Engl J Med 2003; 348:1986–1994.

12. Choi KW, Chau TN, Tsang O, et al. Outcomes and prognostic factors in 267 patients with severe acute respiratory syndrome in Hong Kong. Ann Intern Med 2003; 139:715–723.

13. Fowler RA, Lapinsky SE, Hallett D, et al. Critically ill patients with severe acute respiratory syndrome. JAMA 2003; 290:367–373.

14. Chu CM, Poon LL, Cheng VC, et al. Initial viral load and the outcomes of SARS. Can Med Assoc J 2004; 171:1349–1352.

15. Wang WK, Fang CT, Chen HL, et al. Detection of severe acute respiratory syndrome coronavirus RNA in plasma during the course of infection. J Clin Microbiol 2005; 43:962–965.

16. Leung GM, Rainer TH, Lau FL, et al. A clinical prediction rule for diagnosing severe acute respiratory syndrome in the emergency department. Ann Intern Med 2004; 141:333–342.

17. Knowles SR, Phillips EJ, Dresser L, Matukas L. Common adverse events associated with the use of ribavirin for severe acute respiratory syndrome in Canada. Clin Infect Dis 2003; 37:1139–1142.

18. So LK, Lau AC, Yam LY, et al. Development of a standard treatment protocol for severe acute respiratory syndrome. Lancet 2003; 361:1615–1617.

19. Griffith JF, Antonio GE, Kumta SM, et al. Osteonecrosis of hip and knee in patients with severe acute respiratory syndrome treated with steroids. Radiology 2005; 235:168–175.

20. Anand K, Ziebuhr J, Wadhwani P, Mesters JR, Hilgenfeld R. Coronavirus main proteinase (3CL^{pro}) structure: basis for design of anti-SARS drugs. Science 2004; 300:1763–1767.

21. Loutfy MR, Blatt LM, Siminovitch KA, et al. Interferon alfacon-1 plus corticosteroids in severe acute respiratory syndrome: a preliminary study. JAMA 2003; 290:3222–3228.

Appendix A

Definitions of Common Infections in Long-Term Care Facilities[†]

CONDITIONS APPLICABLE TO DEFINITIONS

A. Only new symptoms or acute changes in chronic symptoms that suggest possibility of an infection should be considered.

B. Potential noninfections causes of the symptoms and signs exhibited by the resident should always be considered before diagnosing an infection.

C. Infection should be diagnosed based on several supporting data and not on a single finding. Microbiological and radiological findings should be used only to confirm clinical evidence of infection.

RESPIRATORY TRACT INFECTION

A. Influenza-like illness
   1. Temperature of 100.4°F (38°C) or higher, and
   2. Presence of at least three of the following clinical manifestations:
      a. Chills
      b. New headache or eye pain
      c. Malaise or anorexia
      d. Sore throat

[†] From McGeer A, Capbell B, Emori TG, et al. Definitions of infection for surveillance in long-term care facilities. Am J Infect Control 1991; 19:1–7.

    e. Myalgia
    f. New or increased dry cough

3. Symptoms or signs must be present during influenza season (e.g., November to April in United States and Canada) to make the diagnosis of influenza.

B. Bronchitis or tracheobronchitis
    1. Presence of at least three of the following clinical manifestations:

        a. New or increased cough
        b. New or increased sputum production
        c. Temperature of 100.4°F (38°C) or higher
        d. Pleuritic chest pain
        e. New or increased rales, rhonchi, wheezes, or bronchial breathing on physical examination of the chest.
        f. Indication of a change in status or breathing difficulty:

            i.   New or increased dyspnea, or
            ii. Respiratory rate higher than 25/min, or
            iii. Worsening mental function, or
            iv. Worsening functional status

C. Pneumonia
    1. Presence of both of the following criteria:

        a. Chest radiograph showing pneumonia, probable pneumonia or presence of a new infiltrate, and
        b. Presence of at least two of the clinical manifestations described for bronchitis and treacheobronchitis

URINARY TRACT INFECTION

A. Noncatheter symptomatic urinary tract infection
    1. Presence of at least three of the following clinical manifestations in the absence of an indwelling urinary catheter:

        a. Temperature of 100.4°F (38°C) or higher or chills
        b. New or increased dysuria, frequency, or urgency
        c. New flank or suprapubic pain or tenderness
        d. Change in urine character (new blood, foul smell, increased sediment grossly or by urinalysis)
        e. Worsening of mental or functional status

B. Catheter-related symptomatic urinary tract infection
    1. Chronic indwelling urinary catheters lead to bacteriuria in almost 100% of cases, and bacteriuria is generally asymptomatic and requires no evaluation or treatment.

2. In the absence of other site(s) of infection, the presence of fever and mental/functional status change meets criteria of symptomatic urinary tract infection.

SKIN INFECTIONS

A. Cellulitis and soft tissue and wound infection
1. Presence of one of the following criteria:
    a. Purulence present at the wound, skin, or soft tissue site, or
    b. Presence of four or more of the following clinical manifestations:
        i. Temperature of 100.4°F (38°C) or higher or worsening of mental/functional status
        ii. New or increasing heat at affected site
        iii. New or increasing redness at affected site
        iv. New or increasing swelling at affected site
        v. New or increasing tenderness at affected site
        vi. New or increasing serous drainage at affected site
B. Herpes zoster
1. Presence of both
    a. vesicular rash, and
    b. physician diagnosis or laboratory confirmation
C. Scabies
1. Presence of both
    a. maculopapular or pruritic rash or both, and
    b. physician diagnosis or laboratory confirmation

GASTROINTESTINAL TRACT INFECTION

A. Gastroenteritis
1. Presence of one of the following must be present:
    a. Two or more loose or watery stools above what is normal for a resident within a 24-hour period, or
    b. Two or more episodes of vomiting in a 24-hour period, or
    c. Both a stool culture positive for an enteric pathogen (e.g., *Salmonella, Shigella, Escherichia coli* 0157:H7, *Campylobacter*) and at least one manifestation compatible with gastrointestinal tract infection (nausea, vomiting, abdominal pain or tenderness, diarrhea)

COMMENTS

Criteria for common upper respiratory tract infections ("cold," pharyngitis), conjunctivitis, ear infection, and oral infections are not described because they are generally of mild consequences and not life-threatening.

Criteria for primary bacteremia or sepsis are omitted because obtaining blood cultures in a long-term care facility has not been documented to be beneficial or cost effective (see Appendix B).

Appendix B

Guide to Evaluating Fever and Infection in Long-Term Care Facilities[†]

CLINICAL EVALUATION

  A. Nursing aide should measure temperature, blood pressure, heart rate, and respiratory rate.
    1. Fever is defined as
       a. one or more rectal temperatures of more than 100°F (3.8°C), or
       b. two or more oral temperatures of more than 99°F (37.2°C), or
       c. a temperature increase of 2°F (1.1°C) over baseline regardless of technique or measurement.
  B. An initial evaluation regarding possible sites of infection should be done by the onsite nurse, and the findings should be communicated to the responsible physician, advance-practice nurse, or physician assistant.
  C. Document the full extent of the evaluation in the medical record. If diagnostic interventions are purposefully withheld, the reasons should be clearly stated in the record.

[†] From Bentley DW, Bradley S, High K, Schoenbaum S, Taler G, Yoshikawa TT. Practice guideline for evaluation of fever and infection in long-term care facilities. Clin Infect Dis 2000; 31:640–653.

LABORATORY TESTS

The diagnostic tests recommended should only be implemented where there are no previous advance directives that limit aggressive medical interventions.

A. Suspected infection: complete blood cell count
   1. A complete blood count, including peripheral white blood cell (WBC) count and differential cell count, on all residents suspected of harboring an infection.
   2. Elevated WBC count is 14,000 WBCs/mm^3 or greater.
   3. A "left shift" is more than 6% band neutrophils or metamyelocytes, or total band neutrophils count of 1500 cells/mm^3 or greater.

B. Urinary tract infection
   1. Diagnostic tests for suspected urinary tract infection should be reserved for only those residents who fulfill criteria for symptomatic urinary tract infection (see Appendix A). Evaluation should not be performed for asymptomatic bacteriuria.
   2. Appropriately collected urine specimens are the following:
      a. Men
         i. Clean catch or midstream specimen, provided resident is functionally capable, or
         ii. Freshly applied clean condom external catheter
      b. Women
         i. Midstream specimen after proper perineal cleansing if resident is functionally capable, or
         ii. In-and-out catheterization
   3. Initial evaluation should be a urine examination for WBCs (pyuria) by leukocyte esterase dipstick and microscopic examination for WBCs.
      a. If no pyuria (<10 WBCs per high-power field of spun urine by light microscopy or negative leukocyte esterase test) is found, urine culture is not indicated.
      b. Presence of pyuria should be followed by performing a urine culture with antibiotic sensitivity tests.
   4. If urosepsis is suspected, resident should be considered for transfer to an acute care facility with blood cultures, urine culture, and urine Gram stain on unspun urine performed at the acute care facility.

C. Sepsis or bacteremia: blood cultures: Blood cultures are not recommended for residents of long-term care facilities (LTCFs) with suspected bacteremia or sepsis. These residents warrant transfer to an acute care facility provided there is approval by resident, resident's family, or person with medical durable power of attorney.

D. Pneumonia

1. Pulse oximetry should be performed on residents with a respiratory rate higher than 25/min to document hypoxemia (oxygen saturation of <90%) as a clue to the diagnosis of pneumonia. Test is also helpful in predicting mortality and impending respiratory failure.

2. Chest radiograph should be performed if hypoxemia is documented or radiograph is suspected to identify the presence of a new infiltrate compatible with pneumonia. Test can also exclude other complicating conditions involving the lungs (e.g., abscess, effusion).

3. Respiratory secretions (expectorated sputum or nasopharyngeal aspirate) should be obtained to assess for presence of purulence. A purulent specimen should be gram stained for organisms and cytological screening for squamous epithelial cells (to determine quality of specimen). If stain of sputum or aspirate demonstrates less than 25 squamous epithelial cells per low-power field by light microscopy, then specimen can be acceptable for culture and sensitivity studies.

E. Respiratory viral infection: Obtain swab samples from throat and nasopharynx from several residents at onset of an outbreak of suspected respiratory viral infection. Place swabs in a single tube containing refrigerated viral transport media and transport them to an experienced laboratory for virus isolation and rapid diagnostic testing for influenza A and other common viruses.

F. Skin and soft tissue infections

1. Cellulitis: Cultures should be performed under select conditions. Surface swabs are not indicated. Fine-needle aspiration of skin lesion is indicated if there is evidence of an abscess, an unusual pathogen is suspected (e.g., gram-negative bacilli in diabetics), or initial antibiotic treatment has been unsuccessful.

2. Pressure ulcers: If a pressure ulcer demonstrates purulence or poor healing, send the purulent drainage or tissue obtained at surgical debridement or biopsy for culture. Surface swabs from pressure ulcers are not clinically useful.

3. Scabies: Scrape several typical scabies burrows and examine by light microscopy for mites, eggs, or mite feces on mineral oil preparations.

G. Infectious diarrhea

1. Stool specimen for diarrhea evaluation is not indicated if the resident has a low-grade fever, new-onset diarrhea, and no

clinical deterioration, and there is no outbreak of diarrhea in the LTCF.

2. If resident develops diarrhea and has received antibiotics within the previous 30 days, suspect *Clostridium difficile* etiology. Submit a stool specimen for *C. difficle* toxin assay. If specimen is negative for toxin and diarrhea persists, submit one or two additional stool specimens.

3. If resident has high fever, abdominal cramps, or bloody diarrhea, or demonstrates WBCs in the stool and there is no history of receiving antibiotics within the previous 30 days, submit stool for culture for isolation of common invasive enteropathogens (e.g., *Salmonella, Shigella, Campylobacter, Escherichia coli* 0157:H7). However, many of these residents will require transfer to an acute care facility because of associated bacteremia, sepsis, or dehydration.

INDICATIONS FOR TRANSFER TO AN ACUTE CARE FACILITY

A. Upon admission of a person to an LTCF, general parameters for considering transfer to an acute care facility for a resident should be recorded in the chart. Advance directives should also be part of this statement.

B. Decisions regarding transfer of an LTCF resident to an acute care facility should ultimately be at the discretion of the attending physician consistent with an existing advanced directive or as informed by the resident, resident's family, or designated person with medical durable power of attorney.

C. In the absence of an advanced directive or directions from the resident, resident's family, or designated person with medical durable power of attorney, the attending physician's decision regarding a transfer should be based on available institutional policies regarding transfer to an acute care facility. If such a policy is not available, then the following parameters should be reviewed when a transfer is considered:

1. Clinical condition, underlying disease(s), and prognosis of the resident

2. Efficacy and cost effectiveness of interventions and acute care

3. Capacity of the LTCF to provide necessary care and support to the resident

Appendix C

Minimum Criteria for the Initiation of Antibiotics in Residents of Long-Term Care Facilities: Results of a Consensus Conference[†]

SKIN AND SOFT TISSUE INFECTIONS

Either new or the purulent drainage increases at a wound, skin, or soft tissue site, or at least two of the following:

    A. Fever [temperature $>37.9°C$ ($100°F$) or an increase of $1.5°C$ ($2.4°F$) above baseline temperatures taken at any time]
    B. Redness
    C. Tenderness
    D. Warmth
    E. Swelling that was new or increasing at the affected site

RESPIRATORY INFECTIONS

    A. If the resident is febrile with a temperature $>38.9°C$ ($102°F$), at least one of the following:
        1. Respiratory rate >25 breaths per minute
        2. Productive cough

[†] From Loeb M, Bentley DW, Garibaldi R, Neuhaus EG, Smith PW. The SHEA Long-Term Care Committee. Antimicrobial use in long-term care facilities. Infect Control Hosp Epidemiol 2000; 21:537–545.

B. If the resident has a temperature $>37.9°C$ (100°F) or 1.5°C (2.4°F) increase above baseline temperature, minimum criteria for initiating antibiotics requires presence of cough and at least one of the following:
    1. Pulse $>100/min$
    2. Delirium
    3. Rigors (shaking chills)
    4. Respiratory rate $>25/min$
C. For afebrile residents known to have chronic obstructive pulmonary disease classified as high-risk because of age ≥65, minimum criteria for initiating antibiotics for a suspected respiratory infection include a new or increased cough with purulent sputum production.
D. For afebrile residents who do have chronic obstructive pulmonary disease, minimum criteria for initiating antibiotics include a new cough with purulent sputum production and at least one of the following:
    1. Respiratory rate >25 breaths per minute
    2. Delirium

URINARY TRACT INFECTION

A. For residents who do not have an indwelling catheter, minimum criteria for initiating antibiotics include acute dysuria alone or fever [$>37.9°C$ (100°F) or 1.5°C (2.4°F) increase above baseline temperature] and at least one of the following:
    1. New or worsening urgency
    2. Frequency
    3. Suprapubic pain
    4. Gross hematuria
    5. Costovertebral angle tenderness
    6. Urinary incontinence
B. For residents who have a chronic indwelling catheter (either an indwelling Foley catheter or a suprapubic catheter), minimum criteria for initiating antibiotics include the presence of at least one of the following:
    1. Fever [$>37.9°C$ (100°F) or 1.5°C (2.4°F) increase above baseline temperature]
    2. New costovertebral tenderness
    3. Rigors (shaking chills) with or without identified cause
    4. New onset of delirium

FEVER IN WHICH THE FOCUS OF INFECTION IS UNKNOWN

Presence of fever [>37.9°C (100°F) or 1.5°C (2.4°F) increase above baseline temperature] and at least one of the following:

A. New onset of delirium
B. Rigors

Index

Acinetobacter, 434
  infections, treatment, 437
Acquired immunodeficiency syndrome
  (AIDS), 99, 315, 349
  and dementia, 360
  residents
    clinical issues in nursing
      home, 359–361
    in LTCF, 356–358
Acquired immunity from aging, changes
  in, 54–56
Acute bacterial sinusitis, 152
Acute bronchitis, antimicrobial therapy
  for, 153
Acute care facility versus long-term care
  facility, 22–25
Acute diverticulitis, diagnosis of, 35
Acute hepatitis, 320–322
  treatment of, 323–324
Acute pyelonephritis, 179
Adenoviral eye infection, 46
Adjuvants, immunotherapeutic, 59
Adverse drug events, 18, 154
Adverse drug reactions, potential
  risk of, 154
Age-related illness, chronic, 51
Aging
  immune system, impact of chronic
    illness on , 57–59

[Aging]
  physiological changes associated
    with, 156
  studies of, 50–52
AIDS. See Acquired immunodeficiency
  syndrome
Allodynia, 279
Alopecia, 458
Alzheimer's disease, 3, 61, 360
Amantadine, 38, 164
  dosing of, 196
  efficacy of, 196
  resistance, 197
  and rimantadine, 195–197
  side effects, 196
Aminoglycosides, 155, 159–160, 183
  resistance, 431
Amoxicillin–clavulanic acid, selection
  of, 152
Amphotericin B (AmBisome), 459–460
  lipid formulations of, 460
  liposomal, 460
Amphotericin B colloidal dispersion
  (Amphotec or Amphocil), 460
Amphotericin B lipid complex
  (Abelcet), 460
Angioplasty, 35
Anorexia, 35, 74
  in older adults, drugs that cause, 83

Anti-cytomegalovirus IgG, 64
Antibiotic resistance, 123
Antibiotic-resistant gram-negative
    bacilli, treatment options for, 436
Antibiotic-resistant gram-negative
    bacteria, prevalence of,
    431–433
Antibiotics
    for bacterial infections, 151
    broad-spectrum, 37
Antibiotic therapy, 34
    intravenous, 92–93
    proportion of, 150
Antifungal agents, 163, 457–460
Antigen presenting cells (APCs), 52, 53
Antigenic drift, 193
Antihistamines, 38
Antimicrobial agents, 159
    absorption of, 155
    cost of inappropriate use of, 154
    criteria for initiation of, 151
    in LTCFs residents, 159–164
    optimal use of, 151–155
    therapeutic utility of, 150
    oral and intramuscular, 150
    prophylactic use of, 187
Antimicrobial clearance, routes of, 157
Antimicrobial-resistant pathogens, 145
    infection and colonization with, 123
    surveillance of, 120
Antimicrobial therapy, 18–19,
    149–151, 152
    drug factors, 155
Antimicrobial use in LTCFs, assessment
    of, 150–151
Antimicrobial utilization, 153
Antituberculous agents, 163
Antiviral agents, 164
APIC. *See* Association of Professionals
    in Infection Control
Apoptosis, 53
Aspergillosis, 461
    pulmonary and sino-orbital, 457
Association of Professionals in Infection
    Control (APIC), 119, 128
Asymptomatic bacteriuria, 81, 171, 174
    prevalence of, 24

[Asymptomatic bacteriuria]
    treatment of, 180
Autoimmune disorders, 55
Azithromycin, 160
Azole(s), 457–459
    effects of, 459
    drugs affecting serum levels of, 458
    prophylactic use of, 462
    types of, 457
Aztreonam, 434

B cells
    in healthy older adults, changes in, 56
    function, 60
Bacteremia, 415
    rates of, 65
Bacterial activity
    in chronic wounds, pyramid schema
        of, 260
    drugs with concentration-dependent,
        158
    drugs with time-dependent, 158
Bacterial infections, antibiotics for, 151
Bacterial products, 109
Bacterial sinusitis, acute, 152
Bacteriuria, asymptomatic, 81, 171, 174
    prevalence of, 24
    treatment of, 180
Basic activities of daily living (BADL),
    37, 41
Benzodiazepines, 40
Beta-lactam antibiotics, 160
    bactericidal activity of, 158
β-Lactamases, 430
    AmpC, inducible chromosomal, 430
    classification of, 429
    inhibitors of, 435
Blood assay for Mtb (BAMT), 236
Blood stream infection (BSI), 412, 415
Blood-borne pathogens, 118
    transmission of, 328
Bloody diarrhea, 301
Body mass index (BMI), 75
Bone metabolism, biochemical
    markers of, 365
Bowel disease, inflammatory, 301

Broad-spectrum antibiotics, 37
Bronchitis, 228
    clinical manifestations, 228
    diagnostic approach, 228–229
    epidemiology and clinical
        relevance, 228
    infection control measures, 229
    therapeutic interventions, 229
Bronchospasm, 203
BSI. *See* Blood stream infection

Candida albicans, 173
Candida infections, 447, 449
    of skin and nails, 450
    systemic, 451
Candida urinary tract infections, 451
    diagnosis of, 453
Candida vaginitis, treatment of, 456
Candida vulvovaginitis, 450–451
    prevention of, 462
Candidiasis, 173
    antimicrobial therapy for, 153
    diagnosis of, 453
    oropharyngeal and vaginal, 453
    therapeutic interventions, 456
Candiduria, 451
    in long-term care setting, approach to
        patient with , 454
    therapeutic interventions, 455–456
Caregivers, informal, significance of, 3
Caspofungin, 460
Cefazolin, 287
Cefepime, 437
Ceftazidime, 434
Ceftriaxone, 150
Cell death, 53
Cell-mediated immune response, 54
Cell-surface receptors, 52
Cellulitis
    antimicrobial therapy for, 153
    clinical manifestations, 285–286
    definition, 284
    diagnosis of, 286–287
    epidemiology and clinical relevance,
        284–285
    infection control measures, 288–289

[Cellulitis]
    prevention, 289–290
    risk factors of, 284
    therapeutic interventions, 287–288
Cephalosporins, 436, 438
Cephamycins, 436
Cerebrospinal fluid (CSF), 454
Certified nursing assistants
    (CNAs), 23, 44
Chicken pox, 386
Cholestasis, 321
Cholesterol-lowering agents, 458
Chromosomal β-lactamases AmpC,
    inducible, 430
Chromosomal enzymes, inducible, 430
Chronic age-related illness, 51
Chronic genitourinary symptoms, 176
Chronic hepatitis, 322, 324
    B and C infection, 325–326
Chronic hyperlactatemia, 363
Chronic inflammatory disease, 51
Chronic liver disease, 327
Ciprofloxacin, 151, 161
Cirrhosis, 314, 323
Cisapride, 458
Clarithromycin, 160
Clindamycin, 161
Clostridium difficile, 42, 106, 154, 269
Clostridium perfringens, 143
Clostridium tetani, 384
Cloudy urine, causes of, 179
Cold-blooded animals, 108
Colonization and infection, difference
    between, 453
Community-acquired pneumonia
    (CAP), 61, 216
Conjunctivitis
    causes of infectious, 337
    clinical manifestations, 336
    clinical presentation of infectious, 337
    diagnostic approach, 336–338
    epidemiology and clinical
        relevance, 336
    prevention, 338
    therapeutic interventions, 338
Coronary heart disease, 34
Coronary ischemia, 35

Coronavirus, 466
  diagnostic approach, 207
  epidemiology and clinical relevance,
      206–207
  incubation period for, 207
  infection control, 208
  treatment of, 207
Corynebacterium diphtheriae, 384
Corticosteroids
  advantasges of, 281
  treatment for SARS, 471
Costovertebral angle (CVA) pain, 176
Cranial neuritis (Ramsay-Hunt
      syndrome), 279
Cryptococcal meningitis, 454
  treatment of, 457
Cryptococcosis, 447–448
  clinical manifestations of, 451
  diagnosis of, 454
  therapeutic interventions, 457
Cryptococcus neoformans, 446
Cumulative illness rating
      scale (CIRS), 58
Cutaneous ectoparasitic infestation, 290
Cytochrome P450 (CYP), 362, 365, 458
  enzymes, 159, 459
  isoenzymes, 156
Cytokines, 52, 54, 365
  proinflammatory, 61
  pyrogenic, 108
  role of, 109
Cytolytic T-lymphocyte, 64
Cytotoxic T cells, 54

Daptomycin (Cubicin®), 162, 163
Deep venous thrombosis, 286
Delirium, 35
  evaluation for, 45
Dementia, 98, 360, 362
Dendritic cells (DCs), 52, 54, 57
  with aging, changes in, 57
Denture stomatitis (chronic atrophic
      candidosis), 450
Dermatophytes infections
  clinical manifestations, 448–449
  diagnosis of, 452–453

[Dermatophytes infections]
  epidemiology and clinical relevance,
      446
  infection control measures, 460–461
  prevention of, 461
  therapeutic interventions, 455–456
Diabetes mellitus, 361
Diarrhea
  antibiotic therapy for, 307
  antimicrobial therapy for, 153
  bloody, 301
  cause of, 302
  clinical manifestations, 300–301
  diagnostic approach, 301–305
    laboratory tests, 304–305
  duration of, 303
  epidemiology and clinical relevance,
      297–300
  etiology, 299
  infection control measures, 307
  management of, 301
  prevention, 308
  therapeutic intervention, 305–307
Digoxin, 458
  intestinal absorption of, 37
Diphtheria, 384–385
  tonsillar and pharyngeal, 385
  vaccine
    administration and
        revaccination, 386
    adverse reactions, 386
    effectiveness, 385
    indications, 385
Diphtheria toxoid (Td), 386
Diverticulosis, 415
DNA probes, 304
Drug(s), 38–40
  absorption, 155
  abuse, 350–352
  causing anorexia in older adults, 83
  classes of, 154
  with concentration-dependent
      bacterial activity, 158
  distribution of, 155
  extrusion, mechanism of, 431
  events, adverse, 154
  interactions, 158–159, 363, 383

[Drug(s)]
metabolism, 82, 156
movement through body, mechanism
of, 155–156
nephrotoxic, 460
pharmacodynamics of, 158
pharmacokinetics of, 155–156
properties, pharmacological, 18
and serum azole levels, 458
side effects, manifestations of, 18
susceptibility test, 243
therapy, 364
monitoring, 243–244
with time-dependent bacterial
activity, 158
tissue penetration of, 158
Drug–nutrient interactions, 82
Dyslipidemia, 361, 365

Echinocandins, 460
Eczematous neurodermatitis, 291
Effector cells, 51, 54
Emphysema, 61
Empirical antimicrobial
therapy, 152–153
Endogenous pyrogens, 108, 109
Endotoxin, 109
Enfuvirtide (Fuzeon), 362
Enterococcal endocarditis, 416
Enterococcus, 411–412
glycopeptide resistance in, significance
of, 412–413
Enzyme(s)
binding sites, 159
chromosomal, inducible, 430
immunoassays (screening assays), 318
inhibition, 159
Epididymoorchitis, 176
Erysipelas, 285
Erythromycin, 160
ESBLs. *See* Extended-spectrum
β-lactamases
Escherichia coli, 173
Esophagogastroduodenoscopy
(EGD), 305
Ethambutol (EMB), 243

Extended-spectrum β-lactamases
(ESBLs), 429, 435
different substitutions in, 430
producing organisms, 432
diagnosis of, 434
prevalence of, 433
role of, 438
risk factors for acquisition of, 433
screening methods for detection
of, 438

Fat accumulation (hyperadiposity), 364
Fat maldistribution, 364–365
Fat wasting (lipoatrophy), 364
Febrile urinary infection, 175
Filamentous fungal infections
clinical manifestations, 451–452
diagnosis of, 454–455
epidemiology and clinical
relevance, 448
infection control measures, 461
prevention of, 462
symptoms, 451
therapeutic interventions, 457
Fluconazole, 163, 457
Flumist™ (MedImmune, Inc.), 373
Fluoroquinolones, 82, 150, 155,
158, 161
Fluvirin™ (Chiron), 373
Fluzone® (Sano. Pasteur, Inc.), 373
Fungal infections
diagnostic approach, 452–455
epidemiology and clinical relevance,
446–448
infection control measures,
460–461
prevention, 461–462
therapeutic interventions, 455–460
Fusion inhibitors, 362

Gastrointestinal infections, 143–144
Gatifloxacin, safety and efficacy of, 343
Genitourinary symptoms, 171
Genitourinary symptoms, chronic , 176
Geriatric nurse practitioners, 97

Geriatric population
  infectious diseases in, 17
  life expectancy in, 5
Geriatric syndromes, 359
  adverse effects of pharmaceuticals
    on, 38–40
Glycopeptide resistance in enterococci,
    significance of, 412–413
Gram-negative bacteria
  antibiotic resistance, mechanisms,
    428–429
  clinical syndromes, 434
  diagnostic approach, 434–435
  epidemiology and clinical relevance,
    428–433
  infection control measures, 438–439
  prevalence of, 431–433
  prevention, 439–440
  therapeutic interventions, 435–438
  treatment options for, 436
Griseofulvin, 290, 455
Guillain–Barré syndrome, 375

Hand hygiene, 124–125
Hand rubs, alcohol-based, 124, 125
Harris–Benedict equation, 74
HAV. *See* Hepatitis A virus
HBV. *See* Hepatitis B virus
HCV. *See* Hepatitis C virus
HDV. *See* Hepatitis D virus
Health-care decision making, 94–97
Health-care workers
    (HCWs), 118, 124
  vaccination of, 387
Heart disease, coronary, 34
Heart failure, symptoms of, 35
Hematuria, 176
Hepatic monoxygenase system,
    inhibitors and inducers
    of, 159
Hepatic steatosis, 363–364
Hepatitis, 458, 459
  acute, 320–322
    treatment of, 323–324
  chronic, 322–324
  B and C infection, 325–326

[Hepatitis]
  clinical manifestations of, 320–323
  complications of, 320–323
  epidemiology and clinical relevance,
    312–320
  infection control and
    prevention, 326–331
  symptoms, 322
  therapeutic interventions, 323–326
  therapy, interferon-based, 324–325
  viral characteristics and
    epidemiology, 313
Hepatitis A virus (HAV)
  diagnosis of, 314
  epidemiology, 312
  incidence of, 312
  infection in LTCFs, frequency
    of, 327
  screening for, 327
  vaccination, indications and schedule,
    327–328
Hepatitis B e-antigen (HBeAg), 316
Hepatitis B surface antigen
    (HBsAg), 316
Hepatitis B virus (HBV), 328
  diagnosis of, 316
  epidemiology, 314
  immunization, 58
  incidence of, 314
  infection, nosocomial, 316
  screening for, 329
  treatment of, 325
  vaccination, indications and schedule,
    329–330
Hepatitis C virus (HCV)
  diagnosis of, 318–319
  epidemiology, 316–318
  infection, postexposure protection
    against, 331
  screening for, 331
  screening assays (enzyme
    immunoassays), 318
  treatment, 325–326
Hepatitis D virus (HDV)
  diagnosis of, 319
  epidemiology, 319
  incidence of, 319

Hepatitis E virus (HEV), 319
Hepatitis G virus (HGV), 320
Hepatobiliary disease, 415
Hepatocellular carcinoma
    (HCC), 314, 323
Hepatotoxicity, 460
Herpes simplex virus, 280
    treatment of, 164, 338
Herpes zoster virus (HZV), 386–387
    clinical manifestations, 279
    complications of, 279
    diagnosis of, 280
    epidemiology and clinical relevance,
        278–279
    infection
        control measures, 282
        treatment, 164
    prevention, 283–284
    therapeutic interventions, 280–281
HEV. *See* Hepatitis E virus
HGV. *See* Hepatitis G virus
High level gentamicin-resistant
        enterococci (HGRE),
        colonization, 413
Highly active antiretroviral therapy
        (HAART), 358
    side effects of, 363–366
HIV. *See* Human immunodeficiency
    virus
Host immunity, impact of age on, 54
Human immunodeficiency virus (HIV),
        66, 99, 237
    epidemiology, 350–356
        general, 350–352
        in older adults, 352–356
    infected patients, bone metabolism
        in, biochemical markers
        of, 365
    infection in nursing
        home, 361–366
    pathogenesis of, 358
    psychosocial concerns and prevention,
        366–367
    treatment, principles, 362
Human metapneumovirus
    clinical manifestations, 209–210
    diagnostic approach, 210

[Human metapneumovirus]
    epidemiology and clinical relevance,
        209–210
Hydrocolloids, 267
Hygiene
    hand, 124–125
    oral, 226–227
Hyperadiposity (fat
        accumulation), 364
Hyperglycemia, 37, 363–364
Hyperlactatemia, chronic, 363
Hyperlipidemia, 364–365
Hypersensitivity responses,
        delayed-type, 79
Hypertension, 34
Hypertriglyceridemia, 365
Hypertrophy, prostatic, 172
Hypoalbuminemia, 304
Hypocalcemia, 470
Hypoglycemic agents, oral, 458
Hypomagnesemia, 470

IL. *See* Interleukin
Immune cells, 52
    effector, 54
Immune dysregulation, 18, 51
Immune function, 63
Immune response
    cell-mediated, 54
    components of, 52–54
    innate versus acquired, 51
Immune system, 51
    aging, impact of chronic illness
        on, 57–59
Immunity
    acquired, 52, 53
    impaired, 57–59, 62–66
Immunization, recommendations for
        adult, 378–381
Immunosenescence, 50–57
Immunotherapeutic adjuvants, 59
Infection(s)
    adenoviral eye, 46
    with antimicrobial-resistant
        organisms, 145
    and aging, importance of, 15–17

[Infection(s)]
clinical features of, in older
persons, 107
and colonization, difference
between, 453
control, 25
components of, 119–127
factors affecting, 116–118
program and plan, 120, 127,
134, 153
regulatory aspects
of, 118–119
in elderly persons
aspects of, 17–19
clinical manifestations of, 17
morbidity and mortality
of, 16
factors increasing susceptibility
for, 33
initial evaluation of, 24–25
manifestations of, 151
nosocomial, reduction of, 121
nutritional interventions, 79
recognition of, 23–24
susceptibility to, 17–18
Infection control professional
(ICP), 119, 120, 127
Inflammatory bowel disease, 301
Inflammatory mediators, 54
clearance of, 61
and immunity, 59–62
Influenza, 62, 142, 371
antiviral agent, dosage, 375
antiviral drugs, prophylactic
dosage of, 197
attack rate, morbidity, and
mortality, 193
clinical manifestations, 194
control, 198–201
diagnostic approach, 194–195
epidemiology and clinical relevance,
192–193
impact of, 193
therapeutic interventions and
infection control, 195–198
treatment and chemoprophylaxis,
195–198

[Influenza]
vaccination, 200–201
administration and revaccination,
373–374
effectiveness, 372–373
indications, 373
vaccines for, 78, 100, 373
viral characteristics, 192–193
Influenza-like respiratory
illnesses (ILI), 199
Instrumental activities of daily living
(IADL), 41
Interdisciplinary teams (IDTs),
role of, 97
Interferon, and oral ribavirin,
combination of, 470
Interferon-alpha, treatment for
SARS, 471
Interferon-gamma (IFN-γ), 54
Interleukin (IL), 365
intracerebroventricular injection
of, 109
Ischemia, coronary, 35
Isoniazid (INH), 238, 243
Itraconazole, 456
oral suspension of, 457

Ketoacidosis, 448, 452
Ketoconazole, 155, 455, 457
Ketolides, 160
Klebsiella pneumoniae, 145, 173

Labyrinthitis, 339
Lactic acidosis, 363–364
Lactobacillus paracasei, 65
Latent TB infection (LTBI),
drug regimens for treatment
of, 239–240
drug therapy for, 237
Legionella pneumophila, 143
Legionnaire's disease, 143
Leukocytosis, 304
Linezolid (Zyvox®), 162, 269, 399, 419
Lipid formulations, of
amphotericin B, 460

Lipoatrophy (fat wasting), 364
Lipodystrophy, 364
Liposomal amphotericin B
    (AmBisome), 460
Live attenuated influenza vaccine
    (LAIV), 373
Liver function tests, 320, 458
Long-term care
    case studies in, 34–37
    definition of, 2
    economics of, 8–11
    evolving changes in, 11–12
    functional assessment in, 42–43, 45
Long-term care facilities (LTCFs)
    AIDS residents in, 356–358
    antimicrobials in, optimal use
        of, 151–155
        prescribing, 152
    characteristics of, 132–133
    epidemiology of fungal
        infections in, 447
    immunization in, 378–381
    infection
        control, 100
        surveillance in, 119
    key components of investigation in
        case ascertainment, 138
        case definition and line
            listing, 136–138
        epidemic curve (time), 139
        geographic assessment (place), 138
        host factors (person), 138
        implementing interventions, 141
        infection control program and plan,
            134–135
        preliminary hypotheses, 139
    residents, 17, 19, 72
        causes of weight loss in older, 75
        diarrhea in, 299, 301
        malnutrition in, 75–77
        micronutrient deficiencies in, 73
        nutritional deficiencies in older, 74
        vitamin A deficiency in, prevalence
            of, 73
    risk factors for outbreaks in, 133–134
    vaccination of health care
        workers in, 387

[Long-term care facilities (LTCFs)]
    vaccine utilization in, 370–371
    epidemiology of VRE in, 413–415
Lovastatin, 458
Lymphocytes (T and B cells), 52
Lysol®, 290

Macrolides, 38, 160
Macrophages, mycobacteriostatic
    activities in, 59–60
Malassezia furfur, 446
Malnutrition
    consequences of, 75–77
    prevalence and causes of, 72–76
Medicaid, 10–11
Medical ethics, elements of, 88–90
Medicare, 6, 9–10
Memory cells, 52, 55
Meningitis, rates of, 65
Metallo-beta-lactamases, 430–431
Methicillin-resistant *Staphylococcus
    aureus* (MRSA), 116, 268, 285
    antibiotics for, 399
    clinical features, 397
    clinical manifestation, 396–397
    colonization
        frequency, 392
        risk factors for, 396
    decolonization, 405–406
    definition of, 392
    diagnostic approach, 398–399
    epidemiology and clinical relevance,
        392–396
    history of, 392–395
    infection, 395–396
        control measures, 400–406
        general considerations, 400–402
        management, 403–406
        precautions, 402–403
        surveillance, 402
    prevention, 406
    syndromes and pathogenesis, 396–397
    therapeutic interventions, 399–400
Methicillin-susceptible *Staphylococcus
    aureus* (MSSA), 395
Metronidazole, 39

Micafungin, 460
Micronutrient deficiency, prevalence, 73
Micronutrient supplementation trials, in older long-term care residents, 80
Mineral supplements, 78–79
Minimum bactericidal concentration (MBC), 158
MRSA. *See* Methicillin-resistant *Staphylococcus aureus*
Mucocutaneous infections
    diagnosis of, 452–53
    therapeutic interventions, 455–456
Mucous membrane infections, diagnosis of, 453
Mycobacteriostatic activities, in macrophages, 59–60
Mycobacterium tuberculosis (Mtb) infection, 233
Mycoplasma pneumoniae, 106
Myelodysplastic syndromes, 452

Nail infections
    diagnosis of, 452–453
    therapeutic interventions, 455
Nasopharyngeal swab, 202
Necrosis, vascular, 365–366
Necrotic tissue, debridement of, 266
Necrotizing fasciitis, 286
Negative pressure wound therapy (NPWT), 266, 267
Nephrotoxicity, 159, 160, 460
Neuraminidase inhibitors, 197
Neurocutaneous disease, 278
Neutropenia, 459
Neutrophils, changes in, with aging, 56–57
NHAP. *See* Nursing home–associated pneumonia
Nitrofurantoin, 151, 183
Non-nucleoside analog reverse transcriptase inhibitors (NNRTIs), 361, 363, 366
Norwegian scabies, 291, 293
Nosocomial infection, 106, 121, 153

Nosocomial viral respiratory infections, control of in nursing home, 205
Nucleoside analog reverse transcriptase inhibitors (NRTIs), 361, 363, 366
Nursing facility care, demand for, 2–8
Nursing homes (NH), 7
    admission, factors involved, 3
    infections, 21, 22
    population, by age, 6
    resident, baseline temperatures in, 110
    usage, rates of, 8
Nursing home–associated pneumonia (NHAP), 215
    clinical manifestations, 218–219
    diagnostic approach, 219–220
    duration of, 221–222
    epidemiology and clinical relevance, 216–218
    etiology of, 217
    incidence of, 216
    management of, 223, 225
    mortality, 217
        risk factors for, 218
    pathogenesis of, 216–217
    pharmacologic interventions, 227
    prevention, 226–227
    risk factors for, 216
    therapeutic interventions, 220–226
    therapy, antibiotic, 224–225
    treatment, location, 220–221
    vaccination for, 226
Nutrient consumption, voluntary, barriers to, 73
Nutritional deficiencies, in older LTCF residents, 74
Nutritional interventions, to reduce infection, 79
Nutritional status, assessment of, 75–77

OBRA. *See* Omnibus Budget Reconciliation Act
Occupational Safety and Health Administration (OSHA), 118
Ocular symptoms, 194
Ofloxacin, 161

Omnibus Budget Reconciliation Act
(OBRA), 118, 127
Onychomycosis, 449, 453
management of, 455
Oral hygiene, 226–227
Oral ribavirin, and interferon,
combination of, 470
Oropharyngeal and vaginal
candidiasis, 453
Oropharyngeal candidiasis, 449
prevention of, 461
theraputic interventions, 455–456
Oropharyngeal flora, aspiration
of, 216
Oseltamivir, 164
dosing, 197
efficacy of, 197–198
resistance, 198
side effects, 198
Osteoarthritis, 365
Osteoclastin levels, 366
Osteonecrosis, 365
Osteoporosis, 365
risk factors for, 366
Otitis externa
clinical manifestations, 341
diagnostic approach, 341
epidemiology and clinical relevance,
340–341
prevention, 342
treatment of, 341–342
Otitis media
clinical manifestations, 339
diagnostic approach, 339–340
epidemiology and clinical relevance,
338–339
therapeutic interventions, 340
Otitis media with effusion (OME),
definition of, 338
Ototoxicity, 159, 160
Oxidative metabolism, by cytochrome
P450 enzymes, 159

Parainfluenza virus (PIV), 142
clinical manifestations, 206
diagnostic approach, 206

[Parainfluenza virus (PIV)]
epidemiology and clinical
relevance, 204
infection control of, 206
serotypes of, 204
treatment of, 206
Paramyxovirus, 201, 204
Parasitic skin infection, 144
Pathogens, blood-borne, 118
PCR. *See* Polymerase chain
reaction
Penicillin-binding protein
2a (PBP2), 392
Penicillins, 418
Permethrin, 292
Phagolysosome, 158
Pharyngitis, antimicrobial
therapy for, 153
Phenytoin, 458
Photopsia, 458
Pityrosporum orbiculare, 446
PIV. *See* Parainfluenza virus
Plasmid DNA, 438
Pleconaril, 209
Pneumococcal disease, 376–386
vaccine, 376–382
antibody response, 382
cost-effectiveness, 382–383
efficacy, 377–382
Pneumococcal immunizations, 125
Pneumococcal infection, 125
incidence of, 65
Pneumococcal vaccination, 66, 125
Pneumonia, 25, 35, 65
antimicrobial therapy
for, 153
community-acquired, 61
Pneumovax®, 377
Pnu-Imune®, 377
Polymerase chain reaction
(PCR), 320, 467
Polymicrobial infection, 173, 415
Polysaccharide vaccines, 382
Polyvalent cation drugs, 40
Porin channels, 431
Postantibiotic effects (PAE),
155, 158

Postherpetic neuralgia
    (PHN), 278, 279
Pressure ulcers, 81
    antibiotic regimens for, 269
    clinical manifestations, 258–259
    contamination, reduction of,
        AHRQ recommendations,
        270–271
    definition of, 252
    diagnostic approach, 259–264
    epidemiology and clinical relevance,
        252–257
    incidence and prevalence,
        252–253
    infection control measures, 270
    pathogenesis of, 257–258
    prevention of, 272–273
        AHRQ recommendations
            for, 271–272
    reducing
        extrinsic risk factors, 265–266
        intrinsic risk factors, 264–265
        therapeutic interventions,
            264–272
    therapy
        adjunctive, 267–268
        antimicrobial, 268–270
    treatment, surgery, 268
Prevnar®, 382
Proinflammatory IL-12 response,
    induction of, 58
Prostaglandin E2, 109
Prostatic hypertrophy, 172
Prostatic infection, 172
Protease inhibitors (PIs), 352,
    362, 365
Protein-energy supplements, 78
Proteus mirabilis, 173
Proton pump inhibitors, 457
Pseudomembranous colitis, 305
Pseudomonas aeruginosa, 144,
    173, 340
Pulmonary aspergillosis, 452
Pulse oximetry, 25
Pyelonephritis, acute, 179
Pylenephritis, 108
Pyrazinamide (PZA), 238, 243

Pyrogenic cytokines, 108
Pyrogens, 108, 109
Pyuria, 174, 178

QuantiFERON® TB Gold test (QFTG),
    236–237
Quinipristin–dalfopristin, 399
Quinolones, 37, 38, 40, 436
    adverse effects of, 162
    resistance, 431
Quinupristin/dalfopristin (Synercid®),
    163, 419

Ramsay-Hunt syndrome (cranial
    neuritis), 279
Receptors, cell-surface, 52
Resource utilization groups
    (RUGs), 10, 12
Respiratory infections, nosocomial
    viral, control of, in nursing
    home, 205
Respiratory syncytial virus (RSV)
    infection, 192
    clinical manifestations, 202
    diagnostic approach, 202–203
    epidemiology and clinical relevance
        of, 201–202
    transmission of, 203–204
    treatment, 203
Respiratory tract disease, causes of, 142
Respiratory tract infections,
    141–143, 152
Respiratory viruses, 142–143
Reverse transcription-polymerase chain
    reaction (RT-PCR), 195, 203
Rhabdomyolysis, 458
Rhinovirus
    clinical manifestations, 208
    diagnostic approach, 208
    epidemiology and clinical
        relevance, 208
    infection control, 209
    treatment, 209
Ribavirin, 470
Rifampin (RIF), 238, 243

Rimantadine, 164
Rotavirus infection, rotazyme
    test for, 304
RSV. *See* Respiratory syncytial virus

Salmonella hadar, 143
Sarcoptes scabiei, 290
SARS. *See* Severe acute respiratory
    syndrome
SARS-CoV. *See* Severe acute
    respiratory syndrome-
    coronavirus
Scabies
    clinical manifestations, 291
    diagnostic approach, 291–292
    epidemiology and clinical relevance,
        290–291
    infection control measures, 293–294
    prevention, 294–295
    symptoms of, 291
    therapeutic interventions, 292–293
    transmission of, 144
SENIEUR protocol, 51, 52, 60
Sepsis, 176
    syndrome, 151
Serological markers, 316
Serum aminotransferase (SGOT), 243
Serum hepatitis, 315
Severe acute respiratory syndrome
    (SARS)
    clinical disease, 468–469
    diagnosis of, 469–470
    epidemiology and clinical
        relevance, 466
    incubation period of, 466
    interferon-alpha treatment for, 471
    prevention, 471
    spread of, 466
    symptoms of, 468
    treatment of, 470–471
Severe acute respiratory syndrome-
    coronavirus (SARS-CoV), 467,
    470, 471
SHEA. *See* Society for Healthcare
    Epidemiology of America
Silicone catheters, 186

Simvastatin, 458
Sino-orbital aspergillosis, 451
Sinus infections, 152
    antimicrobial therapy for, 153
Sinusitis
    acute bacterial, 152
    clinical manifestations, 342–343
    diagnostic approach, 343
    epidemiology and clinical
        relevance, 342
    infection control, 344–345
    prevention, 345
    therapeutic intervention, 343–344
    treatment approach to, 344
Skin infections, 144–145, 284
    diagnosis of, 452
    therapeutic interventions, 455
Skin rashes, complications of, 366
Skin/soft tissue cellulitis, antimicrobial
    therapy for, 153
Society for Healthcare Epidemiology
    of America (SHEA), 119,
    128, 152
Staphylococcus aureus, 18, 173, 412
Staphylococcus epidermidis, 336
Stenotrophomonas maltophilia, 430
Streptococcal screening test, 152
Streptococcus pneumoniae, 106,
    143, 217
Streptococcus pyogenes–associated
    cellulitis, 144
Stevens–Johnson syndrome,
    366, 459
Stool culture, routine, 304
Streptogramin, 419
Sulfonamides, 155
Syndrome(s)
    geriatric, 359
    myelodysplastic, 452
    sepsis, 151
    Stevens–Johnson, 366, 459

TB. *See* Tuberculosis
T cell, 51
    clonal expansion, 54
    cytotoxic, 54

[T cell]
  function, 54–56, 201
  immunity, 58
  phenotype, 52
  proliferation, 58
  response, 56
  surface, 56
T cell–dependent immune response, 58
T-helper 1 and 2 (Th1 and 2)
    response, 54
T-lymphocyte, cytolytic, 64
Teicoplanin, 416, 418
Telithromycin, 160–161
Terbinafine, 290, 455, 459
Tetanus, 384–385
  toxoid, 386
  vaccine, 385–386
Tetanus-diphtheria toxoids (Td), 385
Tetracyclines, 82
Thrombosis, deep venous, 286
Tigecycline, 437
Tinea capitis, 448, 461
Tinea corporis (ringworm), 448
Tinea cruris, 448, 455
Tinea pedis, 285, 449, 461
Tinea versicolor, 446, 449, 455
TMP–SMX. *See* Trimethoprim–
    sulfamethoxazole
Treponema pallidum, 108
Toenail infection, 455
Trimethoprim, 181
Trimethoprim–sulfamethoxazole
    (TMP–SMX), 151, 162, 437
Tuberculin skin test (TST), 235, 236
  criteria for positive reaction, 238
Tuberculosis (TB)
  clinical manifestation of, 236
  diagnosis, 236–237
  drugs, treatment regimens of, 240,
      241–242
  epidemiology and clinical significance,
      234–235
  infection control, 244–247
  latent infection, drug regimens for
      treatment of, 239–240
  pathogenesis, 235–236
  prevention, 244

[Tuberculosis (TB)]
  treatment of, 237–244
Tumor necrosis factor, 365
Tumor necrosis factor-α
    (TNF-α), 57

Upper respiratory tract infection
    (URI), 78, 152
  prevention of, 81
Urinalysis, 178
Urinary retention, 37
Urinary tract infection (UTI), 35, 81,
    151, 415
  antimicrobials for treatment of, 182
  cause of, 412
  clinical manifestations, 175–177
  diagnostic approach, 177–180
  epidemiology and clinical relevance,
      170–175
  febrile, 175
  host response, 174
  infection control measures, 184–185
  microbial etiology of, 107
  prevalence and incidence of, 170–171
  prevention, 185–187
  risk factors, 172
  symptomatic
    clinical presentation of, 180
    diagnosis of, 178, 179
  therapeutic interventions, 180–184
  treatment, 182–184
Urine, cloudy, 179
UTI. *See* Urinary tract infection

Vaccine, 370–371
  influenza, 100
  pneumococcal, 66
  polysaccharide, 382
  varicella, 283
  zoster, 283
Vancomycin, 101, 162, 399
Vancomycin (glycopeptide)-resistant
    enterococci (VRE)
  clinical manifestations of, 415–416
  colonization, 414

[Vancomycin (glycopeptide)-resistant enterococci (VRE)]
control of, 420–421
diagnostic approach, 416–418
epidemiology and clinical relevance, 411–415
infection, 414
control measures, 419–423
treatment, 417
phenotypes of, 416
prevention, 423
screening for, 419–423
therapeutic interventions, 418–419
Varicella vaccine, 386–387
Varicella-zoster immune globulin (VZIG), 282
advantages of, 283
Varicella-zoster virus (VZV), 278, 280
immunity, 283
incubation period of, 282
Vascular necrosis, 365–366
Vestibular neuritis, 339
Viruses, respiratory, 142–143
Vitamin A deficiency, prevalence of, 73
Vitamin and/or mineral supplements, 78–79
Vitek ESBL test, 435
Voriconazole, 457
causes of, 458
oral formulation of, 457

VRE. *See* Vancomycin (glycopeptide)-resistant enterococci
Vulvovaginitis, 450–451
therapeutic interventions, 456
VZV. *See* Varicella-zoster virus

Warfarin, 39, 458
Wound care, local, 266
Wound dressings, 266–267

Xerostomia, 462

Yeast infections, 173, 446–448
clinical manifestations, 449–451
epidemiology and clinical relevance, 446–448
infection control measures, 461
prevention of, 461–462
therapeutic interventions, 456

Zanamivir (Relenza®), 164, 197
dosing, 197
efficacy of, 197–198
resistance, 198
side effects, 198
Zygomycetes, 448
Zygomycosis, 452, 461

About the Editors

Thomas T. Yoshikawa is Provost/Chief Operating Officer and Acting President, Charles R. Drew University of Medicine and Science, Los Angeles, California. Dr. Yoshikawa is a member of several professional organizations within the field of internal medicine, infectious diseases, microbiology, geriatrics, and gerontology. He was a member of the first American Board of Internal Medicine Geriatric Test Committee for (the added qualification in) Geriatric Medicine. He is Editor-in-Chief of the *Journal of the American Geriatrics Society*. He has published over 185 scientific articles, 16 books, and 71 book chapters. Dr. Yoshikawa received the B.A. degree from the University of California, Los Angeles, and the M.D. degree from the University of Michigan Medical School, Ann Arbor. He completed an internship and an internal medicine residency as well as an infectious disease fellowship at Harbor–University of California Los Angeles Medical Center, Torrance, California.

Joseph G. Ouslander is Professor of Medicine and Nursing, Emory University School of Medicine, Atlanta, Georgia. He also serves as the Director of the Division of Geriatric Medicine and Gerontology, Chief Medical Officer of Wesley Woods Center, and Director of the Emory Center for Health in Aging. Dr. Ouslander's primary areas of research interest are geriatric urinary conditions and long-term care quality. He has published more than 100 original research articles and book chapters, as well as edited special volumes on these topics. He is Deputy Editor of the *Journal of the American*

Geriatrics Society. Dr. Ouslander serves or has served as a consultant to Novartis, Pfizer, Watson, Indevus, Esprit, and Amgen. Dr. Ouslander received the B.A. degree from Johns Hopkins University, Baltimore, Maryland, and the M.D. degree from Case Western Reserve University School of Medicine, Cleveland, Ohio, where he completed an internal medicine residency. He also completed a fellowship in geriatric medicine at the University of California Los Angeles School of Medicine, California.